TAYLOR'S DIAGNOSIS MANUAL

SYMPTOMS AND SIGNS IN THE TIME-LIMITED ENCOUNTER

Third Edition

TAYLOR'S DIFFERENTIAL DIAGNOSIS MANUAL

SYMPTOMS AND SIGNS IN THE TIME-LIMITED ENCOUNTER

Third Edition

Editors

Paul M. Paulman, MD
Professor/Predoctoral Director
Department of Family Medicine
University of Nebraska Medical Center
Omaha, Nebraska

Audrey A. Paulman, MD
Clinical Associate Professor
Department of Family Medicine
University of Nebraska Medical Center
Omaha, Nebraska

Jeffrey D. Harrison, MD
Program Director, Rural Residency Program
Department of Family Medicine
University of Nebraska Medical Center
Omaha, Nebraska

Laeth Nasir, MBBS
Professor and Chairman
Department of Family Medicine
Creighton University School of Medicine
Omaha, Nebraska

Kimberly Jarzynka, MD, FAAFP
Associate Program Director, Residency Program
Department of Family Medicine
University of Nebraska Medical Center
Omaha, Nebraska

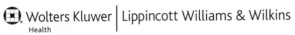
Wolters Kluwer | Lippincott Williams & Wilkins
Health

Philadelphia • Baltimore • New York • London
Buenos Aires • Hong Kong • Sydney • Tokyo

Executive Editor: Rebecca S. Gaertner
Senior Product Manager: Kristina Oberle
Developmental Editor: Red Act Group
Vendor Manager: Alicia Jackson
Manufacturing Manager: Ben Rivera/Beth Welsh
Marketing Manager: Kimberly Schonberger
Designer: Holly McLaughlin
Production Service: Integra Software Services Pvt. Ltd.

© 2014 by **LIPPINCOTT WILLIAMS & WILKINS,** a **WOLTERS KLUWER** business

Two Commerce Square
2001 Market Street
Philadelphia, PA 19103 USA
LWW.com

1st edition, © 1999 Williams & Wilkins
2nd edition, © 2007 Lippincott Williams & Wilkins

Printed in China

Library of Congress Cataloging-in-Publication Data

Taylor's differential diagnosis manual : symptoms and signs in the time-limited encounter / editors, Paul M. Paulman ... [et al.]. — 3rd ed.
    p. ; cm.
Differential diagnosis manual
Rev. ed. of: Taylor's 10-minute diagnosis manual. 2nd ed. c2007.
Includes bibliographical references and index.
    ISBN 978-1-4511-7367-3 (pbk.)
    I. Paulman, Paul M., 1953- II. Taylor, Robert B. III. Taylor's 10-minute diagnosis manual. IV. Title: Differential diagnosis manual.
    [DNLM: 1. Physical Examination—Handbooks. 2. Diagnosis, Differential—Handbooks. 3. Primary Health Care—Handbooks. 4. Signs and Symptoms—Handbooks. WB 39]
    RC69
    616.07'5—dc23

2013008379

CCS0713

The editors of *Taylor's Diagnostic Manual* would like to dedicate this book to our chapter authors who worked hard to provide up-to-date, clinically useful material for our readers.

We would also like to dedicate this book to Makenzie Lind-Olson who was able to keep us all on task and assure successful production of the manual.

Contributors

Riad Z. Abdelkarim, MD, MHCM
Instructor of Medicine
Department of Family Medicine
Johns Hopkins Institutions;
Senior Consultant
Tawam Hospital in affiliation with Johns Hopkins
  Medicine
United Arab Emirates
14.4 Hypothyroidism

Ahmed Salem Al Dhaheri, MBBS
Dermatology Resident
Tawam Hospital in affiliation with Johns Hopkins
  Medicine
United Arab Emirates
13.8 Vesicular and Bullous Eruptions

Nawar Al Falasi, MD
Specialist Dermatology
Medical Services Administration of Abu Dhabi Police
United Arab Emirates
13.5 Pruritis

Fatima Al Faresi, MD
Associate Residency Program Director
Specialist Dermatologist
Tawam Hospital in affiliation with Johns Hopkins
  Medicine
United Arab Emirates
13.4 Pigmentation Disorders

Naama Salem Al Kaabi, MBBS
Dermatology Resident
Department of Dermatology
Tawam Hospital in affiliation with Johns Hopkins
  Medicine
United Arab Emirates
13.3 Maculopapular Rash

Khawla Rashid Alnuaimi, MBBS
Dermatology Resident
Tawam Hospital in affiliation with Johns Hopkins
  Medicine
United Arab Emirates
13.1 Alopecia

Mark D. Andrews, MD
Associate Professor
Director of Procedural Training
Department of Family & Community Medicine
Wake Forest School of Medicine
Winston-Salem, North Carolina
6.1 Halitosis

Alexis M. Atwater, MD
Resident Physician
Department of Family Medicine & Community
  Health
Hospital of the University of Pennsylvania
Philadelphia, Pennsylvania
17.7 Hypercalcemia

Elisabeth L. Backer, MD
Clinical Associate Professor
Department of Family Medicine
University of Nebraska Medical Center
Omaha, Nebraska
  *16.3 Erythrocyte Sedimentation Rate and
  C-Reactive Protein*

Mandeep Bajwa, MD
Resident Physician
Department of Family Medicine
University of Nebraska Medical Center
Omaha, Nebraska
16.7 Thrombocytopenia

Mohammad Balatay, MM, MBBS
Izmir Hospital
Izmir, Turkey
13.6 Rash Accompanied by Fever

Nirmal Bastola, MBBS
Resident Physician
Department of Family Medicine
University of Nebraska Medical Center
Omaha, Nebraska
9.11 Rectal Bleeding

Sandra B. Baumberger, MD
Assistant Professor of Family Medicine
Creighton University School of Medicine
Omaha, Nebraska
7.12 Raynaud's Disease

Ryan Becker, MD
Resident Physician
Department of Family Medicine
University of Nebraska Medical Center
Omaha, Nebraska
4.4 Dementia

Michelle L. Benes, MD, FAAFP
Medical Director of Primary Care
Alegent Creighton Clinic
Omaha, Nebraska
14.2 Gynecomastia

Kevin K. Benson, MD
Clinical Instructor
Department of Family Medicine
Mayo Clinic
Scottsdale, Arizona
12.9 Shoulder Pain

Matt Bogard, MD
Resident Physician
Department of Family Medicine
University of Nebraska Medical Center
Omaha, Nebraska
7.5 Cardiomegaly

Deepa J. Borde, MD
Assistant Professor
Division of Hospital Medicine
University of Florida
Gainesville, Florida
10.6 Oliguria and Anuria

Joshua P. Brautigam, MD
Resident Physician
Department of Family Medicine
University of Nebraska Medical Center
Omaha, Nebraska
17.8 Hyperkalemia

Dorota Brilz, MD
Faculty
Department of Clarkson Family Medicine
Physician
Department of Family Medicine
The Nebraska Medical Center
Omaha, Nebraska
2.1 Anorexia
2.6 Fever

Michael J. Bryan, MD
Instructor of Family Medicine
Mayo Clinic
Scottsdale, Arizona
12.2 Calf Pain

Jennifer J. Buescher, MD, MSPH
Faculty Physician
Clarkson Family Medicine
Omaha, Nebraska
2.3 Edema
2.8 Hypersomnia
2.9 Insomnia
2.10 Nausea and Vomiting

Christopher W. Bunt, MD, FAAFP
Assistant Professor, Associate Residency Program
  Director, Pre-Doctoral Education Director
University of Nebraska Medical Center/Ehrling
  Bergquist Family Medicine Residency
Omaha, Nebraska
8 Respiratory Problems

K. John Burhan, MD
Faculty
Department of Family Medicine
Creighton University Medical Center
Omaha, Nebraska
7.9 Hypertension

Daniela Cardozo, MD
Family Medicine Resident
University of Nebraska Medical Center
Omaha, Nebraska
9.6 Epigastric Distress

Lisa Cassidy-Vu, MD
Assistant Residency Director
Assistant Professor
Department of Family and Community Medicine
Wake Forest School of Medicine
Winston-Salem, North Carolina
6.8 Tinnitus

Frank S. Celestino, MD
Professor and Director of Geriatrics Education
Department of Family & Community Health
Wake Forest School of Medicine
Winston-Salem, North Carolina
6 Ear, Nose, and Throat Problems

Chia L. Chang, PharmD
Clinical Assistant Professor
University of Nebraska Medical Center College
  of Pharmacy;
Pharmacist Coordinator
Nebraska Medical Center
Omaha, Nebraska
7.2 Anticoagulation

Ku-Lang Chang, MBBCh
Assistant Professor
Family Medicine
University of Florida
Gainesville, Florida
10.2 Hematuria

N. Corry Clinton, MD
Resident Physician
Department of Family and Community Health
University of Pennsylvania
Philadelphia, Pennsylvania
17.2 Aminotransferase Levels, Elevated

Curtiss B. Cook, MD
Professor of Medicine
Division of Endocrinology
Mayo Clinic College of Medicine
Mayo Clinic
Scottsdale, Arizona
14.1 Diabetes Mellitus

Lauri Costello, MD
Family Physician
Assistant Professor
Introduction to Clinical Medicine Department
Ross University
Dominica, West Indies
18.2 Bone Cyst

Ronnie Coutinho, MD
Associate Professor
Ross University School of Medicine
Dominica, West Indies
18.3 Mediastinal Mass

Carlton J. Covey, MD, MEd
Assistant Clinical Professor
Uniformed Services University of Health Sciences
Bethesda, Maryland;
Faculty
Nellis Family Medicine Residency
99th Medical Group
Nellis Air Force Base
Las Vegas, Nevada
8.6 Pneumothorax

Peter F. Cronholm, MD, MSCE
Assistant Professor
Department of Family Medicine and
  Community Health;
Affiliate Faculty
Graduate Program in Public Health Studies;
Senior Fellow
Center for Public Health Initiatives;
Senior Scholar
Leonard Davis Center for Healthcare Economics;
Associate
Firearm and Injury Center at Penn;
Associate
Philadelphia Collaborative Violence Prevention
  Center;
Affiliate
Evelyn Jacobs Ortner-Unity Program in Family
  Violence;
Senior Fellow
Center for Health Behavior Research;
University of Pennsylvania
Philadelphia, Pennsylvania
17.1 Alkaline Phosphatase, Elevated
17.2 Aminotransferase Levels, Elevated
17.3 Antinuclear Antibody Titer, Elevated
17.7 Hypercalcemia

Allison M. Cullan, MD
Assistant Professor
Department of Family Medicine
Creighton University
Omaha, Nebraska
12 Musculoskeletal Problems

L. Gail Curtis, MPAS, PA-C
Associate Professor and Vice Chair
Department of P.A. Studies
Department of Family and Community
  Medicine-Clinical
Wake Forest Medical School
Winston-Salem, North Carolina
6.4 Nosebleed

Ophelia E. Dadzie, BSc (Hons), MBBS, MRCP
Consultant Dermatologist and
  Dermatopathologist
Centre for Clinical Science and Technology
University College London Division of Medicine
  (Whittington Campus)
London, United Kingdom
13.2 Erythema Multiforme

Mario P. DeMarco, MD, MPH
Assistant Professor of Clinical Medicine
Department of Family Medicine and Community
  Health
Perelman School of Medicine at the University of
  Pennsylvania
Philadelphia, Pennsylvania
17.7 Hypercalcemia

Michel B. Diab, MD
Clinical Assistant Professor
Department of Community Health and Family
  Medicine
University of Florida College of Medicine;
Medical Director
Eastside Community Practice
Gainesville, Florida
10.3 Erectile Dysfunction

Kristy D. Edwards, MD
Assistant Professor
Department of Family Medicine
University of Nebraska
Nebraska Medical Center;
Omaha, Nebraska
15.1 Lymphadenopathy, Generalized
15.2 Lymphadenopathy, Localized

Richard L. Engle, MD
Assistant Professor of Family Medicine
Mayo Clinic College of Medicine;
Vice Chair
Department of Family Medicine
Mayo Clinic
Scottsdale, Arizona
12.7 Neck Pain

Bradley H. Evans, MD
Senior Resident
Family Medicine Residency
Wake Forest School of Medicine
Winston-Salem, North Carolina
6.7 Stomatitis

Ashley J. Falk, MD
Assistant Professor
Department of Family Medicine
University of Nebraska Medical Center
Omaha, Nebraska
15 Vascular and Lymphatic System Problems

Nathan Falk, MD, CAQSM
Assistant Professor
Department of Family Medicine
University of Nebraska Medical Center
Omaha, Nebraska;
Chief
Primary Care Sports Medicine
Offutt Air Force Base, Nebraska
17 Laboratory Abnormalities: Blood Chemistry and Immunology
17.5 Elevated Creatinine
17.8 Hyperkalemia
17.9 Hypokalemia

Sandra B. Farland, RN, MD
Clinical Instructor
Family & Community Medicine
Wake Forest Baptist Health
Winston-Salem, North Carolina
6.7 Stomatitis

Daniel S. Felix, MS
Behavioral Science Faculty
Department of Family Medicine
Indiana University School of Medicine
Indianapolis, Indiana
3.2 Bipolar Disorder

David B. Feller, MD
Associate Professor
Department of Community Health & Family Medicine
University of Florida
College of Medicine
Gainesville, Florida
10.7 Priapism

Enrique S. Fernandez, MD, MSBD, FAAFP
Senior Associate Dean for Clinical Sciences
Professor of Family Medicine
Ross University School of Medicine
Dominica, West Indies
18 Diagnostic Imaging Abnormalities
18.3 Mediastinal Mass

N. Benjamin Fredrick, MD
Associate Professor
Department of Family and Community Medicine
Penn State Hershey College of Medicine
Hershey, Pennsylvania
5.1 Blurred Vision
5.3 Diplopia

Toby D. Free, MD
Assistant Professor
Department of Family Medicine
University of Nebraska Medical Center;
Medical Director
Bellevue Medical Center
Omaha, Nebraska
4.6 Paresthesia and Dysesthesia
14.6 Thyroid Enlargement/Goiter

Richard Fruehling, MD, FAAFP
Associate Director Rural Training Track
Department of Family Medicine
University of Nebraska Medical Center
Omaha, Nebraska;
St. Francis Medical Center
Grand Island, Nebraska
9 Gastrointestinal Problems
9.1 Abdominal Pain
9.3 Constipation
9.5 Dysphagia

Hassan Galadari, MD, FAAD
Assistant Professor of Dermatology
Dermatology Residency Program Director
Faculty of Medicine and Health Science
United Arab Emirates University;
Consultant Dermatologist
Tawam Hospital in affiliation with Johns Hopkins Medicine
United Arab Emirates
13 Dermatologic Problems
13.1 Alopecia
13.8 Vesicular and Bullous Eruptions

Reshma Gandhi, MBBS, MPH
Resident Physician
Department of Family Medicine
Creighton University School of Medicine
Omaha, Nebraska
14.3 Hirsutism

Kathryn K. Garner, MD
Resident Physician
Family Medicine
Offutt Air Force Base Residency Program
University of Nebraska Medial Center
Omaha, Nebraska
4.8 Stroke

Stephen L. George, MD
Resident Physician
Department of Family Medicine
University of Nebraska Medical Center
Omaha, Nebraska
7.11 Pericardial Friction Rub

Umar Ghaffar, MD, MBBS
Clinical Assistant Professor
University of Florida College of Medicine
Gainesville, Florida
10.5 Nocturia

Nasreen Ghazi, MD
Assistant Professor
Department of Family Medicine & Community
  Health
University of Pennsylvania Health System
Philadelphia, Pennsylvania
17.1 Alkaline Phosphatase, Elevated

Mark D. Goodman, MD
Associate Professor of Family Medicine
Creighton University School of Medicine
Omaha, Nebraska
7.4 Bradycardia

Aaron Goodrich, MD
Resident Physician
Family Medicine
University of Nebraska Medical Center
Omaha, Nebraska
17.5 Elevated Creatinine

Mark D. Goodwin, MD, FAAFP
Assistant Program Director
Clarkson Family Practice Residency
Omaha, Nebraska
2.7 Headaches
2.12 Syncope

David K. Gordon II, MD
Family Physician
Flight Surgeon
Pentagon Flight Medicine Clinic
Arlington, Virginia
8.7 Shortness of Breath

Health A. Grames, PhD, LMFT
Assistant Professor/Program Director
Marriage and Family Therapy Program
Department of Child and Family Studies
The University of Southern Mississippi
Hattiesburg, Mississippi
3.4 Suicide Risk

Michael J. Gravett, MD
Resident Physician
Ehrling Bergquist Family Medicine Residency
Offutt Air Force Base, Nebraska;
Department of Family Medicine
University of Nebraska Medical Center
Omaha, Nebraska
8.2 Cyanosis

Michael L. Grover, DO
Assistant Professor
Vice Chair of Research
Department of Family Medicine
Mayo Clinic
Scottsdale, Arizona
12.4 Knee Pain

John D. Hallgren, MD
55th Medical Group
Offutt Air Force Base, Nebraska;
Adjunct Assistant Professor
Department of Family Medicine
University of Nebraska Medical Center
Omaha, Nebraska
4.5 Memory Impairment

Iriana Hammel, MD, FACP
Associate Professor
Internal Medicine & Geriatrics
Ross University School of Medicine
Dominica, West Indies
18.4 Osteopenia

Thomas J. Hansen, MD
Associate Dean for Medical Education
Creighton University School of Medicine;
Associate Professor
Department of Family Medicine
Creighton University
Omaha, Nebraska
7.1 Atypical Chest Pain

M. Jawad Hashim, MD
Assistant Professor
Department of Family Medicine
Faculty of Medicine and Health Sciences
UAE University
United Arab Emirates
14.7 Thyroid Nodule

Kenisha R. Heath, MD
Chief of Medical Staff
Beale Air Force Base, California;
Uniformed Services University of the Health
  Sciences (USUHS)
Bethesda, Maryland
8.4 Pleural Effusion

Hannah M. Heckart, MD
Resident Physician
Department of Family Medicine
University of Nebraska Medical Center
Omaha, Nebraska
7.13 Tachycardia

Destin Hill, MD
Clinical Physician
Arizona Sports Medicine Center
Scottsdale, Arizona
12.3 Hip Pain

W. Jeff Hinton, PhD, LMFT
Associate Professor & Interim Chair
Department of Child and Family Studies
The University of Southern Mississippi
Hattiesburg, Mississippi
3.4 Suicide Risk

David C. Holub, MD, FAAFP
Assistant Professor of Family Medicine
University of Rochester School of Medicine
   and Dentistry
Rochester, New York
5.7 Pupillary Inequality
5.8 Red Eye
5.9 Scotoma

James E. Hougas, III, MD
Family Medicine Staff Physician
341st Medical Group
Malmstrom AFB
Montana
7.8 Systolic Heart Murmurs

Michael J. Hovan, MD
Associate Professor
Department of Family Medicine
Mayo Clinic College of Medicine;
Inpatient Director and Chair of Education
Department of Family Medicine
Mayo Clinic
Scottsdale, Arizona
14.1 Diabetes Mellitus

Richard H. Hurd, MD
Director
Department of Clarkson Family Medicine;
Physician
Department of Family Medicine
Nebraska Medical Center
Omaha, Nebraska
2 Undifferentiated Problems
2.2 Dizziness
2.11 Night Sweats

John C. Huscher, MD
Assistant Professor of Family Medicine
Associate Program Director Family Practice
   Residency
Norfolk Rural Training Track
University of Nebraska Medical Center;
Hospitalist
Faith Regional Health Services
Norfolk, Nebraska
9.9 Hepatomegaly
9.10 Jaundice

Douglas J. Inciarte, MD
Assistant Professor
Department of Family Medicine
University of Nebraska Medical Center
Omaha, Nebraska
4 Problems Related to the Nervous System
4.2 Coma
7.7 Diastolic Heart Murmurs

Scott Ippolito, MD, FAAFP
Associate Dean of Clinic Sciences and Professor
Ross University School of Medicine
Dominica, West Indies;
Chair
Department of Family Medicine
South Nassau Communities Hospital
Oceanside, New York
18.5 Solitary Pulmonary Nodule

David S. Jackson Jr, MD
Associate Professor
Department of Family and Community Medicine
Wake Forest School of Medicine
Winston-Salem, North Carolina
6.3 Hoarseness

Abbie Jacobs, MD
Clinical Associate Professor
Family Medicine
New Jersey Medical School
Newark, New Jersey
18.1 Abnormal Mammogram

Amy K. Jespersen, MD
Director
Department of Clarkson Family Medicine;
Physician
Department of Family Medicine
Nebraska Medical Center
Omaha, Nebraska
2.5 Fatigue
2.13 Weight Loss

Milton (Pete) Johnson, MD
Associate Director, Rural Training Track
Regional West Medical Center
Scottsbluff, Nebraska;
Rural Training Track
Department of Family Medicine
University of Nebraska Medical Center
Omaha, Nebraska
9.2 Ascites
9.6 Epigastric Distress
9.7 Upper Gastrointestinal Bleeding
9.8 Hepatitis
9.12 Steatorrhea

Rahul Kapur, MD, CAQSM
Assistant Professor
Family Medicine & Sports Medicine
University of Pennsylvania
Philadelphia, Pennsylvania
17.3 Antinuclear Antibody Titer, Elevated

Mark P. Knudson, MD, MSPH
Vice Chair for Education
Family & Community Medicine
Wake Forest University School of Medicine
Winston-Salem, North Carolina
6.2 Hearing Loss

Manoj Kumar, MD, MPH
Hospitalist
Internal Medicine
Regional West Medical Center
Scottsbluff, Nebraska
9.2 Ascites
9.8 Hepatitis

Louis Kuritzky, MD
Clinical Assistant Professor
Family Medicine Residency Program
University of Florida
Gainesville, Florida
10.3 Erectile Dysfunction

Mindy J. Lacey, MD
Assistant Professor
Department of Family Medicine
University of Nebraska Medical Center
Omaha, Nebraska
7 Cardiovascular Problems
7.2 Anticoagulation
11.8 Pap Smear Abnormality

Carol A. LaCroix, MD
Associate Clinical Professor
Department of Family Medicine
University of Nebraska Medical Center
Omaha, Nebraska
16 Laboratory Abnormalities: Hematology
and Urine Determinations
16.1 Anemia
16.2 Eosinophilia
16.5 Polycythemia
16.6 Proteinuria

Zoilo O. Lansang, MD
Resident
Department of Family Medicine
University of Nebraska Medical Center
Omaha, Nebraska
9.9 Hepatomegaly

Brenda Latham-Sadler, MD
Associate Professor
Family and Community Medicine
Wake Forest School of Medicine
Winston-Salem, North Carolina
6.6 Rhinitis

Ernestine M. Lee, MD, MPH
Assistant Professor of Family Medicine
University of Central Florida
Gainesville, Florida;
Faculty
Florida Hospital Family Medicine Residency Program
Winter Park, Florida
10.8 Scrotal Mass

Shou Ling Leong, MD
Department of Family Medicine
Penn State Hershey College of Medicine
Hershey, Pennsylvania
5 Eye Problems

Peter R. Lewis, MD
Professor of Family & Community Medicine
Penn State Hershey College of Medicine
Hershey, Pennsylvania
5.2 Corneal Foreign Body and Corneal Abrasion
5.5 Nystagmus
5.6 Papilledema

Richard W. Lord Jr, MD, MA
Professor
Department of Family and Community Medicine
Wake Forest School of Medicine
Winston-Salem, North Carolina
6.5 Pharyngitis

Safana Anna Makhdoom, MD, BSc
Resident Physician
Department of Family Medicine
University of Nebraska Medical Center
Omaha, Nebraska
9.4 Diarrhea

Anna Maruska, MD
Resident Physician
Family Medicine Residency Program
University of Nebraska Medical Center
Omaha, Nebraska
16.4 Neutropenia

Timothy McAuliff, MD
Resident Physician
Department of Family Medicine
University of Nebraska Medical Center
Omaha, Nebraska
9.3 Constipation

Dana L. McDermott, DO
Lake Erie College of Osteopathic Medicine
Erie, Pennsylvania
17.4 Brain Natriuretic Peptide

Kristina E. McElhinney, DO
Resident Physician
Department of Family Medicine and Community
  Health
University of Pennsylvania Health System
Philadelphia, Pennsylvania
17.3 Antinuclear Antibody Tier, Elevated

Amy L. McGaha, MD, FAAFP
Associate Professor and Residency Program Director
Creighton University Department of Family
  Medicine
Omaha, Nebraska
14.9 Vitamin D Deficiency

Jim Medder, MD, MPH
Associate Professor
Department of Family Medicine
University of Nebraska Medical Center
Omaha, Nebraska
3 Mental Health Problems

Robert C. Messbarger, MD
Associate Program Director
Rural Residency Program Kearney
Department of Family Medicine
University of Nebraska Medical Center
Omaha, Nebraska
9.4 Diarrhea
9.11 Rectal Bleeding

John J. Messmer, MD
Associate Professor
Family & Community Medicine
Penn State Hershey College of Medicine;
Associate Vice-Chair for Inpatient Medicine
Department of Family & Community Medicine
Penn State Hershey Medical Center
Hershey, Pennsylvania
5.4 Loss of Vision

Zachary W. Meyer, MD
Resident Physician
Department of Family Medicine
University of Nebraska Medical Center
Omaha, Nebraska
9.1 Abdominal Pain

Carolyn Carpenter Moats, MD
Consultant Mayo Clinic;
Instructor of Family Medicine
Mayo School of Graduate Education
Mayo Clinic
Scottsdale, Arizona
12.5 Low Back Pain

Lindsey M. Mosel, MD
Resident Physician
Department of Family Medicine
University of Nebraska Medical Center
Omaha, Nebraska
9.7 Upper Gastrointestinal Bleeding

Hamid Mukhtar, MBBS
Family Physician
Pawnee County Memorial Hospital
Pawnee City, Nebraska
11.7 Nipple Discharge in Non-Pregnant Females

Arwa Abdulhaq Nasir, MBBS, MPH
Children's Hospital and Medical Center;
Assistant Professor
Department of Pediatrics
Univeristy of Nebraska Medical Center
Omaha, Nebraska
14 Endocrine and Metabolic Problems

Eddie Needham, MD, FAAFP
Program Director
Florida Hospital Family Medicine Residency;
Associate Professor
University of Central Florida College of Medicine;
Clinical Associate Professor
Florida State University College of Medicine
Tallahassee, Florida
10.8 Scrotal Mass

Susan M. Newman, MD
Resident Physician
Department of Family Medicine
University of Nebraska Medical Center
Omaha, Nebraska
9.5 Dysphagia

Giang T. Nguyen, MD, MPH, MSCE
Assistant Professor
Department of Family Medicine and Community
 Health
University of Pennsylvania;
Medical Director
Penn Family Care
Penn Presbyterian Medical Center
University of Pennsylvania Health System
Philadelphia, Pennsylvania
17.2 Aminotransferase Levels, Elevated

Lisa B. Norton, MD
Staff Family Physician
Wright-Patterson AFB, Ohio
8.5 Pleuritic Pain

Nicole Otto, MD
Clinical Assistant Professor of Family Medicine &
 Community Health
Perelman School of Medicine at the University of
 Pennsylvania;
Primary Care Sports Medicine Chief
University of Pennsylvania Student Health
 Services
Philadelphia, Pennsylvania
17.6 D-Dimer

Jayashree Paknikar, MD, FAAFP
Assistant Professor
Department of Family Medicine
Creighton University School of Medicine
Omaha, Nebraska
11.3 Chronic Pelvic Pain
11.6 Menorrhagia

David Patchett, DO
Assistant Clinical Professor
Midwestern University/AZCOM
Glendale, Arizona
12.6 Monoarticular Joint Pain

Kenneth D. Peters, MD, FAAFP with Added
Qualifications in Geriatrics
Graduate of the University of Nebraska Medical
 Center;
Clinical Instructor
Clarkson Family Practice Residency Program,
 Emeritus
Omaha, Nebraska
2.4 Falls

Layne A. Prest, MA, PhD
Assistant Clinical Professor
University of Washington;
Behavioral Scientist
Peace Health Southwest
Family Medicine Residency
Vancouver, Washington
3.1 Anxiety

David M. Quillen, MD
Associate Professor
Department of Community Health and Family
 Medicine
University of Florida College of Medicine
Gainesville, Florida
10 Renal and Urologic Problems
10.1 Dysuria
10.4 Urinary Incontinence

Naureen Rafiq, MD, MBBS
Assistant Professor
Department of Family Medicine
Creighton University Medical Center
Omaha, Nebraska
7.10 Palpitations
11.9 Postmenopausal Bleeding

Richard Rathe, MD
Associate Dean
Associate Professor
University of Florida College of Medicine
Gainesville, Florida
10.4 Urinary Incontinence

W. David Robinson, PhD, LMFT
Director of Marriage and Family Therapy
 Program
Department of Family, Consumer, and Human
 Development
Utah State University
Logan, Utah
3.3 Depression

Daniel Rubin, MD
Clinical Assistant Professor
Department of Community Health and Family
 Medicine
University of Florida
Gainesville, Florida
10.1 Dysuria

Richard H. Rutkowski, MD
Department of Family Medicine
Mayo Clinic
Scottsdale, Arizona
Instructor
Mayo Medical School;
Clinical Assistant Professor
Family and Community Medicine
University of Arizona College of Medicine
Phoenix, Arizona
12.1 Arthralgia

Amr Salam, MBChB (Hons) BSc (Hons)
Academic Foundation Doctor
North West London Hospitals
Imperial College Healthcare NHS Trust
London, United Kingdom
13.2 Erythema Multiforme

George P. Samraj, MD
Associate Professor
Community Health and Family Medicine
University of Florida
Gainesville, Florida
10.6 Oliguria and Anuria
10.9 Scrotal Pain
10.10 Urethral Discharge

Rodolfo M. Sanchez, MD
Assistant Professor
Department of Family Medicine
Creighton University School of Medicine
Omaha, Nebraska
14.8 Hyperthyroidism/Thyrotoxicosis

Monica Sarawagi, MD
Resident Physician
Department of Family Medicine
University of Nebraska Medical Center
Omaha, Nebraska
9.12 Steatorrhea

Dillon J. Savard, MD
Faculty
Family Medicine Residency
David Grant Medical Center
Travis AFB, California
8.8 Stridor

Shailendra K. Saxena, MD, PhD
Associate Professor
Department of Family Medicine
Creighton University
Omaha, Nebraska
11.2 Breast Mass
11.5 Dyspareunia

Siegfried Schmidt, MD
Associate Professor and Medical Director
Community Health and Family Medicine
University of Florida College of Medicine
Gainesville, Florida
10.2 Hematuria

Shannon C. Scott, DO
Assistant Clinical Professor FM/OMM
Arizona College of Osteopathic Medicine;
Osteopathic Board Certified Family Physician
Midwestern University
Glendale, Arizona
12.8 Polymyalgia

Perry W. Sexton, MD
Clinical Physician
Encinitas Family Care
Encinitas, California
17.4 Brain Natriuretic Peptide
17.6 D-Dimer

Omar Shamsaldeen, MD
Attending Dermatologist
Farwaniya Hospital
Kuwait
13.7 Urticaria

Sanjeev Sharma, MD
Associate Professor
Department of Family Medicine
Creighton University School of Medicine
Omaha, Nebraska
7.3 Chest Pain
11 Problems Related to the Female Reproductive System
11.1 Amenorrhea
11.4 Dysmenorrhea
11.10 Vaginal Discharge

Avery Sides, MD
Resident Physician
Department of Family Medicine
University of Nebraska Medical Center
Omaha, Nebraska
4.3 Delirium

Sumit Singhal, MBBS
Resident Physician
Creighton University
Department of Family Medicine
Omaha, Nebraska
11.1 Amenorrhea

John L. Smith, MD
Associate Professor
Department of Family Medicine
University of Nebraska Medical Center
Omaha, Nebraska
15.3 Petechiae and Purpura

Mikayla L. Spangler, PharmD, BCPS
Assistant Professor
Department of Pharmacy Practice
Creighton University
Omaha, Nebraska
11.2 Breast Mass
11.5 Dyspareunia

Carmen G. Strickland, MD, MPH
Assistant Professor
Department of Family & Community Medicine
Wake Forest University School of Medicine
Winston-Salem, North Carolina
6.6 Rhinitis

Vijaya Subramanian, MBBS
Resident Physician
Department of Family Medicine
University of Nebraska Medical Center
Omaha, Nebraska
9.10 Jaundice

Razan Taha, MD
Family Medicine Resident
Creighton University Medical Center
Omaha, Nebraska
14.3 Hirsutism

Kenji L. Takano, MD
Medical Director
Uniformed Services School of Medicine;
Staff Physician
Family Medicine Clinic
Mike O'Callaghan Federal Hospital
Nellis Air Force Base, Nevada
8.1 Cough

Joseph Teel, MD
Assistant Clinical Professor of Family Medicine &
  Community Health
Perelman School of Medicine
Hospital of the University of Pennsylvania
Philadelphia, Pennsylvania
17.1 Alkaline Phosphatase, Elevated

Christy A. Thomas, MD
Senior Resident
Department of Family Medicine
Wake Forest Baptist Health
Winston-Salem, North Carolina
6.8 Tinnitus

Denae M. Torpey, DO
Chief Resident
Department of Family Medicine
University of Nebraska Medical Center
Omaha, Nebraska
4.7 Seizures

Diego R. Torres-Russotto, MD
Assistant Professor
Department of Neurological Sciences;
Director
UNMC Movement Disorders Program;
Medical Director
TNMC Movement Disorders Center;
Director
Movement Disorders Fellowship Program;
Assistant Director
Neurology Residency Program;
Director
Neurology Clinical Clerkship;
University of Nebraska Medical Center
Omaha, Nebraska
4.1 Ataxia
4.9 Tremors

Alicia C. Walters-Stewart, MD
Clinical Instructor
Department of Family & Community Medicine
Wake Forest Baptist Health
Winston-Salem, North Carolina
6.9 Vertigo

Rebecca Wester, MD
Assistant Professor
Department of Family Medicine/Geriatrics
University of Nebraska Medical Center
Omaha, Nebraska
7.6 Congestive Heart Failure

Katrina N. Wherry, MD
Clinical Professor & Staff Physician
Department of Family Medicine
University of Nebraska Medical Center
Omaha, Nebraska
8.9 Wheezing

Sean P. Wherry, MD
Clinical Professor
Department of Family Medicine
University of Nebraska Medical Center
Omaha, Nebraska
8.3 Hemoptysis

Mohammed Zalabani, MBChB
Family Medicine Resident Physician
Creighton University Medical Center
Omaha, Nebraska
14.5 Polydipsia

Preface

Primary care physicians and other health-care providers including residents, students, physician assistants, and nurse practitioners often face the challenge of diagnosing conditions for patients on the basis of undifferentiated and sometimes confusing presenting complaints or concerns. The increasing "pressure to produce" in the clinical setting and the demands for high-quality health care have made the effective use of time in the clinic essential for primary care practitioners.

Taylor's Differential Diagnosis Manual is designed to support the busy practitioner in the process of diagnosing patient problems in this environment.

The manual is organized around common presenting symptoms, signs, laboratory and imaging findings. Each chapter serves as a stand-alone, concise, clear, and easily read information source for the condition covered. The manual is designed to work at the point of care and to fit inside a lab coat pocket.

The editors are pleased to include in this new edition the latest clinical evidence as well as changes in clinical practice in place since the last edition was published. While adding new content, the editors of this volume have made every effort to maintain the excellent readability and utility that previous authors, editors, and especially Dr. Robert Taylor were able to achieve.

All the authors and editors of *Taylor's Differential Diagnosis Manual* hope that this book is useful to you as you provide care for your patients.

For the authors and editors.

Paul M. Paulman, MD
Omaha, Nebraska
Lead Editor

Acknowledgments

The editors of *Taylor's Differential Diagnosis Manual* would like to acknowledge the work and contributions of the section editors and chapter authors who produced excellent manuscripts. We are also indebted to the editing and production staff at Wolters Kluwer; it truly was a pleasure working with you on this book. The editors are grateful to Dr. Robert Taylor who produced the first edition of *Taylor's Differential Diagnosis Manual*: it provided an excellent template from which to work.

This book would not have been possible without the hard work and incredible organization and management skills of Makenzie Lind-Olson. Makenzie did a great job keeping all members of the team organized and on task and facilitating communication among the many involved in the production of this book. We are very grateful for her efforts.

Paul M. Paulman, MD
Omaha, Nebraska
Lead Editor

Contents

CHAPTER 1

Principles of the 10-Minute Diagnosis

Robert B. Taylor

Principles of the 10-Minute Diagnosis

Paul M. Paulman

Ten minutes for diagnosis? Really?

Yes, really!

If only we had 90 minutes to perform a diagnostic evaluation, as we did as third-year medical students on hospital rotations. Or, if we had even 30 minutes for diagnosis, as I recall from internship. But those days are gone. Today—as clinicians practicing in the age of evidence-based, cost-effective health care—office visits are of much shorter duration than in years past. For example, in a recent study of 4,454 patients seeing 138 physicians in 84 practices, the mean visit duration was 10 minutes (1). Another study of 19,192 visits to 686 primary care physicians estimated the visit duration to be 16.3 minutes (2). Even when the total visit duration exceeds 10 minutes, the time actually devoted to diagnosis—and not to greeting the patient, explaining treatment, doing managed care paperwork, or even the patient's dressing and undressing—is seldom more than 10 minutes.

So, if you and I generally have only 10 minutes per office visit for diagnosis, we need to be focused, while remaining medically thorough and prudent. Actually, such an approach is possible and is how experienced clinicians tend to practice. The following are some practice guidelines to the 10-minute diagnosis *(Dx10)*. And, to illustrate, let us consider a patient: *Joan S., a 49-year-old married woman, in your office for a first visit, whose chief complaint is severe, one-sided headaches that have become worse over the past year.* (For a more complete approach to the diagnosis of headache, see Chapter 2.7.)

SEARCH FOR DIAGNOSTIC CUES THROUGHOUT THE CLINICAL ENCOUNTER

Note how the patient relates to the staff, takes off a jacket, and sits in the examination room. How does the patient begin to describe the problem and what does he or she seem to want from the visit? Who accompanies the patient to the office and who seems to do the talking?

Be sure to use "tell me about" open-ended questions. The inexperienced clinician moves early to closed-ended "Yes" or "No" questions, but the veteran *Dx10* clinician has learned that using narrow questions too early can lead to misleading conclusions, which are in the long run, at the least,

---

This chapter appeared in the first volume of Taylor's Diagnostic Manual. At that time, the title of the book was The 10-Minute Diagnosis Manual. The editing team has elected to maintain Dr. Taylor's chapter in the current version of this book because its message is as pertinent now as it was when Dr. Taylor originally wrote it.

wasteful of time and, at worst, dangerous. An example would be attributing chest pain inappropriately to gastroesophageal reflux disease because the patient has a past history of esophageal reflux and responds affirmatively to questions about current heartburn and intolerance to spicy foods.

Watch the facial reaction to issues discussed. Tune in to hesitation and evasive answers and be willing to follow these diagnostic paths, which may lead to otherwise hidden problems such as drug abuse or domestic violence. *In the case of Joan S., does she answer questions readily or does she seem evasive when addressing some topics, such as family concerns or her home life?*

THINK "MOST COMMON" FIRST

I remind medical students of the time-honored aphorism that "the most common problems occur most commonly." When working with a patient, the physician develops diagnostic hypotheses early in the encounter. When faced with a patient with headache, we should initially consider tension headache and migraine rather than temporal arteritis. Of course, the *Dx10* clinician thinks of special concerns, such as the possibility that the patient with headache might possibly have a brain tumor. The initial history seeks the characteristics and chronology of the symptoms. Then the clinician uses select questions that help rule in or out the diagnostic hypotheses: "What seems to precede the headache pain?" "Has the nature or the severity of your pain changed in any way?" The clinician also seeks important past medical, social, and family history: "What stress are you experiencing that may be influencing your symptoms?" "Does anyone else in your family have a headache problem?"

The physical examination should be limited to the body areas likely to contribute to the diagnosis, and a "full physical examination" is actually seldom needed. *Therefore, for our patient with recurrent headaches, Joan S., the Dx10 examination is likely to be limited to the vital signs, head, and neck, with a screening of coordination, deep tendon reflexes, and cranial nerve function. Examination of the chest, heart, and abdomen is unlikely to contribute to the diagnosis.*

Tests should be limited to those that will help confirm or rule out a diagnostic hypothesis or, later, those that would help make a therapeutic decision. For most patients with headache as a presenting complaint, no laboratory test or diagnostic imaging is needed.

Of course, the uncommon problem occurs *sometimes*. Occasionally, you will encounter the unexpected finding: the patient with headache having unanticipated unilateral deafness or the fatigued individual with an enlarged spleen. Stop and think when you note a cluster of similar unexpected findings; such alertness helped clinicians identify the Muerto Canyon virus as the cause of the 1993 outbreak of the hantavirus pulmonary syndrome in southwestern United States and also the occurrence of primary pulmonary hypertension in patients using dexfenfluramine for weight control. A few times in your career you will have the opportunity to experience a diagnostic epiphany; the *Dx10* clinician will seize this opportunity by staying alert for the unexpected diagnostic clue.

USE ALL AVAILABLE ASSISTANCE

In addition to your professional knowledge, experience, and time, your diagnostic resources include your staff, the patient and his or her family, and the vast array of medical reference sources available.

Your office and hospital staff can be valuable allies in determining the diagnosis. Important clues may be offered when the patient calls for an appointment or when being escorted to the examination room. If a patient remarks to the receptionist or nurse that his chest pain is "just like my father had before his heart attack" or if another wonders if her heartburn could be related to her 15-year-old daughter's misbehavior, the staff member should ask the patient's permission and then share the information with the physician.

The patient and the family generally have some insight into the cause of symptoms such as fatigue, diarrhea, or loss of appetite. In a study of patient's differential diagnosis of cough, Bergh found that while physicians considered a mean of 7.6 diagnostic possibilities, patients reported a mean of 6.5 possibilities, with only 2.8 possibilities common to both (3). *Joan S. and perhaps her family may offer diagnostic suggestions that you have not strongly considered; also, these other hypotheses represent concerns that should eventually be addressed to provide reassurance. For example, might Joan be in the office today chiefly because an old friend has recently been diagnosed with brain cancer and she has become concerned about the significance of her own headaches?*

CONSIDER THE PSYCHOSOCIAL ASPECTS OF THE PROBLEM

To continue the case of the patient with headache, a migraine diagnosis is incomplete if it fails to include the contribution of marital or job stress to the symptoms of family event cancellations, trips to the emergency room, and large pharmacy bills for sumatriptan injections, as well as the impact on others. No diagnosis of cancer or diabetes is complete without considering the impact on the patient's life and the lives of family members (4).

The *Dx10* clinician will be especially wary of the *International Classification of Diseases, Ninth Edition* (ICD-9) diagnostic categories, which facilitate statistical analysis and managed care payments, but lack the richness of narrative and also the personal and family context. For example, compare "diabetes mellitus, uncomplicated, ICD-9 code 250.00" with "type 2 diabetes mellitus in an elderly patient with poor diet, marginal retirement income, and isolation from the family."

Failure to consider the psychosocial aspects of disease invites an incompletely understood or even a missed diagnosis: how many instances of child abuse have been overlooked as busy emergency room physicians care for childhood fractures without also exploring the cause of the injury and the home environment?

When eliciting a medical history from Joan S., it will be important to learn the current stresses at work and at home, and how she thinks her life would be different if the headaches were gone.

SEEK HELP WHEN NEEDED

Today, health care, including diagnosis, must be "evidence based" and not grounded in anecdote or even in your "years of clinical experience." The evidence is, of course, the vast body of medical knowledge, including research reports and meta-analyses found in clinical journals (5), on the World Wide Web (6), and in reference books such as *The 10-Minute Diagnosis Manual*. *When thinking about Joan S., you might search the literature for recent articles on the approach to migraine headaches.*

Help is also available from colleagues. Consider a consultation when you have a diagnosis that is somehow not "satisfying." A personal physician in a long-term relationship with a patient can develop a blind spot, and the diagnosis may be apparent only to someone taking a fresh look. What may be needed at such a time is a rethinking of the problem—almost the antithesis of continuity.

Help can be available from the same-specialty colleague down the hall or from a subspecialist.

THINK IN TERMS OF A CONTINUALLY EVOLVING DIAGNOSIS

You do not always need to make the definitive diagnosis on the first visit; in fact, such an approach tends to foster prolonged visits, excessive testing, overly biomedical diagnoses, and high-cost medicine without adding quality. When faced with an elusive diagnosis, the best test is often the passage of time and a follow-up visit. For example, we all know that headaches are often influenced by stressful life events. Yet, a new patient may not be ready to share his or her personal, often embarrassing, burdens, and it is only when a trustful relationship has been established that the clinician learns about the abusive spouse, the pregnant teenager, or the impending financial disaster.

It is often useful to use the descriptive, categorical diagnosis and seek the definitive diagnosis over time. Examples include the teenage girl with chronic pelvic pain, the young adult with cough for 3 months, the middle-aged person with loss of appetite, and the older person with fatigue or insomnia. Sometimes, on an initial visit, this approach is the only reasonable option.

The *Dx10* clinician will be careful not to "fall in love" with the initial diagnosis and realize that the depressed patient losing weight might also have cancer and that it is too easy to attribute all new symptoms to a known diagnosis of menopause or diabetes mellitus. *If Joan's headaches fail to respond as expected over time, you may wish to reconsider your original diagnosis and perhaps seek further testing that would have seemed excessive on the initial visit. For example, might the "1-year" duration of increased severity merit imaging if a favorable response to initial therapy does not occur?*

In your daily practice, use the time saved in the steps described here to consider and reconsider your diagnoses—as you review chart notes, read medical journals, search medical web sites, and see the patient in follow-up visits. The *Dx10* clinician will remain open to rethinking the patient's diagnostic problem list. In the end, patience and perseverance—often measured in 10-minute aliquots over time—will yield an insightful, biopsychosocially inclusive, and clinically useful diagnosis.

REFERENCES

1. Stange KC, Zyzanski SJ, Jaen CR. Illuminating the black box: a description of 4454 patient visits to 138 family physicians. *J Fam Pract* 1998;46:377–389.
2. Blumenthal D, Causino N, Chang YC. The duration of ambulatory visits to physicians. *J Fam Pract* 1999;48:264–271.
3. Bergh KD. The patient's differential diagnosis: unpredictable concerns in visits for cough. *J Fam Pract* 1998;46:153–158.
4. Taylor RB. Family practice and the advancement of medical understanding: the first 50 years. *J Fam Pract* 1999;48:53–57.
5. Richardson WS, Wilson MC, Guyatt GH, et al. User's guide to the medical literature: how to use an article about disease probability for differential diagnosis. *JAMA* 1999;281:1214–1219.
6. Hersh W. A world of knowledge at your fingertips: the promise, reality, and future directions of on-line information retrieval. *Acad Med* 1999;74:240–243.

CHAPTER **2**

Undifferentiated Problems
Richard H. Hurd

Anorexia
Dorota Brilz

I. BACKGROUND. Anorexia is prolonged appetite loss. It is a common symptom of many medical conditions and should be differentiated from the psychiatric disease "anorexia nervosa."

II. PATHOPHYSIOLOGY

A. General Mechanisms. It is not known exactly how the body regulates appetite stimulation/suppression. It appears that both neural and humoral mechanisms interact. The hypothalamus is believed to regulate both satiety and hunger, leading to homeostasis of body weight in ideal situations. The hypothalamus interprets and integrates a number of neural and humoral inputs to coordinate feeding and energy expenditure in response to conditions of altered energy balance. Long-term signals communicating information about the body's energy stores, endocrine status, and general health are predominantly humoral. Short-term signals, including gut hormones and neural signals from higher brain centers and the gut, regulate meal initiation and termination. Hormones involved in this process include leptin, insulin, cholecystokinin, ghrelin, polypeptide YY, pancreatic polypeptide, glucagonlike peptide-1, and oxyntomodulin (1). Alterations in any of these humoral or neuronal processes can lead to anorexia.

B. Etiology. Causes of anorexia can be divided into the following four categories:

1. **Pathologic.** These include malignancy (particularly gastrointestinal, lung, lymphoma, renal, and prostate cancers); gastrointestinal diseases (including peptic ulcer disease, malabsorption, diabetic enteropathy, dysphagia, inflammatory bowel disease, hepatitis, Zenker's diverticulum, and paraesophageal hernia); infectious diseases (human immunodeficiency virus [HIV], viral hepatitis, tuberculosis, chronic fungal or bacterial disease, chronic parasitic infection, and lung abscess); endocrine disorders (uncontrolled diabetes and adrenal insufficiency); severe heart, lung, and kidney diseases (heart failure; severe obstructive or restrictive lung disease; and renal failure, nephritic syndrome, and chronic glomerulonephritis); neurologic diseases (stroke, dementia, dysphagia, Parkinson disease, and amyotrophic lateral sclerosis); and chronic inflammatory diseases (sarcoidosis, severe rheumatoid arthritis, and giant cell vasculitis).

2. **Psychiatric.** Affective disorders (depression, bipolar disorder, and generalized anxiety disorder) and food-related delusions from other psychiatric disorders (schizophrenia and related conditions).

3. **Pharmacologic.** Decreased appetite may be a side effect of one of these medications: topiramate, zonisamide, selective serotonin receptor inhibitors, levodopa, digoxin, metformin, exenatide, liraglutide, nonsteroidal anti-inflammatory drugs, anticancer and antiretroviral drugs, as well as alcohol, opiates, amphetamines, and cocaine. Withdrawal

from chronic high-dose psychotropic medications and cannabis may cause anorexia. Herbal and nonprescription preparations that cause appetite loss include 5-hydroxy-tryptophan, aloe, caffeine, cascara, chitosan, chromium, dandelion, ephedra, garcinia, glucomannan, guarana, guar gum, herbal diuretics, nicotine, pyruvate, and St. John's wort (2).

4. **Social** factors often cause anorexia. Bereavement, stress, and loneliness may decrease appetite. Moving from one's home, loss of ability to shop for food or to prepare meals, and financial difficulties may also result in appetite changes.

III. EVALUATION

A. **History.** Obtaining detailed history is essential in identifying potential causes of patient's anorexia.

1. **History of Present Illness.** How long has the problem been going on? Is it constant or episodic? Does the patient associate it with anything? Are there are psychological stressors present? How about difficulty or pain with swallowing?

2. **Past Medical History.** Any history of chronic medical problems, malignancies, or past psychiatric problems, including eating disorders.

3. **Medications and Habits.** Use of illicit drugs or any of the above prescription medications that may cause anorexia.

4. **Social History.** Access to food, to include financial and mobility issues. Patients may experience anorexia if their food is prepared in a manner different from their customary fashion (e.g., patients entering an institution). Patients who may be restricted by their medical professionals to a certain health-related diet may experience lack of appetite due to taste preferences.

5. **Review of Systems.** Review of systems should focus on weight changes, as well as gastro-intestinal, psychiatric, and neurologic systems. A food diary is often helpful to quantify patient's intake and analyze for the presence of any patterns.

B. **Physical Examination.**

1. **General Appearance.** Does the patient appear healthy or ill? Review the vital signs for fever, tachycardia, tachypnea, or blood pressure abnormalities as signs of systemic illness.

2. **Head, Eyes, Ears, Nose, and Throat (HEENT).** Examine the oral cavity for lesions or poor dentition. Assess for dysphagia/odynophagia and for the presence of lymphade-nopathy, thyromegaly, or cervical masses.

3. **Cardiovascular System.** Assess the patient for arrhythmias and signs of congestive heart failure, such as rales, jugular venous distention, and lower extremity edema.

4. **Respiratory System.** Auscultate lungs for the presence of wheezes, crackles, or poor air exchange indicating chronic obstructive pulmonary disease or restrictive lung disease.

5. **Gastrointestinal System.** Listen for abnormal bowel sounds. Examine for tenderness, rigidity, ascites, and hepatomegaly. Rectal examination, including guaiac testing, should be performed (3).

6. **Skin.** Jaundice, skin tracks, cyanosis, lanugo, hyperpigmentation, and turgor should be noted.

7. **Neurologic and Psychological Systems.** Examine the functions of cranial nerves, including smell and taste. Look for focal or generalized weakness, gait or balance dis-turbances, or movement disorders. Assess the patient's functional capacity and mental status. Assess for anxiety, depression, dementia, delirium, and psychosis.

C. **Testing.** As in all areas of medicine, diagnostic studies should be guided by the history and physical examination. Tests to consider in anorexia include a complete blood count, electrolyte panel, hepatic panel, and albumin. When assessing nutritional status, measuring prealbumin level may be preferred over albumin level in acute cases of anorexia because prealbumin is the earliest marker of changes in nutritional status (4). Chest x-ray and tuberculosis testing can be helpful in some cases, as might esophagogastroduodenoscopy, colonoscopy, and abdominal computed tomography, or ultrasonography. Other tests to include are HIV, thyroid-stimulating hormone and thyroid hormone, viral hepatitis panel, urine protein, and urinalysis (3), and testing for toxicology and drugs of abuse.

IV. DIAGNOSIS. Although the causes of anorexia are numerous and span the biopsychosocial spectrum, a thoughtful evaluation will generally reveal the underlying cause(s) of the loss of appetite, and specific interventions can then be instituted.

REFERENCES

1. Murphy KG, Bloom SR. Gut hormones in the control of appetite. *Exp Physiol* 2004;89:507–516.
2. Anorexia nervosa in adults: diagnosis, associated clinical features, and assessment. Up To Date 2012. Accessed at http://www.uptodate.com/contents/anorexia-nervosa-in-adults-diagnosis-associated-clinical-features-and-assessment?source-search_result&search=anorexia&selectedTitle=2%7E150 #H549367385 on May 14, 2012.
3. Brooke Huffman G. Evaluating and treating unintentional weight loss in the elderly. *Am Fam Physician* 2002;65:640–651.
4. Beck FK, Rosenthal TC. Prealbumin: a marker for nutritional evaluation. *Am Fam Physician* 2002;65:1575–1578.

2.2 Dizziness
Richard H. Hurd

I. BACKGROUND. Dizziness is a rather imprecise term often used by patients to describe any of a number of peculiar subjective symptoms. These symptoms may include faintness, giddiness, lightheadedness, or unsteadiness. True vertigo, a sensation of irregular or whirling motion, is also included in a patient's complaint of dizziness. Dizziness represents a disturbance in a patient's subjective sensation of relationship space (1).

II. PATHOPHYSIOLOGY

A. Etiology. The causes of dizziness are numerous. It is helpful for the diagnostician to think in general categories of causes when searching for an etiology (see Table 2.2.1).

B. Epidemiology. Dizziness is the complaint in an estimated 7 million clinical visits in the United States each year (2, 3). It is one of the most frequent reasons for referral to neurologists and otolaryngologists. The reasons for frequent referral of this usually benign condition are many. Ruling out potentially serious causes, including those of cardiac and neurologic origin, can be difficult. In addition, the fact that there is no specific treatment for many of the causes of dizziness leads to frustration for both the patient and physician.

III. EVALUATION

A. History. It is extremely important, and can be very difficult, to get patients to describe exactly what they mean when complaining of dizziness. A description of the attack, context, length, duration, and frequency is important. Any precipitating factor should be explored. Concurrent symptoms such as nausea, headache, chest fluttering, or tinnitus can help to direct the clinician to the cause. Any new medication or medication changes should be inquired about.

B. Physical Examination. The physical examination, although thorough, is often focused on a specific system based on the history. It is seldom diagnostic in itself but is more often confirmatory.

  1. Vital signs including orthostatic blood pressures begin the examination.

  2. A neurologic examination must be completed.

TABLE 2.2.1 **Common Causes of Dizziness**

Peripheral vestibular[a]	Central vestibular[b]	Psychiatric[c]	Nonvestibular, nonpsychiatric[d]
Benign positional vertigo	Cerebrovascular disease[e]	Hyperventilation	Presyncope
Labyrinthitis	Tumors[f]	–	Disequilibrium
Meniere's disease	Cerebellar atrophy	–	Medications
Other[g]	Migraine	–	Metabolic disturbances
	Multiple sclerosis	–	Infection
	Epilepsy	–	Trauma
	–	–	Unknown causes[h]

[a]Encompasses 44% of patients.

[b]Accounts for 11% of dizziness cases.

[c]Causes make up 16% of the diagnosis.

[d]Accounts for 37% of the diagnosis.

[e]Stroke or transient ischemic attack and dehydration comprise the largest part of this group.

[f]Usually acoustic neuroma.

[g]Includes drug-induced, ototoxicity, and nonspecific vestibulopathy.

[h]A significant part of this subset and a significant part of all cases of dizziness.

    3. A cardiovascular examination including the heart for murmur or arrhythmia and carotid arterial auscultation should be completed.

    4. An otoscopic examination to assess infection and nystagmus examination including gaze, Dix-Hallpike's maneuvers, and head shaking are important.

    5. An observation of gait to assess cerebellar function is also a part of the examination.

  C. Testing. It is obvious that there is no laboratory test or imaging study directly related to dizziness. Instead, these types of studies are dictated by the etiology that the clinician feels is most likely. They are more to confirm a diagnosis than to actually make it.

    1. Tests might include complete blood count, electrolytes, appropriate drug levels, and thyroid levels.

    2. Imaging studies such as magnetic resonance imaging might be indicated if the concern of tumor is high.

    3. A hearing test as well as maneuvers carried out in a tilt-chair to test labyrinth function may be of value.

  D. Genetics. There does not appear to be any genetic predisposition to dizziness.

IV. DIAGNOSIS

  A. Differential Diagnosis.

    1. The differential diagnosis of dizziness includes all of those conditions mentioned in the preceding text that cause true dizziness (Table 2.2.1). It also includes many other conditions that cause patients to feel abnormal in some vague way, causing them to complain of dizziness. Psychologic conditions such as anxiety, depression, panic disorder, or somatization may all cause a patient to complain of dizziness. Cardiac arrhythmias, ischemic or valvular heart disease, vasovagal anemia, or postural hypotension are some of the conditions leading to cerebral hypoperfusion, and therefore, presyncope.

2. Degenerative changes in the elderly may affect the vestibular apparatus, vision, or proprioception, all of which may be interpreted as dizziness. Finally, peripheral neuropathy or cerebellar disease may also be confused with dizziness.

B. Clinical Manifestations.
The clinical manifestations of dizziness are as varied as those entities included in both the etiologic and the differential diagnosis sections. The fact that dizziness is more often a symptom of some other condition than a separate diagnosis leads to a variety of manifestations that the clinicians must decipher.

REFERENCES

1. M. Bajorek. Night sweats. In: Taylor R, ed. *The 10-minute diagnosis manual.* Philadelphia, PA: Lippincott Williams & Wilkins, 200:31–33.
2. Kroenke K, Hoffman R, Einstadter D. How common are various causes of dizziness? A critical review. *South Med J* 2000;93(2):160–168, Table 2, P7.
3. Sloane PD. Dizziness in primary care: results from the National Ambulatory Medical Care Survey. *J Fam Pract* 1989;29:33–38.

2.3 Edema
Jennifer J. Buescher

I. BACKGROUND. Edema is caused by an abnormality in fluid exchange affecting capillary hemodynamic forces, sodium and water exchange in the kidney, or both (1). Edema is a common symptom in many different medical conditions.

II. PATHOPHYSIOLOGY

A. Etiology. The kidneys maintain a balance between extracellular fluid volume and effective arterial blood volume by adjusting water and sodium excretion (2). Maintaining a plasma volume sufficient for oxygen delivery to the tissues is the most important factor at play. Fluid will move to the extracellular space when the capillary hydraulic pressure is elevated, plasma oncotic pressure decreases, interstitial oncotic pressure increases, or capillary permeability increases. The increase in extracellular (interstitial) fluid causes edema (1).

B. Epidemiology. Edema is a common problem in clinical practice in both acute and chronic conditions.

III. EVALUATION

A. History. Edema is seen in many diverse clinical conditions and therefore a complete history is necessary for an accurate diagnosis. A thorough medication history is also important as many common prescription medications can cause or worsen edema. The history should include the onset of symptoms, associated pain, dietary intake, pregnancy, trauma to the affected area, recent travel, and work history. Acute onset of edema can be indicative of acute lymphatic or venous obstruction, which may require urgent action. Chronic edema is more likely caused by chronic cardiac, liver, or kidney disease (2). Myxedema caused by untreated hypothyroidism can also be a cause of generalized chronic edema.

B. Review of Symptoms. The review of systems must be thorough in the evaluation of edema to differentiate the multiple medical causes of edema. Special attention should be paid to the cardiac, pulmonary, joint, extremity, and gastrointestinal (GI) symptoms.

C. Physical Examination. The physical examination should focus on the location and severity of swelling, skin breakdown, and signs that would help differentiate the many

TABLE 2.3.1	Differential Diagnosis of Edema

Lymphedema
  Postsurgical
  Mass effect from tumor
  Posttraumatic changes
Deep venous thrombosis
Myxedema: hypothyroidism
Acute trauma or fracture
Congestive heart failure
Cirrhosis
Nephrotic syndrome
Iatrogenic edema (excessive standing, tight clothing, etc.)
Medication-induced
  Nonsteroidal anti-inflammatory drugs
  Calcium channel antagonists
  Estrogens
  Vasodilators
  Corticosteroids

Information adapted from O'Brien J. G., Chennubhotle, S. A., & Chennubhotla, R. V. (2005). Treatment of Edema. *American Family Physician*, 2005;71 (11): 2111–2117; Braunwald E, Loscalzo J. In: Anthony EB, Fauci S, eds. *Harrison's principles of internal medicine*, Chapter 36, 17th ed. New York, NY: McGraw-Hill, 2008.

causes of edema. Unilateral or nondependent edema should be evaluated urgently for deep venous thrombosis or lymphatic obstruction from a tumor. Bilateral or dependent edema is most commonly associated with congestive heart failure and abdominal edema is more indicative of hepatic abnormalities. Generalized edema of both the upper and lower extremities and trunk should raise a concern for nephrotic syndrome or other renal abnormalities (1). Dependent edema is common in normal pregnancy, but upper extremity or severe edema in pregnancy can be a sign of preeclampsia and should be evaluated more thoroughly.

   D. Testing. Testing should be directed by the history, review of systems, and examination. Evaluation may include a metabolic panel, liver enzymes, thyroid stimulating hormone, echocardiogram, abdominal ultrasound, vascular ultrasound of the extremity, or other diagnostic tests.

IV. DIAGNOSIS

A differential diagnosis for edema is listed in Table 2.3.1. A complete history and physical examination paired with focused laboratory and radiologic evaluation is necessary for the accurate diagnosis of edema.

REFERENCES

1. O'Brien JG, Chennubhotle SA, Chennubhotla RV. Treatment of edema. *Am Fam Physician* 2005;71(11):2111–2117.
2. Braunwald E, Loscalzo J. Edema. In: Anthony EB, Fauci S, eds. *Harrison's principles of internal medicine*, Chapter 36, 17th ed. New York, NY: McGraw-Hill, 2008:290–295.

2.4 Falls

Kenneth D. Peters

I. **BACKGROUND.** Falls are most common at age extremes. In children older than 1 year of age, injuries are the number one cause of death. Falls account for 25% of these. Bike injuries account for 68% of injuries in children from 5 to 14 years of age (1). In patients older than 65 years of age, the incidence of falls is 30%; in those older than 80 years of age, it is >50%. Accidents are the fifth leading cause of death in patients 65 years of age and older, and falls account for two-thirds of these deaths. Of elderly patients hospitalized for falls, only 50% are alive 1 year later (2).

II. **PATHOPHYSIOLOGY.** Factors that contribute to falls need to be identified and evaluated for preventative measures to be taken. Children fall from heights; elderly fall from level surfaces.

A. **Children and Adolescents.** Fall from heights over 3 feet and falls of infants younger than 1 year of age result in increased risk of skull fracture and intracranial bleeding. Emergent evaluation is needed in cases of loss of consciousness, behavioral changes, seizures, or ongoing vomiting.

B. **Falls in the Elderly.** One half of the falls are secondary to accidents, including factors affecting stability. The other half of the falls are secondary to medical disorders (see Table 2.4.1). If syncope occurred with a fall, it must be determined whether the cause is cardiac or noncardiac (see Table 2.4.2) (Chapter 2.12). Cardiac mortality in falls related to syncope at 1 year is 20% to 30%, whereas noncardiac mortality is <5% (3). There is a strong association between falls and nursing home placement in the elderly; furthermore, specific individualized interventions help prevent falls (4). The risk of hip fracture in the frail elderly can be reduced with the use of an anatomically designed external hip protector (5).

III. **EVALUATION**

A. **History.**

1. **History of the Fall.** An interview of a witness to the fall is essential. This may identify any seizure activity, loss of consciousness, and method of fall. Ask what the patient was doing prior to the fall, including occurrence with positional changes or after voiding, eating, or constipation. Are there associated palpitations implying arrhythmia? Did the patient have a fall or syncope during exercise, which may indicate a cardiac cause? Is there any confusion that is new or changed from the past that suggests central nervous system trauma or seizure? Was urine or bowel incontinence present? Questions concerning home and risk factors should be raised (Table 2.4.1).

2. **Past History.** Explore coexisting illness that may have contributed to the fall (Table 2.4.1). A family history of sudden death can imply arrhythmias. Furthermore, inquire about any family history of prior falls.

B. **Physical Examination.** This should include:

1. Assessment of vital signs, including heart rate and rhythm, orthostatic blood pressure changes, temperature, and respiratory rate.

2. A general body survey for any evidence of trauma.

3. Examination of the eye (fundoscopic, visual acuity, and fields), mouth (tongue lacerations), neck (bruits), lung (congestive heart failure or infection), and cardiovascular (murmurs and rhythm).

4. A neurologic examination that includes mental status, evaluation of balance, gait, mobility, and tests for peripheral neuropathy.

5. The "get up and go test" (rise from a chair, walk 10 feet, return, and sit down), which is a simple rapid way of assessing general condition and musculoskeletal and neurologic status.

TABLE 2.4.1   Factors Affecting Falls

Factors affecting stability	Medical problems contributing to falls
Decreased muscle tone/strength	Arthritis
Changes in gait	Previous stroke
Changes in postural control	Hip fracture
Decreased depth perception	Dementia
Decreased hearing	Osteoporosis
Decreased proprioception	Parkinsonism
Decreased vision	Foot disorders
Slower reflexes	Peripheral neuropathies
Hazardous living arrangements (e.g., poor lighting, slick floors, loose rugs, stairways, unstable furniture)	Hyperthyroidism
	Alcoholism
	Medications
	Hypertension
	Hypotension
	Myocardial infarction
	Arrhythmias
	Congestive heart failure
	Acute stroke
	Internal bleeding
	Infections
	Valvular heart disease
	Seizures

C. Testing

1. **Clinical Laboratory Tests**. Most blood tests are low yield and should be done to confirm clinical suspicion. An electrocardiogram is useful in the elderly to rule out arrhythmia, atrioventricular block, prolonged QT syndrome, or ischemia. A diagnosis of the cause of the fall can be obtained in 50% to 60% of cases based on history, physical, and electrocardiographic study (7).

2. **Diagnostic Imaging.** Skull x-ray (fracture) and computed tomography studies to detect intracranial bleeding are recommended in all infants younger than 1 year of age or if the fall was from >3 feet. Also consider imaging with any loss of consciousness, evidence of head trauma, behavioral changes, seizure disorder, ongoing vomiting, or focal neurologic deficits.

3. Other testing to consider includes echocardiogram (valvular heart disease), electroencephalogram (seizure), carotid ultrasound (bruits), carotid sinus massage (if suggested history), and tilt table testing (if a vasovagal cause of fall is considered). Ambulatory cardiac monitor is considered for sudden infrequent falls.

IV. DIAGNOSIS

A fall by an elderly individual frequently requires a home visit to evaluate factors contributing to falls and to correct unsafe conditions (Table 2.4.1). Symptoms of cardiac disease can occur with exertion or straining. Cardiac arrhythmias tend to be sudden without warning, although

TABLE 2.4.2   Causes of Syncope

Cardiac	Noncardiac
Obstructive	**Vasovagal**
Valvular disease	Pain
Hypertrophic cardiomyopathy	Voiding
Pulmonary hypertension	Increased stress
Pulmonary emboli	Cough
Myxomas	Simple faint
Arrhythmia	Carotid sinus disease
Sick sinus syndrome	**Orthostatic**
Atrial fibrillation	Medication
Arrhythmias	Volume depletion
	Diabetes
	Parkinsonism
	Neurologic
	Stroke
	Seizure
	Migraine

once in a while patients can complain of palpitations. Noncardiac causes include vasovagal reaction where the patient generally complains of dizziness or lightheadedness prior to a fall, often with changes in position or when upright. These can be associated with sweating and nausea. Orthostatic noncardiac causes have gradual onset and resolution. These are most often associated with medications, including antihypertensives, sedatives, anxiolytics, antidepressants, hypoglycemics, psychotropics, histamine-2 blockers, alcohol, over-the-counter cold medicines, and medications with extended half-lives. Neurologic noncardiac events can usually be diagnosed by history and physical examination. A psychiatric cause for falls in less likely, but one should be suspicious in cases of frequent symptoms with no injury.

For the differential diagnosis, refer to Tables 2.4.1 and 2.4.2.

REFERENCES

1. Gruskin KD, Schutzman SA. Head trauma in children younger than 2 years: are there predictors for complications? *Arch Pediatr Adolesc Med* 1999;153:15–20.
2. Steinweg KK. The changing approach to falls in the elderly. *Am Fam Physician* 1997;56:1815–1824.
3. Wiley TM. A diagnostic approach to syncope. *Resid Staff Physician* 1998;44:2947.
4. Tinetti ME, Williams CS. Falls, injuries due to falls, and the risk of admission to a nursing home. *New Engl J Med* 1997;337(18):1279–1284.
5. Kannus P, Parkkari J, Niemi S. Prevention of hip fracture is elderly people with use of a hip protector. *New Engl J Med* 2000:343(21):1506–1513.
6. Albert S, David R, Alison M. Comprehensive geriatric assessment. In: William H, Edwin B, John B, et al. eds. *Principals of geriatrics*, 3rd ed. New York, NY: McGraw-Hill, 1994: Chapter 17:206.
7. Hupert N, Kapoor WN. Syncope: a systemic approach for the cause. *Patient Care* 1997; 31:136–147.

2.5 Fatigue

Amy K. Jespersen

I. BACKGROUND

A. General Considerations. Fatigue is a very common complaint in the primary care office. It may be the primary reason a patient seeks care or a secondary complaint. We are all bothered by fatigue at some point in time. However, for millions of patients each year, it becomes bothersome enough to seek medical attention. True fatigue needs to be distinguished from weakness and from excessive somnolence secondary to sleep disturbances. Fatigue lasting less than a month is considered acute. If symptoms last more than a month, fatigue is considered prolonged.

B. Definitions.

1. Chronic fatigue is diagnosed when symptoms last >6 months. The Center for Disease Control and Prevention has defined chronic fatigue syndrome (CFS) as profound fatigue of 6 months' duration that presents with four of the following eight symptoms:
   a. Impairment in the short-term memory or concentration
   b. Sore throat
   c. Tender lymphadenopathy
   d. Myalgias
   e. Pain in multiple joints
   f. Headaches of a new type, pattern, or severity
   g. Unrefreshing sleep
   h. Postexertional malaise lasting >24 hours (1)

2. Idiopathic chronic fatigue is diagnosed if a patient has been fatigued for >6 months but does not meet the criteria for CFS.

II. PATHOPHYSIOLOGY

A. Etiology. Some of the common causes of CFS are listed in Table 2.5.1. Fatigue may be due to medical disorders, psychiatric disease, or lifestyle factors. In some cases, a cause is never determined. Fatigue that persists for several months or years is more likely to have psychiatric etiology, whereas a shorter duration of fatigue is more likely to have a medical explanation (2). If a medical cause of fatigue is present, it is usually identifiable on the initial history, physical, and laboratory testing (3, 4).

B. Epidemiology. The true incidence of profound fatigue is unknown. It has been estimated that over 7 million office visits per year are for complaints of fatigue (3). The true gender predilection is also unknown; however, women present to the physician's office twice as often as men. Patients younger than 45 years of age are more likely to present for fatigue than patients older than 45 years of age (2).

III. EVALUATION

A. History.

1. A detailed history and review of systems should be performed. The onset, duration, and degree of fatigue should be explored, along with any possible precipitating events. Specific attention should be given to sleep patterns, daytime somnolence, or sleep apnea symptoms.

2. The patient's exercise habits, caffeine intake, and drug or alcohol use should be explored, and medications should be reviewed.

3. A psychiatric history to evaluate symptoms of depression or anxiety should be obtained. Lifestyle issues such as stress at home or in the work place, childcare responsibilities, shift work, or changed work schedules should be addressed.

TABLE 2.5.1	Common Causes of Fatigue		
Medical conditions		**Psychiatric disorders**	**Lifestyle factors**
Hypothyroidism		Major depressive disorder	Sleep deprivation
Anemia		Bipolar disorder	Marital discord
Cardiomyopathy		Alcoholism/substance abuse	Job stress
COPD		Anxiety	Caring for young children
Morbid obesity		Somatoform disorders	Altered work schedule
Sleep disorders			
Medication side effects			
β-Blockers			
Centrally acting α-blockers			
Antidepressants			
Subacute infections			
Viral infections (CMV, EBV, HIV)			
Bacterial endocarditis			
Malignancy			
Fibromyalgia			

COPD, chronic obstructive pulmonary disease; CMV, cytomegalovirus; EBV, Epstein-Barr virus; HIV, human immunodeficiency virus.

B. Physical Examination. A thorough physical examination should be performed. Vital signs should be carefully noted. Attention should be given to the presence of pallor, muscle weakness, goiter, lymphadenopathy, and body habitus. A psychiatric evaluation for signs of depression, anxiety, or other mental illness should be performed. In older adults, a mental status exam to evaluate cognitive function may be appropriate.

C. Testing.
1. Initial laboratory testing should be limited to:
   a. Complete blood count
   b. Comprehensive metabolic profile
   c. Thyroid-stimulating hormone
   d. Erythrocyte sedimentation rate
2. Other tests may be indicated by the history or physical examination:
   a. Antinuclear antibody
   b. Rheumatoid factor
   c. Monospot
   d. Chest x-ray
   e. Colonoscopy
   f. Sleep study
   g. Urine analysis
3. Screening tests appropriate for age and gender should be performed.

IV. DIAGNOSIS

Fatigue is a very commonly encountered complaint. In most cases, a thorough history, physical, and a limited number of ancillary tests reveal a more precise diagnosis. Fatigue is rarely the only presenting symptom in cases of malignancy or connective tissue disease. Studies have shown that among patients with fatigue, approximately 40% have an underlying medical diagnosis, approximately 40% have a psychiatric diagnosis, and 12% have both medical and psychiatric explanations for their fatigue. Approximately 8% of patients have no discernible diagnosis (2). If undiagnosed fatigue persists for >6 months and meets the other criteria for CFS, that diagnosis is applied. If the other criteria for CFS are not met, the term idiopathic chronic fatigue is used. Fatigue that cannot be attributed to a medical or psychiatric diagnosis is often thought to be due to lifestyle factors.

REFERENCES

1. Centers for Disease Control and Prevention. *Chronic fatigue syndrome.* Accessed at National Center for Infectious Diseases (www.cfs.general/index.html) on April 23, 2012.
2. Morrison JD. Fatigue as a presenting complaint in FP. *J Fam Pract* 1980;10:795–801.
3. Epstein KR. The chronically fatigued patient. *Med Clin North Am* 1995;79:315–327.
4. Craig T. Chronic fatigue syndrome: evaluation and treatment. *Am Fam Physician* 2002;65(6): 1083–1091.

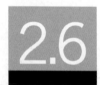

2.6 Fever

Dorota Britz

I. BACKGROUND. Fever is defined as an elevation in core body temperature above the usual daily range for an individual. It is generally accepted as core body temperature of or above 38°C (100.4°F). Hyperpyrexia is extreme elevation of body temperature to above 41.5°C (106.7°F). Fever may be a symptom of various disease processes. A fever without an immediately apparent etiology is generally referred to as fever of unknown origin.

II. PATHOPHYSIOLOGY

  A. Mechanism of Temperature Control. The hypothalamus controls core body temperature. Elevated levels of Prostaglandin E2 (PGE2) in the hypothalamus cause it to reset the body's temperature control to a higher value. This phenomenon leads to peripheral vasoconstriction causing less heat loss, and, if necessary to reach the new temperature goal set by the hypothalamus, also more heat generation in muscles and liver, resulting in fever. In contrast, during hyperthermia the thermostat in the hypothalamus is not reset.

  B. Normal Temperature Variation. Normal body temperature varies by an average of 0.5°C (0.9°F) during the course of the day. Body temperature is generally lowest in the morning and the highest in the evening. Children tend to have higher body temperatures than the elderly. Core temperature will also be higher after eating and for 2 weeks after ovulation.

  C. Temperature Measurement. Rectal measurements are generally 0.6°C (1.0°F) higher than oral (sublingual) readings.

III. EVALUATION

  A. History. Complete history is crucial to establishing the etiology of fever. Particular attention should be paid to the following components:
    1. Duration and pattern of fever
    2. Prescription or over-the-counter medications
    3. Past surgeries, including any implanted devices, and any perioperative complications
    4. Exposure to ill contacts
    5. Travel, especially to foreign countries or remote/wilderness areas
    6. Comprehensive review of systems, to include symptoms sometimes associated with fever, such as weight loss, night sweats, cough, urinary symptoms, abdominal or joint pain, and rashes
    7. Occupational exposures, especially to animals
    8. Family history of illnesses such as malignant hyperthermia

B. Physical Examination.
   1. Particular attention should be paid to skin, HEENT, chest, abdomen, and lymphatics.
   2. Complete set of vital signs should be recorded, to include temperature, heart rate, respiratory rate, and blood pressure. Fever is generally accompanied by tachycardia. Hypotension may be a sign of sepsis.
C. Additional Testing. If the source of fever is not obvious from the history and physical exam, the initial tests would generally include a complete blood count with manual differential, urinalysis, and chest x-ray. Oftentimes cultures of blood, urine, and sputum, as well as testing for pelvic/genital infections may be performed as well. Possible infectious processes within the central nervous system can be investigated with lumbar puncture and obtaining studies of cerebrospinal fluid. Further radiographic studies may be warranted depending on patient's presentation. If these investigations for an infectious process do not yield satisfactory results, further tests may be performed to look for connective tissue diseases with measurements of antinuclear antibodies and rheumatoid factor.

IV. DIAGNOSIS
A. Acute Febrile Illness. Most fevers in the outpatient setting present in the context of acute viral illness. They generally last up to 7 to 10 days and can be treated symptomatically. Common bacterial causes may include pharyngitis/tonsillitis, sinusitis, bronchitis, pneumonia, and urinary tract infection.

TABLE 2.6.1	Most Common Etiologies of Fever of Unknown Origin in Adults and Children
Adults	**Children**
Infectious disease	Infectious diseases
Tuberculosis	Brucellosis
Occult abscess	Cat scratch disease
Osteomyelitis	Leptospirosis
Bacterial endocarditis	Malaria
Sinusitis	Tuberculosis
Dental abscess	Salmonella infections
Connective tissue diseases	Toxoplasmosis
Adult Still's disease	Tularemia
Giant cell arteritis	Viral infections (CMV, EBV, adenovirus, hepatitis, enterovirus)
Malignancy	Bone and joint infections
Drugs	Endocarditis
Antibiotics, antimalarials	Intra-abdominal abscess
Histamine blockers	Liver infections
Anti-seizure medications	Rotavirus
NSAIDs, antiarrhythmics	Urinary tract infections
Antithyroid drugs	Connective tissue disorders
	Juvenile idiopathic arthritis
	Neoplasms
	Drugs
	Kawasaki disease

CMV, cytomegalovirus; EBV, Epstein-Barr virus; NSAID, nonsteroidal anti-inflammatory drug.

B. Postoperative Fever. In the immediate postoperative period fever may often be caused by atelectasis. Pneumonia, urinary tract infection, line infections, wound infections, and abscesses may also cause fever following surgery.

C. Fever of Unknown Origin. Numerous definitions of FUO exist, but most include a fever documented on several different days over 2 or 3 weeks, with no diagnosis found following repeated physical examinations and routine diagnostic tests. Diseases that may cause FUO are listed in Table 2.6.1. One approach to evaluating the patient with FUO is shown in Figure 2.6.1. The underlying etiology is eventually found in over 90% of FUO cases. Historically, the most common cause of FUO was infection, followed by malignancies, and then rheumatologic diseases. In more recent studies, rheumatologic causes have surpassed malignancies as the second most common cause of FUO. FUO is much more likely to be caused by an unusual presentation of a common disease than a common presentation of an unusual disease.

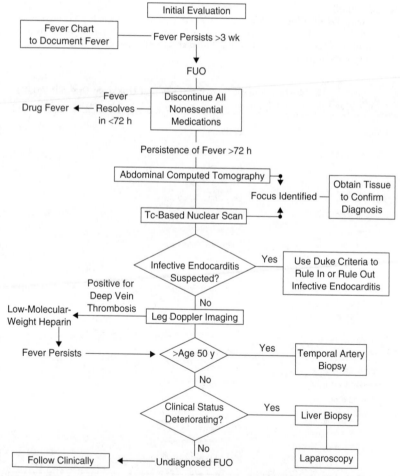

Figure 2.6.1. Approach to the evaluation of fever. FUO, fever of unknown origin.

2.7 Headaches

Mark D. Goodwin

I. BACKGROUND. Headache, or technically cephalgia, is an extremely common phenomenon in the United States and around the globe.

A. Epidemiology. In 2008, headaches were the first-listed diagnosis for over 3 million ED visits (2.4% of all ED visits) and 81,000 inpatient stays (0.2% of all inpatient stays). In developed countries, tension-type headache (TTH) alone affects two-thirds of adult males and over 80% of females.

Migraine prevalence and attack incidence data suggests that 3,000 migraine attacks occur every day for each million of the general population. Current studies have estimated that migraine headache affects 37 million people in the United States, or 12% of the entire population.

The toll of chronic daily headache is not insignificant either as up to one adult in 20 has a headache every or nearly every day. Amazingly though, about 10% of men and 5% of women have never had a headache! The cost is also phenomenal. Migraine headaches cost American employers $13–17 billion a year because of a collective 157 million missed work days, impaired work function, and physician office visits.

II. PATHOPHYSIOLOGY

A. Classifications. Headaches are typically classified into the categories of primary and secondary with the International Classification of Headache Disorders, second edition (ICHD-II) system providing what many consider the gold standard.

B. Diagnosis. Primary headaches include migraines with all the various subsets (with and without aura, retinal, ophthalmoplegic, basilar, etc.), TTH (episodic and chronic), cluster headaches, and other trigeminal autonomic headaches (which includes paroxysmal hemicranias) and finally "other" primary headaches (which include stabbing, cough, exertional, associated with sexual activity, thunderclap etc.). Secondary headaches are far less common (10% of all headaches) but potentially more dangerous. They include headaches related to head and neck trauma and headaches related to cranial or cervical vascular disorders (which include conditions such as transient ischemic attack (TIA), cerebrovascular accident (CVA), arteritis, intracranial/subarachnoid hemorrhage, vascular malformations, cerebral venous thrombosis etc.). Other secondary headaches take in headache attributed to nonvascular intracranial disorder (which includes headaches tied to Chiari malformation Type 1, high or low cerebrospinal fluid (CSF) fluid pressures, increased intracranial pressure or hydrocephalus caused by neoplasm etc.), headache attributed to a substance (which includes medication overuse, medication adverse events, substance withdrawal etc.), headaches attributed to various intracranial and systemic infections (which include meningitis, encephalitis etc.), headaches attributed to disorders of homeostasis (which include hypoxia, hypothyroidism, fasting etc.), headache or facial pain attributed to multiple disorders of the cranium, neck, eyes, ears, nose, sinuses, teeth, mouth, or other facial or cranial structures, and lastly headaches attributed to psychiatric disorders such as somatization and psychotic conditions.

III. EVALUATION. The primary task of the family physician whether they are practicing in a clinic, on a hospital service, or in an emergency room is to determine whether a patient has an organic, potentially life-threatening cause of headache. Fortunately, the majority of headaches do not have a serious cause, but serious causes of headache, such as meningitis and subarachnoid hemorrhage, must be excluded. In the vast majority of cases, the physician can accurately diagnose a patient's headache and determine whether additional laboratory testing or neuroimaging is indicated by considering the various headache types in each category as listed above and obtaining a thorough headache history followed by a focused clinical examination.

A. History. The history is the most important aspect of the evaluation of a patient with headache, especially because primary and secondary headaches can share similar clinical features and associated symptoms. Historical items important to document should include previous similar episodes, the date/time of onset, precipitating and ameliorating factors, character of the pain as well as the level of intensity, the symptom course over time, duration, frequency, location of pain, and associated symptoms such as nausea/vomiting, any autonomic features, fever, chills, and focal neurologic signs/symptoms. A review of the patient's other past medical conditions and current medications is also critical, as this may point to an etiology (such as caffeine or nonsteroidal anti-inflammatory drug [NSAID] withdrawal headaches). The history of the headache can often provide a diagnosis with no further investigation or testing needed.

Certain signs and/or symptoms are often labeled as "red flags" when it comes to headaches. While studies to support the use of these are lacking, the following conditions should prompt additional evaluation—headache beginning after 50 years of age, a sudden onset of the headache, headaches with increasing frequency and severity (especially if they report that this is "this is the worst headache ever"), a new-onset headache in a patient with risk factors for cancer or human immunodeficiency virus (HIV), a headache with signs of systemic infection, headaches with focal neurologic signs or seizure, and a headache subsequent to intracranial hemorrhage.

B. Physical. The physical examination of the headache patient should identify causes of secondary headaches and as such it should target areas identified as abnormal during the headache history. The general physical examination should include vital signs, funduscopic and cardiovascular assessment, and palpation of the head and face. The physician should check for evidence of localized infections such as acute otitis media (AOM) and acute bacterial sinusitis (ABS). A complete neurologic examination is essential. The examination should include mental status, level of consciousness, cranial nerve testing, motor strength testing, deep tendon reflexes, sensation, pathologic reflexes (e.g., Babinski's sign), cerebellar function and gait testing, and signs of meningeal irritation (Kernig's and Brudzinski's signs). It is important to remember that signs like nuchal rigidity and maneuvers such as Kernig's and Brudzinski's all have exceedingly low sensitivities (30%, 5%, and 5%, respectively).

C. Testing. Laboratory and neuroimaging are often not required in the headache patient work-up, especially for patients who present with a primary form of headache. However, if the history and/or physical examination suggest secondary causes, then labs and imaging may be required. Blood counts and cultures would be indicated for those presenting with signs/symptoms of systemic infection. In addition to the complete blood count (CBC) and cultures, a lumbar puncture would be indicated in any patient in whom meningitis is suspected. Urgent scanning is indicated if patients present with new sudden onset of severe headache, headache associated with new abnormal neurologic signs, or a new type of headache in patients infected with HIV and is best achieved using CT. Magnetic resonance imaging (MRI), though more expensive, is better at defining pathologic intracranial changes especially in the posterior fossa. An ESR would be indicated in patients presenting with giant cell arteritis. Lastly, CT scanning without contrast medium, followed by lumbar puncture if the scan is negative, is preferred to rule out subarachnoid hemorrhage.

Consider neurologic consultation if the headache diagnosis is uncertain, if the patient's conscious level is affected or if there is a period of amnesia, if the neurologic examination is abnormal, or if the neuroimaging is abnormal. Neurosurgical consultation is warranted if the patient presents with a subarachnoid hemorrhage or mass lesion (such as tumors or abscess), or if a pituitary lesion is suspected.

IV. SUMMARY. Most primary headaches can be diagnosed by taking a comprehensive history to exclude worrisome symptoms and documenting a normal general and neurologic examination. Diagnostic testing is not necessary in these cases. Secondary headaches usually require additional diagnostic testing.

REFERENCES

1. Jonathan AE. Clinical policy: critical issues in the evaluation and management of adult patients presenting to the emergency department with acute headache. From the American College of Emergency Physicians Clinical Policies Subcommittee; American College of Emergency Physicians; 2008.07.001.
2. ICSI Health Care Guideline-Diagnosis and Treatment of Headache; Jan 2011, 10th edition.

3. Kevin H, Sara W, Marcia R. Direct cost burden among insured US employees with migraine. *Headache* 2008;48(4):553–563.
4. Randall CC. Evaluation of acute headaches in adults. *Am Fam Physician* 2001;63(4):685–692.
5. John RM. Headache in primary care. *Prim Care Clin Office Pract* 2007;34:83–97.
6. Jennifer L. Headaches in U.S. hospitals and emergency departments, 2008. *Agency for Healthcare Research and Quality*, May 2011.
7. *The International Classification of Headache Disorders*, 2nd ed. May 2005.

Hypersomnia

Jennifer J. Buescher

I. BACKGROUND. Hypersomnia, or excessive daytime somnolence (EDS) is defined by the International Classification of Sleep Disorders, Second Edition (ICSD-2) as "the inability to stay awake and alert during the major waking episodes of the day, resulting in unintended lapses into drowsiness and sleep (1)." EDS should be differentiated from generalized fatigue and nonspecific tiredness, as patients often use the terms interchangeably. Generalized fatigue is more subjective and typically related to problems of decreased physical energy, poor concentration and memory, muscle exhaustion, or mood. Due to the prevalence and comorbidities associated with untreated obstructive sleep apnea (OSA), patients with EDS should be considered for an OSA evaluation.

II. PATHOPHYSIOLOGY

    A. Etiology. Hypersomnia can be due to a primary sleep disorder, but is more commonly secondary to disorders that disrupt normal sleep patterns such as sleep deprivation, medication side effects, poor sleep hygiene, sleep-disordered breathing, and other medical and psychiatric conditions (2).

    B. Epidemiology. EDS is a common problem affecting approximately 10% to 20% of adults and children (1, 3) with an even higher prevalence in older adults (4) and patients with psychiatric conditions. EDS is reported as a significant factor in motor vehicle incidents and personal injuries in the United States and has been linked to poor health and reduced cognitive function (2). Narcolepsy (the common tetrad includes sleep paralysis, cataplexy, excessive daytime somnolence, and hypnagogic hallucinations) is an uncommon diagnosis and affects approximately 50/100,000 people (1).

III. EVALUATION

    A. History and Review of Systems. A detailed and complete sleep history is important for determining the appropriate evaluation in patients with EDS. Determining the patient's work schedule, diet, sleep routine, social stressors, home environment and living situation, prescription and nonprescription drug use, as well as the comorbidities and behaviors of bed partners will help in developing a differential diagnosis. A history of sleep attacks or episodes of cataplexy (sudden and transient loss of muscle strength) can be very dangerous and highly suggestive of narcolepsy (1). A full review of systems often highlights other medical and psychiatric disorders that may be causing daytime sleepiness. Abrupt symptom onset should heighten concern for central nervous system tumors, ischemic stroke, or significant metabolic disorders.

    B. Sleep Patterns. Sleep deprivation is probably the most common cause of EDS (2). Sleep deprivation can result from job-related factors (shift work), environmental situations (bed-partner snores loudly, disruptive neighbors, gunshots outside, caring for ill family members), or other medical diagnoses (periodic limb movement disorder, asthma, OSA).

    C. Medication History. Many medications can induce somnolence or interrupt the normal sleep cycle. These are listed in Table 2.8.1 (2, 5).

TABLE 2.8.1   Medications That Can Be Involved in Hypersomnia

Prescription medications causing somnolence

Benzodiazepines

Nonbenzodiazepine sleep aids

Tricyclic antidepressants

Atypical antidepressants

Selective serotonin reuptake inhibitors

Antipsychotics

Lithium

Anticonvulsants

Antiparkinsonian agents

Opiates

Antihistamines

α1-Adrenergic antagonists (prazosin, terazosin)

α2-Adrenergic agonists

Skeletal muscle relaxants

Antimuscarinics and antispasmodics

Barbiturates

Prescription medication causing alertness or insomnia

Amphetamines

Modafinil and Armodafinil

Theophylline

β-Adrenergic agonists

β-Blockers

Corticosteroids

Decongestants

Selective serotonin reuptake inhibitors

Nonprescription and herbal agents affecting sleep

Amphetamines

Alcohol

Nicotine

Illicit drugs

Chamomile

Rosemary

Melatonin

Adapted from Pagel JF. Excessive daytime sleepiness. *Am Fam Physician* 2009;79(5):391–396; Roux FJ, Kryger MH. Medication effects on sleep. *Clin Chest Med* 2010;31:397–405.

TABLE 2.8.2	Differential Diagnosis of Excessive Daytime Somnolence

Primary hypersomnias:

    Narcolepsy with or without cataplexy

    Idiopathic hypersomnia

Secondary hypersomnias:

    Obstructive sleep apnea

    Restless leg syndrome

    Periodic limb movement disorder

    Parkinson's disease

    Insufficient sleep syndrome (behavioral sleep deprivation)

    Head trauma

    Depression

    Anxiety

Medication effects

Illicit drug use

Poor sleep hygiene

Data adapted from Morrison I, Riha RL. Excessive daytime sleepiness and narcolepsy—an approach to investigation and management. *Eur J Int Med* 2012;23:110–117; Pagel JF. Excessive daytime sleepiness. *Am Fam Physician* 2009;79(5):391–396.

D. Physical Examination. A general physical examination may give insight into medical or psychological disorders that require further evaluation, such as OSA, asthma, nocturia/urinary urgency, or anxiety.

E. Testing. The Eppworth Sleepiness Scale can help to quantify sleepiness (1). Intrinsic sleep disorders are best evaluated using a Multiple Sleep Latency Test (MSLT) and the Maintenance of Wakefulness Test (MWT) (2). OSA and limb movement disorders are best evaluated by overnight polysomnography (2).

IV. DIAGNOSIS

A. Differential Diagnosis. The differential diagnosis for hypersomnia is listed in Table 2.8.2.

B. Clinical Manifestations. Hypersomnia may present with significant fatigue, trouble with work or school performance, marital or relationship problems, accidents or personal injury, and can be the first sign of dementia or other neurologic disorders.

REFERENCES

1. Morrison I, Riha RL. Excessive daytime sleepiness and narcolepsy—an approach to investigation and management. *Eur J Int Med* 2012;23:110–117.
2. Pagel JF. Excessive daytime sleepiness. *Am Fam Physician* 2009;79(5):391–396.
3. Calhoun SL, Vgontzas AN, Fernandez-Mendoza J, et al. Prevalence and risk factors of excessive daytime sleepiness in a community sample of young children: the role of obesity, asthma, anxiety/depression, and sleep. *Sleep* 2011;34(4):503–507.
4. Bloom HG, Ahmed I, Alessi CA, et al. Evidence-based recommendations for the assessment and management of sleep disorders in older persons. *J Am Geriatr Soc* 2009;57(5):761–789.
5. Roux FJ, Kryger MH. Medication effects on sleep. *Clin Chest Med* 2010;31:397–405.

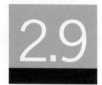

Insomnia

Jennifer J. Buescher

I. **BACKGROUND.** Chronic insomnia is the difficulty of initiating or maintaining sleep that causes significant daytime impairment and has been present for at least 1 month (1). Secondary insomnia is a sleep disturbance caused by an underlying environmental, medical, or psychiatric disorder (1).

II. **PATHOPHYSIOLOGY**
  A. **Etiology.** Primary insomnia is uncommon and is due to an intrinsic disorder of the sleep–wake cycle. Secondary insomnia is much more common. Chronic pain, substance use or abuse, restless legs syndrome, depression, circadian rhythm disturbance (i.e., shift work), and obstructive sleep apnea are common causes of secondary insomnia (1, 2). Poor sleep hygiene, alcohol, caffeine, and nicotine use are also common causes of difficulty with sleep initiation and nonrestorative sleep (2).
  B. **Epidemiology.** Between 10% and 30% of the population is affected by insomnia, but only 10% to 15% of these patients suffer from intrinsic disorders of sleep (1, 3).

III. **EVALUATION**
  A. **History.** A thorough history should focus on determining the cause and duration of insomnia. Precipitating events such as emotional trauma, illness, stress, and prescription or other drug use should be explored with the patient and his or her bed partner.
  B. **Sleep Patterns.** A thorough discussion of the patient's sleep pattern and the sleep patterns of other members of the household should include the timing and the content of evening meals, bedroom environment (temperature, noise, comfort of bed), safety of the outside neighborhood, work schedules, and sleep schedules (including daytime napping).
  C. **Review of Systems.** The review of systems should be directed to the common medical and psychological problems that are associated with insomnia.
  D. **Medications.** Many medications affect sleep by causing or exacerbating restless legs syndrome or periodic limb movements, dreams or nightmares, or by interrupting normal sleep architecture (2). Table 2.9.1 lists some of the more common medications that can interrupt normal sleep patterns.
  E. **Physical Examination.** The physical examination should focus on associated medical conditions associated with insomnia. In primary insomnia, the physical examination is likely to be normal.
  F. **Testing.** Laboratory and diagnostic testing is infrequently useful in the diagnosis of primary insomnia. A detailed sleep diary kept by the patient or a home visit by the physician can be helpful in determining extrinsic factors causing insomnia (1). Polysomnography can assist in the diagnosis of comorbid conditions such as obstructive sleep apnea, restless legs syndrome, and periodic limb movement disorder.

IV. **DIAGNOSIS**
  A. **Differential Diagnosis.** A differential diagnosis of insomnia is listed in Table 2.9.2.
  B. **Clinical Manifestations.** Insomnia can cause significant functional impairment, difficulty in work or school, and marital or relationship problems. Chronic sleep loss from untreated insomnia can cause fatigue-related accidents, poor concentration, decreased memory, and job or school absenteeism and is associated with increased morbidity and mortality from cardiovascular and psychiatric disorders (1, 3).

TABLE 2.9.1	Medications That Interrupt Sleep

Prescription drugs	Non-prescription medications
Carbamazepine	Phenylephrine
Valproate sodium	Pseudoephedrine
Phenytoin	Caffeine
Gabapentin	Stimulant diet pills
Pregabalin	Nicotine
Selective serotonin reuptake inhibitors	Alcohol
Lithium	Illicit drugs
Venlafaxine	
Risperidone	
Clozapine	
Methylphenidate	
Dextroamphetamine	
Albuterol	
Theophylline	
Prednisone	
Beta blockers	

Information from Foral P, Knezevich J, Dewan N, Malesker M. Medication-induced sleep disturbances. *Consult Pharm* 2011;26(5):414–425.

TABLE 2.9.2	Differential Diagnosis of Insomnia

Primary insomnia	Depression
Obstructive sleep apnea	Nightmares or night terrors
Congestive heart failure	Alzheimer's or other dementia
Gastroesophageal reflux disease	Urinary incontinence, nocturia
Chronic pain syndrome	Chronic obstructive pulmonary disease
Fibromyalgia	Illicit drug use
Asthma	Alcohol use or abuse
Restless legs syndrome	Circadian rhythm sleep disorders (shift work, jet lag)
Periodic limb movement disorder	Environmental disturbances (loud noises, bed partner with sleep disorder, uncomfortable or unsafe sleeping conditions)
Anxiety	

Information modified from Foral P, Knezevich J, Dewan N, Malesker M. Medication-induced sleep disturbances. *Consult Pharm* 2011;26(5):414–425; Harsora P, Kessmann J. Nonpharmacologic management of chronic insomnia. *Am Fam Physician* 2009;79(2):125–130; Ramakrishnan K, Scheid DC. Treatments options for insomnia. *Am Fam Physician* 2007;76(4):517–526.

REFERENCES

1. Harsora P, Kessmann J. Nonpharmacologic management of chronic insomnia. *Am Fam Physician* 2009;79(2):125–130.
2. Foral P, Knezevich J, Dewan N, Malesker M. Medication-induced sleep disturbances. *Consult Pharm* 2011;26(5):414–425.
3. Ramakrishnan K, Scheid DC. Treatments options for insomnia. *Am Fam Physician* 2007;76(4): 517–526.

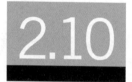

Nausea and Vomiting

Jennifer J. Buescher

I. BACKGROUND. Nausea is the objectionable sensation of abdominal discomfort that produces a sensation that one may vomit. Vomiting is an autonomic response leading to the active and forceful expulsion of gastric contents (1). Nausea may or may not be followed by active vomiting.

II. PATHOPHYSIOLOGY

A. Etiology. Nausea is a subjective symptom experienced in many of the disorders that also cause vomiting. Vomiting is an autonomic response intended to protect humans from the ingestion of harmful or toxic substances (1). Several neurologic abnormalities can trigger the autonomic system and lead to vomiting.

B. Epidemiology. Acute nausea and vomiting are common symptoms and frequently seen in outpatient, inpatient, and emergency settings. Chronic nausea and vomiting are less common but can lead to significant morbidity.

III. EVALUATION

A. History. A thorough history should discuss the duration and frequency of vomiting, the symptoms of other family members, exposure to toxic substances, and the relationship of nausea and vomiting to meals or types of food.

B. Review of Systems. A complete review of systems should specifically address a history of fever, character of abdominal pain, neurologic symptoms, and the signs and symptoms of dehydration.

C. Physical Examination. A complete abdominal exam should first attempt to rule out acute life-threatening or severe problems such as intestinal obstruction, pancreatitis, and acute myocardial infarction. Neurologic exam can help identify vomiting caused by a central nervous system abnormality or vestibular problem (2). The physical exam should also evaluate for complications caused by protracted vomiting, including dehydration and electrolyte disorders.

D. Testing. The evaluation of nausea and vomiting should be directed by the severity, onset, and description of the symptoms and any abnormal findings on physical exam. A flat and upright abdominal radiograph or abdominal CT is helpful in the evaluation of acute and severe nausea or vomiting. Subsequent studies such as barium studies, upper GI series, intracranial CT/MRI, and abdominal ultrasound may be warranted based on the differential diagnosis (1). Laboratory tests including a metabolic panel, pregnancy test, urinalysis, liver function test, lipase, and toxicology screen should be ordered based on the clinical assessment and should be used in the evaluation of the underlying cause and subsequent complications from nausea and vomiting.

IV. DIAGNOSIS

A. Differential Diagnosis. The diagnosis of nausea and vomiting can often be made on clinical history and physical examination without further evaluation (2). Chronic or severe symptoms may be more difficult to diagnose and may require more extensive laboratory and diagnostic testing. Table 2.10.1 provides a list of common causes of acute and chronic nausea and vomiting.

TABLE 2.10.1	Differential Diagnosis of Nausea and/or Vomiting

Acute nausea and/or vomiting	**Chronic nausea and vomiting**
Increased intracranial pressure	Increased intracranial pressure
Meningitis/encephalitis/abscess	Mass lesion
Closed head injury	Hydrocephalus
Cerebrovascular injury	Pseudotumor cerebri
Migraine	Gastroparesis
Vestibular abnormalities	Nonulcer dyspepsia
Labyrinthitis	Irritable bowel syndrome
Motion sickness	Psychiatric disorders
Bowel obstruction	Bulimia nervosa
Intussusception	Anorexia nervosa
Strangulated hernia	Conversion disorder
Volvulus	Anxiety
Cholecystitis/cholangitis	Social phobia disorder
Pancreatitis	Cyclic vomiting
Appendicitis	Uremia
Infectious gastroenteritis	Cirrhosis
Spontaneous bacterial peritonitis	**Medications/toxins**
Pyelonephritis	Alcohol intoxication
Acute myocardial infarction	Chemotherapeutics
Nephrolithiasis	Hormonal contraception
Acute pain	Arsenic
Diabetic ketoacidosis	Organophosphates/pesticides
Pregnancy	Radiation therapy
	Illicit drug use

Modified from Scorza K, Williams A, Phillips D, Shaw J. Evaluation of nausea and vomiting. *Am Fam Physician* 2007;76(1):76–84.

   B. Clinical Manifestations. Many patients with isolated or self-limited nausea and/or vomiting will not seek medical attention; however, their symptoms can lead to temporary functional limitations and missed work or school. Patients with persistent or severe nausea and vomiting can experience significant weight loss, hypokalemia, electrolyte disturbances, dehydration, metabolic alkalosis, dental caries, and esophageal abnormalities, and can experience significant social isolation and missed work or school.

REFERENCES

1. Scorza K, Williams A, Phillips D, Shaw J. Evaluation of nausea and vomiting. *Am Fam Physician* 2007;76(1):76–84.
2. American Gastroenterological Association. Medical position statement: nausea and vomiting. *Gastroenterology* 2001;120(1):261–263.

2.11

Night Sweats
Richard H. Hurd

I. BACKGROUND. Night sweats are drenching sweats that require a change of bedding (1).

II. PATHOPHYSIOLOGY

  A. Etiology. Night sweats that are caused by fever represent a separate entity and are discussed in Chapter 2.6. Night sweats are likely to be an autonomic response to some physical or emotional condition, representing a rather nonspecific symptom that should prompt the clinician to seek a specific cause.

  B. Epidemiology. One study of approximately 800 patients in the practices of several primary care physicians indicated that about 10% were bothered to some degree by night sweats; 70% of patients affected reported some trouble, 20% a fair amount of trouble, and 10% a great deal of trouble (2).

III. EVALUATION

  A. History.

  1. It is helpful to characterize night sweats by determining the onset, frequency, exacerbations, and remissions of symptoms (3). The clinician must thoroughly explore any risk of exposure to infectious causes of night sweats. This history must include questions about behaviors that put the patient at risk of HIV-related infections, sexually transmitted diseases, hepatitis, and tuberculosis. Explorations of travel and occupational exposures should be carried out.

  2. The state of concurrent medical conditions must be determined. Changes in treatment modalities that are both physician driven as well as those initiated by the patient may be a causative factor for night sweats. All the patient's current and recently discontinued medications must be determined.

  3. A thorough review of the systems may point the clinician toward a primary disease that includes night sweats as a symptom. Psychologic factors that might precipitate night sweats in healthy individuals should be discussed.

  4. Interviewing a sleeping partner is an important source of information that must not be neglected. A history of snoring or apneic episodes may point to sleep apnea that has been reported to be a common cause of night sweats (4).

  B. Physical Examination. The fact that night sweats in the absence of any other identifiable cause constitute a physically benign condition makes it imperative that a complete physical examination be carried out in an effort to determine the presence of any concurrent condition. The history may direct the physician toward a more detailed examination of a specific organ system; however, the knowledge that the cause may be multifactorial must be remembered, and no part of the physical examination should be neglected.

  C. Testing. The choice of laboratory tests is guided by the history. For those patients with known medical conditions, appropriate tests for exacerbations should be carried out. The tests might include a complete blood count to assess the status of the infection, erythrocyte sedimentation rate, HbA1C, and C-reactive protein. A history of exposure might suggest an HIV test, a hepatitis panel, or a purified protein derivative skin test for tuberculosis. Thyroid function testing in individuals identified as at risk should also be carried out. Special testing may be required in individuals with travel-related exposure.

  D. Genetics. There is no reported familial cause of primary night sweats.

IV. DIAGNOSIS

  A. Differential Diagnosis. The diagnosis of night sweats is largely historical (see Table 2.11.1).

  B. Clinical Manifestations. Night sweats are most frequently a manifestation of an underlying illness. As such, the manifestation is most often a part of a much larger symptom

TABLE 2.11.1 Causes of Night Sweats

Malignancy	Infectious	Endocrine	Rheumatologic	Drugs	Other
Lymphoma	Human immunodeficiency virus	Hyperthyroidism	Rheumatoid arthritis	–	Sleep apnea
Leukemia	Tuberculosis	Ovarian failure	Lupus	–	Gastroesophageal reflux disease
Other malignancy	Endocarditis	Diabetes mellitus	Juvenile rheumatoid arthritis	–	Angina
	Lung infection	Endocrine tumors	Temporal arthritis	–	Pregnancy
	Other infections				Overbundling
					Extreme heat

complex. The diagnosis centers on discovering the underlying disease entity. When no cause in evident, watchful waiting is useful in an attempt to let the cause become more evident (5).

REFERENCES

1. Smetana GW. Diagnosis of night sweats. *JAMA* 1993;70:2502–2503.
2. Mold JW, Roberts M, Aboshady H. Prevalence and predictors of night sweats, day sweats, and hot flashes in older primary care patients. *Am Fam Med* 2004;2(5):391–397.
3. Bajorek M. Night sweats. In: Taylor R, ed. *The 10-minute diagnosis manual.* Philadelphia, PA: Lippincott Williams & Wilkins, 2000:31–33.
4. Duhon DR. Night sweats: two other causes. *JAMA* 1994;271:1577.
5. Chambliss ML. Frequently asked questions from clinical practice. What is the appropriate diagnostic approach for patients who complain of night sweats? *Arch Fam Med* 1999;2:168–169.

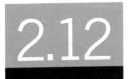

2.12

Syncope
Mark D. Goodwin

I. BACKGROUND. The definition of syncope is a transient and often abrupt loss of consciousness with complete return to the preexisting level of function.

II. PATHOPHYSIOLOGY

A. Epidemiology. Syncope is a common phenomenon occurring in approximately 40% of adults and accounting for 3% to 5% of emergency room visits and 1% to 6% of hospital medical admissions. Presenting in a bimodal pattern, 80% of patients experience their first episode before the age of 30 years and then again as patients age into their 70s and beyond, they experience a second increase in the incidence. A high percentage of patients (30% to 60%) have no causative diagnosis made after even extensive workups. In a large cohort of

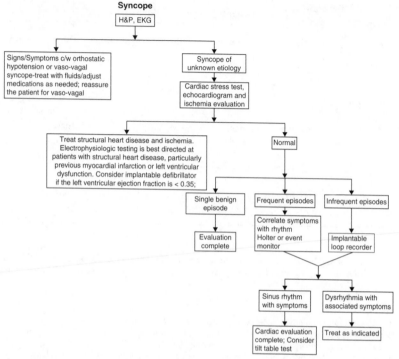

Figure 2.12.1. Causes and Evaluation of Syncope.

patients from the Framingham Heart Study, the most frequently identified causes of syncope were vasovagal (21.2%), cardiac (9.5%), orthostatic (9.4%), medication (6.8%), seizure (4.9%), stroke or transient ischemic attack (4.1%), other causes (7.5%), and unknown (37%).

B. Classification. Syncope can be classified using various systems from malignant and benign conditions to cardiac to noncardiac conditions. However, perhaps the most common classification system employs the following categories: cardiac (which includes structural abnormalities and dysrhythmias or arrhythmias), reflex or neurally mediated (which includes neurocardiogenic, situational, and carotid sinus hypersensitivity etc.), neurologic (which includes seizure, vertebrobasilar TIA, etc.), orthostatic (often grouped into the reflex-mediated category and includes drug effects, volume depletion, and autonomic failure), and miscellaneous (which includes psychogenic, pulmonary embolism etc.) (Figure 2.12.1).

III. EVALUATION

The evaluation of syncope involves developing an appropriate differential diagnosis, determining how much of an evaluation (including laboratory, radiographic, and other testing) is needed, whether or not admission is required, and the patient's overall prognosis.

A. History. Despite the fact that patients will use a variety of terms to describe their signs and symptoms (dizziness, lightheadedness etc.), as is the case in most of medicine, the history and physical examination remains the cornerstone for diagnosing the cause of syncope, with several studies showing a diagnostic yield of approximately 50%. While syncope can be said to be truly distinct from vertigo, seizures, stroke, coma, and other states of altered consciousness, one of the biggest challenges facing clinicians can be discerning between syncope and seizure. Important historical factors to be gleaned include age (with greater age associated with higher risk of serious conditions), position and activity before the episode, prodrome (such as aura with seizures, palpitations with dysrhythmia etc.), triggers (such as pain, fear, or cough, micturition, and defecation common in reflex-mediated syncope), associated symptoms (such as palpitations, chest pain, shortness of breath, headache, paresthesias, slurred speech, aphasia, and focal weakness, associated injury, and duration of symptoms. The patient who presents in a postictal state or with persistent neurologic symptoms did not, by definition, have a syncopal event. Previous episodes and the workup of these can help differentiate benign and malignant causes. Finally family history should be reviewed looking for members with sudden cardiac death, hypertrophic cardiomyopathy, and prolonged or short QT syndromes. Of course a complete past medical and social history (including alcohol, prescription, OTC, and illicit drug use) should also be obtained, as well as any witnesses of the event interviewed.

B. Physical. The physical exam should be complete with a focus on abnormal vitals (such as orthostasis and an abnormal heart rate), the cardiac exam (to rule out murmurs), a complete neurologic exam to rule out focal abnormalities, and examination to exclude any trauma (either as cause of or as a result of the episode). If carotid sinus hypersensitivity is suspected, a carotid sinus massage can be conducted but is contraindicated in the presence of suspected or known carotid artery disease or recent CVA or TIA. Auscultation of the carotids before the procedure is required to rule out an obvious bruit.

C. Testing. Additional testing should include an EKG (although the diagnostic yield is <5%) and *can* include an ECG, electrophysiologic testing, exercise treadmill testing, tilt table testing, short or long term electrocardiographic monitoring, neuroimaging, and EEG if the history and exam dictate. Routine use of laboratory tests is not recommended and only targeted laboratory tests should be ordered as indicated by the history and physical.

IV. DIAGNOSIS

If the primary purpose of the evaluation of the patient with syncope is to determine whether the patient is at increased risk for death then development of a "formula" to establish such risk would be ideal. To that end, various diagnostic point scoring systems have been developed, including the European Guidelines in Syncope Study score, the San Francisco Syncope Rule, and the Risk Stratification of Syncope in the Emergency Department. Each of these has its advantages and disadvantages and none to date has sensitivity rates above 90%. Management of syncope patients and the prognosis are both guided by the specific diagnosis.

The decision whether to admit patients who experience a snycopal episode will depend upon the circumstances of the event as well as the patient's overall risk for injury (including age, history of CAD, suspected cardiac structural abnormality or dysrhythmia, etc.) from the possible cause. The algorithm depicted in Figure 2.12.1, modified from the 2006 AHA/ACCF Scientific Statement on the Evaluation of Syncope, can be helpful in the work-up and evaluation of patients who present with the often confusing condition of syncope.

REFERENCES

1. Gauer RL. Evaluation of syncope. *Am Fam Physician* 2011;84(6):640–650.
2. Angaran P. Syncope. *Neurol Clin* 2011;29:903–925.
3. Ouyang H. Diagnosis and evaluation of syncope in the emergency department. *Emerg Med Clin N Am* 2010;28:471–485.
4. Strickberger SA, Benson DW, Biaggioni I, et al. AHA/ACCF scientific statement on the evaluation of syncope: from the American Heart Association Councils on Clinical Cardiology, Cardiovascular Nursing, Cardiovascular Disease in the Young, and Stroke, and the Quality of Care and Outcomes Research Interdisciplinary Working Group; and the American College of Cardiology Foundation In Collaboration With the Heart Rhythm Society. *J Am Coll Cardiol* 2006;47(2):473–484.

2.13

Unintentional Weight Loss

Amy K. Jespersen

I. BACKGROUND. Unintentional weight loss is generally considered to be significant when greater than 5% of body weight is lost over a period of 6 months or less. It is often associated with increased morbidity and mortality, especially among the elderly. Perceived weight loss should be verified before initiating a workup, because 50% of patients with perceived weight loss do not have true weight loss. Of patients with confirmed weight loss, an explanation is found in approximately 75% of cases. In the remainder, an explanation is never found. The prognosis for patients in whom a diagnosis is not found is generally better. (1) If a physical cause is present it is usually discovered within 6 months (1–3).

II. PATHOPHYSIOLOGY

The various conditions that cause unintentional weight loss do so through one or more of the following mechanisms: inadequate caloric intake, excessive metabolic demands, or loss of nutrients through urine or stool. Other conditions that cause weight loss include:

A. **Malignant Conditions.** Cancer is often the patient's or physician's greatest fear. Malignancy is the cause for unintentional weight loss in 16% to 36% of cases (1–3). Although any cancer can cause weight loss, the more common malignancies to consider are gastrointestinal (GI), leukemia or lymphoma, lung, ovarian, and prostate cancers.

B. **Benign Medical Conditions.** Many chronic medical conditions can cause anorexia, nausea, diarrhea, or postprandial symptoms that discourage the patient from eating. Medical conditions may also necessitate limiting salt, fat, or sugar in the diet, leaving the patient less inclined to eat.

1. GI disorders account for the most common physical cause of weight loss, affecting approximately 17% of patients (4). These include:
   a. Peptic ulcer disease/gastroesophageal reflux disease
   b. Inflammatory bowel disease and malabsorptive illnesses
   c. Hepatitis, cholestasis
   d. Pancreatitis
   e. Atrophic gastritis
   f. Constipation

2. Cardiac diseases, especially congestive heart failure

3. Respiratory diseases, such as chronic obstructive pulmonary disease

4. Renal disease

5. Neurologic or neuromuscular disorders may affect the ability to swallow. Examples include:
   a. Cerebrovascular accident
   b. Parkinson's disease
   c. Scleroderma
   d. Polymyositis
   e. Systemic lupus erythematosus

6. Endocrine disorders can increase metabolic rate or cause nutrient loss. These include:
   a. Hyperthyroidism
   b. Diabetes mellitus
   c. Other causes, such as pheochromocytoma, panhypopituitarism, adrenal insufficiency

7. Chronic infection, especially tuberculosis, fungal infections, or subacute bacterial endocarditis. Any prolonged febrile illness can decrease appetite and increase meta-

bolic demand. Human immunodeficiency virus infection is a special consideration with patients having multiple causes for weight loss.

8. Dementia

9. Medications can cause anorexia, nausea, abdominal pain, or diarrhea, or inhibit gastric emptying.

C. Psychiatric Causes. These are responsible for weight loss in 10% to 20% of patients (1–3).

   1. Depression, bereavement, and anxiety

   2. Paranoia and psychosis

   3. Substance abuse, especially alcoholism

D. Social and Age-Related Causes. These include:

   1. Financial hardship

   2. Diminished sense of taste and smell

   3. Functional inability to shop, prepare food, or feed oneself

   4. Poor dentition or ill-fitting dentures

III. EVALUATION

A. History. A detailed history should be obtained from the patient and caregivers if applicable. Special attention should be given to the types and quantity of food consumed; alcohol use; history of cigarette smoking (current and remote); exercise patterns; medications; presence of nausea, vomiting, diarrhea, early satiety, difficulty swallowing; history of GI illnesses, or previous abdominal surgery; cardiac history; respiratory history; history of kidney disease; depressive symptoms; social situation, including financial resources; and functional ability to shop for groceries and prepare meals.

B. Physical Examination.

   1. Document weight and compare to previous weights

   2. Perform a thorough physical examination, paying special attention to the following areas:

      a. Dentition and oral

      b. Respiratory

      c. Cardiac

      d. GI

      e. Psychiatric

      f. Cognitive

      g. Musculoskeletal

C. Testing. Extensive undirected testing is not indicated and is rarely helpful.

   1. Initial laboratory tests may include

      a. Complete blood count

      b. Comprehensive metabolic profile

      c. TSH and Free T4

      d. Urinalysis

      e. Fecal occult blood testing

   2. Other tests as indicated by history or physical exam may include

      a. Chest x-ray, especially with a history of smoking, cough, or dyspnea

      b. Appropriate age- and gender-based screening (mammography, colonoscopy)

      c. Upper GI endoscopy

IV. DIAGNOSIS

Diagnosis of unintentional weight loss is made by verifying that a loss of more than 5% of body weight has occurred. A thorough history and physical examination and directed laboratory and ancillary tests result in an explanation in three out of four cases. Malignancy is the cause of unintentional weight loss in up to one-third of the cases. Psychiatric illness, usually depression, is another common cause. Benign medical conditions and socioeconomic factors make up the remainder of the identifiable causes. In 25% of cases, no explanation can be found and these patients have a more favorable outcome. Many patients will have a multifactorial reason for weight loss. If a physical cause is responsible, but not identified on initial workup, it usually becomes evident within 6 months (4).

REFERENCES

1. Marton KE, Sox HC Jr, Krupp JR. Involuntary weight loss: diagnostic and prognostic significance. *Ann Intern Med* 1981;95:568–574.
2. Rabinovitz M, Pitlik SD, Leifer M, et al. Unintentional weight loss. A retrospective analysis of 154 cases. *Arch Intern Med* 1986;146:186–187.
3. Thompson MP, Morris LK. Unexplained weight loss in the ambulatory elderly. *J Am Geriatric Soc* 1991;39:497–500.
4. Huffman GB. Evaluating and treating unintentional weight loss in the elderly. *Am Fam Physician* 2002;65:640–650.
5. Stajkovic S, Aitken E, Holroyd-Leduc J. Unintentional weight loss in older adults. *CMAJ* 2011;183(4):443–449.
6. Alibhai S, Greenwood C, Payette H. An approach to the management of unintentional weight loss in elderly people. *CMAJ* 2005;172(6):773–780.

CHAPTER 3

Mental Health Problems
Jim Medder

3.1 Anxiety
Layne A. Prest

I. BACKGROUND. The experience of anxiety is ubiquitous in society. Anxiety can be part of an adaptive or protective response to threat (e.g., the fight–freeze–flight response) or a natural reaction to physical and emotional stress, but it can also be debilitating and a serious health concern. At its core, anxiety is a complex biopsychosocial–spiritual experience that requires comprehensive assessment and treatment. Undiagnosed anxiety disorders contribute to inappropriate or overutilization of health-care resources, but as many as 80% of the individuals with anxiety disorders can be significantly helped through appropriate treatment.

II. PATHOPHYSIOLOGY

  A. Etiology. Many factors contribute to both the development and experience of anxiety. These include genetic/neurologic predisposition, family history, acute and chronic stressors, resources for coping, comorbid conditions, and overall physical health. Extreme anxiety responses, known as *anxiety disorders*, are often comorbid with mood or substance use disorders or other chronic health conditions (e.g., respiratory problems and cancer). Anxiety disorders usually include debilitating physical and emotional symptoms and may be due, at least in part, to primary medical problems such as hyperthyroidism or hypoxia. Consequently, anxious patients present to the emergency room or primary care setting with complaints that can be difficult to assess and diagnose.

  B. Epidemiology. According to the National Institute of Mental Health, 40 million adult Americans (18%) experience an anxiety disorder at any one time. Estimates of the prevalence of the various anxiety disorders vary from study to study but generally are as follows: generalized anxiety disorder (GAD)—6.8 million (women twice as likely as men); obsessive compulsive disorder—3.3 million (equally common among men and women); panic disorder—6 million (women twice as likely as men); posttraumatic stress disorder (PTSD)—7.7 million (women more likely than men); social anxiety disorder—15 million (equally common among men and women); and specific phobia—19.2 million (women twice as likely as men) (1). The various anxiety disorders affect approximately 10% of primary care patients (2).

III. EVALUATION

  A. History

   1. Patients with anxiety disorders frequently describe experiencing physical symptoms such as chest pain, dizziness, palpitations, fatigue, shortness of breath, tremors, sweating, muscle aches or tension, or a variety of gastrointestinal complaints. Common psychologic symptoms can include nervousness and worry, fear of dying or going crazy, or a sense of unreality or detachment from oneself.

2. Some patients attribute their anxiety to their physical symptoms ("Of course, I was anxious. I thought I was having a heart attack"). Consequently, the assessment of anxiety disorders should include the nature, frequency, and duration of the preceding symptoms and the extent to which the symptoms have impacted the individual's life and activity.

3. The patient should also be asked about precipitants of the symptoms, including stressors, specific social contexts, medications (e.g., stimulants), and other drug use (e.g., caffeine and cocaine).

4. Questions about the patient's general medical condition(s) (e.g., hyperthyroidism) are also appropriate.

B. Physical Examination. As with all patients, those whose clinical picture is suspected of including a significant component of anxiety should be examined carefully. The extent of the physical examination should be dictated by the patient's personal health and medical history.

1. The examination may include the following: blood pressure (hypertension and hypovolemia), cardiovascular (angina, arrhythmia, congestive heart failure, and valvular heart disease), respiratory (chronic obstructive lung disease, pulmonary embolism, and pneumonia), and neurologic (tumor, encephalopathy, and vertigo).

2. Patients frequently present with nervous agitation, intermittent eye contact, somewhat pressured speech, and, in the primary care context, a worried focus on the somatic concerns described in the preceding text.

C. Testing. Useful laboratory tests include serum calcium (hypocalcemia), hematocrit (anemia), and thyroid-stimulating hormone (hyperthyroidism/hypothyroidism). Depending on the clinical scenario, an exercise stress test to evaluate chest pain or other tests to rule out organic causes, such as drug screen, oximetry (hypoxia), glucose (hypoglycemia), and electrolytes, may be useful as well.

IV. DIAGNOSIS
A. Differential Diagnosis

1. GAD is characterized by persistent and *excessive* worry about a number of issues on most days for a period of at least 6 months. GAD usually begins by early adulthood, is exacerbated by situational stressors, and usually involves a combination of psychologic and physical symptoms.

2. Panic disorder, with or without agoraphobia, presents with recurrent panic attacks—discrete episodes of anxiety involving shortness of breath, fear of dying, impending doom or losing control, pounding heart, sweating, chest pain, paresthesias, trembling, and nausea. The panic attacks may be provoked by identifiable stressors or situations but often seem to "come out of the blue." Individuals with panic disorder may be so fearful of being in a situation in which they have another panic attack and are unable to escape that they develop agoraphobia (an intense fear of being in open or crowded places, which often contributes to the individuals being reluctant to leave the perceived safety of their home).

3. Acute stress disorder (ASD) and PTSD are characterized by reexperiencing (through intrusive thoughts, flashbacks, and nightmares) an extremely traumatic and possibly life-threatening experience (e.g., rape, murder, motor vehicle accident, and war), followed by hyperarousal, panic, depressed mood, sleep disturbance, and hypervigilance. The individual usually attempts to avoid these memories or the chance of being in danger again through numbing, dissociation, repression, and behavioral changes. The main distinction between ASD and PTSD is the duration of symptoms (i.e., in PTSD, the symptoms last longer than 1 month).

4. Specific phobia is excessive anxiety provoked by exposure to a specific feared object or situation. Common phobias include fear of animals or insects, natural environment (e.g., heights, storms, and water), blood–injection–injury, or situations (e.g., tunnels, bridges, elevators, flying, and driving).

5. Social phobia is an excessive anxiety provoked by exposure to social or performance situations and unfamiliar individuals or surroundings. As a result, individuals with social phobia avoid these types of situations.
6. Obsessive compulsive disorder is characterized by obsessions that cause anxiety (e.g., germs on hands) and compulsions (behaviors aimed at reducing the anxiety such as hand washing). The obsessions usually fall into one or more of the following categories: infection/contagion, safety, religiosity, sexuality, death/dying, and orderliness.
7. Adjustment reaction with anxious features is a condition in which a patient experiences significant anxiety in reaction to a specific stressor such as a major life event or interpersonal conflict. To qualify for this diagnosis, the level of anxiety should be assessed as being more than expected under the circumstances. In addition to these conditions, the clinician should investigate the possibility of mood, substance abuse, and other psychiatric disorders (3).

B. Clinical Manifestations. Most anxious patients present in the primary care setting with a primary focus on their bodies and somatic symptoms rather than "their minds." But inevitably, there is a significant component of worry, fear, and apprehension in the background. Because an exclusive focus on physical complaints (e.g., chest pain and dizziness) can obscure the diagnosis, it is important to ask patients about their psychologic state, living situation, and current stressors as well as evaluate them for underlying medical issues.

REFERENCES

1. National Institute of Mental Health. *Anxiety disorders*. Bethesda, MD: National Institute of Mental Health, 2009. Retrieved from http://www.nimh.nih.gov/health/publications/anxiety-disorders/index.shtml.
2. American Anxiety Disorders Association. Silver Spring, MD. Retrieved from http://www.adaa.org
3. American Psychiatric Association. *Diagnostic and statistical manual of mental disorders*, 4th ed. Washington, DC: American Psychiatric Association, 2000.

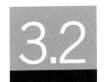

3.2 Bipolar Disorder
Daniel S. Felix

I. BACKGROUND. Bipolar I disorder, formerly known as manic-depressive disorder, is a condition in which a person's mood swings back and forth between two extremes: the highs of mania and the lows of depression. Bipolar disorder is distinguished from other mood disorders by the presence of manic episodes, which typically last for several days or weeks (1, 2) and can lead to risky behaviors (e.g., excessive spending, gambling, sexual carelessness, or infidelity), damaged relationships, poor career or school performance, and even accidental loss of life (2). Bipolar disorder is one of the 10 leading causes of disability worldwide (3) and can be very costly to treat. In most cases, bipolar disorder can be adequately controlled with medications and psychotherapy (1). Like diabetes, bipolar disorder is a long-term illness that must be carefully managed throughout a person's life.

II. PATHOPHYSIOLOGY

A. Etiology. Although the exact causes of bipolar disorder are not known, biologic, psychological, and social factors all play a significant role in its genesis and incidence. Studies of twins give strong evidence for a genetic link, with twins being 40–70% more likely to have bipolar disorder than another sibling (4). However, not every identical twin develops the condition, which suggests that environmental factors are also involved in its origins.

For example, how a person manages their emotions, relationships, and life stresses can influence the frequency and severity of bipolar symptoms.

   B. Epidemiology. Bipolar disorder affects 2.6% of the population, although fewer than half of those affected currently receive adequate treatment (5). Most cases of bipolar disorder start between ages 15 and 25 years (6), and men and women are equally affected, as well as all races, ethnic groups, and socioeconomic classes (1).

III. EVALUATION

   A. History. Assessment for bipolar disorder typically involves gathering a detailed medical history, including past and present medical problems and current medications, as well as a thorough history of past mood swings and manic or depressed behaviors. Patients' families may be consulted to help gather and validate this information inasmuch as patients with bipolar disorder sometimes have trouble recognizing their own manic symptoms (1). A person is much more likely to develop bipolar disorder if one or more of their family members have been diagnosed with it; hence, a comprehensive family history should also be evaluated for the presence of mood disorders in close biologic relatives.

   Manic symptoms of bipolar include
   - Euphoria/elevated mood
   - Inflated self-esteem (false beliefs about self)
   - Decreased need for sleep
   - Rapid and excessive speech
   - Racing thoughts
   - Increased physical energy
   - Increased sex drive/sexual behaviors
   - Spending sprees or unwise financial choices
   - Increased drive to perform or achieve goals
   - Easily agitated/irritated
   - Poor judgment
   - Easily distracted
   - Careless or dangerous use of drugs or alcohol
   - Poor performance at work or school

   Depressive symptoms most often include
   - Persistent low mood or sadness
   - Feelings of worthlessness, hopelessness, or guilt
   - Loss of interest/pleasure in activities that were once enjoyed
   - Fatigue or lack of energy
   - Difficulty concentrating
   - Eating problems
     o Loss of appetite
     o Overeating
   - Sleep problems
     o Difficulty falling asleep or staying asleep
     o Sleeping too much
   - Chronic pain
   - Thoughts of death and suicide

   Both manic and depressive episodes can be triggered by various stressful life events or actions, such as childbirth, marriage, divorce, or the death of a loved one. Antidepressant medications and lack of sleep can often trigger mania in those with bipolar disorder. Excessive use of alcohol or drugs can also trigger bipolar symptoms, although many individuals with bipolar disorder use alcohol and drugs to self-medicate during their high and low moods.

   B. Physical Exam. An evaluative physical exam should be performed to screen for other illnesses associated with mood swings, including signs of thyroid dysfunction and alcohol/drug abuse.

C. Testing. Thyroid hormone levels and tests for alcohol or other drugs may be performed if indicated. Currently, no blood test exists that can specifically detect the presence of bipolar disorder. Valid and reliable screening instruments or questionnaires can be used to assess the presence of both manic and depressive symptoms. More comprehensive assessments can also be used to gather information from patient and nonpatient sources about biologic, psychological, and social behaviors and consequences in the patient's life. Mood charting is also frequently used for bipolar assessment.

IV. DIAGNOSIS

A. Differential Diagnosis. There are various subtypes of bipolar disorder. Bipolar I and bipolar II disorders are distinguishable by the intensity of manic episodes, with bipolar II disorder typically having hypomanic rather than full manic episodes (2). Hypomanic episodes are not as intense, do not include psychosis, and may not impair daily functioning or relationships significantly, but still include a markedly elevated mood and feelings of grandiosity or irritability. Bipolar I and bipolar II disorders include depressive mood episodes of the same severe intensity. Cyclothymia is a form of bipolar disorder with milder depressive and hypomanic moods for at least 2 years (1). These swings can be rapid or slow cycling, but they do not meet the intensity criteria of any other mood disorder. Other mood disorders can appear as bipolar but are actually due to the abuse of substances. A depressed individual, for example, may appear to have swung into a manic state but may in fact be under the influence of mind-altering chemicals taken to self-medicate his or her symptoms of depression.

B. Clinical Manifestations. People seeking help for bipolar disorder most often present to their care providers during episodes of depression. Because of the feelings of euphoria (and damaged relationships) that frequently come with mania and manic behaviors, typically those with whom the person has close relationships (e.g., family members) will seek help for the person when they are manic. Changes in mood are not predictable. It is sometimes hard to tell whether a patient with bipolar is responding to treatment or is naturally coming out of a bipolar phase. Comorbidities with bipolar disorder are many and often include substance abuse disorders (2), although in many cases the abuse of substances occurs to self-medicate feelings of depression or is related to the behavioral control problems associated with mania; conversely, substance abuse may also trigger or prolong bipolar symptoms. People with bipolar disorder are also at higher risk for thyroid disease, migraine headaches, heart disease, diabetes, obesity, and other physical illnesses (7, 8).

REFERENCES

1. National Institute of Mental Health. *Bipolar disorder*. Bethesda, MD: National Institute of Mental Health, 2009. Accessed at http://www.nimh.nih.gov/health/publications/bipolar-disorder/index.shtml.
2. American Psychiatric Association. *Diagnostic and statistical manual of mental disorders-IV-TR*. Washington, DC: American Psychiatric Association, 2000.
3. Jenkins R. Reducing the burden of mental illness. *Lancet* 1997;349:1340.
4. Craddock N, Jones I. Genetics of bipolar disorder. *J Med Genet* 1999;36:585–594.
5. Kessler RC, Chiu WT, Demler O, Walters EE. Prevalence, severity, and comorbidity of twelve-month DSM-IV disorders in the National Comorbidity Survey Replication (NCS-R). *Arch Gen Psychiatry* 2005;62(6):617–627.
6. Kessler RC, Berglund P, Demler O, Jin R, Merikangas KR, Walters EE. Lifetime prevalence and age-of-onset distributions of DSM-IV disorders in the National Comorbidity Survey Replication. *Arch Gen Psychiatry* 2005;62(6):593–602.
7. Krishnan KR. Psychiatric and medical comorbidities of bipolar disorder. *Psychosom Med* 2005;67(1): 1–8.
8. Kupfer DJ. The increasing medical burden in bipolar disorder. *JAMA* 2005;293(20):2528–2530.

Depression

W. David Robinson

I. BACKGROUND

A. Definition. Depression is an illness that affects the mind, body, mood, thoughts, and relationships. It is not just unhappiness but an overwhelming sense of sadness and physical decline that has potential far-reaching deleterious effects.

B. Cost. Within the next 20 years, depression will be the leading cause of disability in the United States (1). Depression costs the United States billions of dollars annually in lost productivity, direct medical costs, and suicide-related mortality expenses (2). Depression also contributes to impaired concentration, failure to advance in education and vocational endeavors, increased substance abuse, impaired or lost relationships, and increased risk of suicide (3).

II. PATHOPHYSIOLOGY

A. Etiology. The biopsychosocial model is an effective way to conceptualize the etiology of anxiety and depression because the factors that create anxiety and depression are varied. The interplay between the biologic, psychological, and social aspects of the particular patient should be assessed to determine the etiology of the disease.

1. Biologic. There is ample information suggesting that genetics plays a role in the development of mood disorders. Studies related to twins have shown that genetics is the biggest underlying factor in the display of depressive symptoms (4). Women are at least twice as likely to suffer from depression as men. Individuals with a family history of mood disorders are at a higher risk for developing a disorder themselves. Other important biologic factors include comorbidities or depression as a result of medical problems and abuse of substances, which may be either the cause or the symptom of the depression.

2. Psychological. Individuals who are continually under a great deal of stress, have a negative outlook on life, or have a passive temperament are more likely to suffer from a mood disorder. These individuals often engage in cognitive distortions, including unrealistic expectations, overgeneralizing adverse events, personalizing negative or difficult events, and overreacting to stressors. Behaviorally, individuals who are continually under stress often believe that any action on their part would be futile, and therefore they continue to repeat self-defeating or problematic behaviors or do nothing at all (learned helplessness).

3. Social. There are many social influences that are related to mood disorders. These include difficult marriages, divorce, problems with children, family and community violence, racism, and economic difficulties. Many individuals do not have the social resources (e.g., friendships, family, and community) or buffers that aid in coping (e.g., spirituality).

B. Epidemiology. Depression is one of the most common conditions seen in primary care (3). Roughly 7% of adults in the United States (over 9 million people) had a major depressive disorder in 2012 (5). However, physicians often underdiagnose patients with depression. Even among patients correctly diagnosed, most patients with depression still do not receive treatment concordant with recommended guidelines. Recent studies have shown that over one-half of individuals diagnosed with depression and over one-third of individuals with severe depression do not receive depression-specific treatment (6). Further, patient adherence to the recommended treatment plan is low (7).

III. EVALUATION

A. History. To be diagnosed with major depression, an individual must have experienced five or more symptoms and must have depressed mood and/or anhedonia over the same 2-week period. The mnemonic SIGECAPS highlights the symptoms of a major depressive episode:

1. Sleep disturbance—early morning awakenings or restless sleep

2. Interest—little interest in activities they used to enjoy (anhedonia)

3. Guilt—feeling guilty or worthless
4. Energy—feeling tired or fatigued
5. Concentration—impaired concentration and/or indecisiveness
6. Appetite—weight change and/or changes in their normal eating patterns (eating less or more than usual)
7. Psychomotor disturbance—any psychomotor agitation or retardation
8. Suicidal thoughts—recurrent thoughts of death, suicidal ideation, and suicide attempt

B. **Physical Examination.** Any patient with depression severe enough to warrant treatment should have both a general screening physical examination (paying particular attention to signs of anemia and endocrinopathies [e.g., hypothyroidism]) and a careful screening neurologic examination. Depression is also often a symptom of many medical conditions (e.g., cardiovascular disease, dementia, multiple sclerosis, cancer, thyroid disorders, acquired immunodeficiency syndrome, and endocrine changes).

C. **Testing.** Laboratory tests should be ordered on the basis of the history and examination findings (e.g., complete blood count for anemia and thyroid-stimulating hormone for thyroid disorders).

1. **Initial Screening**

   The U.S. Preventive Services Task Force recommends screening adults for depression in clinical practice (8). A quick two-question screen for depression can be used to identify individuals at risk: over the past 2 weeks have you (a) felt down, depressed, or hopeless? and (b) felt little interest or pleasure in doing things? If an individual answers yes to one or both of these, he/she should be further evaluated for depression.

2. **Further Screening**

   Multiple screening instruments can be used to detect depression (i.e., Zung and Beck depression inventories). A relatively new, free screening tool that has been found to be efficient and effective in determining depression severity is the Patient Health Questionnaire-9 (PHQ-9) (9). The PHQ-9 is a screening questionnaire chosen because of the ease of administration and scoring and its high sensitivity/specificity. The PHQ-9 is a nine-question form that addresses all the symptoms of major depression (9). Questions are answered using a 4-point Likert scale (0 = not at all and 3 = nearly everyday). Scores of 5 to 9 are associated with mild depression, and scores of 10 or above are associated with moderate or severe depression (10). This tool is meant to be used to monitor treatment response, and recommendations are given that assist primary care physicians to treat to remission. Since depression is often hidden, this tool is often used to screen all patients for depression. More information about this tool can be found at http://www.depression-primarycare.org/clinicians/toolkits/.

IV. DIAGNOSIS

A. **Differential Diagnosis**

1. In addition to the medical conditions related to depression discussed earlier, each individual suspected of depression should also be screened for anxiety disorders, alcohol and drug abuse, suicidality, homicidality, and domestic violence or victims of abuse.

2. There are many types of depressive disorders. It is important to distinguish the specific type of disorder so as to most effectively recommend treatment options:

   a. Major depressive disorder is present when the individual has two or more major depressive episodes.

   b. Dysthymic disorder is characterized by at least 2 years of low-grade depression (does not meet the criteria for a major depressive episode).

   c. Depressive disorder not otherwise specified is used when the individual does not meet criteria for other depressive conditions, but depressive features exist.

   d. Bipolar I disorder is characterized by one or more manic episodes and is usually accompanied by major depressive episodes. It is important to rule out mania in individuals who are depressed because psychopharmacologic treatment of depression can make individuals with bipolar disorder become manic. Screening can be done through various screening instruments (e.g., Mood Disorder Questionnaire). Manic episodes must include at least three of the following symptoms lasting for a period of at least 7 days:

   i. inflated self-esteem or grandiosity
   ii. decreased need for sleep
   iii. more talkative than usual or pressure to keep talking
   iv. flight of ideas or subjective experience of thoughts racing
   v. distractibility
   vi. increase in goal-directed activity (socially, at work, or sexually) or psychomotor agitation
   vii. excessive involvement in pleasurable activities that have a high potential for painful consequences (e.g., spending, gambling, and sexual indiscretions)

  e. Bipolar II disorder is characterized by one or more major depressive episodes and at least one hypomanic episode (lasting at least 4 days). Hypomanic episodes use the same criteria as manic episodes, but hypomania does not cause marked impairment in social or occupational functioning or require hospitalization.

  f. Cyclothymic disorder is characterized by at least 2 years of numerous periods of low-grade depression and hypomanic symptoms.

  g. Mood disorder due to a general medical condition and substance-induced mood disorder are characterized by a mood disturbance caused by the direct physiologic consequence of a general medical condition or substance use, respectively.

  h. Seasonal affective disorder, grief reaction, and adjustment disorder with depressed mood are other disorders that are caused by the time of the year, response to loss, and response to a significant change (e.g., divorce), respectively.

B. Clinical Manifestations.

Depression does not often present in a primary care setting by the patient complaining of depressed mood. It is more likely that the patient will discuss the symptoms of depression (e.g., fatigue, insomnia, and gastrointestinal upset). It is therefore important for the physician to not only attend to the physical complaints but also probe into the emotional symptoms (e.g., dysphoria and anhedonia).

REFERENCES

1. Mathers CD, Loncar D. Projections of global mortality and burden of disease from 2002 to 2030. *PLoS Med* 2006;3(11):e442, doi:10.1371/journal.pmed.0030442\

2. Greenberg PE, Kessler RC, Birnbaum HG, et al. The economic burden of depression in the United States: how did it change between 1990 and 2000? *J Clin Psychiatry* 2003;64(12):1465–1475.

3. Gonzalez HM, Tarraf W, Whitfield K, Vega W. The epidemiology of major depression and ethnicity in the United States. *J Psychiatr Res* 2010;44:1043–1051.

4. Li X, McGue M, Gottesman I. Two sources of genetic liability to depression: interpreting the relationship between stress sensitivity and depression under a multifactorial polygenic model. *Behav Genet* 2012;42(2):268–277.

5. Boenisch S, Kocalevent R, Bramesfeld A, et al. Who receives depression-specific treatment? A secondary data-based analysis of outpatient care received by over 780,000 statutory health-insured individuals diagnosed with depression. *Soc Psychiatry Psychiatric Epidemiol* 2012;47(3):475–486.

6. Kessler RC, Chiu WT, Demler O, Walters EE. Prevalence, severity, and comorbidity of twelve-month DSM-IV disorders in the National Comorbidity Survey Replication (NCS-R). *Arch Gen Psychiatry* 2005;62(6):617–627.

7. Young AS, Klap R, Sherbourne CD, et al. The quality of care for depressive and anxiety disorders in the United States. *Arch Gen Psychiatry* 2001;58(1):55–61.

8. U.S. Preventive Services Task Force. Screening for depression: recommendations and rationale. *Ann Intern Med* 2002;136(10):760–764.

9. Arroll B, Goodyear-Smith F, Hatcher S, et al. Validation of PHQ-2 and PHQ-9 to screen for major depression in the primary care population. *Ann Fam Med* 2010;8(4):348–353.

10. Montano CB, Montano MB. A new paradigm for treating depression in the primary care setting. Medical Education Collaborative. Accessed at http://www.medscape.com.

3.4 Suicide Risk

Health A. Grames and Jeff Hinton

I. BACKGROUND. Suicide is ranked as the tenth leading cause of death in the general US population, the second leading cause of death for young adults between the ages of 25 and 34 years, third for adolescents and young adults from age 15 to 24 years, and fourth for adults between 35 and 54 years (1). In the general US population, males are more likely to commit suicide than females, and American Indian/Alaska Natives and Non-Hispanic Whites have the highest suicide rates (1, 2). Although the risk of suicide can be difficult to assess and predict due to contributing risk factors, comprehensive assessment increases the accuracy of identifying suicidal thoughts and behaviors, allowing the physician to take preventative measures.

Because approximately 75% of those attempting suicide visit a primary care physician (PCP) within 1 month and 10% visit a hospital emergency room within 2 months of their attempt, it is imperative that PCPs are familiar with suicide assessment and intervention protocols (3, 4). PCPs are also in a unique position to provide positive intervention to prevent suicide if they are able to identify and recognize suicide risk factors.

II. PATHOPHYSIOLOGY

A. Etiology. Suicide is often viewed as a moral decision that contradicts many religious and societal values. However, for many individuals who attempt or commit suicide, the quality of life (physical, emotional, and/or spiritual) has become so depleted that they see no other option. Many factors contribute to low levels of quality of life and, therefore, the decision to take one's own life. Both physical and psychiatric disorders are recognized as being among these factors. Physical contributors include chronic illness and changes in neurotransmitters (i.e., serotonin) (5). A disease that is debilitating, painful, and prolonged increases the risk of suicide (6). Psychiatric disorders include major depression, substance abuse, schizophrenia, panic disorder, delirium, bulimia nervosa, bipolar disorder, dysthymia, social phobia, post-traumatic stress disorder, social phobia, and personality disorders (6, 7). Other factors include a history of suicide attempts by the individual or close relatives and friends, violence at home, history of physical or sexual abuse, ownership of a firearm, history of family mental illness, a recent crisis (i.e., loss of income and divorce), illness, and old age. Hopelessness, hostility, negative self-esteem, and isolation have been identified as suicide risk factors in adolescents (8). Use of certain medications has also been shown to increase the risk of suicidal behavior (6). These medications include antidepressants, anticonvulsants, pain medication, smoking cessation medications, and glucocorticoids (6).

B. Epidemiology. The most current data on suicide rates posted by the Centers for Disease Control and Prevention (CDC) indicate that in 2009, 36,909 individuals died by suicide in the United States (1). To put this in perspective, this is higher than the number of individuals who died by homicide and of complications from human immunodeficiency virus/acquired immunodeficiency syndrome. The highest risk age group for committing suicide comprises individuals aged 75 and older (36.1 suicides per 100,000) and the highest risk group is white males aged 85 and over (49.8 per 100,000) (6, 9). Among children, adolescents, and young adults, the latter are at slightly greater risk of committing suicide (12.7 per 100,000) than the national average (10). Among all age groups, males are more likely to commit suicide than females (approximately 4:1), but females are more likely to attempt suicide than males. White males are most likely to commit suicide, accounting for 72% of all deaths by suicide (1). Firearms are the most common mode of suicide by both men and women (10).

III. EVALUATION. A primary care suicide risk assessment should include the completion of a brief patient history and an assessment of suicide risk and protective factors. Although it is not necessary to exhaustively interview all patients, those with identified risk factors should receive further assessment.

   A. History. Because patients rarely talk to their PCPs about suicidal thoughts or past attempts unless asked, it is imperative that physicians briefly screen patients for suicide risk factors. With patients who verbalize suicidal ideation, the PCP must ask patients specific questions to uncover their intentions. Patients at greater risk for suicidal ideation or attempts should be assessed for current thoughts of self-harm. This can be accomplished efficiently as part of an assessment for depression such as the Patient Health Questionnaire-9 (PHQ-9) or by asking the patients direct questions about thoughts of self-harm (7). Some PCPs may feel hesitant to ask such direct questions pertaining to suicide for fear they may be planting an idea in a patient who is already struggling. However, research suggests that talking to a patient about suicide does not increase the level of suicide risk for the patient. At-risk patients must be asked about suicidal thoughts and behavior so that appropriate treatment can follow.

   B. Assessment

   1. The PCP should first assess for suicidal thoughts and risk factors. For patients identifying current suicidal ideation, the PCP should determine if the patient has a detailed suicide plan and how serious the patient is about carrying out the plan. *Level of intent* to carry out the plan can be assessed by asking patients if they have told other individuals of the plan, by asking about specific details of the plan, and by asking patients directly how serious they are about actually harming themselves. Also, the PCP should distinguish between a realistic and an unrealistic plan to commit suicide. A *realistic* plan involves the patient having access and means to complete a suicide, e.g., a patient who threatens to overdose on a medication that has previously been prescribed. An *unrealistic* plan is based on unlikely or impossible means of fulfilling suicidal intentions. For example, a patient may state that he/she wants to shoot herself but does not own or have access to a gun, does not know someone who owns a gun, cannot purchase a gun, and does not consider other more realistic means of suicide to which he/she has access. Although all patients with suicide plans merit preventative actions, such as a suicide management plan, patients with a detailed realistic plan are in more immediate danger and require immediate intervention.

      In addition to conducting a thorough assessment of suicide risk factors, protective factors that may buffer the patient's desires or interest in committing suicide should also be assessed (11). The CDC outlines several protective factors, including the patient having effective clinical care for mental, physical, and substance abuse disorders, easy access to a variety of clinical interventions and assistance in seeking, family and community support (connectedness), support from ongoing medical and mental health care relationships, skills in problem solving, conflict resolution, nonviolent ways of handling disputes, and cultural and religious beliefs that discourage suicide and support instincts for self-preservation (9). These protective factors serve as resources that may be utilized in the suicide prevention treatment plan just as any other medical or mental health component of the plan.

   2. For patients with suicidal ideation and plans, the PCP must assess the *suicide attempt time frame*. Patients should be asked when they plan to attempt suicide and estimate how likely they are to attempt suicide before the next visit to the physician. The answers to these questions are pertinent in determining the level of management. For example, a patient may be very depressed, state a realistic plan of suicide, and offer little reason to live, but say that he/she will not attempt suicide until his/her 3-year-old child has graduated from high school. Although this individual should receive help, he may not be in immediate danger for suicide.

   C. Risk. The PCP's assessment determines the patient's *level of risk* as *minimal, moderate, or severe* (7). The treatment strategy should directly relate to the patient's level of risk.

   1. *Minimal risk.* Patients in this category have likely experienced thoughts of self-harm but have no specific plan, have no history of past attempts, and deny that they would

actually attempt suicide. These patients identify reasons to continue living and are active participants with the PCP in developing a safety plan.

2. *Moderate risk.* Patients in this category have articulated a suicide plan (which may or may not be realistic). However, when questioned directly about their plan, they deny the intent to follow through. While moderate risk patients may have prior suicide attempts in the distant past, they are willing to actively participate with the PCP in developing a safety plan and exploring reasons to live.

3. *Severe risk.* Patients in this category have a specific realistic plan, access to means, and a strong intent to self-harm and are unwilling to work with the PCP to create a safety plan and explore alternative options.

IV. DIAGNOSIS. For patients exhibiting suicidal ideation, the suicide assessment should become the PCP's primary focus of the medical appointment. In these cases, a thorough assessment and treatment plan is warranted. Patients who are considered low risk of committing suicide require follow-up visits and continued monitoring. Patients considered to be at moderate risk for attempting suicide should have a treatment plan that includes contracting with the PCP that he/she will call or otherwise seek medical or mental health intervention if he/she becomes actively suicidal. The PCP should consult with a mental health specialist as needed and refer the patient for mental health intervention. High suicide risk patients need immediate intervention that may include referral for immediate inpatient psychiatric services and/or immediate referral to a mental health professional (7).

REFERENCES

1. Centers for Disease Control and Prevention, National Center for Injury Prevention and Control. Web-based Injury Statistics Query and Reporting System (WISQARS). *10 leading causes of death, 2009, all races, both sexes.* Atlanta, GA. Accessed at http://www.cdc.gov/injury/wisqars/leading_causes_death.html.

2. Centers for Disease Control and Prevention, Injury Center: Violence Prevention. *National suicide statistics at a glance.* Atlanta, GA. Accessed at http://www.cdc.gov/violenceprevention/suicide/statistics/rates02.html.

3. Feldman MD, Franks P, Duberstein PR, et al. Let's not talk about it: suicide inquiry in primary care. *Ann Fam Med* 2007;5(5):412–418.

4. Suicide Prevention Resource Center. *Is your patient suicidal?* Accessed at http://www.sprc.org/library/ER_SuicideRiskPosterVert2.pdf.

5. National Institute of Mental Health. *In harm's way: suicide in America.* Revised ed. [Brochure]. Bethesda, MD: US Department of Health and Human Services, 2003.

6. Soreff S. Suicide. *Medscape reference: drugs, disease, and procedures.* Accessed at http://emedicine.medscape.com/article/2013085-overview#a1.

7. The MacArthur Initiative on Depression and Primary Care. *Tool kit.* Accessed at http://www.depression-primarycare.org.

8. Rutter PA, Behrendt AE. Adolescent suicide risk: four psychological factors. *Adolescence* 2004;39:295–302.

9. National Institute of Mental Health. *Older adults: depression and suicide facts (Facts Sheet).* Bethesda, MD. Accessed at http://www.nimh.nih.gov/health/publications/older-adults-depression-and-suicide-facts-fact-sheet/index.shtml#how-common.

10. National Institute of Mental Health. *Suicide in the U.S.: statistics and prevention.* Bethesda, MD. Accessed at http://www.mentalhealth.gov/health/publications/suicide-in-the-us-statistics-and-prevention/index.shtml.

11. Center for Disease Control and Prevention, Injury Center: Violence and Prevention. *Suicide: risk and protective factors.* Atlanta, GA. Accessed at http://www.cdc.gov/ViolencePrevention/suicide/riskprotectivefactors.html.

CHAPTER 4

Problems Related to the Nervous System

Douglas Inciarte

Ataxia

Diego R. Torres-Russotto

I. BACKGROUND. Ataxia is the type of clumsiness that is produced by dysfunction of the cerebellum and its pathways (1).

II. PATHOPHYSIOLOGY. The usual syndrome includes hand clumsiness, abnormal or unstable gait, and dysarthria. Many movement abnormalities are seen in cerebellar dysfunction (1).

A. Limb Ataxia.

1. Asynergia: decomposition of movements. Instead of the normal smooth performance, there is breakdown of the movement, rendering it irregular.
2. Dysdiadochokinesia: a manifestation of asynergia, this is the breakup and irregularity seen while performing rapid alternating movements.
3. Dysmetria: the misjudging of distance. Dysmetria includes hypermetria (overshooting), hypometria (undershooting), and loss of check (inability to stop a ballistic movement right on target).
4. Intention tremor (see Chapter 9.9, Tremor): Tremor that is characteristically worse during target-directed movements (in comparison with that of posture holding or other actions).
5. Hypotonia: decreased tone is common in cerebellar syndromes.
6. Rebound: sudden displacement of a limb that is holding a posture produces excessive overcorrection.

B. Gait/Truncal Ataxia. Characterized by irregular stepping (worse with tiptoe or heel ambulation), increased lateral sway (not a straight line of ambulation), unstable turns, and inability to walk in tandem. Wide-based ambulation, spontaneous retropulsion, and true postural instability are more advanced signs of ataxia.

C. Ocular Ataxia. Characterized mostly by dysmetric ocular saccades and tends to be associated with nystagmus. Patients might experience diplopia.

D. Ataxic Dysarthria. Global dysarthria but with a very strong component of lingual dysarthria, frequent volume changes (usually with overall hypophonia), and scanning speech.

III. EVALUATION

A. Initial Workup

1. Diagnoses not to miss: medication induced, Wilson disease, thyroid abnormalities, metabolic abnormalities (liver, kidney, or electrolyte/glucose), vitamin B12, D, and E deficiencies, stroke, multiple sclerosis, hydrocephalus, and tumors (medulloblastoma, astrocytoma, ependymoma, metastasis, and others).
2. Paraneoplastic ataxias often precede structural symptoms from the primary tumor and other usual cancer clues; therefore, diagnosis has important implications.

3. Structural myelopathy is one of the most common causes of truncal ataxia, and early diagnosis avoids progression. Upper motor neuron signs can be present on both structural myelopathy and neurodegenerative ataxias.

4. In children, important etiologies for acute ataxia include intoxication, acephalgic migraine, and cerebellitis (usually varicella-zoster virus). Chronic ataxias would point to congenital defects of metabolism and leukodystrophies.

5. Environmental exposure and use of over-the-counter, herbal, or illegal drugs should be ascertained. Consider heavy metal testing.

6. Basic initial workup to consider: peripheral smear (looking for acanthocytes), pregnancy test, ceruloplasmin, thyroid function, complete metabolic panel (CMP), rapid plasma regain (RPR), vitamin B12 level, methyl malonic acid (MMA), homocysteine, folate, 25-OH vitamin D3, vitamin E, antigliadin antibody, urine drug screen, and paraneoplastic panel.

B. Other Tests to Consider in Sporadic Ataxia. Lipoprotein electrophoresis (abetalipoproteinemia), Anti neutrophil cytoplasmic antibody (ANCA), alpha-fetoprotein, HIV, zinc, tissue transglutaminase/endomysial antibody, fragile X-associated tremor and ataxia syndrome (FXTAS) testing, anti-GAD antibody (Stiff person syndrome), quantitative immunoglobulins, human T lymphotrophic virus (HTLV) 1 and 2. Cerebrospinal fluid (CSF) studies should be considered in all acute/subacute cases if not contraindicated.

C. Tests to Consider in Familial Ataxias. FXTAS, Friedreich's ataxia (FA) test, autosomal dominant spino-cerebellar ataxia (SCA) panel.

D. Brain Imaging (MRI Better Than CT). Imaging is needed in most patients to rule out structural abnormalities (like Chiari or Dandy-Walker malformation), especially in those with rapid or unusual progression or with associated abnormal neurologic examination.

E. Cervical and Thoracic Spine Imaging (Usually through MRI). Needed to rule out structural myelopathy as the cause of truncal ataxia.

IV. DIAGNOSIS

A. Sporadic Ataxia. If initial workup is negative (see above), other etiologies include multiple systems atrophy, celiac disease, Creutzfeldt-Jacob disease, genetic ataxias (like Friedrich ataxia, SCA 2, 3 and 6), and paraneoplastic syndromes (false-negative panel tests are expected). One of the most common causes of ataxia is alcohol abuse. Cerebellar degeneration due to alcohol can be global, but a particular alcohol syndrome, dorsal vermial atrophy, is associated with severe truncal ataxia.

B. Genetic Ataxia. A good source of genetic ataxia information includes the Online Mendelian inheritance in Man (OMIM) and the Washington University in St. Louis Neuromuscular web sites (2). Special mention is needed for a relatively new, highly prevalent, commonly undiagnosed disease called FXTAS (3). This syndrome is seen in those carriers of the fragile X premutation who might also have parkinsonism and dementia. MRI of the brain tends to be revealing, including the MCP sign (bilateral T2-hyperintense middle cerebellar peduncle).

1. Dominant ataxias: These include the SCAs, dentatorubral pallidoluysian atrophy (DRPLA), and the episodic ataxias. There are more than 25 SCAs and their differentiation is difficult, rendering the SCA panel genetic testing an option (proper patient genetic counseling is needed).

2. Recessive ataxias: These include FA, abetalipoproteinemia, ataxia telangiectasia syndrome, and the treatable, isolated vitamin E deficiency (TTP1 gene mutation). FA is the most common one and presents with upper motor neuron signs, neuropathy, and cardiomyopathy. It is caused by an expanded GAA repeat on the *Frataxin* gene.

REFERENCES

1. Fahn S, Jankovic J. *Principles and practice of movement disorders.* Philadelphia, PA: Churchill Livingstone Elsevier, 2007.

2. Pestronk A. *Neuromuscular Diseases Division.* Accessed at Washington University in St. Louis Department of Neurology (http://www.neuro.wustl.edu/neuromuscular) on July 1, 2012.

3. Hagerman PJ, Hagerman R. Fragile X-associated tremor/ataxia syndrome. *Ment Retard Dev Disabil Res Rev* 2004;10(1):25–30.

4. Torres-Russotto D and Perlmutter J. Task-specific dystonias: a review. *Ann N Y Acad Sci* 2008;1142:179–199.

5. Louis ED. Essential tremor. In: Lewis PR, Timothy AP, eds. *Merritt's neurology*, 12th ed. Philadelphia, PA: Lippincott Williams & Wilkins, 2010:594–596.

6. Fahn S. Involuntary movements. In: Lewis PR, Timothy AP, eds. *Merritt's neurology*, 12th ed. Philadelphia, PA: Lippincott Williams & Wilkins, 2010:50–53.

4.2 Coma

Douglas J. Inciarte

I. BACKGROUND. Coma is a sustained period (>1 hour) of unconsciousness that is distinguished from sleep by the inability to arouse the patient (1, 2).

II. PATHOPHYSIOLOGY. Coma is a nonspecific manifestation of central nervous system (CNS) impairment that may be due to any number of insults. There is a large differential of possible causes that may be subdivided into focal (e.g., stroke) versus nonfocal (e.g., hypoxia), traumatic versus nontraumatic, or CNS versus systemic causes. The end result is that there is a global dysfunction of both the cerebral hemispheres or the ascending brain stem and diencephalon activating systems (2).

III. EVALUATION. The history and physical examination can often elicit the potential causes of coma.

  A. History. After ensuring the stability of the airway, breathing, and circulation (ABCs), it is essential to gather pertinent history from friends, family members, and any medical personnel. A sudden loss of consciousness would suggest causes such as intracerebral hemorrhage, seizure, cardiac arrhythmias, or drug overdose. A slower progression implies a much larger list of differential diagnoses.

  B. Physical Examination. The examination of coma is essentially done by scales; there are several scales used to assess the state of consciousness, such as Jouvet, Moscow, Glasgow, Bozza-Marrubini, and Full Outline of UnResponsiveness (FOUR) score. The most common scale used in practice is the Glasgow scale, which is useful especially on trauma patients and continues to be the most widely used. The FOUR score is easy to use and gives more detail than the Glasgow and is a better tool for monitoring in the ICU; it provides a better prognosis and could be used in primary care (Tables 4.2.1 and 4.2.2).

  C. Testing. Imaging of the head using either a computed tomography (CT) scan or a magnetic resonance imaging (MRI) should be done as quickly as possible to rule out structural causes and to guide emergent treatment (e.g., hemorrhage or herniation). Laboratory testing should include an arterial blood gas, a complete blood count, a comprehensive metabolic profile, toxicology (including ethanol, commonly abused drugs, acetaminophen, and salicylates), ammonia, and lactate. Blood and cerebrospinal fluid should also be cultured. An electroencephalogram (EEG) should be performed to look for unrecognized seizures. The EEG can also give clues to the cause and the prognosis (2).

IV. DIAGNOSIS

  A. Differential Diagnosis. The differential diagnosis of coma is broad but is usually established based on the history, physical examination, laboratory findings, EEG, and imaging. The differential diagnosis, subdivided based on normal versus abnormal CT scan or MRI, includes

    1. Normal CT scan or MRI

      a. Drugs/overdose: alcohol, sedatives, opiates

      b. Metabolic: anoxia, electrolyte disturbances, glucose abnormalities, thyroid disorders, hepatic coma

      c. Severe infections: pneumonia, meningitis, encephalitis, sepsis

TABLE 4.2.1	Glasgow Coma Scale	
Clinical Parameter		**Points**
Eyes	Open spontaneously	4
	To verbal command	3
	To pain	2
	No response	0
Best motor response	To verbal command Obeys	6
To painful stimulus	Localizes pain	5
	Flexion withdrawal	4
	Flexion abnormal	3
	Extension	2
	No response	1
Best verbal response	Oriented	5
	Confused	4
	Inappropriate speech	3
	Incomprehensible speech	2
	No response	1
Total		(3–15)

TABLE 4.2.2	FOUR (Full Outline of UnResponsiveness) Score	
	Findings	**Score**
Eye response	Eyelids open or opened, tracking or blinking to command	4
	Eyelids open but not tracking	3
	Eyelids closed but open to loud voice	2
	Eyelids closed but open to pain	1
	Eyelids remain closed with pain	0
Motor response	Makes sign (thumbs up, fist)	4
	Localizing to pain	3
	Flexion response to pain	2
	Extension response to pain	1
	No response to pain or generalized	0
Brain stem reflexes	Pupil and corneal reflexes present	4
	One pupil wide and fixed	3
	Pupil or corneal reflexes absent	2
	Pupil and corneal reflexes absent	1
	Absent pupil, corneal and cough reflex	0

(Continued)

TABLE 4.2.2	**FOUR (Full Outline of UnResponsiveness) Score** *(Continued)*	
	Findings	**Score**
Respiration	Not intubated, regular breathing pattern	4
	Not intubated, Cheyne-Stokes breathing pattern	3
	Not intubated, irregular breathing pattern	2
	Breathes above ventilator rate	1
	Breathes at ventilator rate or apnea	0
Total		(0–16)

    d. Shock
    e. Seizure-related conditions
    f. Severe hypothermia or hyperthermia
    g. Concussion
  2. Abnormal CT scan or MRI
    a. Hemorrhage or infarction
    b. Infection: abscess, empyema
    c. Brain tumor
    d. Traumatic injuries
    e. Others (3)
  B. Clinical Manifestations. The patient lacks self-awareness and makes no purposeful movements. Vital signs, including the ability to maintain respiratory function, may be impaired; so, immediate attention to ensuring stable ABCs is essential. Coma must be distinguished from other similar clinical entities such as vegetative state, catatonia, severe depression, neuromuscular blockade, or akinesia plus aphasia (1, 2).

REFERENCES

1. Burst JCM. Coma. In: Rowland LP, ed. *Merritt's neurology*, 11th ed. Philadelphia, PA: Lippincott Williams & Wilkins, 2005:20–28.
2. Michelson DJ, Ashwal S. Evaluation of coma and brain death. *Semin Pediatr Neurol* 2004;11(2):105–118.
3. Ropper AH. Acute confusional states and coma. In: Braunwald E, Hauser SL, et al. eds. *Harrison's principles of internal medicine*, 15th ed. Philadelphia, PA: McGraw-Hill, 2001:132–140.
4. Bordini AL, Luiz TF, Fernandez M, et al. Coma scale: a historical review. *Arch Neuropsychiatr* 2010;68(6):930–937.
5. Wijidicks E, Bamlet WR, Maumatten BV, et al. Validation of a new coma scale: the FOUR score. *Ann Neurol* 2005;58:585–593.

4.3 Delirium

Avery Sides

I. BACKGROUND. According to the American Psychiatric Association's *Diagnostic and Statistical Manual of Mental Disorders*, Fourth Edition (DSM-IV-TR) (1), delirium has the following key features: disturbance of consciousness with a reduced ability to focus, sustain, or shift attention; change in cognition or the development of a perceptual disturbance that is not better accounted for by a preexisting, established, or evolving dementia; disturbance developing over a short period of time (usually hours to days) and tending to fluctuate during the course of the day;

evidence from the history, physical examination, or laboratory findings that the disturbance is caused by the direct physiologic consequence of a general medical condition, substance intoxication or withdrawal, a medication side effect or toxin exposure, or a combination of these factors.

II. PATHOPHYSIOLOGY

A. Etiology. The neurobiologic mechanism of delirium is poorly understood, but one hypothesis includes a relationship with decreased acetycholine activity. However, a multitude of causes for delirium have been identified, often with more than one present (see Table 4.3.1).

B. Epidemiology. A systemic review of occurrence notes delirium to range between 11% and 42% of medical inpatients per admission. The prevalence at admission ranges from 10% to 31%, while the incidence of new delirium at admission ranges from 3% to 29% (2).

Delirium is common in a multitude of settings. Of those admitted to the ICU, studies indicate that >70% of patients over the age of 65 will experience delirium, while >50% under the age of 65 will also experience delirium (3). A total of 25% of the elderly undergoing cardiac surgery in the prior 7 days were found to have delirium, with the same percentage experiencing delirium within 3 days of a stroke (4). Delirium is not just found in the inpatient setting. Many patients leave the hospital with persistence of delirium. In those over 50 years old with delirium, 44% were found to have persistance at discharge, 32% continued at 1 month, 25% continued at 3 months, and over 21% can have persistance for 6 months following discharge (5).

TABLE 4.3.1   Common Causes of Delirium

Cardiac
  Congestive heart failure, chronic obstructive pulmonary disease, shock

Infections
  Pneumonia, septicemia, meningitis, urinary tract infection

Central nervous system disorders
  Stroke, seizure, nonconvulsive status epilepticus, postictal state, intracranial hemorrhage, meningitis, encephalitis, hypertensive emergency, superimposed on dementia, Wernicke encephalopathy, sensory deprivation, migraine—treatment of acute attack

  Increased intracranial pressure

Withdrawal from substances
  Alcohol, benzodiazepines, opiates

Metabolic disorders
  Renal failure, fluid/electrolyte disorder hypoxia, hypercarbia, hyponatremia, hypernatremia, uremia, hypovolemia, hypervolemia, acidosis, alkalosis, hypercalcemia, hypocalcemia, hypomagnesemia

  Hypoglycemia, Hypothyroidism, hyperthyroidism, adrenal dysfunction, niacin deficiency

  Hepatic failure (hepatic encephalopathy), anemia, hyperglycemia, thiamine deficiency

Environmental
  Bladder catheterization, stress, change in environment, surgery, anesthesia, sleep loss, pain, fever

  Urinary retention, hypothermia, physical restraints, fecal impaction

Medications by class
  Psychotropic drugs, antiepileptics, antiparkinson drugs, corticosteroids, histamine H2-blockers

  Drugs with anticholinergic effects, nonsteroidal anti-inflammatory drugs, opioids

  Tricyclic antidepressants, barbiturates (withdrawal), benzodiazepines (withdrawal)

  Illicit drugs, beta-blockers (rare), ETOH (withdrawal), chronic alcoholism

III. EVALUATION

A. History. Evaluation begins with the history of present illness. In delirium, it is important to note the presence of prodromal anxiety or hypersensitivity as well as time of day the individual is affected. Over 50% of those affected experienced psychiatric symptoms, with half affected by hypoactivity while half experience hyperactivity. Other important aspects of those affected include a large percentage with emotional disturbances, and nearly half experiencing pychosis (6).

Determining that a cognitive impairment or perceptual disturbance is not due to a preexisting or progressing dementia or other mental disorder requires knowledge of the patient's baseline mental status, and level of functioning. If this is not known, information should be sought from family, friends, and other care providers. Other medial history can yield insite into the cause of delirium. Important aspects to note include history of delirium, history of prior brain damage, post operative states, and history of previous substance use.

Because drug toxicity accounts is the number one cause of reversinle delirium, clinicians should not neglect considering over-the-counter drugs, drugs belonging to other family members, drugs prescribed by other physicians, or illicit drugs. Because the features of delirium fluctuate during the course of the day, a review of nursing notes, especially from the evening and night shifts, can be very helpful for discovering or documenting changes in consciousness and cognition.

B. Physical Examination. The examination must focus on two issues: (i) confirming that delirium is present, and (ii) uncovering the medical illness that has likely caused the delirium. A comprehensive examination is often difficult in a confused and uncooperative patient. Clinicians should perform a focused examination guided by the history and context, keeping in mind the multifactorial nature of delirium.

C. Testing. The history and physical examination should guide most of the diagnostic investigation. First-line investigations should include electrolytes, complete blood count, urinalysis, liver and thyroid function tests, glucose, creatinine, calcium, chest x-ray, and electrocardiogram. Blood gas determinations are often helpful. Drug levels can be obtained when appropriate, but the clinician should be aware that delirium can occur even with therapeutic levels. The following diagnostic tests may be indicated when a cause of delirium is not apparent after the initial evaluation: urine and blood toxicology screen, syphilis serology, human immunodeficiency virus antibody, autoantibody screen, vitamin B_{12} level, head computed tomography or magnetic resonance imaging, a lumbar puncture with cerebrospinal analysis, and electroencephalogram testing.

IV. DIAGNOSIS

A. Differential Diagnosis. The most common issue in the differential diagnosis is whether the patient has dementia rather than delirium, has delirium only, or a delirium superimposed on a preexisting dementia. Careful attention to the key features (disturbed consciousness, change in cognition or perceptual disturbance, acute onset, and fluctuating course) should readily distinguish delirium from dementia and other primary psychiatric disorders such as depression, psychosis, or mania. Nonconvulsive status epilepticus and several lobar or focal neurologic syndromes (Wernicke's aphasia, transient global amnesia, Anton's syndrome, frontal lobe tumors) can result in features that may overlap with those of delirium.

B. Clinical Manifestations. Engaging in conversation with a patient in delirium can be difficult because he or she may become easily distracted, unpredictably switch from subject to subject, or persevere with answers to a previous question. In more advanced cases of delirium, the patient may be drowsy or lethargic. Cognitive changes may include memory impairment (most commonly short-term memory), disorientation (usually to time and place), difficulty with language or speech (dysarthria, dysnomia, dysgraphia, or aphasia), and perceptual disturbances (illusions, hallucinations, or misperceptions). The patient may be so inattentive and incoherent that it may be difficult or impossible to assess cognitive function. Other associated features of delirium may include sleep disturbance or a reversal of the night–day sleep–wake cycle, hypersensitivity to light and sound, anxiety, anger, depressed affect, and emotional lability. Because of confusion, disorientation, and agitation, patients with delirium may harm themselves by climbing over bedrails or pulling out their intravenous line or Foley catheter.

REFERENCES

1. American Psychiatric Association. *Diagnostic and statistical manual of mental disorders*, 4th ed, Text Revision. Washington, DC: American Psychiatric Association, 2000.
2. Siddiqi N, House AO, Holmes JD. Occurrence and outcome of delirium in medical in-patients: a systematic literature review. *Age Ageing* 2006;35(4):350–364.
3. Moller JT, Cluitmans P, et al. Long-term postoperative cognitive dysfunction in the elderly ISPOCD1 study. ISPOCD investigators. International Study of Post-Operative Cognitive Dysfunction. *Lancet* 1998;351(9106):857–861.
4. Sheng AZ, Shen Q, Cordato D, Zhang YY, Yin Chan DK. Delirium within three days of stroke in a cohort of elderly patients. *J Am Geriatr Soc* 2006;54(8):1192–1198.
5. Cole MG, Ciampi A, Belzile E, Zhong L. Persistent delirium in older hospital patients: a systematic review of frequency and prognosis. *Age Ageing* 2009;38(1):19–26.
6. Sandberg O, Gustafson Y, Brännström B, Bucht G. Clinical profile of delirium in older patients. *J Am Geriatr Soc* 1999;47(11):1300.

4.4 Dementia

Ryan Becker

I. BACKGROUND. Dementia is characterized by cognitive or behavioral symptoms that interfere with the patient's ability to function at work or socially, a decline from previous functioning, and cognitive or behavioral impairments detected through a combination of history and cognitive assessment. The National Institute on Aging and the Alzheimer's Association guidelines state that cognitive or behavioral impairments must be present in at least two of the following domains: ability to recall new information, reasoning, visuospatial ability, language, or personality (1).

II. EPIDEMIOLOGY. Dementia is rare in the young and middle aged, but increases in prevalence as age increases. After 65 years of age, the lifetime risk of developing dementia is approximately 17–20%; 70% of patients with dementia have Alzheimer disease (AD), about 17% have vascular dementia, and 13% have a combination of dementia with Lewy bodies, Parkinson-related dementia, alcoholic dementia, frontal lobe dementia, or other forms of secondary dementia. AD affects 5.3 million Americans and is the sixth leading cause of death. Median survival time after diagnosis of dementia is 4.5 years (1).

III. RISK FACTORS. Increasing age is the most prominent and consistent risk factor for dementia. Presumably, this is secondary to a lifetime of exposures to the brain in various forms such as minor vascular events, white matter disease, and inflammation. In persons 71–79 years of age, the prevalence is approximately 5%, increasing to 37% in persons older than 90 years (1, 2).

A lower education level has been associated with an increased risk of dementia. Having a college education has been shown to delay cognitive dysfunction by 2 years compared with having less education. A family history of a first-degree relative with AD increases the risk of Alzheimer by four times; two first-degree relatives increase the risk by eight times. Genetic factors play a role in dementia risk. Persons with an apolipoprotein E4 genotype have a six to eight times higher risk of developing AD than non-E4 carriers. Other genotypes include amyloid precursor protein, presenilin 1 (PS-1), and PS-2 (1, 2).

Vascular risk factors play a role in dementia. Hypertension, hypercholesterolemia, and diabetes mellitus have all been associated with an increased risk of AD and vascular dementia. Chronic anticholinergic use is associated with a small increased risk (2).

IV. DIFFERENT TYPES OF DEMENTIA.
Dementia is a syndrome rather than a disease. Etiology and pathophysiology can vary greatly. Most of the more common types of dementia are progressive, but some are due to reversible causes.

A. AD is the most common form of dementia. AD is multifactorial with a familial and genetic predisposition. Clinical diagnosis will find an impairment in two or more cognitive domains that interfere with activities of daily living (ADLs) and with a progressive decline from a previous level of functioning. Cognitive domains include the ability to recall new information, reasoning, visuospatial ability, language, and personality. Later in life, patients may present with confusion, depression, delusions, or visual hallucinations (2).

B. Vascular dementia patients have cognitive deficits with a history of vascular damage discovered during a history, clinical examination, or brain imaging. These patients usually have risk factors such as hypertension, hypercholesterolemia, diabetes mellitus, smoking, or atrial fibrillation. Clinically recognizable cognitive deficits will present in a stepwise or even fluctuant progression. Focal neurologic deficits may also be present (2).

C. Frontotemporal dementia (FTD), formally known as Pick's disease, is the most common form of dementia in persons younger than age 65 years. Behavioral and language manifestations are core features of FTD, whereas memory is typically preserved, which differs from AD. Common behavioral features include loss of insight, social inappropriateness, and emotional blunting. Language features include loss of comprehension and object knowledge and nonfluent or hesitant speech. Atrophy and neuronal loss are present in the frontal and temporal lobes of the brain. The etiology of FTD is unknown (3).

D. Dementia with Lewy bodies is characterized by dementia accompanied by delirium, visual hallucinations, and parkinsonism. Other symptoms may include syncope, falls, sleep disorders, and depression. The presence of both Lewy bodies and amyloid plaques with deficiencies in acetylcholine and dopamine neurotransmitters suggests that dementia with Lewy bodies is on a spectrum of dementia between Parkinson's disease and AD (4).

E. Normal pressure hydrocephalus is a potentially reversible form of dementia characterized by the triad of cognitive deficits, gait instability, and urinary incontinence in combination with enlarged ventricles seen on computed tomography (CT) or magnetic resonance imaging (MRI) of the brain (2).

F. Dementia can be found in association with other degenerative neurologic diseases such as Parkinson's disease with dementia, Huntington's disease, and progressive supranuclear palsy (2).

G. Infectious diseases such as neurosyphilis, human immunodeficiency virus (HIV), and Creutzfeldt-Jakob disease can present with associated cognitive deficits (2).

H. Alcohol-related dementia presents with anterograde and retrograde amnesia with confabulation. Long-term memory and other cognitive skills usually remain spared (2).

I. Other causes that are treatable include hypo- and hyperthyroidism, vitamin B12 deficiency, hyponatremia, hypercalcemia, medication induced (sedatives and analgesics), and intracranial space-occupying lesions such as chronic subdural hematoma, meningioma, glioma, and metastasis (2).

V. EVALUATION
A. History and Physical Examination.
1. When dementia is suspected, a detailed history should be taken from the patient and family/caregiver. Questions regarding the time of onset and speed of progression are important. Also ask about the level of impairment in the instrumental activities of daily living (IADLs) such as managing money and medications, shopping, housekeeping, cooking, and transportation. Early in dementia, IADLs that require calculation and planning such as managing finances are often the first to be impaired. ADLs such as dressing, eating, toileting, and grooming generally remain intact until the later stages of dementia (1).

2. A Mini-Mental State Examination, complete neurologic examination, and depression screen should be performed. A referral for formal neuropsychologic testing may be considered in patients who are difficult to evaluate because of a language barrier, patients with suspected psychiatric diagnosis, patients with less education level, or upon request (1).

B. Testing
1. The American Academy of Neurology recommends routing testing only for (5)
   a. Vitamin B12 deficiency
   b. Thyroid-stimulating hormone level for hypothyroidism
2. The American Geriatrics Society recommends (1)
   a. Vitamin B12/folate
   b. Thyroid-stimulating hormone level
   c. Complete blood count
   d. Complete metabolic panel
   e. Calcium level
   f. Non-contrast head CT or MRI
3. Tests recommended in patients with specific risk factors
   a. Cerebrospinal fluid analysis
   b. Lyme titer
   c. HIV testing
   d. Rapid plasma reagin test
4. Investigational studies in the future
   a. Positron emission tomography scan
   b. Apolipoprotein E4 genetic studies
C. Clinical Manifestations. Dementia, whether mild or advanced, often presents as a complaint from the family or caregiver of the patient. If the patient happens to present with the chief complaint of memory loss, consider depression, factitious disorders, mild cognitive impairment, sleep deprivation, or normal age-related cognitive decline. A good history and physical examination will help make the diagnosis.

REFERENCES

1. Simmons BB, Hartmann B, Dejoseph D. Evaluation of suspected dementia. *Am Fam Physician* 2011;84(8):895–902.
2. Kester MI, Scheltens P. Dementia: the bare essentials. *Pract Neurol* 2009;9(4):241–251.
3. Cardarelli R, Kertesz A, Knebl JA. Frontotemporal dementia: a review for primary care physicians. *Am Fam Physician* 2010;82(11);1372–1377.
4. Neef D, Walling AD. Dementia with Lewy bodies: an emerging disease. *Am Fam Physician* 2006;73(7):1223–1229.
5. Petersen RC, Stevens JC, Ganguli M, et al. Practice parameter: early detection of dementia: mild cognitive impairment (an evidence-based review). Report of the quality standards subcommittee of the American Academy of Neurology. *Neurology* 2001;56(9):1133–1142.

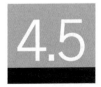

4.5 Memory Impairment
John D. Hallgren

I. BACKGROUND. Memory impairment indicates the degradation of the ability to store or recall information for use by the brain. It sometimes presents in an obvious manner, such as in delirium or dementia. Patients can also present with much subtler symptoms, which either they or a close contact notices. This chapter will address the more subtle memory complaints and how to differentiate normal decline from more concerning levels of loss.

II. PATHOPHYSIOLOGY

A. Etiology

1. Memory is a complex cognitive process, involving both conscious and unconscious aspects of recall. It can be functionally divided into four types: episodic, semantic, procedural, and working. Episodic memory refers to the brain's record of events and semantic memory is the recall of isolated facts or concepts; these memory types are consciously formed and recalled. Procedural memory is the recall of motor functions such as playing a piece of music or typing and may be consciously or unconsciously formed and recalled. Finally, working memory refers to keeping objects, words, and concepts available to complete complex tasks and is synonymous with executive function. It is also a conscious recall. Each memory type shows evidence of processing within different areas of the brain, indicating that each is a separate function (1).

2. Many pathologic processes can cause memory loss. Subtle memory loss often first affects the complex processes involved in working memory; in progressive illnesses, this will begin affecting episodic and semantic memory as well. Dementias of all types will often affect different areas of memory in different stages. Less common diseases associated with motor dysfunction more typically affect procedural memory, such as Parkinson's disease and Huntington's chorea (1). Concussion and other traumatic brain injury, encephalitis, medication effects, mood disorders, thought disorder, attention deficit-hyperactivity disorder, and primary amnestic disorders such as transient global amnesia all cause memory problems.

B. Epidemiology.
The frequency with which patients volunteer memory problems as a presenting complaint is poorly reported. However, a study of over 4,000 persons in North Carolina showed that 56% of persons reported memory complaints when surveyed (2). Mild cognitive impairment (MCI) has an estimated prevalence of 10–20% in persons older than 65 years of age. In the general population, the annual incidence of MCI in a primary care setting was 5–10% (3).

III. EVALUATION

A. History.
A thorough history of memory complaints to establish timing, surrounding events, newly introduced medications, comorbid conditions, and other factors is of paramount importance. It is significant to note whether the complaint originated from the patient or from another informant, both to corroborate information and to know whether the patient has insight into the problem.

B. Physical Examination.
As with the history, physical examination should be utilized to rule out whether existing or new-onset disease processes could be affecting memory. Assessment for injury, stigmata of infectious or rheumatologic disease, and careful neurologic assessment to determine whether there is any motor or sensory dysfunction will assist in determining primary memory problems from those caused by other diseases.

C. Testing

1. The first task is to separate acceptable age-associated cognitive decline from MCI. The gold standard for memory complaints is formal neuropsychiatric testing, but the comprehensive nature and cost of the test precludes its ready use for all memory complaints. Several short tests for memory intended for use at the bedside or office visit exist, such as Folstein's Mini-Mental State Examination. However, most were developed for dementia and are generally insensitive for detecting MCI. The Montreal Cognitive Assessment (www.mocatest.org) has been validated for MCI at a score cutoff of 26. It has a positive likelihood ratio (LR) of 6.9 and a negative LR of 0.11 (4). A computerized test with a positive LR of 14 and a negative LR of 0.14 is also validated for MCI, but is restricted in its use for approved research applications only (5). There is no specific chemical, serologic, or imaging testing specific for MCI. Value for these tests lies in ruling out other conditions.

2. If MCI is detected by memory assessment, clinical judgment must be used to guide testing for potentially reversible conditions. Current guidelines for dementia from the American Geriatric Society are summarized in Figure 4.5.1 (6).

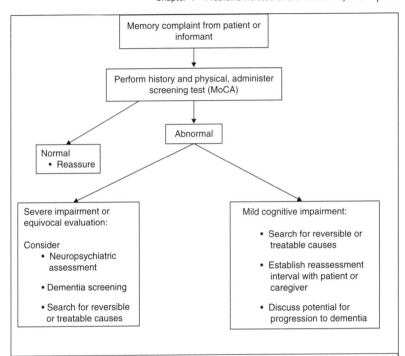

American Geriatric Society recommendations for evaluation of suspected dementia

Laboratory evaluation:

- Hematologic: complete blood count

- Serum chemistry: hepatic and renal function panels, calcium, glucose, vitamin B12, folate, thyroid-stimulating hormone

- Serology: rapid plasma reagin, human immunodeficiency virus

Radiologic evaluation:

- Magnetic resonance imaging or computerized tomography of the brain

    o Higher utility for <60 y of age, focal signs/symptoms, abrupt onset/decline, predisposing conditions (metastatic cancer, anticoagulant use)

- 18F-fluorodeoxyglucose positron emission tomography (approved by Medicare to assess for frontotemporal dementia in atypical cases of dementia)

(Adapted from "A Guide to Dementia Diagnosis and Treatment" at http://dementia.americangeriatrics.org/#eval)

Figure 4.5.1. Algorithm for assessment of memory loss with American Geriatric Society recommendations for laboratory and imaging assessment of suspected dementia (6). MoCA, Montreal cognitive assessment.

IV. DIAGNOSIS

A. Patients with memory complaints, whether self-reported or reported by an informant, should have a thorough history and physical and laboratory and imaging studies to evaluate for reversible or treatable causes. Equivocal evaluations can be further assessed with formal neuropsychiatric testing. More profound memory loss indicative of dementia or delirium is addressed elsewhere in this book.

B. Some mild memory loss associated with aging is considered normal. The phenomenon has many names, including age-associated cognitive decline and age-associated memory impairment. It also lacks definition, but can be characterized by isolated memory deficits without impact on daily functioning (3).

C. MCI is a separate, if still poorly defined, clinical entity. It is characterized by cognitive and memory decline that is more severe than seen with age-associated cognitive decline but less severe than dementia, with overall preserved independent function. Patients with MCI are at higher risk for progression to dementia, at a rate of approximately 10% per year (3). For patients with MCI, the physician should establish a plan for periodic reevaluation and discuss the risk for progression to dementia, the role of emerging testing, and potential strategies to prevent further decline.

REFERENCES

1. Budson AE, Price BH. Memory dysfunction. *N Engl J Med* 2005;352:692–699.
2. Blazer DG, Hays JC, Fillenbaum GG, Gold DT. Memory complaint as a predictor of cognitive decline: a comparison of African-American and white elders. *J Aging Health* 1997;9:171–184.
3. Peterson RC. Mild cognitive impairment. *N Engl J Med* 2011;364:2227–2234.
4. Nasreddine ZS, Phillips NA, Bédirian V, et al. The Montreal Cognitive Assessment, MoCA: a brief screening tool for mild cognitive impairment. *J Am Geriatr Soc* 2005;53:695–699.
5. Saxton J, Morrow L, Eschman A, et al. Computer assessment of mild cognitive impairment. *Postgrad Med* 2009;121(2):177–185.
6. American Geriatrics Society. *A guide to dementia diagnosis and treatment.* Accessed at American Geriatrics Society (http://dementia.americangeriatrics.org/) on August 22, 2010.

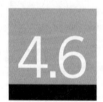

Paresthesia and Dysesthesia

Toby D. Free

I. BACKGROUND.
Paresthesia is a skin sensation, such as burning, prickling, itching, or tingling, with no apparent physical cause. Dysesthesia is defined as either the impairment of sensation, especially that of touch, or a condition in which an unpleasant sensation is produced by ordinary stimuli.

II. PATHOPHYSIOLOGY

A. Etiology. Paresthesias and dysesthesias are due to dysfunction of the nervous system that can occur anywhere along the pathway of sensation between the cortex and the sensory receptor. Dysfunction can be related to either lack of function (e.g., numbness due to carpal tunnel syndrome) or excess function (e.g., pain from postherpetic neuralgia) (1).

B. Epidemiology. The most common source of paresthesia is peripheral neuropathy. The most common causes in the United States are diabetes and alcoholism. Other common causes include hypothyroidism, vitamin B12 deficiency, postherpetic neuralgia, and nerve entrapments such as carpal tunnel syndrome (2).

III. EVALUATION

A. History. The history should include time of onset, duration, and location. Past medical history should be obtained for illnesses that can cause paresthesias or dysesthesias (e.g., diabetes, human immunodeficiency virus [HIV], hypothyroidism, and rheumatoid arthritis). Social history may reveal substance abuse (e.g., alcoholism, or intravenous drug use, which would raise the suspicion of HIV) or occupational exposures (e.g., exposure to lead or mercury, or mechanical repetition). Family history may disclose a hereditary neuropathy (2).

B. Physical Examination. The patient should have a general physical examination and complete neurologic examination, paying particular attention to the sensory portion of the examination. Complicating the physical examination is the fact that the examiner must rely on the patient's subjective response to the examination. The examination should test for pain (using a pin or needle), light touch (using a cotton-tipped swab or wisp of cotton), vibration (using a tuning fork), temperature, and position sense (performed with the eyes closed). The examination should delineate the distribution of abnormal sensation as this may be enough to establish a diagnosis. The patient may be asked to map the affected area. Other aspects of the neurologic examination should include testing of muscle strength and reflexes. Muscle wasting may be noted (1, 2). Flexion of the patient's neck (Lhermitte's sign) causing electric shock-like pain in the back or extremities may be present in patients with multiple sclerosis, cervical spinal cord disease, or vitamin B12 deficiency. Tinel sign, which is a reproduction of the paresthesia with percussion on or just proximal to the carpal tunnel, and Phalen's maneuver, involving full flexion of the wrist for greater than 60 seconds, can aid in the diagnosis of carpal tunnel syndrome.

C. Testing. If clinical examination does not reveal a cause for the patient's symptoms, then initial laboratory workup should include complete blood count, renal function, fasting serum glucose, vitamin B12 level, urinalysis, thyroid-stimulating hormone, and erythrocyte sedimentation rate. Further laboratory testing might include folate, the Venereal Disease Research Laboratory or rapid plasma reagin test, antinuclear antibody, serum immunoelectrophoresis, purified protein derivative, and blood levels of heavy metals (e.g., lead) (2, 3). Electromyography and nerve conduction testing are often helpful in delineating either the anatomic source of the neuropathy (e.g., carpal tunnel syndrome) or the systemic cause (e.g., paraneoplastic syndromes) (3). Radiologic studies such as computed tomography or magnetic resonance imaging may be indicated for specific causes, such as a suspected lumbar disc herniation.

D. Genetics. There are several hereditary causes of neuropathies. These include Charcot-Marie-Tooth disease, Denny-Brown's syndrome, and familial amyloidotic polyneuropathy (2).

IV. DIAGNOSIS

A. Differential Diagnosis. The differential diagnosis of paresthesias and dysesthesias is broad (see Table 4.6.1).

B. Clinical Manifestations. The cause of paresthesias and dysesthesias can frequently be determined clinically. Distal sensory loss is the most common and is frequently due to metabolic or toxic causes such as diabetes, alcoholism, vitamin B12 deficiency, or heavy metal exposure. Some causes, such as diabetes or alcoholism, can have various clinical patterns. Diabetes most commonly causes a symmetric distal sensory loss, but can also cause multifocal neuropathies, autonomic neuropathies, or even symmetrical proximal motor neuropathies (3).

Most nerve entrapments are distinguished by an examination consistent with their nerve distribution (e.g., loss of sensation of the fifth finger and adjacent half of the fourth finger in ulnar neuropathies, which are usually caused by compression at the cubital tunnel in the elbow).

Dermatomal distributions would point to either a radiculopathy or postherpetic neuralgia. Neuropathies involving the cranial nerves are rare, but may be caused by Guillain-Barré syndrome, diabetes, HIV, or Lyme disease (3).

TABLE 4.6.1	Causes of Paresthesia and Dysesthesia
Endocrine	Diabetes, hypothyroidism, acromegaly
Nutritional	Vitamin B12/folate deficiencies
Toxic	Chemotherapy, heavy metals, chronic overdose of pyridoxine, alcohol, medications such as nitrofurantoin
Connective tissue disorders	Polyarteritis nodosa, rheumatoid arthritis, lupus
Entrapment syndromes	Carpal and cubital tunnel syndromes, thoracic outlet syndrome, lateral femoral cutaneous syndrome, tarsal tunnel syndrome, spinal disc herniations
Trauma	
Central nervous system	Cerebrovascular accident, tumors
Infectious	Syphilis, Lyme disease, postherpetic neuralgia, human immunodeficiency virus, leprosy
Malignancy	Paraneoplastic syndromes from small cell carcinoma of the lung and cancers of the breast, ovary, and stomach
Miscellaneous	Guillain-Barré syndrome, multiple sclerosis, critical illness polyneuropathy (2, 3)

REFERENCES

1. Asbury AK. Numbness, tingling, and sensory loss. In: Braunwald E, Hauser SL, et al. eds. *Harrison's principles of internal medicine*, 15th ed. New York, NY: McGraw Hill, 2001:128–132.
2. McKnight JT, Adcock BB. Paresthesias: a practical diagnostic approach. *Am Fam Physician* 1997;56(9):2253–2260.
3. Poncelet AN. An algorithm for the evaluation of peripheral neuropathy. *Am Fam Physician* 1998;57(4):755–760.

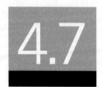

4.7 Seizures

Denae M. Torpey

I. **BACKGROUND.** A seizure is characterized as temporary neurologic signs or symptoms as a result of abnormal, transient, synchronous neuronal activity in the cerebral cortex. Epilepsy is a group of disorders characterized by recurrent seizures that are unprovoked and not caused by an easily reversible condition.

II. **PATHOPHYSIOLOGY**

A. **Etiology.** Causes of seizures include primary central nervous system (CNS) dysfunctions as well as metabolic derangement or systemic disease. Distinguishing between the two is vital since therapy must be directed at correcting the underlying condition as well as at seizure control. However, over two-thirds of new onset seizures are idiopathic (1).

1. **Primary CNS dysfunctions.** Head trauma, stroke or vascular malformations, mass lesions (tumors), intracranial hemorrhage, CNS infections, encephalitis, meningitis, febrile seizures, primary epilepsy disorders, and dementia.

2. **Systemic disease or metabolic.** Hypoglycemia, hyponatremia, hypocalcemia, hypomagnesemia, uremia, hepatic encephalopathy, eclampsia, drug toxicity or withdrawal, porphyria, hyperthermia, and genetic disorders.

The age of the patient may help in establishing a cause of the seizure. In the elderly, they are more likely to result from dementia, cerebrovascular disease, or tumors. Children and infants are more likely to experience seizures caused by trauma and infection or idiopathic seizures.

B. **Epidemiology.** The incidence of epilepsy is bimodal with a peak high in childhood, decreases in midlife, then peaks again in the elderly. The overall lifetime risk of having a seizure is 10%; however, only 3% will go on to develop epilepsy (2). The annual incidence of epilepsy is 50 per 100,000 population, with a prevalence of about 5–10 per 1,000 (2).

III. EVALUATION

A. **History.** Care should be taken to elicit risk factors for seizures pertinent to the patient's age (including a family history of seizures and developmental history), possible seizure precipitants (medication, alcohol or drugs of abuse, sleep deprivation, intense exercise, flashing lights, trauma, and fever), and the clinical features, setting, chronology, and duration of the seizure. In many cases, information about the seizure must be obtained from a witness because of the patient's age or level of consciousness. Given that 20% of childhood seizures occur only at night, it is important to inquire about early morning behavior in children, including disorientation and transient neurologic dysfunction (1). The following questions are especially important in determining the etiology of the seizure:

1. Was there an aura prior to the seizure?
2. Was there a fall or injury prior or during the seizure?
3. Was there a loss or impairment of consciousness?
4. Was there staring, eye blinking, vocalizations, or automatisms (repetitive purposeless movements such as lip smacking, chewing, or facial grimacing)?
5. Was there a loss of bowel or bladder continence?
6. Was there rhythmic muscular jerking and/or rigidity?
7. Was there a postictal period?

The two features most indicative of a seizure include the presence of an aura associated with seizures of focal onset and postictal confusional state following a generalized tonic–clonic seizure. Having urinary incontinence or a few tonic or jerking movements is not sufficient to discern seizures from other causes of transient loss of consciousness (1).

B. **Physical Examination.** The examination is usually normal in patients with epilepsy, but occasionally shows signs of trauma, an underlying systemic or neurologic disorder, or stigmata of chronic alcoholism may be evident. Additionally, it is important to look for cutaneous manifestations of some genetic disorders (facial nevus flammeus of Sturge-Weber syndrome, adenoma sebaceum of tuberous sclerosis, or *café au lait* macules and cutaneous neurofibromas of neurofibromatosis).

C. **Testing.** Laboratory studies in adults and children should be ordered on the basis of suggestive historical or clinical findings. In children with a first simple febrile seizure (<10 minutes, isolated, and generalized), laboratory testing should be directed toward identifying the cause of the fever. Studies that may be appropriate for evaluation of a first seizure include a complete blood count, glucose, electrolytes, calcium, magnesium, renal, liver and thyroid function tests, urinalysis, pregnancy screen, and drug and heavy metal toxicology screening (if there is a question of substance abuse or possibility of exposure).

1. A lumbar puncture should be performed if there is a concern about meningitis or encephalitis or if the patient is immunocompromised. The American Academy of Pediatrics suggests that a lumbar puncture be "strongly considered" when a febrile seizure occurs in an infant younger than 12 months of age or all children on prior antibiotic treatment, "considered" in infants 12–18 months of age, and "recommended" if meningeal signs are present in infants older than 18 months of age (3). If increased intracranial pressure is suspected, the lumbar puncture should be preceded by computed tomography (CT) scan or magnetic resonance imaging (MRI) of the head.

2. An electroencephalogram (EEG) is essential in the evaluation of epileptic seizures. An abnormal EEG may confirm the diagnosis, but a normal or nonspecifically abnormal EEG does not exclude the diagnosis of a seizure. Sleep deprivation and provocative measures such as hyperventilation and photic stimulation may increase the yield of an EEG.

3. Neuroimaging is often necessary to rule out a structural lesion of the brain. Any patient with neurologic findings on examination, with mental deficiency, or older than 25 years of age when presenting with new-onset seizure warrants neuroimaging. A brain MRI is more sensitive and is preferred over a CT scan. An EEG and neuroimaging need not be performed in the evaluation of an otherwise neurologically healthy child with a simple febrile seizure.

IV. DIAGNOSIS

A. Differential Diagnosis. A variety of events, either physiologic or psychogenic, can often be mistaken as seizures. These include syncope, complex migraines, breath-holding spells, transient ischemic attacks, sleep disorders (parasomnias and narcolepsy), transient global amnesia, movement disorders, and psychiatric disorders (panic attacks, anxiety with hyperventilation, dissociative states, and psychogenic seizures).

B. Clinical Manifestations. The clinical expression of a seizure depends on the location and extent of propagation of the discharging neurons.

1. **Partial seizures.** A partial (focal) seizure begins in a localized area of the cortex. The signs and symptoms of a partial seizure depend on the cortical region involved and may range from a subjective perception (aura) to motor, autonomic (flushing and hypersalivation), somatosensory, or psychic phenomena.

   a. **Simple partial seizures.** Consciousness is preserved with simple partial seizures. However, they may evolve into a complex partial seizure, and both may evolve into a generalized seizure.

   b. **Complex partial seizures.** A complex partial seizure implies spread of the seizure discharge to allow impairment of consciousness. Usually, they arise in the temporal lobe or medial frontal lobe. Patients with complex partial seizures usually exhibit automatisms or some other complex coordinated motor activity that is not directed or purposeful.

2. **Generalized seizures.** A generalized seizure involves both the cerebral hemispheres at the onset. Generalized seizures begin with an abrupt loss of consciousness (except myoclonic seizures). They are subdivided based on the presence or absence and character of ictal motor manifestations.

   a. **Generalized tonic–clonic seizures (Grand mal).** Consciousness is lost and usually is not preceded by an aura. Tonic contractions of limb muscles occur first, producing flexion and extension, followed by clonic phase characterized by rhythmic muscular jerking.

   b. **Absence seizures (Petit mal).** Absence seizures are characterized as brief (5–10 seconds) loss of consciousness without loss of postural tone. These may be exhibited with staring, blinking, or slight head turn and are usually inducible by hyperventilation.

   c. **Other.** This includes tonic (not followed by clonic phase), clonic (not preceded by tonic phase), atonic (sudden collapse due to loss of postural tone), and myoclonic (sudden, brief muscular contractions affecting any group of muscles).

REFERENCES

1. Simon RP, Greenberg DA, Aminoff MJ, eds. Seizures & syncope. In: *Clinical neurology*, 7th ed. New York, NY: McGraw-Hill, 2009:270–291.
2. Middleton DB. Seizures. In: South-Paul JE, Matheny SC, Lewis EL, eds. *Current diagnosis & treatment: family medicine*, 2nd ed. New York, NY: McGraw-Hill, 2008:88–102.
3. American Academy of Pediatrics. Practice parameter: the neurodiagnostic evaluation of the child with a first simple seizure. *Pediatrics* 1996;97(5):769–772; discussion 773–775.

Stroke
Kathryn K. Garner

I. BACKGROUND. Stroke is defined as an acute neurologic deficit that lasts more than 24 hours. Events lasting <24 hours are referred to as transient ischemic attacks.

II. PATHOPHYSIOLOGY
A. Etiology. Stroke is caused by occlusive vascular disease (thrombotic or embolic) leading to ischemia 85% of the time and hemorrhagic vascular disease 15% of the time.

B. Epidemiology. Risk factors for stroke include uncontrolled hypertension, hyperlipidemia, diabetes mellitus, tobacco smoking, cardiac disease, coagulopathies, obesity, and hormone therapy. Stroke is the fourth most common cause of death (1) and the most common acute neurologic event in the United States.

III. EVALUATION (2, 3)
A. History. Historical factors of note include
1. Time of abrupt onset of symptoms, last time at previous baseline
2. Unilateral change in motor control, vision, gait, strength, or sensation
3. Other neurologic disorders such as migraine, systemic lupus, vasculitis, seizure disorder, previous brain hemorrhage, or recent head trauma
4. Sudden onset of unusual headache
5. Presence of one or more risk factors

B. Physical Examination. Physical findings include
1. Alteration of mental status and/or consciousness
2. Slurred or inappropriate speech, aphasia
3. Hemiparalysis, hemiparesis
4. Altered sensation
5. Visual field defect, diplopia, nystagmus
6. Hypertension
7. Cardiac dysrhythmia
8. Ataxia and other gait abnormalities
9. Vascular tenderness to palpation or bruit, temporal and carotid arteries
10. Document findings in standard fashion with the National Institutes of Health (NIH) Stroke Scale initially and serially during evolution of stroke

C. Testing. Studies and laboratory tests include
1. Computed tomography (CT) scan of the head to identify hemorrhage. CT perfusion and angiography as well as magnetic resonance imaging diffusion weight images are promising for the detection of smaller strokes earlier.
2. Complete blood count, with platelet count, basic metabolic panel, cardiac enzymes, prothrombin time, international normalization ration (INR), and partial thromboplastin time for underlying diseases and baseline if thrombolytic or anticoagulant therapy is anticipated.
3. Special studies such as hepatic function panel, toxicology screen, blood alcohol level, antiphospholipid antibodies, protein S and C, antithrombin III, and others if indicated by history or physical examination.
4. Electrocardiogram to help diagnose dysrhythmias or preceding myocardial infarction.
5. Echocardiogram to visualize structural defects such as patent foramen ovale or mural thrombi. Transesophageal echocardiography may possibly be appropriate if concern for patent foramen ovale or valve vegetations.
6. Carotid/intracranial Doppler studies to find occlusive vascular disease or source of artery to artery emboli.

IV. DIAGNOSIS

A. Differential Diagnosis. The differential diagnosis of stroke includes aberrant migraine, seizure disorder, metabolic disorders, psychogenic condition (hysterical conversion reaction and hyperventilation), and tumor with hemorrhage.

B. Clinical Approach. With the availability of thrombolytic therapy, a rapid diagnosis upon presentation has become critical. A history and physical examination should be completed as quickly as is practical, with special attention to the neurologic examination. Quantitative assessment of strength and function on the affected side should be documented for comparison with subsequent examinations (NIH Stroke Scale is preferred). Laboratory studies are ordered to assess for stroke mimickers and a noncontrast head CT scan is obtained to rule out hemorrhage, provided the patient is clinically stable. Appropriate interventions to control blood pressure, seizures, hyperglycemia, and cardiac dysrhythmias should proceed concomitantly with the evaluation. Acetyl salicylic acid (ASA) and dipyridamole therapy are superior to ASA alone for secondary prevention but equivocal to clopidogrel alone. Full anticoagulation is appropriate only for cardiac emboli causing a stroke. Statin administration and lipid measurement should be considered for all stroke patients. Optimal LDL levels are <100 mg/dl or <70 mg/dl if the patient has multiple stroke risk factors including diabetes mellitus, history of previous stroke, hypertension, hypercoagulability, or tobacco smoking.

REFERENCES

1. CDC FASTATS: www.cdc.gov/nchs/fastats/stroke.htm, 2009.
2. American Heart Association Stroke Outcome Classification. Executive summary. *Circulation* 1998:97:2474–2478.
3. Harrison's Online: Part 15. Neurological disorders. Section 2. Diseases of the Central Nervous system. Chapter 349. Cerebrovascular diseases.
4. Update to the AHA/ASA recommendations for the prevention of stroke in patients with stroke and transient ischemic attack. *Stroke* 2008;39:1647–1652.

4.9 Tremors

Diego R. Torres-Russotto

I. BACKGROUND. Tremor is one of the most common movement disorders and is characterized by an *oscillatory* and usually rhythmic movement. The first step in the evaluation of any movement disorder is to recognize the movement phenomenology, to be able to generate a list of different etiologies (1). Jumping straight to the differential leads to misdiagnoses. Thirty to fifty percent of cases with action tremor are misdiagnosed and do not have essential tremor (2).

II. PATHOPHYSIOLOGY. Assessment of patients with tremor still depends upon the history and physical examination. This chapter will review only a few of the many types of tremors.

A. Resting Tremor. Resting tremor is one in which the amplitude decreases or disappears as soon as the muscles involved with the tremor get voluntarily contracted. Therefore, this is predominantly present during rest. This tremor might also appear after the patient has been holding arms up in front for a while (usually in the wrist or fingers), the so-called re-emergent tremor. Re-emergent tremor will usually disappear by contracting the involved muscles, helping differentiate this tremor from other postural tremors.

B. Action/Kinetic/Postural Tremors. These tremors are those that appear or in which amplitude increases as soon as the muscles involved get voluntarily contracted.

C. Intention Tremor. Intention tremor is a posture-kinetic tremor in which amplitude increases with target-directed movements (e.g., while comparing the tremor during finger-to-nose-finger maneuver vs. just holding the arms straight). Intention tremor is regarded as a sign of disturbed function of the cerebellum and its pathways.

D. Posture-specific or task-specific tremor. This is commonly due to dystonia. Examples include the tremor present during flexion of a limb but not during extension; or the *intermittent, jerky, irregular, arrhythmic* head tremor of patients with cervical dystonia. Particular features that differentiate dystonic tremor from other tremors include the presence of abnormal posturing, muscle hypertrophy, null point (a place in the range of motion of the joint involved where tremor amplitude significantly decreases), and sensory tricks (aka geste antagoniste, a sensory stimulus like touching the area can improve the dystonic tremor). This category includes the task-specific tremors (e.g., those present only during writing or while playing an instrument) (2).

III. EVALUATION AND DIFFERENTIAL DIAGNOSIS
A. Initial Workup
1. Diagnoses not to miss: medication induced, pregnancy, Wilson disease, thyroid abnormalities, liver, kidney, or electrolyte/glucose abnormalities, vitamin B12, D, and E deficiencies. Psychogenic tremors are rare and always a diagnosis of exclusion.
2. Basic initial workup to consider: pregnancy test, ceruloplasmin, thyroid function, CMP, vitamin B12 level, MMA, homocysteine, folate, 25-OH vitamin D3, and vitamin E. Environmental exposures and use of over-the-counter, herbal, or illegal drugs should be ascertained. Consider heavy metals and urine drug screen testing.
3. Structural imaging (usually with magnetic resonance imaging of the brain) could be considered in cases suspicious for multiple sclerosis (MS), strokes, ataxia, primary and metastatic tumors; in those with rapid or unusual progression; or with associated abnormal neurologic examination.
4. Functional imaging (like positron emission tomography (PET) or single photon emission computed tomography (SPECT)) can help differentiate between Parkinson disease and essential tremor. Referral to a movement disorders center might be the most cost-effective measure.

B. Resting Tremor. Differential includes parkinsonism of any cause (idiopathic, secondary to dopamine blockers [anti-psychotics, anti-emetics], lithium, amiodarone, and strokes), Wilson disease, dystonia, midbrain/Holmes tremor (trauma, strokes, and MS), etc. Ascertainment of presence of rigidity and bradykinesia is very important as it would complete the triad for parkinsonism.

C. Action/Kinetic/Postural Tremor. The two most common etiologies are medication induced and essential tremor.
1. Medication-induced action/kinetic tremor: almost all drugs that affect the CNS have the potential to cause or worsen tremors. Most common drugs include anti-depressants, anti-epileptics, benzodiazepines, opioids, anesthetics, and dopamine blockers (both anti-psychotics and anti-emetics).
2. Essential or primary tremor: tends to be a familial action tremor of hands (can also have tremor in face, neck, voice, and lower limbs), slowly progressive and responsive to alcohol (in some). Currently, the definition of essential tremor is under debate, as it is felt to encompass multiple diseases under the same umbrella term. The prevalence is about 2% to 6%. Essential tremor is underdiagnosed, misdiagnosed, and undertreated, leading to inadequate patient satisfaction. Treatment options include propranolol, primidone, and topiramate. After treatment failure with two drugs, referral to a deep brain stimulation surgery center should be offered to the patient.

D. Intention Tremor. Etiologies for ataxia should be entertained, although medications and essential tremor remain important causes. Fragile X-associated tremor and ataxia syndrome is a high-prevalence condition, a common cause for tremor and ataxia, and can also display parkinsonism (please refer to Chapter 4.1, Ataxia).

REFERENCES
1. Fahn S. Involuntary movements. In: Lewis PR, Timothy AP. *Merritt's neurology*, 12th ed. Philadelphia, PA: Lippincott Williams & Wilkins, 2010:50–53.
2. Louis ED. Essential tremor. In: Lewis PR, Timothy AP. *Merritt's neurology*, 12th ed. Philadelphia, PA: Lippincott Williams & Wilkins, 2010:825–826.
3. Torres-Russotto D, Perlmutter J. Task-specific dystonias: a review. *Ann N Y Acad Sci* 2008;1142:179–199.

CHAPTER **5**

Eye Problems
Shou Ling Leong

5.1 Blurred Vision
Norman Benjamin Fredrick

I. BACKGROUND. Blurred vision is the most common visual complaint (1). "Blurred vision is the loss of sharpness of vision and the inability to see small details" (2).

II. PATHOPHYSIOLOGY

    A. Etiology. The causes of blurred vision range from mild to potentially catastrophic. Most causes involve the orbit (anterior and posterior segments), although a number of extraocular causes must be considered (medications, viral infections such as herpes simplex virus, systemic causes such as sarcoidosis, and cerebrovascular events) (see Table 5.1.1).

    B. Epidemiology. In younger patients, blurred vision is often acquired through trauma, occupational exposures, and infections. Certain age-related eye disorders such as macular degeneration, cataracts, and temporal arteritis may cause blurred vision, potentially contributing to the risk of falling (3).

III. EVALUATION

    A. History. Careful attention should be paid to the rapidity of the onset, associated eye pain, and whether the blurring is unilateral or bilateral. Blurred vision that worsens at night may indicate a cataract (4). Intermittently blurred vision may be caused by excess tearing, allergies, uncontrolled diabetes, acute glaucoma, transient ischemic attacks, cerebrovascular insufficiency, and multiple sclerosis (5). Other important factors include a family history of eye disorders (macular degeneration and glaucoma), any work exposures (chemicals and prolonged computer use), medications (such as corticosteroids and antibiotics), and past medical history (diabetes and hypertension) (6).

    B. Physical Examination. The physical examination should include the following elements:

        1. Conjunctival erythema and discharge should be noted. The corneal light reflex should be symmetric and sharp; fluorescein staining should be performed to evaluate for the evidence of trauma, ulcers, or herpetic lesions. The anterior chamber (space between the cornea and the iris) should be evaluated with a penlight for blood (hyphema) and pus (hypopyon).

        2. Careful documentation of visual acuity (corrected and uncorrected) is important to monitor the progression of the disease. If the patient is unable to discern letters on the Snellen eye chart, the examiner should determine the extent of acuity impairment by testing the distance from the patient's eyes at which the patient can first see the examiner's fingers.

        3. Visual field testing may indicate an underlying stroke (homonymous field defect) or retinal detachment (quadrant or hemispheric loss of vision).

        4. Ocular muscle involvement may be detected by testing the cardinal positions of the orbit through range of motion.

TABLE 5.1.1	Causes of Blurred Vision			
	Painless		**Painful**	
	Sudden onset	**Gradual onset**	**Sudden onset**	**Gradual onset**
Unilateral	Vitreous hemorrhage, macular degeneration, retinal detachment, retinal-vein occlusion, amaurosis fugax, cataracts	Cataracts, "dry" macular degeneration, tumor	Corneal abrasion, infection or edema, uveitis, traumatic hyphema, acute glaucoma, temporal arteritis, optic neuritis, orbital cellulitis	Rare
Bilateral	Poorly controlled diabetes, medications (anticholinergics, cholinergics, corticosteroids), migraines, psychological trauma	Cataracts, macular degeneration, medications (hydrochloroquine, ethambutol, digoxin toxicity), optic chiasm mass, fatigue, computer vision syndrome (7), refractive errors (myopia, hyperopia, astigmatism, presbyopia); incorrect eyewear	Trauma, chemical spill, welder's exposure	Rare (sarcoidosis, collagen vascular disease)

Compiled from Shingleton BJ, O'Donoghue MW. Primary care: blurred vision. *N Engl J Med* 2000;343(8):556–562.

5. In up to 20% of the cases, *pupillary examination* may be the only clue to serious underlying pathology. Using a penlight, the abnormalities of pupillary size or shape (the pupils should be symmetric; a unilateral miotic pupil may indicate iritis) or color (black is normal) may be detected. Other findings may include cataracts, ruptured globes (with eccentric pupils), and optic nerve disease (afferent papillary defect—paradoxical papillary dilatation in response to light).

6. Direct ophthalmoscopy may reveal an abnormal red reflex that suggests a hemorrhage, cataract, or retinal detachment. Papilledema warrants further evaluation.

C. **Testing.** An elevated sedimentation rate may suggest a diagnosis of temporal arteritis. Computed tomography is appropriate to evaluate blurred vision following trauma or when there is concern for mass effect (1).

D. **Genetics.** Macular degeneration, glaucoma, collagen vascular diseases, diabetes, and multiple sclerosis (optic neuritis) are potentially heritable conditions.

IV. DIAGNOSIS

A. **Differential Diagnosis.** See Table 5.1.1.

B. **Clinical Manifestations.** A careful history and physical examination often limit the differential diagnosis. Conditions that require immediate ophthalmologic referral include acute glaucoma, retinal detachment, vitreous hemorrhage, retinal-vein occlusion, herpes simplex infection, and orbital cellulitis.

REFERENCES

1. Shingleton BJ, O'Donoghue MW. Primary care: blurred vision. *N Engl J Med* 2000;343(8):556–562.
2. Hart JA. Diplopia. *Medline plus encyclopedia.* Accessed at Medline Plus.com (http://www.nlm.nih.gov/medlineplus/ency/article/003029.htm), 2004.
3. Buckley JG, Heasley KJ, Twigg P, Elliott DB. The effects of blurred vision on the mechanics of landing during stepping down by the elderly. *Gait Posture* 2003;21(1):65–71.
4. Pavan-Langston D. *Manual of ocular diagnosis and therapy.* Philadelphia, PA: Lippincott Williams & Williams, 2002.
5. WrongDiagnosis.com. Blurred vision. Accessed at *Wrong diagnosis symptoms* (http://www.wrongdiagnosis.com/sym/blurred_vision.htm#possible), 2003.
6. Vaughan DG, Asbury T, Riordan-Eva P. *General ophthalmology.* New York, NY: McGraw-Hill Medical, 2003.
7. Rosenfield M. Computer vision syndrome: a review of ocular causes and potential treatments. *Opthal Physiol Opt* 2011;31(5):502–515.

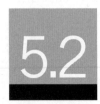

Corneal Foreign Body and Corneal Abrasion

Peter R. Lewis

I. BACKGROUND. Macroscopic and/or microscopic material from the external environment may lodge in the cornea—the anterior and transparent part of the eye that overlies the anterior chamber and is continuous with the sclera—potentially resulting in injury—abrasion—that can cause pain and lead to vision loss/disability.

II. PATHOPHYSIOLOGY

   A. Etiology. Commonly involved materials resulting in a corneal foreign body and/or abrasion include sand, dirt, leaves, and other organic materials in the environment as well as additional occupational and/or recreational exposure to materials such as metal shavings or glass particles. Added risk factors for corneal abrasion include surgery with general anesthesia, infancy, and a prior history of corneal abrasion.

   B. Epidemiology. Among symptomatic patients, a corneal foreign body represents a common cause of eye-related complaints for adult and pediatric patients presenting to primary care physicians, nurse practitioners, physician assistants, ophthalmologists, optometrists, and emergency departments (1). The frequent association between a corneal foreign body and occupational (including the medical profession) or leisure-time exposure highlights the preventable nature of this condition with protective eyewear (2). Contact lens represent another common source of corneal abrasion. Given the potential for a corneal foreign body to lead to a corneal abrasion, prompt recognition and removal is warranted.

III. EVALUATION

   A. History. A patient with a corneal foreign body is frequently self-evident by history. "Foreign-body" sensation, pain, photophobia, and increased lacrimation are commonly associated patient complaints, which are likely to be heightened in the patient with a related corneal abrasion. The patient frequently notes redness in the eye. As a result, corneal foreign body with or without abrasion should be included in the differential diagnosis of any patient presenting with a "red eye." Decreased vision may be reported depending on whether or not the corneal foreign body and related inflammation are in the region of the patient's visual axis. Individuals with corneal foreign bodies and abrasions who are victims of significant industrial accidents, motor vehicle trauma, or gunshot wounds may be unable to communicate or may primarily complain of pain at sites of more substantial injury. The patient and/or family member should be asked to identify the source(s) and composition of any suspected corneal foreign body. The treating clinician should determine whether or not a workman's compensation claim is being filed in relation to any eye complaint/injury. Tetanus immunization status should be determined. By contrast, some patients with corneal foreign bodies may have no symptoms. A history of metal grinding or welding should raise the clinician's suspicion for an asymptomatic foreign body. This is an important detail to consider for the patient undergoing magnetic resonance imaging (MRI) in which case a plain film x-ray of the orbits should first be obtained.

B. Physical Examination. For the pediatric or adult patient with a suspected corneal foreign body and potential for associated corneal abrasion, the physical examination should commence with general inspection/observation of the patient and vital signs to include visual acuity—uncorrected and (as the case may be) corrected. If not previously done, contact lens wearers should remove their contact lens. The family physician or other clinician should observe for facial asymmetry and investigate accordingly to include cranial nerve testing. If the patient's complaint and injury are clearly confined to the eye, then a comprehensive ocular examination should continue with added gross inspection to evaluate for asymmetry in the periorbital region, conjunctiva, cornea, sclera, and pupils. Extraocular movements and pupillary responsiveness should be assessed. A sufficiently large foreign body may be visible by gross inspection with a penlight on physical examination. Magnification should be used, including a slit lamp, where available. The eyelids should be everted, because foreign bodies may lodge in multiple locations including under the eyelid. An undilated funduscopic examination should also be performed.

1. A topical anesthetic may be required. As noted above, visual acuity should be determined before the use of any topical anesthetic. Altered visual acuity may be due to a corneal foreign body interfering with the visual axis and may be associated with penetrating ocular trauma.

2. Screening for a corneal infiltrate or hyphema (blood in the anterior chamber) is necessary. The presence of a rust stain is highly suggestive of a metallic foreign body causing abrasion that may lead to ulceration.

3. Fluorescein staining and examination with cobalt-blue light or Wood's lamp should be used to search for an associated corneal abrasion (3). A vertically oriented corneal abrasion suggests the presence of an associated foreign body in the upper tarsal region.

C. Testing. For patients with suspected associated penetrating foreign body, computed tomography or ultrasound may be required and urgent ophthalmology consultation should be obtained, likely in a hospital's emergency department. An MRI should be avoided in the setting of a suspected or a confirmed metallic foreign body.

IV. DIAGNOSIS. In the event of serious and/or multiple injuries, an expedited and detailed trauma survey should be conducted and plans made for ambulance transport to the closest emergency department. Severe corneal trauma related to a foreign body, especially in children, may require examination under general anesthesia in the operating room by an ophthalmologist. Other reasons for prompt ophthalmologic referral include corneal infiltrate (increased association with infection), corneal laceration, hyphema, and any suspicion for a penetrating injury. For the patient suitable for evaluation in the outpatient setting, the differential diagnosis for anterior eye pain includes corneal ulceration, keratitis (including that caused by shingles), cluster or migraine headache, giant cell arteritis, and glaucoma. If the cause of the patient's complaint of anterior eye pain is not readily discernible in the primary care clinician's office, then referral to an ophthalmologist or optometrist is warranted.

REFERENCES

1. Shields T, Sloane PD. A comparison of eye problems in primary care and ophthalmology practices. *Fam Med* 1991;23:544.

2. Work Loss Data Institute. Eye. Encinitas (CA): Work Loss Data Institute; 2010. Accessed at National Guideline Clearinghouse– http://guideline.gov/content.aspx?id=25694&search=work+loss+data+institute.+eye on May 29, 2012.

3. Wilson SA, Last A. Management of corneal abrasions. *Am Fam Physician* 2004;70(1):123–128.

Diplopia
Norman Benjamin Fredrick

I. BACKGROUND. Diplopia means double vision. Patients complain of seeing the same view as two overlapping images (1). The images may be horizontal, vertical, or diagonal to one another (2).

II. PATHOPHYSIOLOGY

A. Etiology. Diplopia occurs when the scene before the patient is sent as two different images to the visual cortex. The normal mapping process cannot occur and the brain perceives two overlapping images. There are two main types of diplopia: monocular and binocular. Monocular diplopia implies a problem with only one of the eyes. These are often refractive abnormalities and disorders of the globe itself (i.e., cornea, lens, and retina). Binocular diplopia is primarily due to disorders of ocular motility (i.e., either the muscles or the innervation of the ocular muscles). Monocular diplopia is readily distinguished from binocular diplopia by the fact that the diplopia persists despite covering the unaffected eye (1).

B. Epidemiology. Binocular diplopia is more common than monocular diplopia. Patients primarily complaining of diplopia are adults. Children younger than 10 years of age tend to compensate for visual disturbances by suppressing one of the images.

III. EVALUATION

A. History. Standard history is required with an emphasis on the following points:

1. Distinguishing between double vision and blurry vision is important. Patients complain of seeing two images with diplopia.

2. Most complaints of diplopia are due to a binocular abnormality arising from incoordination of the ocular muscles. Asking whether the images are side by side, vertical to each other, or diagonal to each other may help determine which ocular muscle group is involved. Complaints of vertical diplopia (which includes diagonal diplopia) are due to muscle groups associated with the cranial nerves (CNs) III and IV. The abnormality may stem from these nerves or, more distally, from the muscles themselves (i.e., myasthenia gravis and muscle entrapment). Complaints of horizontal diplopia indicate an abnormality with the lateral/medial rectus muscles and/or CN VI (binocular vertical diplopia).

3. A sudden onset of diplopia may suggest a vascular etiology.

4. A history of any instigating events such as facial trauma, sinus infection, or migraine headache may provide important diagnostic information.

5. The review of symptoms should include questions about a history of fever, headache, sinus congestion, and associated neurologic complaints.

6. A family history of thyroid disorders, myasthenia gravis, or diabetes may suggest an autoimmune cause.

7. Other significant past medical history includes diabetes (retinopathy and third CN palsy), hypertension, and underlying vascular diseases (2).

8. Ask the patient whether the symptom improves with gazing in a certain direction. If the gaze improves (although it is unlikely to resolve), the cause is usually due to a neuromuscular problem or a mechanical restriction (1).

B. Physical Examination. The examination should include the following:

1. **Observation.** Look for any evidence of strabismus (malalignment of the globes as indicated by an abnormal corneal light reflex), cataracts, corneal abnormalities such as scars, evidence of cellulitis, eyelid ptosis (myasthenia gravis and CN III palsy), eyelid retraction (thyroid ophthalmopathy), or periorbital ecchymoses (trauma). If the patient's head is being held at a tilt, consider a lesion involving the superior oblique muscle (and its corresponding CN VI).

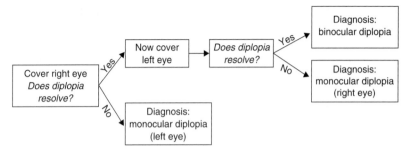

Figure 5.3.1. The diplopia cover test.

2. **Auscultation.** Listen over the closed eye for a carotid cavernous fistula bruit.
3. **Palpation.** Palpate for a step-off or any tenderness to suggest a periorbital fracture.

C. **Testing.** The following office-based testing should be considered:
   1. Visual acuity should include testing the patient's uncorrected and corrected vision.
   2. Cover test—cover each eye sequentially. If the diplopia persists when one eye is covered (i.e., the diplopia persists with just one eye open), the patient has monocular diplopia. Monocular implies an abnormality of just one eye (the "bad" eye). When the offending eye is covered, the diplopia resolves. When the good eye is covered, the diplopia persists. If the patient's vision returns to normal when either the left or right eye is covered, the patient has binocular diplopia. This is an extremely useful test to help narrow the causes of diplopia (Figure 5.3.1). Further evaluation for the causes of monocular diplopia can be focused on the abnormal eye (2).
   3. Visual acuity with a pinhole is most helpful for patients who have monocular diplopia. If the offending eye is covered with a pinhole, the visual acuity in that eye often improves. This points to a problem with refraction (3).
   4. Range of ocular movements and visual field testing—these tests may be used to further narrow the differential diagnosis. In orbital trauma, for example, entrapment (or contusion) of the inferior rectus and/or the inferior oblique muscles or their nerves may worsen the diplopia (4).
   5. Pupillary evaluation may reveal asymmetric pupils. Consider a CN III palsy.
   6. An abnormal corneal reflex indicates a problem with the alignment of the globes themselves. This produces a binocular diplopia (although not exclusively). Further imaging, such as with a computed tomography (CT) scan or a magnetic resonance imaging (MRI; with contrast), may be warranted (2).
   7. If an ocular muscle group is suspected in binocular diplopia, a Parks 3-step test is used to determine the particular muscles. Consult an ophthalmology text or see references 2 and 3.
   8. Fatigability of ocular muscles suggests myasthenia gravis.
   9. Consider a CT scan or an MRI of the skull and orbits if there is concern for mass, fracture, increased intracranial pressure, sinus disease, or vascular abnormality. A Tensilon test may be ordered if myasthenia gravis is suspected.

IV. DIAGNOSIS

A. **Differential Diagnosis.** The differential diagnosis for diplopia, which can often be substantially narrowed based on the history and the physical examination, is broken into two main groups—monocular and binocular diplopia.
   1. **Causes of monocular diplopia.** Monocular diplopia is usually due to refractive errors. Specific causes may include corneal distortions (scars and keratoconus), multiple openings in the iris, cataract, lens displacement (e.g., Marfan's syndrome), advanced astigmatism, pseudophakos (artificial intraocular lens) subluxation, vitreous abnormalities, retinal conditions, contact lens complication, intraocular foreign body, herpes zoster

ophthalmicus, orbital cellulitis, orbital fracture (floor and medial wall), orbital tumors (rhabdomyosarcoma), and arteriovenous malformations (carotid cavernous fistula).

2. **Causes of binocular diplopia.** Nerve palsies (abducens, oculomotor, and trochlear), migraine headache, myasthenia gravis, thyroid ophthalmopathy, mononeuritis multiplex (CN VI—abducens), diabetic CN III palsy (normal pupil, headache, or pain around the orbit), and diabetic palsies (CN IV or V).

B. **Clinical Manifestations.** Diplopia may cause difficulty with depth perception, especially with balance, and activities such as driving or operating machinery. Patients with diplopia should not perform these activities (2).

REFERENCES

1. Vaughan DG, Asbury T, Riordan-Eva P. *General ophthalmology.* New York, NY: McGraw-Hill Medical, 2003.
2. Wessels I. Diplopia. Accessed at *Medline plus encyclopedia* (http://www.nlm.nih.gov/medlineplus/ency/article/003029.htm), 2004.
3. Brazis PW, Lee AG. Binocular vertical diplopia. *Mayo Clin Proc* 1998;73:55–66.
4. Webb LA. *Manual of eye emergencies.* Philadelphia, PA: Butterworth-Heineman, Bartley, 2004.
5. Rucker JA, Kennard C, Leigh, RJ. *The neuro-opthalmological examination. Handbook of clinical neurology.* Amsterdam, The Netherlands: Elsevier B.V., 2011.

5.4 Loss of Vision

John J. Messmer

I. **BACKGROUND.** Vision is perhaps one of the most valued senses and when disturbed it becomes a significant concern for the patient. Determining the cause and providing treatment is a corresponding concern for the physician.

Visual loss can be sudden or gradual, monocular or binocular, partial or complete and may be a solitary symptom or part of a complex syndrome. Other sections of this manual deal with blurring of vision, reduced visual acuity, and segmental loss of the visual field (scotomata). This section will address abrupt loss of the entire visual field or visual field deficits in one or both eyes occurring in a short time.

II. **PATHOPHYSIOLOGY**

A. **Etiology.** Abrupt visual loss or visual deficits developing over minutes to hours rather than weeks or years fall into three categories: vascular, neurologic, and mechanical.

Vascular causes can be ischemic or inflammatory. Ischemic vascular events can be atherosclerotic, embolic, infectious, or obstructive. Inflammatory causes include the arteritides and autoimmune causes, although the latter groups tend to be subacute (days to weeks) rather than acute.

Neurologic causes include demyelinating diseases, occipital lobe seizures (more typical in children), migraine, and functional etiologies.

Mechanical causes include trauma, retinal and vitreous detachment, and damage to the ocular structures due to facial injury or infection.

B. **Epidemiology.** Incidence and prevalence is based on the etiology of the vision loss.

III. **EVALUATION**

A. **History.** Due to the multiple and varied causes of visual loss, the history is critical to delineate etiology and to guide evaluation, treatment, or referral. Knowledge of the anatomy and vascular supply of the eye, optic nerve, and optic tracts aids in taking a thorough history.

1. Binocular, total visual loss (complete blindness). Unless there has been trauma to the face causing extensive damage to the globes, this is almost always due to severe atherosclerotic

disease of the posterior circulation to the brain. Approximately 5–10% of ischemic strokes are in the posterior circulation. Vision is lost over minutes to days and returns slowly with varying degrees of homonymous hemianopsia. The patient might also have other symptoms of posterior circulation deficits: reduced level of consciousness, denial of blindness ("Anton's syndrome"), and "blindsight" in which some visual processing continues.

Bilateral vision loss can also occur from bilateral lesions in the optic radiations posterior to the lateral geniculate nuclei ("cortical" or "cerebral" blindness); however, the likelihood of bilateral lesions localized to these pathways is relatively low.

2. Monocular partial or complete visual loss. Anatomically this must be due to some event anterior to the optic chiasm. Ischemic causes include arteritis, non-arteritic anterior ischemic optic neuropathy (NAION), central retinal vein, or arterial occlusion. Neurologic etiology includes optic neuritis.

Arteritis is typically preceded by weeks or months of headache and myalgias and often amaurosis fugax and jaw claudication. Patients are typically older than 50 years, with 2:1 female to male ratio. NAION is usually in patients over 50 years, with predominance in women. Incidence is 2–10 per 100,000 in the United States. It can be bilateral and may not cause total visual loss, but the entire eye may be affected. It is thought to be an ischemic process causing swelling of the optic nerve vessels as the nerve exits the eye. Typically painless and often present upon arising, it is often associated with hypertension, diabetes, and the presence of other atherosclerotic diseases.

Central retinal artery occlusion typically causes painless monocular blindness. Incidence is estimated at 0.85 per 100,000 per year. Etiology is typically embolic and is associated with smoking and cardiovascular disease. Patients are usually in the 7th decade or older but can be young adults. Branch retinal artery occlusion has the same associations as central retinal artery occlusion, but a smaller branch is affected and visual loss is partial. Emboli can originate from atheromata or can result from other etiologies of embolism.

Central retinal vein occlusion (CRVO) is a fairly common cause of abrupt monocular blindness, typically in men older than 65 years, occurring in slightly more than 2 per 1,000 in patients over 40 years and 5.4 per 1,000 in patients over age 64 years. Men and women are affected in roughly equal numbers. Most CRVO is ischemic from an intramural thrombus and is associated with cardiovascular disease, hypertension, diabetes, and open angle glaucoma. The occlusion is posterior to the cribriform plate.

Branch retinal vein occlusion (BRVO) occurs at arteriovenous crossings. The artery compresses the venule inducing thrombosis. Predisposing problems include hypertension, cardiovascular disease, and glaucoma. The degree of visual loss is dependent on the amount of retina affected.

Optic neuritis is not as abrupt as other causes of monocular visual loss. It usually develops over 2–5 days with loss of color vision and depth perception, progressing to decreased visual acuity rather than blindness and it can be bilateral. Causes include multiple sclerosis, Lyme disease, and neurosyphilis and may be idiopathic. Idiopathic optic neuritis affects women more than men; typically patients are in their thirties and usually one eye is affected.

Retinal detachment typically begins in the periphery and is noted as loss of peripheral vision, often described as a curtain across the side vision. Central vision is affected if the detachment of the macula is involved. Detachment can occur due to fluid accumulating in the subretinal space from a number of etiologies including in association with a posterior vitreous detachment, more commonly seen in male myopes over 45 years. In a vitreous detachment, condensations of the vitreous cast shadows on the retina perceived as shadows or "floaters." As the vitreous pulls at the retina, peripheral flashes of light (photopsia) are seen.

Secondary retinal detachment is associated with severe hypertension, chronic glomerulonephritis, retinal venous occlusions, retinal angiomatosis, papilledema, postoperative inflammation, tumors, granulomatous uveitis, and vasculitis.

Retinal migraine differs from common or classic migraine because headache is not a prominent part of the symptom complex. Recurrent unilateral vision loss lasting minutes to approximately an hour is the pattern. It must be differentiated from ischemic etiologies.

Trauma is usually apparent from history and examination and can include blunt or sharp trauma, chemical or thermal burns, and foreign bodies.

3. Binocular, partial visual loss. Pathology in the optic tract rostral to the chiasm posteriorly will be involved in binocular visual loss that is relatively abrupt or rapid in onset. Chronic visual loss, such as diabetic retinopathy, glaucoma, and macular degeneration will not be covered in this section.

Retrochiasmal lesions are localized to the occipital lobes 43% of the time, the optic radiation 31%, the lateral geniculate nucleus 1.2%, the optic tract 10%, and multiple areas 11.1%. Infarction and hemorrhage account for 70% of the lesions; the remainder includes trauma, tumors, neurosurgical procedures, demyelinating diseases, and miscellaneous causes.

History alone may not distinguish between small artery strokes and small neoplasms. The presence of risk factors for stroke and known atherosclerotic disease in other organs increases the likelihood of this etiology. A history of malignant neoplasm will make metastatic disease a possibility. A primary brain neoplasm might be associated with headache or other neurologic deficits.

Often the patient will not recognize the visual loss, which will only be determined by physical examination for another complaint. The larger the field deficit and the more congruous in shape and position, the more posterior in the visual axis the lesion is located.

B. Examination. Examine for evidence of trauma. Perform visual acuity, examine extraocular movements and visual fields by confrontation. Evaluate papillary equality and direct and consensual response. Examine the fundus by direct ophthalmoscopy. In some cases, a detailed eye examination may be needed.

If the history is suggestive of systemic disease, the appropriate examination should also be included, e.g., vital signs, auscultation of the carotids and heart if emboli or atherosclerotic disease is considered, palpation of temporal arteries if temporal arteritis is suspected, and general neurologic examination when considering stroke or multiple sclerosis.

C. Testing. Computed tomography is useful for the evaluation of trauma and in the diagnosis of cerebral tumors. For purposes of diagnosis of visual loss, MRI will likely be a more useful imaging study as long as no intraocular ferrometallic foreign bodies are suspected. Soft tissues are well delineated, tumors and vascular accidents and anomalies are seen well and when combined with magnetic resonance angiography can evaluate for atherosclerosis. Sedimentation rate is important in the diagnosis of arteritis.

IV. DIAGNOSIS

A. Differential Diagnosis and Clinical Manifestations

1. **Temporal arteritis** may include myalgias, amaurosis fugax, headache, tender and/or palpable temporal arteries, and monocular blindness with an afferent papillary defect.
2. **Retinal artery occlusion** should be suspected when there are risk factors for emboli, painless monocular blindness, afferent papillary defect, pale fundus, and cherry red macula (except in 15% of the population with a cilioretinal artery supplying the macula; this may preserve the afferent limb of the papillary response). If the visual loss is partial and a bright embolus is seen in a branch artery or an artery is seen to stop abruptly, it is likely a branch retinal artery occlusion. Branch occlusions may be difficult to see with direct ophthalmoscopy.
3. **Central retinal vein occlusion** presents with monocular loss, hemorrhage and edema, obscuration of the disc, and afferent papillary defect. Partial loss, normal pupil response, hemorrhage limited to a small area distal to an arteriovenous crossing in patients with atherosclerosis risks is likely a BRVO.
4. **Non-arteritic ischemic neuropathy** presents with monocular loss without hemorrhage or emboli and a pale disc, often in a middle-aged person.
5. **Demyelinating disease** may present with waxing and waning visual blurring and/or loss, usually partial, and often monocular loss, particularly if there is a history of multiple sclerosis or the patient is in the usual age group.

6. **Retinal detachment** presents with partial monocular loss with new floaters and photopsia. If blurring of the retina is seen on examination, there may be a retinal detachment, although this may be difficult to determine with direct ophthalmoscopy.

7. **Bilateral occipital lobe damage** will cause total binocular blindness and is likely due to a stroke, especially if the onset is abrupt.

8. **Optic tract lesions** cause various visual field defects. Total monocular loss without vascular change in the fundus may be due to optic nerve injury. Bitemporal hemianopsia points to an optic chiasm lesion. Homonymous lesions are rostral to the chiasm; the more congruous the defect, the more posterior the lesion.

B. **Clinical Approach.** The primary care physician's role in loss of vision is to evaluate the associated conditions once ophthalmologic urgent consultation is made.

REFERENCES

1. Pavan PR, Burrows AF, Pavan-Langston D. Retina and vitreous. In: Pavan-Langston D, ed. *Manual of ocular diagnosis and therapy*. Philadelphia, PA: Lippincott Williams & Wilkins, 2008:176–205.
2. Fraser JA, Newman NJ, Biousse V. Disorders of the optic tract, radiation, and occipital lobe. In: Kennard C, Leigh RJ, eds. *Handbook of clinical neurology*, Vol. 102 (3rd series) Neuro-ophthalmology. Amsterdam: Elsevier, 2011:205–221.
3. Younge BR. Anterior ischemic optic neuropathy. Accessed at http://emedicine.medscape.com/article/1216891-overview on April 22, 2012.
4. Dafer RM, Jay WM. Headache and the eye. *Curr Opin Ophthalmol* 2009;20:520–524.

5.5 Nystagmus

Peter R. Lewis

I. **BACKGROUND.** Nystagmus is an involuntary, rhythmic oscillation of one or both eyes in any or all fields of gaze. It may be continuous or intermittent. Nystagmus can be classified into two basic types, jerk (the more common classification) and pendular.

A. **Jerk Nystagmus.** This consists of an initial slow phase, followed and named for the direction (upbeat, downbeat, horizontal, torsional—also referred to as rotary, or mixed) by the corrective saccade or fast phase ("jerk") in the opposite direction.

B. **Pendular Nystagmus.** This consists of smooth back and forth ("pendular") movements (horizontal, vertical, torsional, or mixed) of the eye(s).

II. **PATHOPHYSIOLOGY.** The appropriate development, function, and integration of the visual/ oculomotor and vestibular systems are required for optimal focus and tracking of visual objects (1, 2). Nystagmus may be associated with abnormalities of the central or peripheral nervous system, although in many instances a precise cause may not be identified (3). Any form of vision loss may be associated with nystagmus. Extreme-gaze evoked nystagmus is effectively physiologic, occurring normally in approximately one-half of the population.

A. **Etiology.** Jerk or pendular nystagmus may be characterized as being either congenital/ infantile or acquired.

1. Congenital/infantile nystagmus is most commonly associated with underlying sensory (efferent) visual abnormalities. It may not become evident until several months of age. If no efferent defect is identified, the nystagmus is judged to be idiopathic, presumably due to a defect in the oculomotor complex.

2. Acquired nystagmus (not including the extreme-gaze evoked form noted above) that develops later in life is more likely to be pathologic and associated with a life-threatening disorder.

   a. Two forms of acquired nystagmus when seen in children should raise the clinician's suspicion for an underlying tumor and prompt referral for neuroimaging.

    i. **Opsoclonus** is characterized by repetitive, irregular, and multidirectional ("dancing eyes" or saccadomania) eye movements. Opsoclonus may be associated with cerebellar or brain stem disease, postviral meningitis, or neuroblastoma.

    ii. **Spasmus nutans** is the rare triad of torticollis (head turn or "wry neck"), nystagmus, and head bobbing. The nystagmus can be monocular or binocular and dissociated; of low amplitude and high frequency; and with horizontal or vertical pendular movements. It most commonly develops between 6 months and 3 years in otherwise healthy children and if of a benign etiology usually resolves between the ages of 2 and 8 years. Of note, an identical clinical picture can be produced by a glioma of the optic chiasm or nearby structures.

  b. Acquired forms of nystagmus that are more common in adults also frequently point to a serious underlying neurologic cause and include the following:

    i. **Seesaw nystagmus**, in which the movements are pendular. One eye rises and rotates inward, whereas the other descends and rotates outward. This is frequently seen with lesions of the optic chiasm or third ventricle, as may occur with a parasellar mass (e.g., craniopharyngioma or pituitary adenoma).

    ii. **Downbeating nystagmus**, in which the fast phase beats down and may be associated with a lesion of the cervicomedullary junction at the level of the foramen magnum. Arnold-Chiari malformation and spinocerebellar degeneration are the most common causes. Oscillopsia (an intermittent or constant sensation of the environment moving back and forth) may be present.

    iii. **Upbeating nystagmus**, in which the fast phase beats up and is of large or small amplitude. The associated lesion commonly involves the brain stem or vermis of the cerebellum as occurs in stroke, tumor, or degeneration.

    iv. **Convergence–retraction nystagmus**, which is marked by the convergence of the eyes with jerk nystagmus and the retraction of the globe on upgaze, eyelid retraction, limitation in upgaze, and large unreactive pupils. This is caused by midbrain abnormalities.

    v. **Periodic alternating nystagmus**, in which the fast phase occurs in one direction with a head turn for 60 to 90 seconds and then reverses direction with an intermediate "neutral zone." This can be seen with vestibulocerebellar disease (stroke, multiple sclerosis, and spinocerebellar degeneration), severe bilateral visual loss (optic atrophy and dense vitreous hemorrhage), or it can be congenital.

    vi. **Gaze-evoked nystagmus**, which is a type of jerk nystagmus that appears only when the eyes look to the side. Pathologic forms are most commonly seen with alcohol or other central nervous system (CNS) depressants. Cerebellar brain stem disorders can also be associated with this type of nystagmus.

    vii. **Vestibular nystagmus**, which is caused by the dysfunction of the inner ear, auditory nerve, or the central nuclear complex. Peripheral vestibular disease (e.g., labyrinthitis, Ménière's disease, neuronitis, vascular ischemia, trauma, or drug toxicity) produces unidirectional jerk nystagmus with a fast phase opposite the lesion that is usually horizontal. Common associated symptoms include vertigo, tinnitus, hearing loss, and vomiting. Central (nuclear) disease (e.g., demyelinating disorder, tumor, trauma, or stroke), by contrast, is characterized by unidirectional or bidirectional nystagmus that may be purely horizontal, vertical, or rotatory and is characteristically toward the side of the lesion. Vertigo, tinnitus, and deafness are mild, if present, and symptoms are not relieved with eye fixation as in peripheral disease.

    viii. **Torsional nystagmus**, which is usually constant and due to an associated midbrain (e.g., pons and medulla) lesion involving the vestibular nuclei as may occur in stroke or multiple sclerosis. The nystagmus may be superimposed on horizontal or vertical nystagmus and directed toward or away from the side of the associated **lesion.**

      ix. ***Dissociated nystagmus***, in which nystagmus in one eye is different from the other. This is seen in posterior fossa lesions. If an abduction nystagmus is present with an internuclear ophthalmoplegia, consider multiple sclerosis with a lesion involving the medial longitudinal fasciculus.

  B. Epidemiology. Precise data regarding the prevalence of nystagmus are unavailable.

III. EVALUATION

  A. History. Age of onset, self-identified precipitants, time course, associated symptoms, family history of visual impairment and/or associated neurologic disorders, and functional impairment should be elicited from the patient or parent. In children, it is necessary to inquire about a history of prematurity and related visual impairment(s). Blurred vision, if present, is characteristic of an acquired nystagmus. Vertigo implies vestibular disease. Associated weakness, numbness, or loss of vision may be suggestive of multiple sclerosis. Eliciting a history of medication and substance use may provide helpful clues as to potential etiology for the patient's nystagmus. Medications that can induce nystagmus (usually downbeat or upbeat) include lithium, barbiturates, phenytoin, salicylates, and benzodiazepines. Nystagmus may also be seen with PCP (phencyclidine) use. Acute alcohol intoxication can produce a gaze-evoked nystagmus, as does the chronic alcohol-induced thiamine (Vitamin B1) deficiency common to Wernicke's encephalopathy.

  B. Physical Examination. This should begin with a developmental assessment followed by a visual examination. Loss of visual acuity is typically worse in acquired nystagmus. The ability to track moving objects with the head in a fixed position (optokinetic reflex) takes a number of months to mature and typically fails to develop in congenital nystagmus. The direction, plane, and amplitude of the eye movement should be characterized. It is necessary to evaluate any cause of poor vision that may contribute to the nystagmus. Aniridia (absence of iris) or iris transillumination as seen in albinism may be observed. Congenital cataracts or corneal opacities have poor red reflexes. It is important to analyze the optic nerve to assess for hypoplasia or atrophy. Latent nystagmus (seen only when one eye is covered—the basis of the screening "cover–uncover" test) is present in infantile strabismus (4). Altered head position and head bobbing may be associated with congenital nystagmus and spasmus nutans. If benign paroxysmal positional vertigo is suspected, the Dix-Hallpike's maneuver may be performed in an effort to reproduce the patient's symptoms (5). A complete neurologic assessment should be performed. Appropriate neurology and ophthalmology consultation(s) should be requested as indicated.

  C. Testing. Urine drug screening for alcohol or barbiturates should be considered when significant gaze-evoked nystagmus is observed. Serum drug levels of phenytoin or lithium should be obtained as indicated. Additional blood tests to be considered include vitamin B12, magnesium, and toxoplasmosis and/or human immunodeficiency virus serologies. If a CNS infection is suspected (e.g., herpes simplex), then cerebrospinal fluid analysis is indicated. Magnetic resonance imaging (MRI) should be obtained before the lumbar puncture. Ocular albinism can be associated with a bleeding disorder secondary to platelet dysfunction (Hermansky-Pudlak syndrome) or white blood cell dysfunction with increased susceptibility to infection and lymphoma (Chédiak-Higashi syndrome). Respectively, a bleeding time or a polymorphonuclear leukocyte function test should be ordered. Urinary vanillylmandelic acid should be obtained in a patient with opsoclonus to evaluate for the possibility of a neuroblastoma. Associated hypertension related to this catecholamine secretion may be observed.

  D. Genetics. Variable patterns of inheritance have been associated with congenital nystagmus (6). Certain autosomal dominant ataxias are associated with downbeat nystagmus. Symptoms usually do not begin until late adulthood.

IV. DIAGNOSIS

  A. Differential Diagnosis. Other involuntary ocular oscillations include the following:

    1. ***Oculogyric crisis*** consists of nonrhythmic, sustained, and irregular eye deviations. This is seen in phenothiazine (e.g., certain antipsychotic and antihistaminic drugs) toxicity.

2. **Ocular bobbing** is characterized by fast, conjugate, downward movement of the eye, followed by a slow drift to the primary position of gaze. This is seen in comatose patients with large pontine lesions (e.g., hemorrhage, stroke, or tumor). Obstructive hydrocephalus or metabolic encephalopathy can also cause this type of eye movement.

3. **Superior oblique myokymia** is characterized by small unilateral, vertical, and rotatory movements of one eye. Symptoms of oscillopsia worsen when looking downward and inward. This is usually benign and self-limited, but has been noted with multiple sclerosis.

4. **Essential head tremor.** Nystagmus may occur with essential head tremor in which case there is often a family history of same. The head tremor and related nystagmus may be extinguished by fixing the head position or by utilizing a β-blocker.

B. **Clinical Manifestations.** The clinical manifestations of nystagmus were discussed in Section II.A. Because many forms of nystagmus localize to the posterior fossa or are associated with a demyelinating disorder, an MRI is the imaging modality of choice if the cause is otherwise not identified. In a patient with opsoclonus, an abdominal computed tomography (CT) scan or an MRI should be done to look for a neuroblastoma involving the adrenal glands. An abdominal ultrasound or CT scan is needed to evaluate the kidneys if aniridia is present, as there is a significant incidence of associated Wilms' tumor. As noted above, neurology and ophthalmology consultation(s) should be requested as indicated.

REFERENCES

1. Leigh RJ, Zee DS. *The neurology of eye movements*, 4th ed. Oxford: Oxford University Press, 2006.
2. Straube A, Bronstein A, Straumann D. Nystagmus and oscillopsia. *Eur J Neurol* 2012;19:6–14, doi: 10.1111/j.1468-331.2011.03503.x
3. Serra A, Leigh RJ. Diagnostic value of nystagmus: spontaneous and induced ocular oscillations. *J Neurol Neurosurg Psychiatry* 2002;73(6):615–618.
4. Simon JW, Kaw P. Commonly missed diagnoses in the childhood eye examination. *Am Fam Physician* 2001;64(4):623–628.
5. Swartz R, Longwell P. Treatment of vertigo. *Am Fam Physician* 2005;71(6):1115–1122.
6. Gottlob I. Nystagmus. *Curr Opin Ophthalmol* 2001;12(5):378–383.

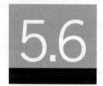

5.6 Papilledema

Peter R. Lewis

I. **BACKGROUND.** Papilledema is an optic disc swelling produced by increased intracranial pressure. It may be detected in the asymptomatic pediatric or adult patient during the course of a screening funduscopic examination with a non–life-threatening cause. Conversely, it may be identified in initially asymptomatic or gravely symptomatic patients (including pregnant women) as a marker of a life-threatening condition such as subarachnoid hemorrhage, meningitis, or brain tumor (1).

II. **PATHOPHYSIOLOGY**

A. **Etiology.** True papilledema is always associated with increased intracranial pressure. The differential diagnosis for papilledema includes trauma, primary or metastatic intracranial tumor, aqueductal stenosis (as is seen in certain types of congenital hydrocephalus), pseudotumor cerebri (idiopathic intracranial hypertension; frequently misdiagnosed as migraine headache) (2), subdural hematoma, subarachnoid hemorrhage, arteriovenous malformations, brain abscess, meningitis, encephalitis, and sagittal sinus thrombosis.

B. **Epidemiology.** Most patients with papilledema are adults. Many of the causes of papilledema (e.g., subarachnoid hemorrhage and cancer) are more common with advancing age.

Pseudotumor cerebri is most commonly discovered in adolescent females and young women. Individuals with immunosuppression (e.g., human immunodeficiency virus [HIV]/ acquired immunodeficiency syndrome, chemotherapy, chronic prednisone therapy) are at heightened risk for central nervous system (CNS) infections (e.g., meningitis, encephalitis, and brain abscess) that may be associated with papilledema.

III. EVALUATION. The history and physical examination are tailored to the age, setting, and urgency of the patient presentation. Patients with an acute and rapid increase in intracranial pressure with associated papilledema may be moribund and comatose, requiring emergent and expedited assessment and care. In less urgent situations, patients may present with nonspecific symptoms (e.g., headache) (1) that prompt an investigation, initially on the basis of the history and physical examination, for associated intracranial pressure and its cause. Alternatively, the search for clues to the presence and the cause of increased intracranial pressure only begins subsequent to the discovery of papilledema during the course of a screening funduscopic examination.

A. History. In the symptomatic patient, headache, nausea, vomiting, diplopia, focal weakness, fever, neck stiffness, photophobia, and/or fleeting loss of vision (obscurations)—especially with the head in dependent positions—raise the clinician's index of suspicion for increased intracranial pressure. Parents of infants or children may report increased head size or decreased alertness. After probing patient complaints and associated symptoms, the clinician should determine the presence or risk factors for vascular disease (including prior stroke), cancer, trauma, or immunosuppression. A thorough medication and drug use history should also be obtained. Prescription medications which may result in papilledema include tetracycline, lithium, and corticosteroids. Toxins which may lead to papilledema include methanol and ethylene glycol. A family history of conditions related to increased intracranial pressure should be elicited.

B. Physical Examination

1. This commences with a general assessment of the patient and vital signs, including blood pressure and visual acuity. Rarely is a decrease in visual acuity seen in association with increased intracranial pressure; if present, it typically suggests other causes (e.g., vein occlusion, anterior ischemic optic neuropathy, or optic neuritis).

2. Additional components of a detailed ophthalmologic examination, including funduscopic assessment, should be performed. If present, sixth nerve palsies are evidenced by limited lateral gaze and may be associated with horizontal diplopia, whereas third nerve palsies demonstrate a limitation in medial gaze, elevation, and accompanying eyelid depression. Regarding the funduscopic examination in the asymptomatic patient, it is necessary to take care to first determine if there is true disc edema or only pseudopapilledema (this may well require consultation with an ophthalmologist). Pseudopapilledema is optic nerve head elevation caused by hyaline deposition ("drusen") within the optic nerve head itself and is reported to be more common in Caucasians (3). There is no associated increased intracranial pressure or CNS pathology. When true papilledema is present, it is typically bilateral. There are optic disc findings common to early versus later stages of papilledema as well as acute versus chronic papilledema. Disc edema produces an obscuring of the blood vessels' margins. Tiny splinter hemorrhages are seen in and around the optic nerve. An absence of spontaneous venous pulsations (SVPs) may be seen in conjunction with true papilledema due to increased intracranial pressure. If SVPs are present, there is normal intracranial pressure. Prominent retinal hemorrhages suggest malignant hypertension or central retinal vein occlusion.

3. A complete head and neck examination to check for neck stiffness, temporal artery tenderness, pain in and around the eyes, and sinus tenderness is also important. Thorough vascular and neurologic examinations of the head and neck are to be included. Measure head circumference in infants and young children; check for bulging or prematurely closed fontanels in the former group.

C. Testing. If true papilledema is found, laboratory testing and clinical imaging should be directed at determining the cause and the severity of the associated increased intracranial pressure. In urgent clinical presentations, patients should be referred to the Emergency Department of the nearest hospital. Suggested laboratory tests include sedimentation rate,

C-reactive protein, and white blood count if CNS infection is suspected. Serologies for HIV, syphilis, and herpes should be obtained as indicated. A lumbar puncture for the measurement of opening pressure and a cerebrospinal fluid (CSF) examination to evaluate for evidence of meningitis, tumor, or hemorrhage should be performed only after ruling out a compressive lesion with a computed tomography (CT) scan or magnetic resonance imaging (MRI). If true papilledema is suspected by the primary care clinician and/or confirmed in consultation with an ophthalmologist, then diagnostic imaging is mandatory. A CT scan with and without contrast should be ordered. If the CT scan is inconclusive, an MRI will be particularly helpful to evaluate for brain stem and cerebellar lesions, which can obstruct CSF flow—thereby leading to papilledema—in children and adults. An MRI angiography may be required to identify a related vascular abnormality such as an aneurysm. A consulting ophthalmologist may perform fluorescein angiography to assist with diagnosis and subsequent management. A CT scan is the preferred technique to evaluate for acute intracranial bleeding. Neurology and/or neurosurgical consultation(s) may also be indicated depending on the cause of the patient's papilledema. An ultrasound of the optic disc may be used if the diagnosis of pseudopapilledema is uncertain.

D. Genetics. Many of the underlying conditions associated with papilledema have genetic contributions.

IV. DIAGNOSIS

A. Differential Diagnosis. Disc swelling without increased intracranial pressure may be caused by the following conditions:

1. **Optic Neuritis.** An afferent pupillary defect exists along with decreased vision and pain on extraocular movement. Color vision will be decreased in this normally unilateral condition. It may be seen with multiple sclerosis.

2. **Malignant Hypertension** (of essential or secondary causes, including severe preeclampsia). Blood pressure is markedly elevated and the patient is symptomatic. The eye findings may include bilateral prominent disc edema, flame hemorrhages that extend peripherally, and cotton wool spots.

3. **Central Retinal Vein Occlusion.** This is characterized by a unilateral disc swelling with very prominent flame and blot hemorrhages, without increased systemic blood pressure.

4. **Anterior Ischemic Optic Neuropathy.** This may be due to arteritis (e.g., temporal/"giant cell") presenting with headache, stiff neck, temporal tenderness, jaw claudication, and elevated sedimentation rate. If undetected and untreated, severe visual loss in one eye followed by visual loss of the other eye may occur. When arteritis is absent, typically no symptoms are present except decreased vision. Associated conditions include systemic hypertension, diabetes mellitus, and collagen vascular disorders.

5. **Infiltration of the Optic Nerve.** Tuberculosis granuloma, leukemic infiltrate, sarcoidosis, and metastatic disease are more common examples of infiltrative processes that may involve the optic nerve. The infiltration can be unilateral or bilateral and can lead to rapid loss of vision.

6. **Leber's Hereditary Optic Neuropathy.** This usually affects males in the second or third decade and is characterized by unilateral progressive loss of vision with disc swelling.

7. **Diabetic Papillitis.** This represents an ischemic infarction to the optic nerve in advanced diabetics. This is often bilateral and causes mild disc elevation.

B. Clinical Manifestations. Chronic papilledema can result in optic atrophy (with decreased optic nerve swelling) and progressive visual loss (initially peripheral) that may progress to frank blindness. Such patients should be followed with serial perimetry (visual field testing) by an ophthalmologist.

REFERENCES

1. Clinch CR. Evaluation of acute headaches in adults. *Am Fam Physician* 2001;63(4):685–692.
2. Brazis PW, Lee AG. Elevated intracranial pressure and pseudotumor cerebri. *Curr Opin Ophthalmol* 1998;9(6):27–32.
3. Giovannini J, Chrousos G. *Papilledema.* Accessed at eMedicine www.emedicine.com/oph/topic187.htm, on June 4, 2012.

Pupillary Inequality

David C. Holub

I. BACKGROUND. Anisocoria is defined as an inequality of pupillary size (diameter).

II. PATHOPHYSIOLOGY

A. Etiology

1. The pupil is a hole or aperture in the iris that permits the passage of light through to the retina. Two muscles within the iris control pupillary size. The *sphincter pupillae* is a circular muscle that controls pupillary constriction, or miosis. The *dilator pupillae* is a radial muscle that controls pupillary dilation, or mydriasis.

2. The pupillary constrictor is innervated by fibers from the parasympathetic autonomic nervous system. These fibers originate in the midbrain and travel to the Edinger-Westphal nucleus in the dorsal midbrain, and then with the third cranial nerve (CN III, the oculomotor nerve) through the cavernous sinus to the orbit. They diverge from CN III to synapse in the orbit with the ciliary ganglion. Postganglionic short ciliary nerves then innervate the pupillary constrictor muscle. Lesions at any anatomic site along this pathway lead to pathologic mydriasis (1).

3. The pupillary dilator muscle is innervated by fibers from the sympathetic autonomic nervous system. These neurons originate in the hypothalamus, descend through the brain stem to the C8-T2 lateral horn, and then travel with the cervical sympathetic trunk to the superior cervical ganglion. Postganglionic long ciliary nerves travel with the internal carotid artery until the superior orbital fissure, where they diverge and continue to the dilator pupillae muscle. These fibers both stimulate the dilator pupillae and inhibit the pupillary constrictor and ciliary muscles. They also innervate the levator palpebrae muscle and therefore contribute to eyelid elevation. Lesions at any anatomic site along this pathway lead to pathologic miosis (1).

B. Epidemiology. Physiologic anisocoria is common, affecting perhaps as many as 20% of normal individuals. The difference in pupillary size is small, usually <1 mm (2).

III. EVALUATION

A. History. In most patients, anisocoria is discovered incidentally; presenting symptoms are relatively uncommon. It is necessary to inquire about ocular symptoms such as pain, redness, tearing, or photophobia. Any past history of eye disease, injury, surgery, or medications should be elicited.

B. Physical Examination. The pupils should be examined in both dim and bright lights, assessing both direct and consensual pupillary light reflexes. An afferent pupillary defect (Marcus Gunn pupil) permits a consensual light reflex, but no pupillary constriction or paradoxical pupillary dilation to direct light. In an efferent pupillary defect, pupillary constriction to both direct and consensual light reflexes is absent.

1. The critical first step in assessing a patient with anisocoria is to determine which is the abnormal pupil (i.e., Is one pupil abnormally constricted or is the other pupil abnormally dilated?). It is necessary to examine the pupillary responses in both bright and dim lighting. The pupil that does not dilate in dim light or constrict in bright light is the abnormal one.

2. Extraocular movements should be tested. In patients with third nerve palsy, the affected eye shows outward deviation during primary gaze. It is able to come to midline only with attempts at inward gaze, and downward gaze leads to inward rotation.

C. Testing. Computed tomography or magnetic resonance imaging is valuable for suspected intracranial mass lesions or bleeding. Angiography is indicated for suspected cerebral aneurysm or carotid dissection. Consider obtaining chest radiography to evaluate for occult lung malignancy in patients with Horner's syndrome (triad of miosis, ptosis, and unilateral facial anhidrosis).

IV. DIAGNOSIS
A. Differential Diagnosis
1. The differential diagnosis of miosis includes Horner's syndrome, unilateral anterior uveitis, Lyme disease, or syphilis.
2. The differential diagnosis of mydriasis includes palsy of or damage to CN III, Adie's pupil, the use of certain medications (with anticholinergic effects), trauma, and acute angle closure glaucoma.

B. Clinical Manifestations
1. Pathologic miosis may be caused by a lesion or disease state that affects any anatomic site from the brain to the pupil itself. Horner's syndrome is the triad of miosis with ptosis and ipsilateral facial anhidrosis (variably present depending on the level of the lesion). It is caused by damage to the cervical thoracic sympathetic fibers. A brain stem stroke may lead to these findings. Disease of the internal carotid artery, such as dissection, may also interrupt the signals normally carried by these nerves. Horner's syndrome also frequently occurs due to tumors that compress these nerve fibers. These may include parotid gland tumors, carotid body tumors, lymphoma with enlarged cervical adenopathy, mediastinal tumors, or apical lung tumors (typically in the superior sulcus). Direct trauma can also damage the sympathetic nerve fibers (3). Miosis may also be caused by unilateral ocular disease such as anterior uveitis, in which inflammation leads to the development of adhesions (synechiae) between the iris and the anterior lens capsule. Lyme disease and neurosyphilis may involve the eye as well, leading to an Argyll Robertson pupil—an irregular pupil that reacts poorly to light but normally to accommodation.
2. Pathologic mydriasis is typically caused by disease states that affect the oculomotor nerve (CN III) and thereby the parasympathetic fibers that travel with this nerve. Other clinical manifestations of a third nerve palsy include abnormalities of ocular movement and ptosis. Neurologic diseases such as multiple sclerosis may cause third nerve palsy. Nerve compression can occur from vascular phenomena (posterior communicating artery aneurysm), increased intracranial pressure due to head trauma with bleeding, or an intracranial mass. In the comatose patient with head trauma, a temporal lobe herniation compressing the midbrain may also lead to unilateral mydriasis. Unilateral mydriasis may also be an isolated finding in Adie's pupil, caused by damage to the ciliary ganglion through infection, ischemia, or trauma. Patients are typically women, 20–50 years of age, and usually asymptomatic. They present with anisocoria, diminished or absent light reflexes (both direct and consensual), and an exaggerated and prolonged (tonic) pupillary constriction during accommodation.
3. Unilateral pharmacologic mydriasis may occur with anticholinergic medications.
4. Acute angle closure glaucoma is a crucial consideration in the evaluation of unilateral mydriasis. Patients present with eye pain, redness, and visual impairment. An examination reveals a fixed, mid-dilated pupil and elevated intraocular pressure.

REFERENCES

1. Mosenthal W. *A textbook of neuroanatomy*. London: Parthenon Publishing, 1995.
2. Eggenberger E. *Anisocoria*. Accessed at http://emedicine.medscape.com/article/1158571-overview on May 2012.
3. Bardorf C. *Horner syndrome*. Accessed at http://emedicine.medscape.com/article/1220091-overview on May 2012.

Red Eye
David C. Holub

I. BACKGROUND

A. The red eye is one of the most common ocular complaints encountered in primary care. Although many causes of the red eye are benign, some are true emergencies. Failure to act accordingly may pose an immediate threat to the patient's vision.

B. Anatomically, almost any structure in the eye or its surrounding tissues may manifest with redness.

II. PATHOPHYSIOLOGY

A. Etiology. The primary causes of a red eye are infection or trauma to the various anatomic structures of the eye. Occasionally, connective tissue disease or a primary ocular disease can also manifest with a red eye. Causes include the following:

1. **Scleritis** is an inflammation of the sclera, the fibrous outer envelope of the eye.
2. **Episcleritis** is an inflammation of the connective tissue that lies between the sclera and the conjunctiva.
3. **Conjunctivitis** is an inflammation of the conjunctiva, the mucous membranes that line the anterior surface of the eye and the posterior surface of the eyelid.
4. **Blepharitis** is an inflammation of the eyelid, which may itself appear red and make the eye appear red as well.
5. A **hordeolum** is a superficial inflammatory granuloma of the eyelid that develops acutely from an obstruction of the ocular sebaceous glands (Zeiss or meibomian glands).
6. A **chalazion** manifests similarly, but is a deeper-seated granulomatous obstruction of these glands.
7. **Acute dacryocystitis** results from an obstruction and secondary infection of the lacrimal system.
8. **Iritis** or **anterior uveitis** involves an inflammation of the anterior part of the eye (iris and ciliary body).
9. **Keratitis** occurs when the cornea, the transparent outer covering of the anterior eye, becomes inflamed, infected, or traumatically injured, resulting either in a **corneal abrasion** or a **corneal foreign body**.
10. **Hyphema**, or hemorrhage into the anterior chamber, which also results from trauma, may manifest with visible redness if the amount of bleeding is significant. Even relatively minor trauma may lead to a **subconjunctival hemorrhage**, evident as a prominent red area in the normally white sclera.
11. **Acute angle closure glaucoma** leads to a rapid rise in intraocular pressure and may manifest as redness along with ocular pain, visual loss, headache, and nausea.
12. **Contact dermatitis**, **atopic dermatitis**, **preseptal (periorbital) cellulitis**, or **orbital cellulitis** cause the skin and soft tissues surrounding the eye or involving the eyelid to become inflamed or infected.

B. Epidemiology. Conjunctivitis is the most common eye complaint in the United States, accounting for 30% of all acute ocular complaints (1).

III. EVALUATION

A. History. An assessment of the red eye begins with questions regarding its location (unilateral, bilateral, or unilateral spreading to bilateral); onset (sudden or gradual); duration (acute, subacute, or chronic); inciting factors (such as trauma); and associated signs and symptoms. Ocular pain, swelling, photophobia, or disturbances in visual acuity are frequently signs of a more emergent condition. Other associated symptoms may include crusting, discharge, itching, burning, tearing, dry eyes, or a foreign body sensation. Systemic symptoms such as fever, headache, abdominal pain, nausea/vomiting, rhinorrhea, or cough should be elicited. A past history of similar ocular complaints is important. The patient should be asked about the use of contact lenses or eye drops. The past medical history may include certain systemic diseases that produce ocular involvement, such as syphilis, inflammatory bowel disease, and some collagen vascular diseases (sarcoidosis, ankylosing spondylitis, reactive arthritis, rheumatoid arthritis, and Sjögren's syndrome). There may also be a history of allergic or atopic disorders such as asthma, eczema, or allergic rhinitis.

B. Physical Examination

1. The physical examination of the eye should always begin with an assessment of visual acuity with a wall-mounted or handheld Snellen's eye chart. Visual acuity should always be measured either with the patient's corrective lenses or through pinhole testing. Visual disturbances owing solely to refractive error improve with the use of lenses or pinhole testing. Visual impairment due to organic eye disease does not.

2. Once this has been completed, a significant portion of the physical examination can then be easily accomplished in the primary care office setting without specialized equipment. A visual *inspection* of the eye and its surrounding soft tissues is essential to determine where the redness is located anatomically (i.e., sclera, conjunctiva, anterior chamber, eyelid, or periorbital tissues). Other notable findings include the presence of any lid swelling or crusting, purulent discharge, tearing, erythema or swelling of the periorbital tissues, or proptosis. Vesicular skin lesions near the eye suggest a herpes infection, which can have severe consequences on any infected structures within the eye. A palpation of the globe and surrounding soft tissues for firmness or tenderness should then be performed. A limitation of or pain with extraocular movements should be assessed. Eyelid eversion should be carried out to look for retained foreign bodies. Finally, a pupillary examination should be undertaken to assess size, shape, and reactivity.

3. Further examination of the eye requires both the appropriate equipment and the skill to use this equipment and interpret the findings correctly. Although this is feasible in the primary care setting, clinicians should obtain ophthalmologic consultation at this time if needed.

4. A slit lamp examination should be performed to assess for abnormalities of the anterior chamber, such as the presence of red or white blood cells or visible floating particulate matter (flare). The slit lamp is a more precise method for measuring anterior chamber depth than lateral visual inspection of the eye with a penlight. The cornea, with the application of fluorescein staining and the cobalt blue light source on the slit lamp, can be assessed for abrasion, ulceration, or a foreign body. Some patients may be unable to tolerate this examination due to pain or photophobia. In this instance, a topical anesthetic may be applied to the eye.

5. The measurement of intraocular pressure is important in the evaluation for acute angle closure glaucoma. This can be accomplished with a Schiötz tonometer or a handheld electronic tonometer pen in the primary care setting. In the ophthalmologist's office, gonioscopy (a visual inspection of the angle between the iris and cornea) can also be performed.

6. A funduscopic examination should be undertaken, ideally after pupillary dilatation has been effected through the installation of a mydriatic solution. As pupillary dilatation can precipitate an attack of acute angle closure, it is essential that this diagnosis be excluded prior to attempting this. Under direct ophthalmoscopy, the cornea, lens, and vitreous humor can be assessed for pathology.

C. Testing. Relatively few studies are useful in the differential diagnosis of the red eye. Cultures of purulent discharge are occasionally helpful if bacterial conjunctivitis is suspected. Blood cultures and a complete blood count with differential are prudent in cases of suspected orbital cellulitis. Computed tomography or magnetic resonance imaging should be considered if true orbital cellulitis is suspected (as opposed to preseptal cellulitis involving only the eyelids) to rule out serious complications including abscess or cavernous sinus thrombosis. Workup for rheumatologic disease may be considered in patients with iritis, episcleritis, or scleritis (2).

IV. DIAGNOSIS

A. Differential Diagnosis. Given the potential severity of some of the causes of red eye, the primary care physician's first priority is to determine if immediate intervention or ophthalmologic referral is warranted. The most serious causes of the acute red eye that need to be ruled out include acute angle closure glaucoma, hyphema, orbital cellulitis, acute keratitis, corneal ulcer, scleritis, and iritis/uveitis. Less serious causes include conjunctivitis (other than gonococcal), lid disorders, and subconjunctival hemorrhages.

B. Clinical Manifestations

1. **Acute angle closure glaucoma** presents with severe unilateral eye pain and blurry vision, often accompanied by visual halos, headache, abdominal pain, and nausea and vomiting. The physical examination reveals a shallow anterior chamber either by penlight or slit lamp examination, partially dilated pupils that respond poorly to light, a hazy cornea, firmness of globe on palpation, and elevated intraocular pressure on tonometry (3).

2. **Scleritis** typically presents with pain, tearing, photophobia, and decreased visual acuity. Visible swelling accompanies the redness. Discharge is typically absent. Fifty percent of the cases are bilateral.

3. **Iritis** or **uveitis** usually presents as blurred vision, pain, and photophobia affecting a single eye. Discharge is typically absent, although occasionally patients may have watery discharge. Physical examination reveals a sluggishly reactive pupil with pain and photophobia on both direct and consensual pupillary testing. Slit lamp examination also reveals proteinaceous or cellular matter in the anterior chamber (cell and flare).

4. **Keratitis** commonly presents with severe eye pain, photophobia, and blurry vision. A slit lamp examination with fluorescein staining identifies any disruption in the corneal epithelium. Owing to its serious nature, this must be regarded as a corneal infection until proven otherwise.

5. **Hyphema** may be preceded by a history of ocular trauma. Vision is impaired only with a large quantity of blood in the anterior chamber. Physical examination shows visible blood on slit lamp examination, a dilated pupil, and elevated intraocular pressure.

6. **Orbital** or **preseptal (periorbital) cellulitis** presents with visible erythema, swelling, warmth, and tenderness of the skin and soft tissues surrounding the eye. The eyelid is typically involved. Orbital cellulitis, a more serious infection, may manifest with fever, proptosis, and abnormalities of vision or pupillary response. Extraocular movements may also be limited. These findings are absent in preseptal cellulitis.

7. **Conjunctivitis** is the most common cause of eye redness and may be bacterial, viral, or allergic in etiology. Allergic conjunctivitis usually begins bilaterally, as opposed to infectious conjunctivitis, which often begins unilaterally and is then spread to the other eye due to manipulation by the patient. Itching and tearing are common. A discharge is ubiquitous—clear or watery in allergic or viral etiologies but purulent in bacterial cases. Allergic conjunctivitis may be accompanied by other allergic symptoms or physical examination findings. Although cultures of purulent discharge are often negative, it is difficult to clinically distinguish between viral and bacterial conjunctivitis. Typically, either cultures or empiric treatment with topical antibiotics was warranted. A 10-minute in-office immunoassay for adenovirus, the most common etiologic agent of viral conjunctivitis, is now available. It has high sensitivity and specificity compared with polymerase chain reaction (4). Notable exceptions to the typically benign course of infectious conjunctivitis are cases of gonococcal and chlamydial conjunctivitis. A history of exposure to genital secretions is critical, as the course of the illness and the treatment differ significantly.

8. **Episcleritis** appears similar to simple conjunctivitis. The redness may be deeper and more localized than seen in conjunctivitis. Discharge is typically absent (1).

9. **Blepharitis** presents as redness, crusting, and often as a swelling of the eyelid. It commonly occurs in combination with conjunctivitis, a **hordeolum** (with associated eyelid tenderness and possibly a visible abscess), or a **chalazion** (without associated eyelid tenderness or abscess).

10. **Dacryocystitis** presents with unilateral redness, swelling, and tenderness over the lacrimal sac, which is located inferonasal to the eye along the side of the nose. This condition is seen almost exclusively in children and in patients over the age of 40 years.

11. **Corneal abrasions**, **ulcerations**, and **foreign bodies** manifest with a foreign body sensation, eye pain, photophobia, and tearing. An examination with a slit lamp under fluorescein reveals dark green staining in areas where the corneal epithelium has been disrupted. Lid eversion is essential to search for retained foreign bodies. Corneal infections must first be excluded.

12. **Subconjunctival hemorrhage** appears as a localized reddish discoloration of the sclera due to minor trauma (including sneezing or coughing).

REFERENCES

1. Silverman MA. *Conjunctivitis.* Accessed at http://emedicine.medscape.com/article/797874-overview on May 2012.
2. Farina GA. *Red eye evaluation.* Accessed at http://emedicine.medscape.com/article/1216540-overview on May 2012.
3. Porter RS, ed. *The Merck manual of diagnosis and therapy*, 19th ed. West Point, PA: Merck & Co, 2011.
4. Sambursky R, Tauber S, Schirra F, et al. The RPS Adeno Detector for diagnosing adenoviral conjunctivitis. *Ophthalmology* 2006;113(10):1758–1764.

5.9 Scotoma

David C. Holub

I. BACKGROUND. A scotoma is a focal area of vision loss in the patient's visual field. Patients commonly refer to a scotoma as a "blind spot." Scotomata may be further categorized in several different ways.

A. A scotoma may be classified by its location in the visual field. A **central** scotoma occurs at the point of fixation and causes significant and immediately noticeable visual impairment to the patient. A **paracentral scotoma** occurs near the point of fixation and is also usually noticeable to the patient. A **peripheral scotoma** occurs away from the point of fixation at the edge of the visual field. Peripheral scotomata may be asymptomatic and only discovered on visual field testing performed for a different reason.

B. A **positive scotoma** manifests as a black spot in the patient's visual field. A **negative scotoma** manifests as a blank spot in the patient's visual field. Patients are nearly always aware of positive scotomata, but negative scotomata may only be detected during an ophthalmologic examination.

C. An **absolute scotoma** indicates a complete loss of visual perception, whereas a **relative scotoma** involves diminished but not absent light perception in the affected area. A **color scotoma** defines diminished or lost color vision only.

D. The term scintillating scotoma has come into common usage by both patients and clinicians, typically in the context of a migraine with aura. This is something of a misnomer, because scintillations and scotomata are distinct visual phenomena. That they frequently occur together in a migraine with aura has led to the origin of this term.

II. PATHOPHYSIOLOGY

A. **Etiology.** Everyone has a physiologic scotoma at the optic disc, the site where the optic nerve enters the retina. Diseases that affect the optic nerve may cause an enlargement of this scotoma to the point that it interferes with visual acuity. This manifests as a central scotoma. Diseases that affect the macula may also present with central scotoma as a prominent

TABLE 5.9.1	Causes of Central and Peripheral Scotomata	
Cause	**Optic nerve/macula**	**Retina**
Ocular disease	Primary open angle glaucoma	Retinal detachment
	Age-related macular degeneration	
Neurologic disease	Optic neuritis (secondary to multiple sclerosis)	
	Optic neuritis (idiopathic)	
Vascular disease	Temporal arteritis	Retinal vasculitis
		Retinal artery occlusion
		Retinal vein occlusion
Rheumatologic disease	Sarcoidosis with ocular infiltration	Diabetic retinopathy
Endocrine disease	Thyroid ophthalmopathy	Cytomegalovirus retinitis
Infectious disease	Ocular syphilis	
Malignancy	Optic nerve glioma	
	Optic nerve sheath meningioma	
	Intracranial tumor with optic nerve compression	
	Paraneoplastic syndromes	
Nutritional deficiency	Thiamine deficiency	
	Vitamin B12 deficiency	
	Folate deficiency	
Toxin exposure	Lead exposure	Chloroquine toxicity
	Methanol exposure	
	Ethylene glycol exposure	
	Ethambutol toxicity	
	Isoniazid toxicity	
	Digitalis toxicity	
	Amiodarone toxicity	
	Nutritional amblyopia (due to chronic tobacco or alcohol use)	

symptom. Peripheral scotomata result from disease processes that affect either the retina or the optic nerve at any point along the visual pathways. Table 5.9.1 lists the common causes of both central and peripheral scotomata.

B. Epidemiology. The incidence of scotoma varies depending upon the associated disease state. The strongest association is with optic neuritis. Sixty percent of patients with scotoma due to optic neuritis will eventually develop multiple sclerosis (1).

III. EVALUATION

A. History. Patients with a central scotoma report a visual field defect as a primary complaint. Elucidating the exact type of scotoma, as outlined in the definitions above, is important in anatomically localizing the responsible lesion. A focused history should assess for other visual disturbances such as diminished visual acuity, diminished color vision, or ocular pain. Neurologic symptoms may be found in patients with multiple sclerosis. Systemic symptoms may indicate an underlying connective tissue disease or vasculitis. The past medical history may include known neurologic or connective tissue diseases or vasculitis. A history of current and past medications is very important. Certain medications such as chloroquine/hydroxychloroquine, isoniazid, ethambutol, digitalis glycosides, and possibly amiodarone can be directly toxic to the retina or optic nerve (2). Immune suppressant medications can predispose to infections such as cytomegalovirus retinitis. A human immunodeficiency virus (HIV) infection can also predispose the patient to these infections. A history of risk factors for HIV infection should be obtained. A history of ingestion or exposure to toxins such as lead, methanol, or ethylene glycol should be obtained (2). Certain dietary practices, poor nutrition, or excessive alcohol intake may lead to thiamine or vitamin B12 deficiency.

B. Physical Examination

1. No ocular physical examination should be undertaken for any condition without first performing a test of visual acuity. This may be done with a handheld or wall-mounted Snellen eye chart. Once visual acuity has been documented, the rest of the eye examination may be undertaken.

2. Color vision should be tested with pseudoisochromatic plates (Ishihara plates are most commonly used). Diminished color vision is common in optic nerve disease, particularly red desaturation. In this condition, red-colored objects appear washed out or faded. Patients may report the color of these objects as pink or orange.

3. Pupillary testing is important, because the presence or absence of a relative afferent pupillary defect is helpful in evaluating for unilateral optic neuritis. A relative afferent pupillary defect is also known as a Marcus Gunn pupil. The testing is performed in a dimly lit room with the patient's eyes fixated on a distant object. The examiner shines a bright light into the asymptomatic eye and should observe bilateral pupillary constriction due to the consensual light reflex. The examiner then swings the flashlight across the nasal bridge to the affected eye. If there is optic nerve dysfunction in the affected eye, the pupil paradoxically dilates due to the inadequate transmission of direct light stimulation to the brain. In patients with systemic disease causing bilateral optic neuritis, an afferent pupillary defect may be absent (3).

4. A funduscopic examination is best performed after pupillary dilatation. A pale or white optic disc indicates optic neuropathy. However, the disc will not be pale in the acute setting of a first event. Only after weeks or months will the disc appear pale. Retinal hemorrhages, exudates, or retinal vasculature abnormalities may be visualized.

5. After the ocular examination is complete, a general physical examination including a complete neurologic examination should be undertaken.

6. Visual field analysis is critical in the evaluation of scotoma. Primary care clinicians seldom have the office equipment to perform this testing properly. Visual field testing by confrontation or by tangent screen examination is inadequate; patients should be referred to an eye specialist for testing with the appropriate equipment.

C. Testing. The selection of appropriate laboratory and radiographic studies should arise from the history and physical examination findings, including formal visual field testing. Blood tests such as antinuclear antibodies, rheumatoid factor, or levels of angiotensin-converting enzyme should be ordered if there is a clinical suspicion for a vasculitis or connective tissue disease. Temporal arteritis requires urgent diagnosis and an erythrocyte sedimentation rate should be ordered if this is suspected. If markedly elevated, temporal artery biopsy may be indicated. Serum vitamin B12 and red blood cell folate levels are indicated in patients with bilateral central scotoma. Serologic testing for syphilis or HIV is indicated in patients with risk factors for these infections. Thyroid function tests are appropriate in patients with ocular or systemic physical examination findings that suggest thyrotoxicosis. Serum lead levels should be measured in patients with a history of occupational or domestic lead exposure. In patients with suspected multiple sclerosis, a lumbar puncture should be considered to obtain cerebrospinal fluid for analysis of myelin basic protein and oligoclonal bands. Magnetic resonance imaging (MRI) with gadolinium is both sensitive and specific for optic neuritis. An MRI may also be useful in establishing a diagnosis of multiple sclerosis or in visualizing intracranial tumors. Some central nervous system tumors, such as optic nerve sheath meningioma, are also well visualized by computed tomography with contrast. Again, tests should be ordered only if there is a significant pretest clinical suspicion for these conditions based on the patient's history and physical examination findings.

IV. DIAGNOSIS

A. Differential Diagnosis. The approach to scotoma begins with classifying central versus peripheral scotomata. Central scotomata are attributable to optic nerve or macular disease. Peripheral scotomata are caused by retinal disease.

B. Clinical Manifestations. Scotoma presents with a visual field defect as the primary complaint. Patients with retinal diseases and glaucoma have few, if any, symptoms, except for vision loss. Patients with multiple sclerosis may also present with symptoms such as gait abnormalities, speech difficulties, difficulties with bowel and/or bladder control, weakness, or paresthesias. Jaw claudication and headache are seen in temporal arteritis. Sarcoidosis may cause fever, arthralgias, lymphadenopathy, or skin lesions.

REFERENCES

1. Riordan-Eva P. Eye. In: Tierney LM, McPhee SJ, Papadakis MA, eds. *Current medical diagnosis and treatment,* 44th ed. New York: Lange Medical Books, 2005:166.
2. Zafar A. *Toxic/nutritional optic neuropathy.* Accessed at http://emedicine.medscape.com/article/1217661-overview on May 2012.
3. Ing E. *Neuro-ophthalmic examination.* Accessed at http://emedicine.medscape.com/article/1820707-overview on May 2012.

CHAPTER 6

Ear, Nose, and Throat Problems

Frank S. Celestino

Halitosis

Mark D. Andrews

I. BACKGROUND. Halitosis (fetor oris) refers to unpleasant or offensive odors emitted from the mouth into the expired air. It may merely be a social handicap related to poor oral hygiene or oral cavity disease. Rarely, it can represent a marker of more serious systemic illness requiring diagnosis and treatment (1–3). The Greeks and Romans wrote about bad breath and it was discussed in the Jewish Talmud. Today, oral malodor has been stigmatized, giving rise to a commercial market for mints/breath fresheners exceeding $1.5 billion annually in the United States (4). Despite this publicity, patients seek help only rarely and are generally unaware of the problem, although it can severely affect interpersonal relations and self-confidence.

II. PATHOPHYSIOLOGY

A. Etiology. Physiologic halitosis, such as with eating onions and garlic or with morning breath, is temporary. These odors are reversible, transient, and responsive to traditional oral hygiene practices (3, 5). In contrast, pathologic halitosis is more intense and not easily reversible. It may arise from similar mechanisms but results more frequently from regional or systemic pathology, leading to persistent odors that ultimately may require treatment (1–4).

Persistent halitosis (usually noted by individuals around the patient) is more severe than physiologic halitosis. The most important task initially is to categorize the halitosis as either localized to the oral cavity or originating systemically. In 80–90% of patients, halitosis is due to bacterial activity from disorders of the oral cavity, and in the remainder of patients, the condition is attributed to nonoral or systemic sources (2). Volatile sulfur compounds arising through the microbial degradation of amino acids are the presumed source of most offending odors (1, 5, 6). The list of offending bacteria is extensive, including many gram-negative obligate anaerobes (1, 2). The tongue with its malodorous colonizing bacteria sheds cellular debris and decaying food and is often the chief source of oral malodor (4). Nonoral sources include nasal passages (5–8%), tonsils (3%), and other sites (2–3%) (7). In addition, the causes of halitosis can be subcategorized into pathologic and nonpathologic types.

1. Nonpathologic Causes

    a. Morning breath is due to decreased salivary flow overnight along with increased fluid pH, elevated gram-negative bacterial growth, and volatile sulfur compounds production (1, 5).

    b. Xerostomia of any cause (e.g., sleep, diseases, medication, mouth breathing, and especially age-related declines in salivary quantity and quality) can contribute to halitosis.

    c. Missed meals can lead to halitosis secondary to decreased salivary flow and the absence of the mechanical action of the food on the tongue surface to wear down filiform papillae (7).

d. Tobacco or alcohol can be a contributing cause of halitosis.

e. Metabolites from ingested food (onions, garlic, alcohol, pastrami, and other meats) are absorbed into the circulation and then excreted through the lungs.

f. Medications such as anticholinergic drugs can cause xerostomia, especially in the elderly. Other implicated agents include amphetamines, antipsychotics, antihistamines, decongestants, narcotics, antihypertensives, anti-parkinsonian agents, chemotherapy, and radiation therapy.

2. Pathologic Causes

   a. Local Oropharynx. Chronic periodontal disease and gingivitis are common sources through the promotion of bacterial overgrowth (2, 3). In their absence, the most likely oral source is the posterior dorsum of the tongue, with posterior nasal drainage being a frequent contributing factor to local bacterial overgrowth. Stomatitis and glossitis caused by systemic disease, medication, or vitamin deficiencies can lead to trapped food particles and desquamated tissue. An improperly cleaned prosthetic appliance can be a local contributor, as can primary pharyngeal cancer. Other conditions associated with parotid dysfunction (e.g., viral and bacterial infections, calculi, drug reactions, and systemic conditions including Sjögren's syndrome) are also important. Tonsils infrequently cause halitosis (found in 3% of the population), even with crypt tonsilloliths. These may alarm patients but are usually asymptomatic and not associated with any pathology.

   b. Gastrointestinal Tract. Gastrointestinal sources occasionally contribute to intermittent bad breath. Potential sources include gastroesophageal reflux disease, gastric outlet obstruction, diverticulae, gastrointestinal bleeding, gastric cancer, malabsorption syndromes, and enteric infections (1, 6, 8).

   c. Respiratory Tract. Chronic sinusitis, nasal foreign bodies or tumors, postnasal drip, bronchitis, pneumonia, bronchiectasis, tuberculosis, and malignancies may cause halitosis.

   d. Psychiatric. Halitophobia is imaginary halitosis associated with psychiatric disorders and may account for 5% of cases (1, 5).

   e. Systemic sources include diabetic ketoacidosis (sweet, fruity, acetone breath), renal failure (ammonia or "fishy" odor), hepatic failure ("fetor hepaticus"—a sweet amine odor), high fever with dehydration, and vitamin or mineral deficiencies leading to a dry mouth (1, 2, 6). Trimethylaminuria, a rare genetic disorder, causes a severe rotten fish odor from the mouth and body (1).

B. Epidemiology. The prevalence of halitosis is not known, with estimates ranging from 2 to 25% (2, 3). Most adults who worry about halitosis are not found on objective testing to have malodor (2, 3, 7); 25–40% of individuals seeking help for halitosis may be halitophobic or suffering from pseudohalitosis (7).

III. EVALUATION

A. History. Focus should be on the characteristics of the bad breath, although the patient is often unable to describe his or her condition accurately because of olfactory desensitization. Is the odor transient or constant? Constant odor suggests chronic systemic disease or serious disorders of the oral cavity. What are the precipitating, aggravating, or relieving factors? Ask about smoking habits, diet, drugs, dentures, mouth breathing, snoring, hay fever, and nasal obstruction. Because the therapy for halitosis of oral origin, beyond the limitation of aggravating factors, is proper oral hygiene and tongue brushing/scrapping, an evaluation of the patient's tooth brushing and flossing regimen is imperative.

B. Physical Examination. Ideally patients should refrain from eating, drinking, smoking, or gargling for 2 hours before examination. Emphasis is on the oral cavity, particularly looking for ulceration, dryness, trauma, postnasal drainage, infections, craniofacial anomalies, inflamed cryptic tonsils, or neoplasms. Since the primary reference standard for detecting oral malodor is the human nose, direct sniffing of expired air ("organoleptic assessment") is the most common evaluation method (3). Techniques for localizing the odor source (systemic vs. oral cavity) include (3) the following:

   1. Seal the lips and blow air through the nose. If a fetid odor is noted at a distance of 5 cm, but not detected from mouth-only testing (see point 2), then a primary nasal source is likely.

2. Pinch the nose with the lips initially closed. Hold respiration and, with nares closed, exhale gently through the mouth. Odors detected from this maneuver at a distance of 10 cm, but not from nose-only expiration, are generally mouth related.
3. If a similar odor is noted from both maneuvers above, then a systemic source should be suspected.
4. The spoon test assesses tongue-related odors. A plastic spoon is used to scrape and collect debris from the posterior tongue; 5 seconds later, spoon odor is evaluated at a distance of 5 cm.
5. The dental floss maneuver tests for interdental plaque odor. After unwaxed floss is passed between the posterior molars, smell is assessed at a distance of 3 cm.

C. **Testing.** For most patients, laboratory testing and diagnostic imaging are unnecessary and should only be pursued based on specific findings from the history and physical examination. The Schirmer's test can help to identify xerophthalmia and associated xerostomia seen with Sjögren's syndrome and other rheumatologic conditions. If indicated, radiologic studies and imaging procedures of the sinuses, thorax, and abdomen are used to identify infectious processes and neoplasms. Advanced odor detection methods—gas chromatography, sulfide detectors, and bacterial polymerase chain reaction techniques—are best reserved for research settings (7).

IV. DIAGNOSIS

A. **Differential Diagnosis.** The key is a thorough history and focused physical examination to distinguish local oral from systemic processes. Because nearly 90% of all malodorous conditions can be traced to oral causes, simple maneuvers can be diagnostically helpful in excluding the likelihood of more distant or complex systemic sources.

B. **Clinical Manifestations.** In addition to fetid odor, there may be ulceration, dryness, trauma, postnasal drainage, infections, inflamed cryptic tonsils, or neoplasms.

REFERENCES

1. Porter SR, Scully C. Oral malodour (halitosis)—clinical review. *BMJ* 2006;333(7569):632–635.
2. Hughes FJ, McNab R. Oral malodor—a review. *Arch Oral Biol* 2008;53(S1):supp S1–S7.
3. ADA Council on Scientific Affairs. Oral malodor. *J Am Dent Assoc* 2003;134:209–214.
4. Lee SS. Halitosis update—a review of causes, diagnosis and treatments. *J Calif Dent Assoc* 2007;35(4):258–268.
5. Rosenberg M. The science of bad breath. *Sci Am* 2002;286(4):58–65.
6. Armstrong BL, Sensat ML, Stoltenberg JL. *J Dent Hygiene* 2010;84(2):65–74.
7. Van den Broek AM, Feenstra L, de Baat C. A review of the current literature on management of halitosis. *Oral Dis* 2008;14(1):30–39.
8. Moshkowitz M, Horowitz N, Leshno M, Halpern Z. Halitosis and gastroesophageal reflux disease: a possible association. *Oral Dis* 2007;13(6):581–586.

6.2 Hearing Loss
Mark P. Knudson

I. **BACKGROUND.** Hearing loss (HL) occurs when there is an interruption of the complex path in which sound waves are converted to electrical impulses, transmitted to the brain, and interpreted as sound. Identification of the point of interruption is critical to the evaluation of HL.

II. **PATHOPHYSIOLOGY**

A. **Etiology.** HL can be divided into three etiologic categories: conductive hearing loss (CHL), sensorineural hearing loss (SNHL), and mixed hearing loss (MHL) (1–3). CHL results from the blockage of the canal, impairment of the tympanic membrane (TM), or the excessive impedance in the middle ear (effusion) or ossicles (otosclerosis). SNHL results from impaired function of the inner ear or cochlea, the eighth cranial nerve, or the central nervous system. MHL involves deficits in both components of hearing.

B. Epidemiology. Recent studies suggest that roughly 16% of adult Americans and more than 8% of 20- to 29-year-olds have documented HL (4). At birth, 1 in 1,000 newborns have profound HL, with an equal number having moderate HL affecting speech (4, 5). Among individuals older than 65 years of age, 7–8% report HL; yet, more than twice that number have evidence of HL when screened (3, 4). As many as 50% of Americans have evidence of HL by the time they reach 75 years of age (1, 3). Risk of HL is greatest among men, whites, certain occupations (military, firefighters, and factory workers), and in certain recreational activities (loud music and target shooting) (3, 4).

III. EVALUATION

A. History. Progression, severity, laterality, asymmetry, and associated symptoms (tinnitus, vertigo, and pain) are key differentiating features (2, 3). While patients with acute HL may present with decreased hearing, most patients with chronic loss have no specific hearing concern. They may present with social isolation, affective disorder, impaired function, and even confusion (3). Family members report slow, overly loud, or inappropriate answers as well as a tendency to monopolize or disrupt conversation or to tilt the head in conversation. CHL, while often of sudden onset from occlusion of canal or rapid collection of fluid, tends to be mild in nature. SNHL can be abrupt and severe (idiopathic and vascular), or gradual (Ménière's syndrome and acoustic neuroma) (1–3). CHL often affects the quality of hearing first, with a muffled "head in a drum" sensation. The patient may lose high-frequency and voice discrimination; however, they are still capable of detecting subtle sounds. SNHL of "sensory type" (such as impairment of the organ of Corti) results in elevated hearing threshold but maintenance of speech discrimination, while "neural type" (such as acoustic nerve damage) impairs speech discrimination (2, 3). Both types of SNHL tend to be more profound than CHL. Tinnitus is more often associated with SNHL. Vertigo reflects disturbance of the inner ear or eighth cranial nerve (e.g., Ménière disease, labyrinthitis, neoplasm, brain stem ischemia, and perilymphatic fistula). Pain or pressure may indicate trauma, infection, effusion, and rarely eighth nerve neoplasia.

B. Physical Examination

1. A simple hearing challenge may confirm HL or detect significant hearing asymmetry. Having the patient cover one ear, ask them to identify soft sounds such as the tick of a watch, the scratching of two fingers rubbed together, or a softly spoken word. Whispered voice was 90% sensitive for the detection of HL (2, 3). Inspect the ear, canal, and TM to rule out the obvious causes of CHL such as cerumen. Pneumatoscopy to demonstrate normal movement of the TM helps rule out perforation, atelectasis, Eustachian tube dysfunction, stiffened TM, and middle ear effusion (1–3).

2. Weber's test is performed with a vibrating tuning fork placed on the top of the patient's head and asked to describe the sound heard. Sound is perceived to be louder in the affected ear in CHL, because the background noise is absent on that side. The sound in the unaffected ear is perceived as louder in SNHL. Rinne's test is conducted with the vibrating tuning fork placed on the mastoid to detect bone conduction (BC) and when the patient can no longer hear the sound, the tuning fork is held next to the ear to test for air conduction (AC). In an individual with normal hearing, AC is significantly better than BC. CHL reduces AC and has little effect on BC. Recently, the accuracy and predictive values associated with these traditionally taught maneuvers has been questioned (3).

C. Testing

1. **Laboratory Testing.** A now well-established approach to childhood testing involves the use of routine screening in newborns. Auditory brain stem response and otoacoustic emissions can reliably identify early newborn HL (5, 6). For other age groups, an audiogram performed at several frequency responses is the standard to detect individuals with HL. Although the sensitivity is good (93–95%), the poor specificity (60–74%) can result in many false-positive findings (3, 5). Audiography may detect pure tone loss but may also identify impairment in speech discrimination. Pure tone testing documents

the lowest decibel sound heard at a given frequency. Unfortunately, it does not identify one's ability to discriminate language. On the other hand, speech detection can estimate the impairment of actual language function in a cooperative and attentive patient. Ultimately, audiography is recommended for anyone with a normal ear examination who endorses hearing difficulty or who fails a simple hearing challenge such as detection of whispered speech (1, 3).

Auditory-evoked response detects the electroencephalographic stimulation caused by repetitive sounds and can be useful in the obtunded, uncooperative, or very young patient.

In unexplained cases, tests for autoimmune disease, syphilis, and thyroid disease may be done.

2. Imaging. Computed tomography (CT) is fast, less expensive than magnetic resonance imaging (MRI), and is able to detect bleeding or traumatic abnormalities such as fracture within the petrous ridge (7). CHL from middle ear anomalies, myringosclerosis, and cholesteatoma may also be seen with CT. MRI with gadolinium is used in patients with SNH and is superior to a CT scan for white matter disease, vascular events, acoustic neuromas and labyrinth disorders (2, 7). High-resolution CT with contrast may be used in cases where MRI is contraindicated. Sudden profound HL or distinctly asymmetric loss with a normal ear examination requires urgent imaging (2, 3, 7).

D. Genetics. Since 1992 when the first genetic link to hearing loss was demonstrated, several hundred genetic loci have been isolated that are linked to HL (5). With the advent of universal newborn screening for HL, we have a better understanding of the frequency and onset of genetic HL (5, 6). Of newborns with proven HL, 25% are due to CHL, with roughly 15% of these from microtia or atresia of the outer or middle ear. Among the larger number with SNHL, about 25% are genetic (with more of these being nonsyndromic in nature). Most cases of genetic nonsyndromic HL are inherited in an autosomal recessive manner, and the majority result in SNHL due to cochlear defects. Common forms of adult HL such as otosclerosis and Ménière's disease may also follow a genetic pattern of inheritance.

IV. DIAGNOSIS

A. Differential Diagnosis. Common causes of SNHL include idiopathic HL, acoustic neuroma, multiple sclerosis, hypothyroidism, vertebrobasilar insufficiency, stroke, Ménière's syndrome, and rarely drug toxicity (1–3). CHL is most frequently caused by impacted cerumen, TM perforation, middle ear effusion, and otosclerosis. Rarely, tumors (e.g., squamous cell cancer, exostoses, or cholesteatoma) can cause CHL. MHL most commonly is secondary to presbycusis and noise-induced loss.

B. Clinical Manifestations. Adult patients with CHL typically present with sudden onset of unilateral and often high-frequency HL, at times associated with external ear symptoms. Patients with SNHL present more insidiously, but may progress to more complete and profound HL, and be associated with diseases of a more serious nature. As a result, screening has been advocated to detect treatable forms of HL and to identify serious underlying conditions associated with hearing impairment (1, 3). However, population-based screening recommendations vary widely among national organizations and remain controversial due to the lack of convincing evidence supporting its effectiveness (1, 3).

REFERENCES

1. Walling AD, Dickson GM. Hearing loss in older adults. *Am Fam Physician* 2012;85(12):1150–1156.
2. Isaacson B. Hearing loss. *Med Clin N Am* 2010;94:973–988.
3. Pacala JT, Yeuh B. Hearing deficits in the elderly patient. *JAMA* 2012;307(11):1185–1194.
4. Agrawal Y. Prevalence of hearing loss and differences by demographic characteristics among US adults: data from the National Health and Nutrition Examination Survey, 1999-2004. *Arch Intern Med* 2008;168(14):1522–1530.
5. Jerry J, Oghala JS. Towards an etiologic diagnosis: assessing the patient with hearing loss. *Adv Otorhinolaryngol* 2011;70:28–36.
6. U.S. Preventive Services Task Force. Universal Screening for hearing loss in newborns: U.S. Preventive Services Task Force recommendation statement. *Pediatrics* 2008;122:143–148.
7. Martin M, Hirsch B. Imaging of hearing loss. *Otol Clin N Am* 2008;41:157–178.

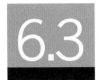

Hoarseness

David S. Jackson, Jr.

I. BACKGROUND. Hoarseness is a vocal disorder characterized by alterations in quality, pitch, loudness, or vocal effort that can impair communication and reduce quality of life (1). Vocal quality may be described as breathy, strained, rough, raspy, tremorous, strangled, or weak (2). It is a common presenting complaint to primary care providers and affects all ages. Hoarseness is a symptom and not a diagnosis. Therefore, while most cases of hoarseness are self-limiting, significant pathologic etiologies must be considered, especially in those cases lasting more than a few weeks.

II. PATHOPHYSIOLOGY. Human voice is produced by passive vibrations of the vocal folds during an airstream. Normal voice production requires several elements: an adequate air flow, intact vocal fold edges, normal vocal fold elasticity, proper fold apposition, and maintenance of internal vocal fold tension during speech (3). Hoarseness results when any of these factors are dysfunctional.

A. Etiology (1–3)

1. **Inflammatory Response.** Exposure to environmental irritants, infection, gastric secretions, and allergic response
2. **Disruption of Normal Vocal Cord Anatomy.** Vocal cord nodules, malignancy, and contact ulcers
3. **Malfunction of the Larynx**
   a. Systemic. Hypothyroidism, aging, neurologic diseases including Parkinson's disease, and multiple sclerosis
   b. Traumatic. Postintubation, direct neck trauma, and postsurgery (thyroidectomy and carotid endarterectomy)
4. **Psychogenic.** Laryngeal conversion disorder

B. Epidemiology. Hoarseness is a very common problem with a lifetime prevalence of at least 30% and a point prevalence of 7–8% (1). It is more frequent in women than in men, with a 60:40 ratio. It occurs more often at the extremes of age, with up to 23.4% of children and 47% of older adults having hoarseness at some point. Up to 7.2% of adults missed work each year related to voice problems (1). Those who extensively use their voice (e.g., teachers, singers, aerobic instructors, politicians, and telemarketers) have even higher incidences of voice abnormalities (1, 3).

III. EVALUATION

A. History. Hoarseness may be an isolated symptom, but most often is accompanied by other symptoms such as cough, runny nose, sore throat, dysphagia, and even fever. Associated symptoms such as hemoptysis, severe dysphagia, weight loss, stridor, or odynophagia are "red flags" often indicating serious underlying disease (1–3). The amount of history needed to elucidate a diagnosis is dependent on whether the symptoms are acute or chronic. The differential for acute hoarseness has a limited number of etiologies, and with a few probing questions, a diagnosis can usually be made. Chronic hoarseness has a much broader list of possibilities. More extensive inquiry including a more exhaustive review of systems is necessary. Particular attention should be paid to alcohol and smoking habits, work environment exposure to irritants (fumes, dust, etc.), reflux symptoms, and any history of environmental allergies. Review of prescription and over-the-counter medication use is necessary. Delineation of any self-therapy that the patient may have tried can be helpful (use of acid-suppressing medication for reflux symptoms).

B. Physical Examination

1. Listening to the patient's voice during the history component of the visit may give a hint as to the etiology (such as the typical "hot potato" voice of peritonsillar abscess).

A complete head and neck exam with particular attention to the oropharyngeal exam (especially the tonsillar area and posterior oropharynx), cervical lymph nodes, and the thyroid gland is essential. Auscultation of the lungs and heart can be helpful. If a more systemic process is suspected (such as Parkinson's disease or hypothyroidism), a more complete exam may be needed.

2. If there are red flag components of the history or findings on exam that suggest possible malignancy such as nontender cervical nodes, prompt visualization of the larynx is necessary. Otherwise, laryngoscopy is reserved for those patients with chronic hoarseness showing no improvement with appropriate therapy after 10–12 weeks (1). Office-based procedures described below are first options (1, 3). Operative laryngoscopy requires anesthesia and is reserved for complex cases not amenable to outpatient evaluation.

   a. Indirect visualization by mirror or rigid endoscope has a degree of patient intolerance, but with the advent of fiber-optic technology is less often used.

   b. Fiber-optic nasopharyngolaryngoscopy (with or without stroboscopic light application) allows excellent view of the larynx with simple preparation (local nasal lidocaine) and few side effects.

C. **Testing.** Specific thyroid laboratory testing is indicated if hypothyroidism is in the differential, but typically there are no other clinical lab tests needed. Scanning modalities, primarily magnetic resonance imaging, should be reserved for further evaluation of possible malignancies found on laryngoscopy or for concern for mass effects in the laryngeal area (1). Chest x-ray and computed tomography scans would be indicated for lung pathology if recurrent laryngeal nerve involvement is suspected.

IV. DIAGNOSIS

A. Differential Diagnosis (1–3)

1. **Acute.** Self-limited and lasting less than 2–3 weeks.

   a. Upper respiratory illness, typically viral. Often with associated nasal congestion, postnasal drip, sore throat, and irritative cough

   b. Voice strain. Acute (yelling, screaming, protracted coughing, frequent clearing of the throat, or episodic prolonged talking)

   c. Acute exposure to irritants (chemical fumes in the home [cleaning materials] or workplace, environmental dust, or smoke)

   d. Foreign body

2. **Chronic**

   a. Irritants
   - Exposure to chemical fumes, particulate matter (dust) in environment (home or workplace)
   - Tobacco smoke. Increased risk of neoplastic change
   - Laryngopharyngeal reflux. May have associated symptoms of cough, heartburn, or throat clearing, but often have no reflux symptoms (4).

   b. Allergic phenomenon. Direct cord edema or postnasal drainage

   c. Medication effects. May cause excessive mucosal dryness and subsequent vocal cord edema (nasal or pulmonary inhaled corticosteroids, antihistamines, decongestants, and anticholinergics)

   d. Neurologic diseases: Parkinson's disease (70–90% of patients) (5), myasthenia gravis, multiple sclerosis, and vocal cord paralysis from stroke or injury to recurrent laryngeal nerve (operative injury or irritation from Pancoast tumor)

   e. Sjögren syndrome. Related to mucosal dryness and subsequent irritation/edema of the cords

   f. Spasmodic dysphonia

   g. Hypothyroidism

   h. Benign vocal cord lesions. Nodules and polyps may be related to voice abuse, smoking, or reflux

   i. Laryngeal malignancy. It is often related to smoking and alcohol use. May wax and wane before becoming more chronic. Male to female incidence 5:1 (6)

   j. Presbyphonia (the aging voice). Vocal cord atrophic changes (7)

B. Clinical Manifestations. Patients presenting with acute hoarseness typically exhibit no overt signs other than the typical appearance of someone with an upper respiratory illness. The patient with chronic hoarseness may manifest the signs of an underlying chronic illness such as the tremor and bradykinesia of Parkinson's disease, the body habitus of the chronic bronchitic or emphysematous patient, or the edematous, depressed appearance of hypothyroidism. Red flag symptoms or painless cervical adenopathy raises the possibility of malignant disease. Laryngoscopy can define structural abnormalities including benign, premalignant, or malignant lesions as well as vocal cord dysfunction.

REFERENCES

1. Schwartz S, Cohen S, Dailey S, et al. Clinical practice guideline: hoarseness (dysphonia). *Otolaryngol Head Neck Surg* 2009;141(3S2):S1–S31.
2. Feierabend RH, Malik SN. Hoarseness in adults. *Am Fam Physician* 2009;80(4):363–370.
3. Mau T. Diagnostic evaluation and management of hoarseness. *Med Clin N Am* 2010;94:945–960.
4. Koufmann JA, Amin MA, Panetti M. Prevalence of reflux in 113 consecutive patients with laryngeal and voice disorders. *Otolaryngol Head Neck Surg* 2000;123:385–388.
5. Sewall GK, Jiang J, Ford CN. Clinical evaluation of Parkinson's-related dysphonia. *Laryngoscope* 2006;116:1740–1743.
6. Howlander N, Noone AM, Krapcho M, et al. (ed) *SEER cancer statistics review, 1975-2009 (Vintage 2009 populations)*. Retrieved from National Cancer Institute, Bethesda, MD. Accessed at http://seer.cancer.gov/csr/1975_2009_pops09/ on May 24, 2012.
7. Kendall K. Presbyphonia: a review. *Curr Opin Otolaryngol Head Neck Surg* 2007;15(3):137–140.

6.4 Nosebleed

L. Gail Curtis

I. BACKGROUND. Nosebleed, or epistaxis, is a common primary care problem, defined as the loss of blood from the mucous membranes lining the nose. Though usually mild to moderate and from a single nostril, rarely epistaxis can be life threatening. Over half the population will experience a nosebleed in their lifetime but less than 10% need or seek medical care (1).

II. PATHOPHYSIOLOGY. The nasal mucosa is highly vascularized. The blood supply to the nose arises from the internal maxillary and facial arteries as branches from the external carotid artery as well as the anterior and posterior ethmoid arteries originating from the internal carotid (2, 3). The anteroinferior septum (Little's area) is supplied by a confluence of both systems known as "Kiesselbach's plexus." Little's area is the site of >90% of epistaxis because it is ideally placed to receive environmental irritation (cold, dry air, and cigarette smoke) and is easily accessible to digital trauma (3). Fortunately, this area is easy to access and treat.

A. Etiology. Epistaxis results from an interaction of factors that damage the nasal epithelial (mucosal) lining and vessel walls. Some are local, some systemic, and some a combination of both (1–4):

1. **Environmental.** Dry air and cold ambient temperature
2. **Local.** Accidental or digital trauma, infection, allergies, foreign body, anatomic abnormalities (deviated septum), iatrogenic (surgery), and neoplasms; 80% of patients with deviated septums experience epistaxis (5).
3. **Systemic.** Hypertension, platelet and coagulation abnormalities, blood dyscrasias, disseminated intravascular coagulation, renal failure, and alcohol abuse. The role of hypertension in causing nose bleeds is controversial, with no clear independent association being established (2, 3). However, elevations in blood pressure may make epistaxis harder to control.

4. **Drugs and Herbs Affecting Clotting.** Aspirin, nonsteroidal anti-inflammatory drugs, warfarin, heparin, ticlopidine, dipyridamole, clopidogrel, ginseng, garlic, and ginkgo biloba.

5. **Other Drugs.** Thioridazine, anticholinergics (drying), corticosteroids, antihistamines, cocaine, and especially nasal steroids.

6. **Hereditary.** Hemophilia, von Willebrand's disease (VWD), and hereditary hemorrhagic telangiectasia (HHT) (Osler-Weber-Rendu). Epistaxis is the most common symptom of HHT (6).

B. **Epidemiology.** Though epistaxis is a common problem with a lifetime prevalence of 60%, <6% of people seek medical care and only a few require hospitalization (1). Nosebleeds are more common in men than in women and are increased in children less than 10 years of age and adults over age 35 years (1, 4). There is also an increased incidence during winter months (1, 2).

III. EVALUATION

A. **History.** Initial history should include onset, duration, quantity, and location, particularly whether one or both nostrils are affected. A detailed personal and family history looking for possible precipitating factors (see Section II.A) should be taken (1, 2, 7). It is also important to inquire about chronic medical conditions that could be contributory, including a history of blood dyscrasias, hypertension, liver disease, alcohol, and drug use (especially inhaled drugs). In children with epistaxis with unilateral nasal discharge or foul odor, suspect an intranasal foreign body.

B. **Physical Examination.** The nasal examination should focus on identifying the bleeding site. Topical sprays of anesthetics and vasoconstrictors can be used to help control the bleeding and allow for visualization (1). As mentioned, Little's area accounts for most epistaxis, but approximately 10% of nosebleeds originate from a posterior nasal source and often manifest as bilateral bleeding with posterior drainage (1, 3). It can be far more challenging to identify a source of epistaxis in this area. Providing effective treatment for obstinate bleeding in this area may also be more uncomfortable for the patient and more formidable for the health provider.

1. When examining the patient with epistaxis, first assess the vital signs for hypotension, orthostasis, and hemodynamic instability. After examining the face for any obvious signs of recent injury, it is important to visualize as much of the nasal vestibule as possible. It is imperative to keep the patient's head upright, for if he or she tilts backward, only the roof of the nasal cavity is seen. The nasal speculum should be utilized and held in a horizontal position to avoid iatrogenic trauma from the speculum blades and to allow an optimal view of the nasal septum.

2. Illumination of the area is key for visualization of the bleeding. This can be performed by the direct illumination of the area or if available by indirect illumination using a head mirror. Suction may be needed to remove clots, fresh blood, or mucus to help visualize the bleeding site. Endoscopic exam provides the best visualization. In addition to aiding diagnosis particularly of posterior bleeds or unexpected etiologies, endoscopy can allow cauterization of bleeding sites and avoidance of nasal packing (3).

3. Depending on the patient's history, a more general examination may be needed with a focus on the skin to look for petechiae, telangiectasias, hemangiomas, and ecchymoses.

C. **Testing**

1. **Laboratory Tests.** If bleeding is minor and not recurring, no testing is needed. For vigorous bleeding or recurrent epistaxis, order a complete blood count (CBC) with platelet count, and possibly blood type and crossmatch for hypovolemic shock or severe anemia. Unless dictated by the patient's history, coagulation tests such as bleeding time, prothrombin time, and partial thromboplastin time, though often obtained, have no evidence-based support in working up epistaxis (8). The CBC can also detect blood dyscrasias. If concern for VWD exists, specific VWD factors should be tested.

2. **Imaging.** Limited computed tomography of the nose and sinuses is appropriate if concern exists for benign neoplasms or malignancy. Rarely, angiography may also be indicated for diagnosing (and treating) vascular lesions.

IV. DIAGNOSIS

A. Differential Diagnosis. For unexplained and poorly responsive persistent or recurrent nosebleeds, it is important to look further for the underlying cause. In this circumstance, further evaluation with expedient laboratory testing, nasal endoscopy, appropriate imaging, or further consultation is needed to rule out more serious or malignant causes. Rare causes of epistaxis include potentially life-threatening posttraumatic pseudoaneurysm of the internal carotid artery. This entity presents from days to weeks after initial trauma to the base of the skull with a classic triad of unilateral blindness, orbital fractures, and massive epistaxis (9). Finally, although the obstruction of air movement is the most common presenting symptom of intranasal neoplasms, patients may also present with epistaxis and/or nasal pain (2, 3).

B. Clinical Manifestations. Bleeding from one or both nostrils occurs, with associated frequent swallowing and sensation of fluid in the back of the nose and/or throat. If there is severe bleeding or marked anemia, patients may experience weakness, presyncope, fatigue, and even hemodynamic instability (2, 3, 7).

REFERENCES

1. Schlosser RJ. Epistaxis. *N Engl J Med* 2009;360:784–789.
2. Manes RP. Evaluation and management of the patient with nosebleeds. *Med Clin N Am* 2010;94: 903–912.
3. Gifford TO, Orlandi RR. Epistaxis. *Otol Clin N Am* 2008;41:525–536.
4. Kucik C, Clenney T. Management of epistaxis. *Am Fam Physician* 2005;71(2):305–311.
5. O'Reilly BJ, Simpson DC, Dharmeratnam R. Recurrent epistaxis and nasal septal deviation in young adults. *Clin Otolaryngol* 1996;21:82–84.
6. Sharathkumar A, Shapiro A. Hereditary haemorrhagic telangiectasia. *Haemophilia* 2008; 14(6): 1269–1280.
7. Mulla O, Prowre S, Sanders T, Nix P. Epistaxis. *BMJ* 2012;344:e1097.
8. Shakeel M, Trinidade A, Iddamalgoda T, Supriya M, Ah-See KW. Routine clotting screen has no role in the management of epistaxis. *Eur Arch Otorhinolaryngol* 2010;267:1641–1644.
9. Fontela PS, Tampieri D, Atkinson JD, Daniel SJ, Teitelbaum J. Posttraumatic pseudoaneurysm of the intracavernous internal carotid artery presenting with massive epistaxis. *Pediatr Crit Care Med* 2006;7(3):260–262.

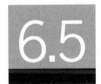

Pharyngitis
Richard W. Lord

I. BACKGROUND. Pharyngitis, commonly called sore throat (ST), is a painful infectious, inflammatory, or irritative process of the pharynx that is composed of the oropharynx (including tonsils), nasopharynx, and hypopharynx. ST is one of the most common reasons for adults and children to seek care from a primary care physician (1). Although the differential diagnosis of ST includes a wide range of entities, the most common cause in immunocompetent individuals is acute infectious pharyngitis, predominantly viral (2, 3). Despite this fact, pharyngitis is a too frequent reason for antibiotic prescription (2, 4). Inappropriate use of antibiotics can have negative consequences for individuals and the public's health. Therefore, it is important for clinicians to develop an approach for identifying the minority of individuals with pharyngitis caused by group A beta-hemolytic streptococcus (GABHS) who require antibiotics.

II. PATHOPHYSIOLOGY. Sensory innervation to the pharynx is provided by the glossopharyngeal and vagus nerves that also supply sensation to the ear; hence, referred otalgia can be seen even though the primary process involves the throat (2). As noted below, a variety of pathologic processes can result in stimulation of the throat's nociceptive nerve endings.

A. **Etiology** (2–4)

1. **Infectious**. Viral (many types), influenza, human immunodeficiency virus, mononucleosis, herpangina, nonstreptococcal bacterial (diphtheria in unimmunized, gonorrhea, syphilis, fusospirochetal infection/Vincent's angina), chlamydia pneumoniae, and mycoplasma pneumoniae), group A streptococcal, pertonsillar abcess, tonsillitis, thrush, retropharyngeal abscess, epiglottitis, and fungal laryngitis.

2. **Inflammatory/Mechanical.** Laryngopharyngeal reflux, allergic rhinitis with postnasal drip, chronic mouth breathing, foreign body (globus pharyngeus), vocal cord granuloma, mucositis, granulomatous disease, pemphigus, and Kawasaki disease.

3. **Neoplastic.** Squamous cell carcinoma, lymphoma, and sarcoma.

Most of the pathologies mentioned above are quite rare. In contrast, depending on the age group studied, 50–80% of ST is due to common respiratory viruses while 5–30% (5–15% in adults and 15–30% in children) results from GABHS (2, 4, 5); 1–10% of pharyngitis cases are due to infectious mononucleosis (IM) and nonstreptococcal bacteria. The early identification and treatment of GABHS helps prevent rheumatic fever, provide symptomatic relief, reduces suppurative complications, and decreases infectivity (4, 5).

B. **Epidemiology.** Pharyngitis is the sixth most common reason for seeing a physician and accounts for approximately 5% of all primary care office visits (1). In 2006, there were 15 million visits for ST at a cost of over $300 million (2, 4). Data show that the probability of GABHS pharyngitis in primary care peaks between 5 and 15 years of age (4, 5); 43% of families with an index case of GABHS will have a secondary case. IM as a cause of ST peaks between 15 and 30 years of age (2, 6).

With infectious ST, transmission occurs mostly by hand contact with nasal discharge rather than by contact with oral secretions (2, 3). Symptoms typically occur 48– 72 hours later. Although pharyngitis can occur at anytime during the year, there is a peak in the winter and early spring in temperate climates (2).

III. **EVALUATION.** The goal of the evaluation is to differentiate those patients who are likely to have an infectious cause of pharyngitis and need laboratory testing and those who have noninfectious causes. A secondary goal is to identify those few patients with serious and potentially life-threatening processes like abscesses and neoplasms. A rigorous history, physical examination, and appropriate diagnostic laboratory tests are used to accomplish these goals.

A. **History**

1. **The onset and duration** of the ST can help differentiate infectious from noninfectious causes. Typically, the onset of infectious causes is abrupt and lasts for 7–10 days. Often with noninfectious causes, the onset of symptoms is unclear and often persists for more than 3 weeks.

2. **Associated symptoms** can also give clues to the cause of the ST (2, 3). Fever, cough, headache, and other constitutional symptoms are the hallmarks of an infectious etiology. Symptoms of allergies, heartburn, and depression point to noninfectious causes. Any history of seasonal allergies, trauma, malignancy, radiation therapy, inhalation, ingestion, or thyroid dysfunction also suggests noninfectious causes.

3. **GABHS features** (4, 5). If infection is believed to be the cause of the ST, the focus is then on trying to differentiate GABHS from other bacterial and viral causes. Classically, GABHS pharyngitis is severe and of acute (<1 day) onset and accompanied by fever (temperature >101°F [38.33°C]), painful swallowing, tender anterior cervical adenopathy, and sometimes myalgias, but not by cough or rhinitis. Headache, nausea, vomiting, and abdominal pain may be seen as well, especially in children. Conversely, the gradual onset of mild ST accompanied by rhinorrhea, cough, hoarseness, conjunctivitis, or diarrhea in an afebrile patient speaks strongly for a viral cause. Despite these broad generalizations, classic symptom complexes alone are neither sensitive nor specific enough to rely on for judging the need for antibacterial treatment (3, 5, 7, 8).

4. **Red flags** (2, 3). Severe underlying illness is suggested when ST is accompanied by stridor, unstable vital signs, weight loss, "hot potato" voice, and immunocompromised state.

B. **Physical Examination.** The physical examination should include assessing vital signs (especially temperature) and examining the head, eyes, ears, nose, throat, neck, and skin.

Findings classically associated with GABHS infection include palatal petechiae, intense ("beefy red") tonsillopharyngeal erythema with exudates, tender anterior cervical adenopathy, and a scarlatiniform rash. Conversely, the absence of these features, along with the presence of rhinitis, hoarseness, conjunctivitis, stomatitis, discrete ulcerative lesions, or a typical viral exanthem, points toward a viral cause. In IM, the classic features of GABHS are often combined with posterior cervical or generalized lymphadenopathy and hepatosplenomegaly. However, once again, none of these physical findings in and of themselves have sufficiently high sensitivity and specificity to rely on for accurate diagnosis (7, 8). An abdominal examination is dictated either by gastrointestinal symptoms or by the presence of severe fatigue with posterior cervical adenopathy (suggesting IM). A cough or a fever should lead to a pulmonary examination. A cardiac examination is important for toxic-appearing patients.

C. **Testing.** The two tests typically used in the diagnosis of pharyngitis are the throat culture (TC) and the rapid streptococcal antigen detection test (RSADT) (4, 5). Recently, polymerase chain reaction (PCR) testing has become available for diagnosing GABHS (3, 4, 6). PCR may ultimately replace culture, but for now is relegated to research studies.

   1. The sensitivity of an appropriately obtained (vigorously swabbing both tonsils and posterior pharynx) TC is 90–95% (2, 4, 5). Unfortunately, the TC does not reliably distinguish between an acute GABHS infection and a streptococcal carrier state with concomitant viral infection. A negative TC does permit the withholding of antimicrobial therapy (i.e., specificity = 0.99) (2, 4, 5).

   2. Although methods vary, RSADTs do have high degrees of specificity (92–95%) (4, 5). Their sensitivity in routine clinical practice is variable (60–85%) (4, 5). Therefore, in the past, the recommendation had been to follow up a negative antigen test with a backup TC. Newer guidelines (2–6) have been developed that base treatment decisions only on the RSADTs without follow cultures for negative rapid tests. RSADTs suffer the same limitation as TCs in the presence of carrier states.

   3. Streptococcal antibody titers are of no immediate value in the diagnosis of acute GABHS pharyngitis. If IM is suspected, a complete blood count and heterophil antibody testing can reliably confirm the diagnosis if the patient is in the second week of illness.

   4. Generally, no other testing is needed unless a serious suppurative sequela is suspected (e.g., retropharyngeal abscess), in which case radiologic imaging should be pursued (2, 3).

IV. DIAGNOSIS
A. Differential Diagnosis
   1. Recent guidelines (2–6) have called for the use of specific criteria to estimate the probability of diagnosing GABHS. One popular set, the Centor criteria (4, 5), includes the following: tonsillar exudates, tender anterior cervical lymphadenopathy, and absence of cough and history of fever. The positive predictive value of three or four of these criteria is 40–60%. The absence of three or four of these criteria has a negative predictive value of 80% (3–5). The following principles are put forth in these guidelines.
      a. Clinically, screen all adult patients with pharyngitis using the Centor criteria.
      b. Do not test or treat patients with none or only one of these criteria.
      c. For patients with two or more criteria, the following options have been defined.
         i. Test patients with two, three, or four of the criteria and treat only those with positive RSADTs.
         ii. Test patients with two or three criteria and treat those with positive RSADTs or those with four criteria.
         iii. Do not use any diagnostic tests and only treat patients with three or four criteria.
      d. Do not perform follow-up TCs on patients with negative RSADTs when the sensitivity is >80%.
   2. Other scoring systems have also been developed that incorporate the patient's age generalizing the use of these to children and adults (2–5). This system gives 1 point for each of the Centor criteria present, and then adds 1 point for age less than 15 years, 0 points for age 15–45 years, and –1 for age greater than 45 years. This guideline recommends the following strategy: 0–1 points, no treatment or testing is needed; 1–3 points, treat

those with positive RSADTs; 4–5 points, treat empirically. Note that for a score of 1, clinicians are given two options under this guideline.

3. The goal of these scoring systems is to help reduce the overuse of antibiotics in treating pharyngitis. Studies estimated that use of these scoring rubrics could decrease inappropriate antibiotic use by 60–88% (2–4). Simply trying to use clinical judgment without a clinical prediction rule is not considered good practice (3, 7, 8).

B. Clinical Manifestations. The primary manifestation is throat and anterior neck pain accompanied by some degree of painful swallowing. Other symptoms, depending on the underlying etiology, may include fever, nausea, vomiting, fatigue, rash, ear pain, and even abdominal discomfort. Signs may range from minimal or no pharyngeal erythema and exudate to severe suppurative findings, including marked cervical adenopathy. Tonsillar abscess formation causes swelling and deviation of the soft palate with malodorous breath. Epiglottitus, peritonsillar abscesses, and retropharyngeal abscesses are often associated with a "hot potato" voice.

REFERENCES

1. Woodwell DA, Cherry DK. National ambulatory medical care survey: 2002 summary. Hyattsville, MD: National Center for Health Statistics. *Adv Data* 2004;346:1–44.
2. Chan TV. The patient with sore throat. *Med Clin N Am* 2010;94:923–943.
3. Pelluchi G, Grigoryan L, Galeone C, et al. European Society for Clinical Microbiology and Infectious Diseases: guideline for management of acute sore throat. *Clin Microbiol Infect* 2012;18(Supp 1): S1–S27.
4. Wessels M. Streptococcal pharyngitis. *N Engl J Med* 2011;364:648–655.
5. Choby BA. Diagnosis and treatment of streptococcal pharyngitis. *Am Fam Physician* 2009;79(5): 383–390.
6. Institute for Clinical Systems Improvement (ICSI). Diagnosis and treatment of respiratory illness in children and adults, Jan 2011. Accessed at http://www.icsi.org on July 8, 2012.
7. Shaikh N, Swaminathan N, Hooper EG. Accuracy and precision of the signs and symptoms of streptococcal pharyngitis in children: a systematic review. *J Pediatr* 2012;160(3):487–493.
8. Aalbers J, O'Brien KK, Chan WS, et al. Predicting streptococcal pharyngitis in adults in primary care: a systematic review of the diagnostic accuracy of symptoms and signs and validation of the Centor score. *BMC Med* 2011;9:67–77.

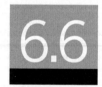

Rhinitis

Carmen G. Strickland and Brenda Latham-Sadler

I. BACKGROUND. Rhinitis refers to a constellation of symptoms including rhinorrhea, nasal congestion, sneezing, nasal pruritus, and postnasal drainage. Although often viewed mistakenly as a trivial illness, rhinitis is responsible for significant morbidity, medical costs, reduced work productivity, and lost school days. There is also increasing recent evidence that aggressive management of rhinitis improves asthma therapy outcomes (1).

II. PATHOPHYSIOLOGY. Regardless of the triggers, the nose has a limited repertoire of responses that primarily serve to protect the lower respiratory track. Symptoms of allergic rhinitis (AR) result from a complex allergy-driven mucosal inflammation caused by interaction between inflammatory cells and a number of vasoactive and proinflammatory mediators including cytokines (1, 2). Sensory nerve activation, plasma leakage, and venous sinusoid congestion contribute. In contrast, nonallergic rhinitis (NAR) is not an immunoglobulin E (IgE)-dependent or primarily inflammatory process. The exact stimulus in NAR causing excessive cholinergic glandular secretion is unknown, but enhanced vagal activity is important. Ultimately, rhinitis involves pathologic interplay between vascular and neurologic systems (2, 3).

A. Etiology (1, 3–5)

1. **Allergic. (AR)** Seasonal, perennial, episodic
2. **Infectious.** Acute versus chronic, viral versus bacterial
3. **Nonallergic. (NAR)**
   a. **Drug-induced.** Oral contraceptives, hormone replacement therapy, erectile dysfunction drugs, some antihypertensives, ophthalmic β-blockers, local decongestants or intranasal cocaine (rhinitis medicamentosa), aspirin and nonsteroidal anti-inflammatory drugs (especially in patients with asthma and/or chronic rhinosinusitis), some antidepressants, and benzodiazepines
   b. **Atrophic rhinitis.** Extensive surgery
   c. **Gustatory rhinitis.**
   d. **Physical/chemical exposures.** Occupational, pollution, dry air, bright light
   e. **Vasomotor rhinopathy.** Irritant triggers (strong odors, tobacco, alcohol), cold air, exercise
   f. **Associated with a systemic condition.** Menstrual cycling, pregnancy, hypothyroidism, autoimmune disorders, amyloidosis, acquired immunodeficiency syndrome, primary mucociliary defects, cystic fibrosis, antibody deficiency, granulomatous disease, sarcoidosis
   g. **NARES**. (nonallergic rhinitis with eosinophilia syndrome)
   h. **Miscellaneous.** Foreign body, nasal polyp, septal deviation, neoplasm, enlarged adenoids or tonsils, recent head trauma with cerebrospinal fluid leak, autonomic dysfunction, senile rhinitis
4. **Mixed**. AR and NAR components

B. Epidemiology. Rhinitis affects 1 in 5 adults and nearly one-third of children (1). It is associated with an average of 5.67 missed days of work annually (6). For all age groups, the rate of AR to NAR is 3:1. In adults, the most common form is AR (43%) followed by NAR (34%) (1); 27% of adults will have mixed causes (2). In 2002, total direct and indirect costs of care were nearly 12 billion dollars (1). Worldwide, the prevalence of all forms of rhinitis is increasing.

III. EVALUATION. The goal of evaluation is to determine whether rhinitis symptoms are caused by allergy, infection, nonallergic triggers, anatomic abnormalities, systemic processes, or some combination of these.

A. History. What are the specific symptoms (i.e., stuffiness, itching, clear, or purulent drainage), and what does the patient believe is causing the symptoms? Are the symptoms unilateral or bilateral? Allergy and viral infections produce bilateral nasal complaints, whereas most rhinitis relating to the structural problems of the nose is unilateral. When did the symptom(s) begin? How often and when do the symptoms occur? Do they predominate at certain times of the year? What other symptoms are associated? What makes the symptoms better or worse? Associated complaints (e.g., frank fatigue, irritability, depression, or chest symptoms) suggest untreated allergic causes, systemic disease, or drug-induced illness. Include questions about atopic disease, history of allergies, asthma, nasal surgery, and prescription medication use. Address tobacco (personal or secondary exposure), alcohol or recreational drug use, over-the-counter medication, herbal remedies, and pets in the home. Are there suspected environmental irritants? Is there a family history of allergies or other relevant systemic diseases?

B. Physical Examination. A general inspection of the patient frequently offers clues to the cause. "Allergic shiners" (infraorbital, bluish discoloration of the skin) or a crease at the lower part of the nose from repeated rubbing are common physical findings of AR. Assessing vital signs and examining the ears, nose, and throat along with cervical lymph nodes and the thyroid will help sort out the source of symptoms. Perform anterior rhinoscopy of nasal passages using a nasal speculum (a 4–5 mm ear speculum on a handheld otoscope is acceptable) and a good light source. Assess for nasal patency, mucosal color (pale, red, or bluish), the degree and location of edema, the presence and type of nasal drainage (thin, clear, thick, purulent, unilateral, or bilateral), anatomic deformities (bone spurs and septal deviation), and the presence of polyps or other masses. Examine the lungs and the skin for signs of atopic disease (wheezing or eczema). If systemic illness is suggested after focused examination, a thorough multisystem exam is necessary.

C. Testing. Rhinitis is typically diagnosed and treated on the basis of history and exam findings without need for additional testing. Skin testing for IgE-mediated sensitivity is reserved for resistant AR, diagnostic uncertainty, confirmation of avoidance measures, or prior to desensitization immunotherapy (1, 2). Fiber-optic nasal endoscopy can help in difficult diagnostic cases or with anatomic variants. Nasal smears for eosinophils are best used in patients positive for AR but skin test is negative (1). Referral is indicated if serious pathology is suspected or found, if physical examination is difficult secondary to nasal obstruction, or if the symptoms do not improve with empiric treatment. If an anatomic abnormality or chronic sinus pathology is suspected, limited computed tomography of the face sinuses is recommended (1, 6).

IV. DIAGNOSIS

A. Differential Diagnosis. Allergic and other noninfectious causes of rhinitis are typically associated with clear rhinorrhea. To distinguish between AR and NAR, focus on the symptoms of sneezing, clear drainage, postnasal drip, itching, nasal congestion, specific irritants or allergens, and family and personal history of atopy and allergy (1, 6). Next, consider seasonal, perennial, or geographic relationships. The presence of blue or pale boggy turbinates with clear drainage suggests an allergic process. A physical examination should confirm the patient's story and help identify any anatomic defects or systemic disease. Response to therapy is also helpful in confirming the suspected diagnosis. Remain vigilant for contributing conditions such as polyps, structural abnormalities, neoplasia, severe reflux, and systemic diseases. Several follow-up visits may be necessary to assess, treat, and educate patients with rhinitis and to confirm any need for further evaluation or treatment by an otolaryngologist or allergist (6).

Infectious viral rhinitis produces nasal drainage with associated symptoms of generalized head or body aches, nasal congestion, diffuse sinus pressure, and sneezing. Viral etiology explains the vast majority of infectious rhinitis; only 0.5–2.0% of acute infectious rhinitis has a bacterial etiology (1). Complicating bacterial infection (rhinosinusitis) is associated with facial pressure and localized pain over a maxillary sinus or the upper teeth. Edematous, erythematous turbinates are suggestive of an infectious etiology of rhinitis. Expert panels have concluded that neither nasal mucus color nor the presence of fever is useful in differentiating bacterial from viral disease (1, 2).

B. Clinical Manifestations. In addition to the classical symptoms of rhinitis, patients may manifest an array of associated symptoms to include cough, itchy eyes, facial pressure, voice changes, headaches, fatigue, irritability, poor concentration, and sleep disordered breathing (1).

REFERENCES

1. The Joint Task Force on Practice Parameters in Allergy, Asthma and Immunology. The diagnosis and management of rhinitis: an updated practice parameter. *J Allergy Clin Immunol* 2008;122:S1–S84.
2. Weber RW. Allergic rhinitis. *Primary Care Clin Office Pract* 2008;35(1):1–10.
3. Fletcher R. An overview of rhinitis. Accessed at http://www.UpToDate.com on March 26, 2012.
4. Kaliner MA. Non allergic rhinopathy (vasomotor rhinitis). *Immunol Alllergy Clin N Am* 2011;31(3): 441–455.
5. Settipane RA. Other causes of rhinitis: mixed rhinitis, rhinitis medicamentosum, hormonal, rhinitis of the elderly and gustatory rhinitis. *Immunol Allergy Clin N Am* 2011;31(3):457–467.
6. Quillen DM, Feller DB. Diagnosing rhinitis: allergic vs. nonallergic. *Am Fam Physician* 2006;73(9):1583–1590.

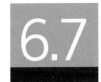

6.7 Stomatitis

Sandra B. Farland and Bradley H. Evans

I. BACKGROUND. Stomatitis, generally referred to as lesions or inflammation in the mouth, represents a broad category of oral mucosal infections, inflammatory conditions, and other oral lesions. Because of possible malignancy, persistent lesions require definitive diagnosis.

II. PATHOPHYSIOLOGY

A. Etiology. Causes of oral lesions include the following: (i) premalignant or malignant lesions related to tobacco or alcohol use (leukoplakia, erythroplasia, and oral cancer); (ii) human immunodeficiency virus (HIV)-related lesions (e.g., Kaposi's sarcoma and oral hairy leukoplakia); (iii) infections that may be bacterial (e.g., necrotizing ulcerative gingivitis, syphilis), viral (e.g., herpes simplex virus [HSV], hand-foot-and-mouth disease, and herpangina), or fungal (e.g., thrush, angular cheilitis, and denture stomatitis); (iv) ulcerative and erosive conditions (e.g., recurrent aphthous ulcers, Behçet's disease, inflammatory bowel related, and Reiter's syndrome); (v) traumatic and irritant lesions (chronic cheek biting, chemical exposures, and burns from hot food); (vi) drug-related eruptions (Stevens-Johnson syndrome, chemotherapy-associated mucositis); and (vii) non-ulcerative lesions related to more generalized disease (e.g., discoid lupus, Darier's disease, lichen planus, pemphigus, and pemphigoid) (1–4).

B. Epidemiology. Oral lesions are more common in the adult population than tension headaches, phlebitis, or arthralgias. In the third National Health and Nutrition Examination survey, oral lesions were found in 27.9% of the adult population and 10.3% of children (5).

III. EVALUATION

A. History. The history should describe the lesion and the potential risk factors for its etiology. Describe the onset: was it abrupt, suggesting an infection, or insidious, suggesting an inflammatory or neoplastic origin? Are there associated signs and symptoms? Many oral infections are associated with pain, malaise, and fever. Behçet's disease has associated ocular and genital lesions, whereas other autoimmune diseases such as systemic lupus erythematosus (SLE) or ulcerative colitis may have systemic symptoms (1–3). Describe the lesions: are they painful or painless? Infections, inflammatory lesions, and aphthous ulcers are usually painful (1, 2, 4), whereas premalignant and malignant lesions may be painless (3, 6). Are there vesicles or bullae? Pemphigoid and pemphigus may cause bullae and/or ulcers. HSV starts as vesicular lesions and then ulcerates. Varicella zoster lesions can occur in the mouth (1, 4, 6). Did vesicles precede the lesions suggesting HSV or was there ulceration without vesicles, suggesting aphthous ulcers (1, 2, 4)? Are the lesions that will not wipe off the mucosa white? Leukoplakia, a premalignant lesion, is white and will not wipe off. Any coexisting red component, called *erythroplasia*, greatly increases the malignant potential of the lesion (2, 3, 7). Lichen planus also produces a striated white lesion, usually on the buccal mucosa (1). Where are the lesions? HSV tends to occur on periosteally bound mucosa (gingiva and hard palate), whereas recurrent aphthous ulcers occur on nonperiosteally bound mucosa (buccal, lip, or tongue mucosa) (1, 2, 4). The floor of the mouth under the tongue, the lateral aspects of the tongue, the retromolar regions, and the soft palate are worrisome areas for malignancy to develop (3, 7), but malignancy can occur anywhere.

Past medical history is also important. Systemic inflammatory conditions such as SLE or lichen planus can produce oral ulcerations. Recurrence suggests aphthous ulcers and HSV. Dentures increase the susceptibility to denture stomatitis or angular cheilitis, both caused by *Candida* species (1, 3, 7). HIV increases the likelihood of oral hairy leukoplakia, Kaposi's sarcoma, and severe oral candidiasis. Exposure to individuals with similar symptoms suggests enteroviral infections such as herpangina and hand-foot-and-mouth disease.

Medications such as sulfonamides and many other drugs can cause Stevens-Johnson syndrome, whereas chemotherapy for the treatment of cancer can produce severe mucositis. Social history should focus on alcohol and tobacco use, exposures to oral irritants, and sexual activity, including oral-genital sexual contact (1, 2, 7).

B. **Physical Examination**

1. **Head, eyes, ears, nose, throat (HEENT).** Based on the history, a focused physical examination of the HEENT is necessary. Look for signs of trauma. Examine the conjunctiva and nasal mucosa for inflammatory changes or ulcerations. Evaluate the patient for coexisting upper respiratory signs and symptoms such as rhinorrhea, sinus tenderness to palpation, and otitis media. Inspect facial skin for vesicles from HSV or varicella zoster or other lesions such as ecchymoses, a malar rash, or a viral exanthem. Evaluate preauricular, postauricular, and cervical lymph node chains. Finally, evaluate the oral cavity, documenting the size, location, and appearance of the lesion.

2. **Additional Physical Examination.** Based on the results of the HEENT examination and the patient's specific history, additional physical examination might include (i) pulmonary examination for viral pneumonitis or findings in autoimmune diseases; (ii) abdominal and rectal examination for Crohn's disease or ulcerative colitis; (iii) genitourinary examination for mucosal ulcers in Behçet's disease and Stevens-Johnson syndrome, as well as signs of syphilis or gonorrhea; (iv) a skin examination looking for viral exanthems, drug eruptions, lichen planus, pemphigus, pemphigoid, and SLE; and (v) a musculoskeletal examination for signs of SLE, Reiter's syndrome, or other autoimmune diseases (7).

C. **Testing**

1. Clinical laboratory testing should be guided by the history and physical findings. A potassium hydroxide wet mount is useful in the diagnosis of candidiasis. Viral and bacterial cultures can be obtained from swabs of oral lesions, but viral cultures are usually more helpful than bacterial cultures. Darkfield microscopy can be performed from swabs of syphilis chancres or plaques. Incisional biopsy, as well as direct or indirect immunofluorescence, may be helpful to delineate desquamative gingivitis and vesiculobullous lesions (1, 3). Cytologic scrapings of premalignant or malignant lesions, prepared in a manner similar to a Papanicolaou smear, are not a substitute for a biopsy of suspected oral neoplasia (1, 3, 6, 7). The presence of leukoplakia, erythroplakia, or any non-healing persistent ulcer mandates biopsy (2, 3, 6).

2. Diagnostic imaging is rarely indicated. It may prove useful in selected cases such as complicating sinus disease ("mini" sinus computed tomography [CT] scan), coexisting neck mass or lymphadenopathy suspicious for malignant disease (head and neck CT scan), suspected metastatic disease (chest x-ray, CT scan of the head, abdomen, and chest), or trauma (cervical spine series, cranial CT scan, dental Panorex films) (2, 3). A chest x-ray is indicated in suspected viral or autoimmune pneumonitis or in secondary bacterial pneumonia.

D. **Genetics** may play a role in the susceptibility to aphthous ulcers and autoimmune disorders.

IV. DIAGNOSIS

A. **Differential Diagnosis** of stomatitis includes lesions in the six categories listed in Section II.A. The diagnosis depends on the synthesis of the key historical and physical examinations, as well as the laboratory and imaging elements. All oral ulcers that do not heal, as well as white or reddish-white lesions that do not resolve in 2–3 weeks, require biopsy to rule out malignancy (2, 3, 6).

B. **Clinical Manifestations.** Stomatitis manifests as lumps, ulcerations, or discolored patches that may be painful or painless depending on the underlying pathology.

REFERENCES

1. Bruce AJ, Rogers RS III. Acute oral ulcers. *Dermatol Clin* 2003;21:1–15.
2. Aragon SB, Jafek BW, Johnson, S. Stomatitis. In: Bailey BJ, Johnson JT, eds. *Head & neck surgery—otolaryngology.* Lippincott Williams & Wilkins, 2006:579–599.

3. Chan MH. Biopsy techniques, diagnosis and treatment of mucocutaneous lesions. *Dent Clin N Am* 2012:56(1):43–73.
4. Gonsalves WC, Chi AC, Neville BW. Common oral lesions: part 1. superficial mucosal lesions. *Am Fam Physician* 2007;75(4):501–506.
5. Shulman JD, Beach MM, Rivera-Hidalgo F. The prevalence of oral mucosal lesions in U.S. adults: data from the third national health and nutrition examination survey, 1988-1994. *J AM Dent Assoc* 2004;135(9):1279–1286.
6. Gonsalves WC, Wrightson AS, Henry RG. Common oral conditions in older persons. *Am Fam Physician* 2008;78(7):845–852.
7. Porter SR, Leao JC. Review article: oral ulcers and its relevance to systemic disorders. *Aliment Pharmacol Ther* 2005;21:295–306.

6.8 Tinnitus

Lisa Cassidy-Vu and Christy J. Thomas

I. BACKGROUND. Tinnitus is sound perceived by a patient in the absence of an external acoustic stimulus. Tinnitus, meaning "to ring," can be described as buzzing, humming, ringing, whistling, or hissing (1, 2). The perceived noise can be described as being within or around the head, in one or both ears or from a distant point, and can be continuous or intermittent, steady or pulsatile (1, 3, 4). Pulsatile tinnitus raises more concerns for underlying significant pathology than does non-pulsatile. Bilateral intermittent non-pulsatile tinnitus is rarely associated with serious disease, whereas unilateral ringing is more worrisome (1, 2, 4). Because tinnitus is usually a subjective experience, evaluation and monitoring rely heavily on self-report by the patient.

II. PATHOPHYSIOLOGY

A. Etiology. Tinnitus is not a disease in itself, but rather a symptom of some other ongoing process, pathologic or benign. Many theories have been proposed as to the pathogenesis of this phenomenon, including but not limited to disruption of normal auditory feedback loops, repetitive discharging of injured cochlear hair cells causing continuous stimulation of auditory nerve fibers, and hyperactivity in the brain stem auditory nuclei (1, 2, 5). The precise mechanism remains to be explained. However, based on recent research, the most compelling of these theories is that tinnitus occurs as a result of spontaneous and aberrant nerve activity within central auditory pathways (1, 2, 5). To aid in diagnosis and treatment, it is important to first characterize tinnitus as objective or subjective (2, 3, 5). Objective tinnitus can be heard through a stethoscope placed near the patient's ear, over the head and neck structures. Subjective tinnitus, which is far more common, is heard only by the patient.

1. Objective (somatosounds). These sounds generally fall into three categories: vascular abnormalities, neurologic diseases, or Eustachian tube dysfunction (1, 3). These sounds are commonly pulsatile in nature. They are real sounds, mechanical in origin, and can be heard by the examiner as well as the patient. Sources include (1, 3, 5) the following:

   a. Venous hums may be heard in patients with intracranial or systemic hypertension, due to currents in the venous system, commonly the jugular vein.

   b. Arteriovenous fistulas are more likely to be symptomatic than arteriovenous malformations and can be associated with dural venous thrombosis, which may occur spontaneously or in association with trauma, infection, tumor, or surgery.

   c. Arterial bruits near the temporal bone, most commonly the petrous carotid system, may transmit sounds associated with turbulent blood flow.

d. Paragangliomas are vascular glomus tumors arising from paraganglia cells around the carotid bifurcation, along the tympanic arteries in the middle ear, or within the jugular bulb. As the tumor enlarges, it may cause hearing loss.

e. Myoclonus of nearby structures, most commonly the palatine muscles, the stapedius muscle, and the tensor tympani. These sounds may be clicking or banging, rapid and intermittent, worsened by stress, or accentuated by external noises such as running faucets, music tones, and voices.

f. A patulous or abnormally patent Eustachian tube can cause tinnitus by allowing in concert with respiration too much and too little aeration of the middle ear cavity. This syndrome may occur after significant weight loss and usually presents as an ocean wave sound synchronous with respiration or sometimes as a popping sound.

2. Subjective. While much more common than objective tinnitus, this type is less easily definable. Causes of subjective tinnitus can be divided into various subcategories as below (1, 3, 5):

a. Otologic. Can be conductive: inhibition of sound transmission caused by cerumen impaction, tympanic membrane perforation, swelling of external auditory canal due to otitis externa, middle ear fluid, otosclerosis. Can be sensorineural: disease or abnormality of the inner ear caused by noise-induced hearing loss, presbycusis, Ménière's disease.

b. Ototoxic. Medication or substance related (see Section IIIA5).

c. Neurologic. Head injury, whiplash, multiple sclerosis, acoustic neuroma, and other cerebellopontine angle tumors.

d. Infectious. Otitis media, sequelae of Lyme disease, meningitis, syphilis.

e. Metabolic. Hyper- or hypothyroidism, hyperlipidemia, anemia, vitamin B12 deficiency, zinc deficiency.

f. Psychogenic. Depression, anxiety, fibromyalgia; can be worsened if sleep disturbances are present.

g. Other. Temporomandibular joint dysfunction; other mandibulodental disorders.

B. Epidemiology. In the United States between 1999 and 2004, approximately 50 million adults reported having any tinnitus, with peak incidence of frequent tinnitus falling between 60 and 69 years of age (6). Women are more likely to report any tinnitus; however, the prevalence of any or frequent tinnitus is higher in males, and non-Hispanic whites are more commonly affected compared with other racial groups (6). Patients who smoke or formerly smoked and those with a BMI >30, diagnosis of high blood pressure, diabetes mellitus, and dyslipidemia have an increase in reported tinnitus (3). The prevalence of frequent tinnitus is also highest in persons who are exposed to loud occupational or leisure noises and firearms; 60% of patients with noise-induced hearing loss experience tinnitus (3). Patients with marked tinnitus often have associated morbidities such as sleep deprivation, emotional disturbances, decreased social interaction, and overall poor health (6); 25% of those with ringing report that it regularly interferes with their daily activities, while 3% say they are disabled (3).

III. EVALUATION

A. History. Pulsatile unilateral tinnitus especially if associated with other unilateral otologic symptoms should raise concern for potentially serious underlying disease. With this in mind, the following historical features should be explored (2, 4, 5, 7).

1. Onset of tinnitus. When rapidly progressive or sudden, pay attention to any recent illness, injury, noise exposure, or change in drug regimen. Progressive bilateral onset in conjunction with advanced aging suggests presbycusis.

2. Location and pattern. Is it unilateral or bilateral? Explore whether the tinnitus is continuous or episodic; steady or pulsatile. Cerumen impaction, otitis, and acoustic neuroma are associated with unilateral symptoms.

3. Characteristics and detailed description of the tinnitus may help differentiate between objective or subjective sources. Is the pitch high or low? Low-pitch rumbling sounds are often associated with Ménière's disease, whereas high-pitched patterns suggest sensorineural hearing loss. What is the degree of loudness? Is there associated hearing loss, aural fullness, vertigo? Are there any exacerbating or ameliorating factors? If the tinnitus changes with position or varies with respiration, this may point to a patulous Eustachian tube.

4. Exposure to ototoxic occupational or avocational noise levels.
5. Medication history. Medications that commonly cause or exacerbate tinnitus include aspirin, non-steroidal anti-inflammatory drugs, aminoglycosides, erythromycin, tetracycline, vancomycin, cisplatin, methotrexate, vincristine, bumetanide, furosemide, quinine, chloroquine, heavy metals such as mercury and lead, calcium channel blockers, benzodiazepines, antidepressants, lidocaine, and ethanol.
6. Significant weight loss can lead to a patulous Eustachian tube.
7. Concurrent medical/psychiatric conditions to be considered include hypertension, diabetes mellitus, thyroid disorders, hyperlipidemia, anemia, B12 deficiency, infection, anxiety, and depression. Venous hums may be caused by systemic hypertension or increased intracranial pressures. Atherosclerotic plaques in the vasculature can also contribute to symptoms. Tinnitus may be a contributing factor to the development of depression and anxiety. In turn, psychiatric disturbances may heighten the awareness of tinnitus, especially in those with concurrent sleep disturbances. Auditory hallucinations must be ruled out by history.
8. **Concurrent symptoms.** Ask about ear pain or drainage, fever, hearing loss, vertigo, and nasal congestion.
B. **Physical examination.** A complete head and neck exam should be performed, focusing on otologic and neurologic aspects including bedside assessment of hearing, balance, and gait (2, 4, 5, 7). Test cranial nerves 5, 7, and 8 and look for any nystagmus (2, 4). In cases where vascular etiology is suspected, clinicians should auscultate over the orbits, supraclavicular areas, carotid arteries, mastoids, periauricular area, neck, and temples in various positions. If psychiatric contributions are suspected, include an evaluation of mood, affect, and perception.
C. **Testing.** All patients experiencing tinnitus should undergo a comprehensive audiometry evaluation (2, 4, 5, 7). This will determine the presence of hearing loss, distinguish between conductive and sensory hearing impairments, aid in ruling out retrocochlear auditory dysfunction, and thoroughly evaluate the characteristics of the tinnitus. An audiometry test battery usually includes tympanometry, measurements of acoustic reflex, pure tone and high-frequency audiometry, and speech recognition. Often the combination of history, physical exam, and audiometry leads to an etiologic diagnosis. When indicated, laboratory testing may be needed with a complete blood count, thyroid function studies, serum glucose, lipid profile, syphilis serology, and autoimmune panel including rheumatoid factor, sedimentation rate, and antinuclear antibodies (4, 5, 7). In patients with short duration, infrequent episodes of mild pulsatile tinnitus, reassurance, and observation is a reasonable initial step in the setting of a normal physical exam and audiometry. However, all cases of constant or frequent pulsatile tinnitus and persistent unilateral non-pulsatile tinnitus that is unexplained mandate obtaining a magnetic resonance imaging (MRI) study with contrast (4, 7, 8). Further evaluation by an otolaryngologist or neurologist is strongly recommended in these situations (2, 4, 7). Likewise, any significant asymmetry on hearing or acoustic reflex testing requires MRI and consultation (7, 8). Computed tomography (CT) or CT angiography can be substituted when MRI cannot be used or to further evaluate cases where otosclerosis, trauma, or hereditary hearing loss is suspected (8).

IV. DIAGNOSIS
A. **Differential diagnosis.** Tinnitus can rarely be idiopathic. Such a diagnosis is largely one of exclusion. The key to the diagnosis of tinnitus is a thorough history eliciting the specific characteristics of the tinnitus coupled with a focused physical exam and routine audiometric testing.
B. **Clinical manifestations.** Because tinnitus cannot be heard by others with the naked ear, there are no outward manifestations. The impact of tinnitus on quality of life can be significant, however. Given the fact that approximately one-fourth of tinnitus sufferers report an increase in symptoms over time, it may be prudent to periodically assess the impact of tinnitus using standardized instruments such as the Tinnitus Handicap Inventory or the Tinnitus Reaction Questionnaire (1).

REFERENCES

1. Dinces EA. Etiology and diagnosis of tinnitus. Accessed at http://www.UpToDate.com on May 25, 2012.
2. Lockwood AH. Tinnitus. *Neurol Clin* 2005;23:893–900.
3. Bauer CA. Tinnitus and hyperacusis. In: Flint PW, Haughey BH, Lund VJ, Niparko JK, Richardson MA, Robbins KT eds. *Cummings otolaryngology head and neck surgery*. Philadelphia: Mosby, 2010;2131–2139.
4. Crummer RW, Hassan GA. Diagnostic approach to tinnitus. *Am Fam Physician* 2004;69(1):120–126.
5. Ahmad N, Seidman M. Tinnitus in the older adult: epidemiology, pathophysiology and treatment options. *Drugs Ageing* 2004;21(5):297–306.
6. Shargorodsky J, Curhan GC, Farwell WR. Prevalence and characteristics of tinnitus among US adults. *Amer J Med* 2010;123(8):711–718.
7. Hannan SA, Sami F, Wareing MJ. Tinnitus. *BMJ* 2005;330:237–238.
8. Kang M, Escott E. Imaging of tinnitus. *Otol Clin N Am* 2008;41:179–193.

6.9 Vertigo
Alicia C. Walters-Stewart

I. BACKGROUND

A. True vertigo is characterized by the illusion of movement—a feeling that the body or environment is moving. Patients often report rotation or spinning, although occasionally they describe a sensation of linear acceleration or tilting. This sensation often begins abruptly and, if severe, is accompanied by nausea, vomiting, and staggering gait (1). Vertigo represents one of the four major symptom categories that account for patients' complaints of dizziness (2, 3). The other three categories are

1. **Presyncope.** This is a sensation of impending faint ("severe light-headedness") and implies a temporary decrement of cerebral circulation. Common causes include postural hypotension, vasovagal reactions, cardiac arrhythmias, impaired cardiac output, and hypoglycemia.

2. **Disequilibrium.** This is a feeling of unsteadiness of gait or imbalance in the absence of any abnormal head sensation indicating a disturbance of the motor control system. Causes include alcoholism, drugs, cervical facet joint arthropathy, stroke, multiple sclerosis, and multiple neurosensory deficits (e.g., a combination of visual impairment, vestibular hypofunction, peripheral neuropathy, and medications).

3. **Light-headedness.** Patients often describe a vague or mild wooziness, or heavy headedness, or a swimming or floating sensation as if disconnected with the environment. This category has a high association with both hyperventilation syndrome and psychologic disturbances such as anxiety, depression, and panic (2).

B. Careful interviewing allows the placement of patient complaints into one of the four categories, each implying certain pathophysiologic mechanisms and, therefore, specific differential diagnoses (2–5). The remainder of this chapter will primarily focus on evaluating patients with the symptom complex of true vertigo in an effort to determine specific underlying causes.

II. PATHOPHYSIOLOGY

A. **Etiology.** The vestibular system monitors the motion and position of the head in space by detecting angular and linear acceleration. The sensory receptors in the utricle and saccule detect linear acceleration, and it is the cristae of the semicircular canals that detect angular acceleration (head turning) (3). Information from the peripheral receptors is relayed through the vestibular portion of the eighth cranial nerves to the brain stem nuclei and portions of the cerebellum. Additional important connections are made with the ocular motor nuclei and spinal cord. True vertigo represents an asymmetry or imbalance of neural activity between the left and right vestibular nuclei. Abnormal activity in this system can arise either from peripheral lesions (labyrinth or vestibular nerve) or from central lesions (brain stem or cerebellum) (1).

B. Epidemiology. The overarching complaint of "dizziness" accounts for 5% of all primary care office visits and is the chief complaint in nearly 3% of all non–pain-related emergency department visits (2). In young adults (<30 years of age), psychologic causes account for most cases of dizziness, whereas vestibular lesions become more common in midlife. In the elderly, cerebrovascular and cardiac disorders, combined with multiple sensory deficits, outweigh simple vestibular causes. Approximately one-half of these dizziness-related visits are related to true vertigo (2). Therefore, many patients with dizziness have nonvestibular underlying processes. Of those with vertigo, central lesions are found in approximately 1% of all patients (2). Dizziness and vertigo are usually benign, self-limited processes not associated with excess mortality, although some individuals suffer impaired quality of life because of recurrent or persistent symptoms.

III. EVALUATION

The key task for the clinician is distinquishing peripheral from central vertigo (3–5).

A. History. The patient's age, underlying comorbidities (especially hypertension, diabetes, heart disease, and psychiatric illness), and symptom classification category help limit the diagnostic possibilities. Further specificity is gained by eliciting the following:

1. **Temporal pattern.** Are the symptoms episodic or continuous? If episodic, how long do they last? Peripheral origin vertigo is often intermittent and of sudden onset compared with the usual, more gradual onset of central vertigo. A continuous history suggests central nervous system (CNS) pathology, drug or toxin effects, metabolic dysfunction, or psychiatric disease. Benign paroxysmal positional vertigo (BPPV) episodes last less than a minute; vertebrobasilar transient ischemic attacks last for several minutes up to an hour; Ménière's disease persists for 1–24 hours; and vestibular neuronitis or acute labyrinthitis continues for several days.

2. **Precipitating or exacerbating factors.** Has there been recent head trauma (implying perilymphatic fistula) or viral illness (labyrinthitis)? What is the relationship to sudden head movement or turning over in bed (BPPV), coughing or sneezing (perilymphatic fistula), postural changes (orthostasis), exercise (arrhythmias), foods (salty meals exacerbating Ménière's), walking and turning (multiple sensory deficits), micturition or pain (vasovagal reaction), and emotional upset (hyperventilation) (4–6)?

3. **Associated symptoms.** Marked nausea, vomiting, diaphoresis, aural fullness, and recruitment (perception of sounds being too loud) are typical of peripheral vestibular disorders. Episodic vertigo associated with tinnitus and gradual (unilateral) hearing loss involving low frequencies preferentially suggest Ménière's disease. Asymmetric weakness, cranial nerve or cerebellar dysfunction, significant new headache, diplopia, numbness, or dysarthria suggests brain stem or CNS disease. Headache, scotomata, or tunnel vision points to vestibular migraine (2, 5). Numbness or paresthesias may indicate neuropathy contributing to multiple sensory deficits. A single, abrupt episode of severe vertigo with negative Dix-Hallpike (DH) testing (see Section IIIB) that gradually subsides over days implies labyrinthitis (if hearing is affected) or vestibular neuronitis (if hearing is unaffected). Mild vertigo with prominent tinnitus, unilateral hearing loss, and loss of corneal reflex is worrisome for an acoustic neuroma (4, 6).

4. **Medications or toxins.** Many medications can cause "dizziness," although only a few (aminoglycosides, lead, mercury, quinolones, anticonvulsants, and neuroleptics) cause vertigo (3). Assess toxin exposure by exploring job and recreational activities, including illicit drug use.

B. Physical examination. This emphasizes orthostatic vital signs, the eyes, ears, and neurologic and cardiovascular systems. As mentioned below, two provocative maneuvers should be a routine part of the physical examination (3, 5).

1. **Detection of nystagmus** is critical because it is the only objective sign of vertigo (3, 5, 7). Nystagmus can occur spontaneously or in response to changes in eye or body position. It represents vestibular dysfunction mediated through the vestibular optic reflex (VOR). Peripheral vestibular disorders usually cause horizontal or rotatory nystagmus, whereas CNS pathology is reflected by vertical nystagmus—an ominous sign. Two provocative maneuvers, DH testing and head thrust testing, further help distinquish central from peripheral vertigo (3, 5, 7).

   a. **DH test.** In true vertigo caused by BPPV, DH maneuvers (the gold standard test) often confirm the diagnosis (sensitivity 50–90%, specificity 70–95%) (7). The patient is moved rapidly from a sitting to a supine position 30° below horizontal with the head turned at a 30° angle, first to one side and then to the other. A positive DH test includes precipitation of vertigo, latency of onset by a few seconds, rotational nystagmus, resolution within a minute, and lessened symptoms and nystagmus with prolonged latency on repeated testing (i.e., fatigability) (3, 7). The lack of latency and fatigability as well as nonsuppression of nystagmus by gaze fixation characterize vertigo caused by serious central lesions.

   b. **Head Thrust** (3, 5). The examiner stands in front of the patient and grasps the head with both hands. The patient is asked to focus on the examiner's nose as a very quick 20° thrust to one side is done. When there is dysfunction of the VOR on one side (as in peripheral lesions), a corrective eye movement (corrective saccade) back to the examiner's nose is seen. Normally, in contrast, the eyes easily stay fixated on the nose. Specificity is over 95% while sensitivity is variable around 50% (3, 5).

2. **Neurologic examination** serves to detect brain stem or CNS pathology. It is important to focus on the patient's motor coordination and sensory function to detect the presence of an unsteady gait, past-pointing, ataxia, or abnormal Romberg test.

3. **Otoscopy** can detect otitis media or cholesteatoma. Nystagmus with vertigo following positive or negative pressure applied to the tympanic membrane (pneumatic otoscopy) suggests a perilymphatic fistula (4, 6).

4. **Other provocative tests** (forced hyperventilation, laboratory-based VOR testing, and vigorous horizontal head shaking) are not routinely helpful and are best left to consultants.

C. Testing

1. **Clinical laboratory tests.** Most (80–90%) patients need no laboratory testing (4–7). Audiometry is suggested if tinnitus or hearing loss is present. Blood tests are dictated by appropriate clinical indications only. Brain stem auditory-evoked responses can help detect multiple sclerosis or acoustic neuroma. Holter monitoring is indicated if arrhythmias are suspected. Specialized testing—posturography, rotational chair testing, electronystagmography—is best ordered by a consultant when the diagnosis remains unclear after initial evaluation.

2. **Diagnostic imaging.** Consider Doppler ultrasound for suspected transient ischemic attack and magnetic resonance imaging if CNS lesions are suspected. In patients with acute persisting vertigo and headache in whom the head impulse test is normal (that is, a peripheral cause is excluded), the differential diagnosis is between a cerebellar stroke and acute migrainous vertigo and here neuroimaging is mandatory (unless the patient is a previously investigated migraineur) (5).

D. Genetics. There are no significant genetic or familial influences related to vertigo.

IV. DIAGNOSIS

A. Differential diagnosis. Peripheral causes of vertigo (in approximate order of frequency in primary care) include BPPV, viral labyrinthitis or vestibular neuronitis (acute unilateral vestibulopathy), serous otitis, perilymphatic fistula, Ménière's disease, and drugs (alcohol and aminoglycosides) (6, 7). Central causes of vertigo include vertebrobasilar transient ischemic attack, cerebellar infarction or neoplasm, multiple sclerosis, brain stem infarction or neoplasm, cerebellopontine angle tumors, migraine, hyperventilation, seizures, spinocerebellar degeneration, and certain systemic disorders (infections, vasculitis, and syphilis) (4, 6). Red flags indicative of probable central vertigo include new headache (especially occipital), central neurologic symptoms and signs, acute deafness, and vertical nystagmus (5). The cervical spine can rarely be the source of vertigo, either by osteoarthritic spur occlusion of the vertebral arteries or by proprioceptive overstimulation by facet joint arthropathy. Even rarer is the MAL de Debarquement syndrome characterized by a prolonged (years) sense of swaying and dysequilibrium after a long sea voyage (3).

B. Clinical manifestations. The common features of vestibular dysfunction are vertigo, nystagmus, and postural instability. The clinician's chief task is to distinguish between usually benign peripheral causes and more ominous central processes by attending to the historical and physical examination characteristics outlined in Section III. Central vertigo is associated with moderate nausea and vomiting, ataxia, neurologic signs and symptoms, rare hearing loss, and very slow compensation (3). Peripheral vertigo manifests combinations of severe nausea and vomiting, tinnitus, fluctuating hearing loss, milder postural imbalance, a lack of neurologic signs and symptoms, positive provocative testing, and rapid compensation (4).

REFERENCES

1. Dieterich M. Dizziness. *The Neurologist* 2004;10:154–164.
2. Post RE, Dickerson LM. Dizziness: a diagnostic approach. *Am Fam Physician* 2010;82(4):361–368.
3. Kutz JW. The dizzy patient. *Med Clin N Am* 2010;94:989–1002.
4. Chawla N, Olshaker JS. Diagnosis and mangement of dizziness and vertigo. *Med Clin N Am* 2006;90:291–304.
5. Barraclough K, Bronstein A. Vertigo. *BMJ* 2009;339:b3493.
6. Labuguen RH. Initial evaluation of vertigo. *Am Fam Physician* 2006;73:244–251, 254.
7. Bhattacharyya N, Baugh RF, Orvidas L, et al. Clinical practice guideline: benign paroxsymal positional vertigo. *Otolaryngol Head Neck Surg* 2008;139:S47–S81.

CHAPTER 7

Cardiovascular Problems

Mindy J. Lacey

7.1 Atypical Chest Pain

Thomas J. Hansen

I. **BACKGROUND.** "Typical" chest pain is pain that is typical of anginal pain. This pain is usually described as substernal, radiating to the left neck and arm, and is pressurelike or has a squeezing sensation. "Atypical" chest pain is defined as the absence of this typical presentation.

II. **PATHOPHYSIOLOGY.** Atypical chest pain can originate in any of the thoracic organs, as well as from extrathoracic sources (e.g., thyroiditis or panic disorder).

III. **EVALUATION.** The approach to the evaluation of acute chest pain, whether typical or atypical, should be to rapidly assess whether the pain is due to cardiac disease. Atypical chest pain does not rule out an acute myocardial infarction (AMI), especially in women (1), patients with diabetes, and the elderly, in whom an AMI may present in an atypical fashion. A clinical history of the chest pain and an electrocardiogram (ECG) should be obtained within 5 minutes after presentation (2). The ECG is critical for guiding initial therapy and decisions regarding diagnosis and treatment.

   A. **History.** The clinical history should focus on the time of onset, the characteristic of the pain, the location (retrosubsternal, subxiphoid, diffuse), the frequency of the pain (constant, intermittent, acute onset), the duration of the pain, precipitating factors (exertion, stress, food, respiration, movement), the quality of the pain (burning, squeezing, dull, sharp, tearing, heavy), and any associated symptoms (shortness of breath, diaphoresis, nausea, vomiting, jaw pain, back pain, radiation, palpitations, weakness, fatigue).

   Other pertinent questions include assessing risk factors for coronary artery disease (diabetes, smoking, hypertension, hypercholesteremia, family history), anorexia, anxiety, cough and/or wheezing, drug use, fever, previous history of deep vein thrombosis or pulmonary embolism, pain increased with recumbency or relieved by leaning forward, presence of a mass, lesion, or rash on the chest, previous history of cancer, pregnancy/postpartum, oral contraceptive use, or trauma, relationship of pain with eating, and syncopal or near-syncopal episodes.

   B. **Physical examination.** The physical examination should include a rapid assessment of vital signs, as well as oxygen saturation and electrocardiographic evaluation. Following this, an examination of the chest should be performed. Cardiac examination should focus on pericardial rubs, systolic and diastolic murmurs, third or fourth heart sounds, and distended jugular veins. Auscultation of the lungs should focus on diminished breath sounds, a pleural rub, rales, rhonchi, and wheezes. Examination of the legs should focus on edema and poor perfusion of a limb, which may indicate an aortic dissection. Examination of the musculoskeletal system should focus on reproducible or localized pain. Examination of the skin should assess for lesions, masses, or rashes.

   C. **Testing**
      1. **Oxygen saturation.** Oxygen saturation below 92% may indicate a myocardial infarction, spontaneous pneumothorax, pulmonary embolism, or pneumonia. An arterial blood gas is warranted.

2. **ECG.** Always compare with an old ECG when available. The presence of T wave inversion is consistent with *myocardial ischemia*. ST elevation is consistent with *myocardial injury*, and ST depression is consistent with *subendocardial infarction*. A Q wave is diagnostic of a *myocardial infarction* (3). A *pulmonary embolism* is classically associated with the $S_1Q_3T_3$ pattern, representing a large S wave in I, an ST depression in II, and a large Q wave in III with T wave inversion. Sensitivity of this is less than 20%, however. *Acute pericarditis* demonstrates diffuse ST-segment elevation, in which the ST segment is flat or slightly concave, and PR depression.

3. **Other laboratory tests**
   a. **Comprehensive metabolic profile.** Used to detect metabolic abnormality as the cause of chest pain as well as abnormalities of the liver
   b. **Complete blood count.** Used to detect infection and inflammatory disorders
   c. **Creatine kinase-MB and troponin.** High positive predictive value for an AMI if elevated, but may be negative initially
   d. **D-dimer.** Sensitive but not specific for a pulmonary embolism
   e. **Liver function tests, amylase, *Helicobacter pylori*.** Used to determine a gastrointestinal etiology of the pain, such as liver distention, pancreatitis, and gastric or duodenal ulcers due to *H. pylori*
   f. **Toxicology screen.** Recommended if cocaine use is believed to be the cause of the chest pain

4. **Imaging studies**
   a. **Chest x-ray.** Useful in diagnosing pneumonia, pneumothorax, aortic dissection, acute pericarditis, and esophageal rupture
   b. **Ultrasound.** Helpful to diagnose pericardial, valvular disease and to demonstrate cardiac wall motion abnormalities
   c. **Stress echocardiogram.** Used for stable patients who have been ruled out for infarction to determine if cardiac disease is present
   d. **Computed tomography.** Used to diagnose aortic dissection in stable patients and may identify pulmonary embolism or cardiac effusion

IV. DIAGNOSIS

A. **Differential diagnosis.** The differential diagnosis for atypical chest pain includes (4)
   1. **Breast lesions.** Abscess, carcinoma, fibroadenosis, mastitis
   2. **Cardiovascular.** AMI, angina pectoris, aortic dissection, aortic valvular disease, hypertrophic cardiomyopathy, mitral valve prolapse, myocarditis, pericarditis, primary pulmonary hypertension, thoracic aortic aneurysm, neoplasm
   3. **Gastrointestinal disease.** Esophageal rupture, esophagitis, foreign body presence, gastric distention, gastritis, liver distention, Mallory-Weiss syndrome, pancreatitis, peptic ulcer disease, Plummer-Vinson syndrome, splenic infarct, subphrenic abscess, Zenker's diverticulum
   4. **Musculoskeletal disorder.** Bruised or fractured rib, cervical disc herniation, costochondritis, intercostal muscle cramp, intercostal myositis, pectoral strain, osteoarthritis, thoracic outlet syndrome
   5. **Neuralgia.** Herpes zoster, neurofibroma, neoplasm, tabes dorsalis, sensitization of dorsal horn spinal neurons in the territory of the intercostobrachial nerve (5)
   6. **Psychogenic causes.** Anxiety, panic attack
   7. **Pulmonary disease.** Bronchitis, neoplasm, pleuritis, pneumonia, pulmonary hypertension, pulmonary embolism
   8. **Thyroid.** Thyroiditis

B. **Clinical approach.** Once a cardiac etiology for atypical chest pain has been eliminated, a careful history and physical examination usually yield a diagnosis. The aforementioned tests are useful in making the diagnosis and determining an appropriate treatment plan.

REFERENCES

1. DeCara JE. Noninvasive cardiac testing in women. *J Am Med Womens Assoc* 2003, 58(4):254–263.
2. Lee TH, Goldman L. Evaluation of the patient with acute chest pain. *JAMA* 2000;342:1187–1195.
3. Braunwald B, Fauci A, Kasper D, et al., eds. *Harrison's principles of internal medicine*, 15th ed, New York, NY: McGraw-Hill, 2001.

4. Adler SN, Gasbarra DB, Adler-Klein D, eds. *A pocket manual of differential diagnosis,* 4th ed. Philadelphia, PA: Lippincott Williams & Wilkins, 2000.
5. Rasmussen J, Grothusen J, Rosso AL, et al. Atypical chest pain: evidence of intercostobrachial nerve sensitization in complex regional pain syndrome. *Pain Physician* 2009;12:E329–E334.

7.2 Anticoagulation

Mindy J. Lacey and Chia L. Chang

I. **BACKGROUND.** Pharmacologic modulation of coagulation is commonly employed to prevent inappropriate thrombosis or end-organ pathology in various disease entities, often atherosclerotic in origin. The basic premise of therapy with agents that hinder the normal clotting machinery involves sufficiently inhibiting the formation of new thrombi while avoiding hemorrhagic complications (1). The principal uses of anticoagulation in common clinical practice involve the prevention and treatment of myocardial infarction, stroke, pulmonary embolus, deep venous thrombosis, and other states of acquired and hereditary hypercoagulability (2).

II. **PATHOPHYSIOLOGY.** Coagulation involves both primary and secondary hemostasis: primary referring to the formation of a platelet plug at the site of endothelial injury within minutes, and secondary referring to the generation of fibrin to cross-link the platelet plug, ensure tensile strength, and long stability in blood flow. Secondary hemostasis is the result of a complex interconnected cascade of serine protease-mediated reactions allowing for simultaneous amplification and regulation. Pharmacologic anticoagulation usually alters one of these pathways preferentially (Table 7.2.1). The therapeutic effects, as well as the complications of excesses (i.e., platelet vs. coagulation factor type bleeding), are a result of a given agent's target.

Table 7.2.1	Physiologic Targets of Commonly Used Anticoagulants	
Agent	**Target**	**Mechanism**
Aspirin	Platelets	Cyclooxygenase inhibition
Clopidogrel	Platelets	Glycoprotein IIb/IIIa blocking
		Prevents the activation of glycoprotein IIb/IIIa (platelet aggregation) via inhibition of adenosine diphosphate (ADP) receptors
Warfarin	Coagulation cascade	Vitamin K antagonist
Heparin (high and low molecular weight)/ heparinoids	Coagulation cascade	Heparin combines with antithrombin III to accelerate its activity to inactive thrombin and then inactivates Factor X and inhibits prothrombin's conversion to thrombin. This also prevents fibrin formation from fibrinogen during active thrombosis
		Low molecular weight heparin (LMWH) (Lovenox) similar as heparin but its effect is more selective as anti-factor Xa and anti-factor IIa (anti-thrombin)
Dabigatran	Coagulation cascade	Direct thrombin inhibitor
Rivaroxaban	Coagulation cascade	Factor Xa inhibitor

III. EVALUATION. A thorough clinical history and physical examination are critical in the diagnosis of thrombosis and states of anticoagulant overdose, as well as guiding the choice of therapy. Briefly, the clinical phenotype is often that of the underlying disease process prompting anticoagulation (i.e., cerebrovascualr accident), and evaluation of these patients treated with anticoagulation often centers on the identification of hemorrhagic complications such as easy bruising, prolonged bleeding, and other bleeding diathesis. It is critical to obtain a history of current/chronic anticoagulation therapy (including herbals) prior to invasive procedures or the initiation of treatment with other drugs that may alter the metabolism of drugs affecting hemostasis.

III. DIAGNOSIS. Barring overt clinical stigmata of abnormalites of coagulation, laboratory evaluation is the cornerstone of regulating therapy. The three main assays utilized include the international normalized ratio (INR), partial prothrombin time (PTT), and less frequently bleeding time. INR, a standardized system for reporting prothrombin time, is a tool used for monitoring the function of the extrinsic coagulation cascade and is typically a measure of the effects of warfarin. PTT is a marker of the degree of inhibition of the intrinsic coagulation cascade by heparin and other related compounds, with the exception of low-molecular-weight heparins that often do not require routine laboratory monitoring. While bleeding time is a measure of primary hemostasis/platelet function and related drugs, the test is often cumbersome to use in daily practice and clinical features (bruising, etc.) are more commonly employed to assess the effects of antiplatelet agents.

IV. TREATMENT. See Table 7.2.2.

Table 7.2.2	Pharmacotherapy of Commonly Encountered Conditions Requiring Anticoagulation		
Condition	**Common treatment**	**Therapeutic target**	**Duration of therapy**
Atrial fibrillation	Treatment based on CHADS 2 score: Aspirin (ASA), ASA+Plavix, Warfarin, Pradaxa, Xarelto	Warfarin: INR 2–3	Lifelong
Deep venous thrombosis	Warfarin Heparin/LMWH during acute treatment	Warfarin: INR 2–3	Warfarin: Depending on factors: provoking vs. non-provoking, and risks of bleeding 3 mo to lifelong
Pulmonary embolus	Warfarin Heparin/LMWH during actue treatment	Warfarin: INR 2–3	Warfarin: Depending on factors: provoking vs. non-provoking, and risks of bleeding 3 mo to lifelong
Cerebrovascular accident	Thrombotic type: ASA, Plavix, Aggrenox Cardioembolic type: Warfarin	Warfarin: INR 2–3	Lifelong
Myocardial infarction	ASA, Plavix	None	Lifelong
Mesenteric/visceral thrombosis	LMWH: acute tx Warfarin	Warfarin: INR 2–3	Lifelong

(Continued)

Table 7.2.2	Pharmacotherapy of Commonly Encountered Conditions Requiring Anticoagulation*(Continued)*		
Condition	**Common treatment**	**Therapeutic target**	**Duration of therapy**
Prosthetic heart valve—mechanical	Aortic: Warfarin	Aortic: INR 2–3	Lifelong
	Mitral: Warfarin	Mitral: INR 2.5–3.5	
Prosthetic heart valve—biomechanical	Aortic: ASA	Warfarin: INR 2–3	Lifelong
	Mitral: Warfarin × 3 mo then ASA		
Antiphospholipid antibody syndrome	Warfarin	Wafarin: INR 2–3	Lifelong
	LMWH for actue siturations		
Factor V Leiden	ASA or warfarin depending on risks	Warfarin: INR 2–3	Lifelong
	LMWH for acute situations		

INR, international normalized ratio.

REFERENCES

1. Lee A, Crowther M. Practical issues with vitamin K antagonists: elevated INRs, low time-in-therapeutic range, and warfarin failure. *J Thromb Thrombolysis* 2011;31(3):249–258.
2. Houbballah R, LaMuraglia GM. Clotting problems: diagnosis and management of underlying coagulopathies. *Semin Vasc Surg* 2010;23(4):221–227.
3. American College of Chest Physicians. *Antithrombotic therapy and prevention of thrombosis*, 9th ed. American College of Chest Physicians Evidence-Based Clinical Practice Guidelines. February 2012; 141 (2 suppl).

7.3 Chest Pain

Sanjeev Sharma

I. BACKGROUND. Chest pain accounts for approximately 5.6 million emergency department visits annually. It is second only to abdominal pain as the most common reason for an emergency department visit. More than 3 million patients are hospitalized yearly in the United States for chest pain. The etiology of chest pain is usually benign and noncardiac in nature. A standardized approach to addressing the management of these patients is essential, given the adverse consequences of missing a life-threatening condition.

II. PATHOPHYSIOLOGY. Cardiac pain is usually due to low perfusion to the myocardium through the coronary arteries that are completely or partially blocked by atherosclerotic plaque. This leads to tissue hypoxia, anaerobic metabolism, lactic acidosis, and abnormal prostaglandin secretion. Pain originating from the lungs or pleura is caused by the irritation or inflammation of the lungs and/or the pleura or diaphragm. Gastrointestinal pain arises from mucosal inflammation or structural abnormality, such as stricture or obstruction. Referred pain can be from diseases of gallbladder, pancrease, or stomach. Injury, inflammation, or other pathologies of chest wall structures including ribs, muscles, spine, and skin can give rise to chest pain.

III. EVALUATION. The patient should be evaluated to determine the diagnosis and to formulate an immediate management plan. Priority should be given to rule out life-threatening cardiovascular causes. In patients with acute pain, the clinician must assess the patient's hemodynamic and respiratory status. If either is compromised, management should focus on stabilizing the patient.

A. History. Description of the chest pain is critical for diagonising the etiology of the chest pain. Other factors that help determine the cause are patients's age, sex, and other medical comorbid conditions. Questions should be asked about the exact location, quality, severity, onset, duration, exacerbating factors, and radiation of pain. Radiation of pain to the left arm is common in myocardial ischemia. Pain of aortic dissection radiates between the scapulae. It is necessary to inquire about cardiac risk factors, including smoking, hypertension, diabetes mellitus, hyperlipidemia, cigarret smoking, and a family history of coronary artery disease (1). It is also important to ask about gastrointestinal symptoms.

B. Physical examination. A rapid physical assessment of the patient should include a full set of vital signs, determination of the presence or absence of cyanosis, dyspnea, and diaphoresis, examination of the neck, thorax, and abdomen, and palpation of the major peripheral arteries for the presence of and the characteristics of the pulse. Local tenderness over chest wall points toward chest wall pathologies.

C. Testing

1. **Laboratory tests.** Pulse oximetry should be ordered to assess oxygen status. Cardiac enzymes, creatinine phosphokinase (CK, CK-MB), and troponin T or I should also be ordered in patients suspected of cardiac pain (2). C-reactive protein, brain natriuretic peptide, and serum myoglobin have been used in the management of patients with chest pain. The possibility of life-threatening cardiac pain cannot be excluded based upon a single negative value of any of these markers; three sets of cardiac enzymes should be used (3). A complete metabolic profile including liver function tests, amylase, and lipase should be ordered if a gastrointestinal cause is suspected (4).

2. **Electrocardiogram (ECG).** An electrocardiogram (ECG) is essential. An ECG showing changes consistent with ischemia or infarction is associated with a high probability of acute myocardial infarction or unstable angina.

3. **Echocardiogram.** This is helpful if valvular abnormality is suspected.

4. **Chest X-ray.** Pulmonary diseases such as pneumonia, pleural effusion, and pneumothorax can be diagnosed. Widened mediastinum is seen in patients with aortic dissection.

5. **Computed tomography (CT) scan or magnetic resonance imaging.** If the patient's history and examination are consistent with aortic dissection, these imaging studies should be performed to evaluate the aorta. A transthoracic echocardiogram can be performed to assess cardiac function.

6. **Ventilation–perfusion scan/spiral CT scan of the chest.** These are appropriate initial tests in patients with a history of venous thromboembolism or coagulation abnormality.

7. **Cardiac stress testing.** These tests are indicated in patients with intermediate to high risk of coronary heart diseases. Options available are Bruce protocol that includes 3 minutes of incremental walk on treadmill. Stress test with imaging includes echocardiogram with exercise or dobutamine stress test. Pharmacologic stress testing such as adenosine cardiolite and dobutamine are some of the tests that can be done.

8. **Other testing.** If the patient with chest pain shows no evidence of life-threatening conditions, the clinician should focus on serious chronic conditions with the potential to cause major complications in the future; the most common of these is stable angina. Cost-effective and noninvasive tests for coronary disease such as exercise electrocardiography or stress echocardiography should be performed for low-risk patients. Gastrointestinal causes can be evaluated by endoscopy. As many as 10% of patients with chest pain may have emotional or psychiatric conditions. These patients should be appropriately evaluated by an expert (5).

IV. DIAGNOSIS. The differential diagnosis of chest pain is presented in Table 7.3.1. The initial step when a patient presents with chest pain is to exclude life-threatening conditions including acute coronary syndromes, pneumothorax, pulmonary embolism, and aortic dissection. Good history and physical examination and ECG and chest X-ray will help exclude these causes. Once life-threatening causes are ruled out, other tests can be ordered to determine the cause of chest wall abnormalities.

TABLE 7.3.1	Differential Diagnosis of Chest Pain

Cardiac

Ischemic disease
  Acute myocardial infarction
  Stable angina
  Unstable angina
Myocarditis
Pericarditis
Valvular heart disease
  Aortic stenosis
  Mitral valve prolapse
  Hypertrophic cardiomyopathy
Aortic dissection

Noncardiac

Pulmonary
  Pneumonia
  Pleuritis
  Pulmonary embolism
  Pleural effusion
  Pneumothorax

Gastrointestinal
  Esophageal spasm
  Esophagitis/gastritis
  Peptic ulcer disease
  Gallstone

Musculoskeletal
  Costochondritis
  Muscle spasm
  Cervical radiculopathy

Neurologic
  Herpes zoster
  Nerve root compression

Psychiatric
  Anxiety state

REFERENCES

1. Rich EC, Crowson TW, Harris IB. The diagnostic value of the medical history. *Arch Intern Med* 1987;147:1957.
2. Hamm CW, Goldmann BU, Heeschen C, et al. Emergency room triage of patients with acute chest pain by means of rapid testing for cardiac troponin T or troponin I. *N Engl J Med* 1997;337(23): 1648–1653.
3. Caragher TE, Fernandez BB, Jacobs FL, et al. Evaluation of quantitative cardiac biomarker point-of-care testing in the emergency department. *J Emerg Med* 2002;22(1):1–7.

4. Eslick GD, Fass R. Noncardiac chest pain: evaluation and treatment. *Gastroenterol Clin North Am* 2003;32(2):531–552.
5. Ho KY, Kang JY, Yeo B, et al. Non-cardiac, non-oesophageal chest pain: the relevance of psychological factors. *Gut* 1998;43(1):105–110.

7.4 Bradycardia

Mark D. Goodman

I. BACKGROUND. Bradycardia, which is defined as a heart rate less than 60 beats/minute, results from abnormalities in impulse formation or failure of conduction. It may or may not be a cause for concern. For the well-conditioned athlete, bradycardia may carry no underlying risk or morbidity, but for the patient with a cardiac or neurologic condition, bradycardia can be deadly.

The most important initial assessment is whether the slow heart rate is pathologic or innocent. In the presence of syncope, neurologic changes, myocardial ischemia/angina, fatigue, or dyspnea, one can safely assume that bradycardia adversely impacts health (1).

II. PATHOPHYSIOLOGY

A. Etiology. Conditions that can manifest as bradycardia include exposure, electrolyte imbalance (hypokalemia), infection, hypoglycemia, hypothyroid/hyperthyroid, inferior wall myocardial infarction, cardiac ischemia, increased intracranial pressure, medications (e.g., β-blockers, calcium channel blockers, antiarrhythmics, lithium, and digoxin), atrial fibrillation, long QT syndrome, and sick sinus syndrome. Reversible causes include profound bradycardia, which often develops in patients with obstructive sleep apnea and hypoxia, but may be eliminated with appropriate apnea treatment.

1. Long QT syndrome
   a. This condition was first described in 1957 in a family with recurrent syncope and sudden death. Several different familial syndromes manifest as QT prolongation on an electrocardiogram (ECG), with a predilection for malignant ventricular arrhythmias and possible syncope or sudden death. If the presenting event is syncope, a clinical evaluation that includes an ECG almost always reveals the prolongation of the QT interval, the clinical hallmark of this disorder. Several drugs can prolong the QTc interval, and it is important to distinguish drug-induced QTc prolongation from the inherited form of long QT syndrome (2).
   b. Life-threatening cardiac events tend to occur under specific circumstances in a gene-specific manner: some during exercise, some with arousal/emotion, some at sleep/rest, and some with loud noises.

2. Sick sinus syndrome
   a. Sick sinus syndrome comprises a variety of conditions involving sinus node dysfunction (more common in the elderly). Multiple manifestations on ECG include sinus bradycardia, sinus arrest, sinoatrial block, and bradytachycardia syndrome, characterized by alternating periods of sinus bradycardia and supraventricular tachycardia. The mainstay of treatment is an atrial or dual-chamber pacemaker (3, 4).
   b. Causes can include cardiomyopathies, collagen-vascular disease, ischemia, infarction, pericarditis, myocarditis, rheumatic heart disease, electrolyte disorders (especially hypokalemia or hypocarbia), and medications. The most common cause is idiopathic degenerative fibrotic infiltration. Coronary artery disease can coexist with sick sinus syndrome. The syndrome occurs in 1/600 cardiac patients older than 65 years and accounts for 50% of pacemaker placements in the United States.

B. Epidemiology. The incidence of bradycardia in the general population is unknown, but among cardiac patients and those older than 50 years, it is present in 0.6/10,000 individuals. Peak incidence occurs in the sixth and seventh decade.

III. EVALUATION

A. History

1. **Symptoms.** Elicit evidence of cardiac neurologic or respiratory compromise, such as dyspnea, palpitations, angina, decreased exercise tolerance, tachypnea, light-headedness, or syncope.

2. **Cardiac risk factors.** Inquire about family history, tobacco use, hyperlipidemia, diabetes mellitus, and hypertension.

3. **Underlying conditions.** Are underlying bradycardia risk factors present? Ask about cardiomyopathies, alcohol dependence/misuse, rheumatic heart disease, and any other coexisting medical conditions.

4. **Medications.** Bradycardia can be induced by digoxin, phenothiazine, quinidine, procainamide, β-blockers, calcium channel blockers, clonidine, lithium, and antiarrhythmic medications. β-Blocker bradycardia is especially common, because β-blockers are not only used for hypertension and angina prophylaxis but also for migraine prevention, essential tremor, thyrotoxicosis, glaucoma, and anxiety. β-Blockade can also manifest as QT interval prolongation.

B. Physical examination.
Resting pulse and blood pressure, temperature, respiratory rate, and, if there is concern for hypovolemia, blood pressure and pulse in both lying and standing positions (orthostatic evaluation) should be taken. Cardiac auscultation follows the palpation of the thyroid gland, and the search for other evidence of thyroid disorder (skin, hair, eye proptosis). The presence or absence of pulses, and search for bruits and abdominal aneurysm should follow. Is edema present? Are lung fields clear? Is there jugular venous distention? Cyanosis?

C. Testing

1. Obtain cardiac enzymes, congestive heart failure peptide, electrolytes, calcium and magnesium, thyroid-stimulating hormone, thyroxine, and triiodothyronine levels, as well as drug levels of digoxin and antiarrhythmics if indicated.

2. Obtain an ECG and if necessary an event monitor (for patients reporting rarer intermittent symptoms) or a Holter monitor (in those patients who report more frequent symptoms).

IV. DIAGNOSIS

A. Differential diagnosis.
The different types of bradycardia include

1. **Sinus bradycardia (5).** Normal P-QRS-T sequence at a rate less than 60 beats/minute.

2. **Sinus nodal block: a missing P wave.** This can be incomplete, where the occasional sequence of P-QRS-T is lost, or complete, where P waves are completely absent, and QRS-T proceeds at a slow "escape" rate from the ventricular pacemaker.

3. **Sick sinus syndrome.** Generalized abnormality, as previously described, of cardiac impulse formation that can manifest as varying combinations of bradycardia and tachycardia.

4. **First-degree atrioventricular (AV) block: common ECG finding.** The PR interval represents the conduction time from the sinus node through the atrium, AV node, and His-Purkinje system to the development of ventricular depolarization. Values over 0.2 qualify (by convention).

5. **Second-degree AV block.** This occurs when an organized atrial rhythm fails to conduct to the ventricle in a 1:1 ratio. There are several types, including the following:

   a. Mobitz type 1 (Wenckebach), in which the ECG shows a stable PP interval but a progressive increase in the PR interval until a P wave fails to conduct

   b. Mobitz type II, which is characterized by a stable PP interval with no measurable prolongation of the PR interval before an abrupt conduction failure

6. **Third-degree AV block: referred to as complete heart block.** Atrial and ventricular activity are independent of each other.

B. Clinical approach. There are few indications for intervention in patients with bradycardia who are truly asymptomatic. Where possible, and if symptoms or considerable cardiac risk is present, offending medications can be changed or reduced, underlying conditions (e.g., thyroid abnormalities) should be treated, pacing can be considered, and patient education and prevention strategies should be tried.

REFERENCES

1. Mangrum JM, Dimarco JP. The evaluation and management of bradycardia. *JAMA* 2000;342(10): 703–709.
2. Moss AJ. Long QT syndrome. *JAMA* 2003;289(16):2041–2044.
3. Roth B. *Beta-blocker toxicity eMedicine.* (www.emedicine.com) updated April 15, 2005.
4. Adan V, Crown LA. Diagnosis and treatment of sick sinus syndrome. *Am Fam Physician* 2003;67(8):1725–1732.
5. Baustian GH, Hodgson JM. *Sinus bradycardia.* FIRSTConsult (www.firstconsult.com) updated May 19, 2005.

Cardiomegaly

Matt Bogard

I. BACKGROUND. Cardiomegaly is an enlargement of the heart. This is a physical finding, is often the result of other diseases, and is almost always abnormal. Heart size is easily and most commonly determined radiographically on chest X-ray by the cardiothoracic ratio (CTR). This is measured as the ratio of the widest horizontal measurement of the heart to the widest horizontal measurement of the internal thorax (1). The CTR is normally 50–55% in adults and up to 60% in infants and children. The heart may appear falsely enlarged due to abnormalities of the chest wall or to improper radiographic technique.

II. PATHOPHYSIOLOGY

A. Etiology. Most cardiac enlargement is due to pressure overload and muscle hypertrophy of one or more chambers of the heart, volume overload with dilation of cardiac chambers, or cardiomyopathy. Therefore, cardiomegaly is typically the result of other cardiovascular disorders (hypertension, ischemic disease, valvular heart disease, or familial structural abnormalities) but can also be caused by systemic diseases (anemia, viral or rickettsial infections, bite or sting toxins, medications, anabolic steroids (2), hyperthyroidism or hypothyroidism, hyperparathyroidism, acromegaly (3), diabetes, autoimmune and infiltrative [amyloid or sarcoid] diseases, and metastases). Ventricular aneurysm and pericardial effusion can also enlarge the cardiac silhouette. Significant athleticism can cause cardiomegaly, termed "athlete's heart" (4). In many cases, particularly with left ventricular hypertrophy, cardiomegaly is reversible with treatment of the underlying cause.

B. Epidemiology. Cardiomegaly can be an incidental finding when discovered early in the disease process. It can occur in children and young adults as a result of rheumatic heart disease, infections, or in familial cardiomyopathies where the presenting symptom may be sudden death from arrhythmias, often brought on by heavy physical exertion. Due to the higher prevalence of ischemia, hypertension, and autoimmune disorders as a function of age, most cases of cardiomegaly are in older adults.

III. EVALUATION

A. History. Past medical history may include congestive heart failure, coronary disease, hypertension, rheumatic fever, and systemic diseases. Family history may reveal hypertension, hyperlipidemia, or sudden death. Social history might include alcohol or substance abuse or an exposure to a cardiac toxin. System review could include fatigue, dizziness, dyspnea, angina, cough, edema, nocturia, and loss of weight with cardiac cachexia, as well as symptoms more specific to any systemic underlying disease.

B. Physical examination

1. **Cardiac.** Inspection may note a chest deformity causing apparent cardiomegaly or a visible heave lateral to the midclavicular line. Palpation of the point of maximal impulse (PMI) below the fifth intercostal space and lateral to the midclavicular line is highly specific for left ventricular enlargement in the absence of chest wall abnormalities. The PMI may be diffuse (2–3 cm) and may be hyperdynamic in states of increased sympathetic tone, or it may feel weak in dilated cardiomyopathy. The PMI may be nonpalpable with pericardial effusion. If the PMI cannot be appreciated by palpation, the location of the left border of the heart may be ascertained by dullness to percussion. Dullness beyond the midclavicular line and fifth intercostal space is abnormal. Peripheral pulses may be weak and pulsus alternans detectable with decreased left ventricular function. Heart murmurs of abnormal valves responsible for the cardiomegaly may be auscultated, as well as the regurgitant murmurs resulting from dilated chambers. Diminished heart sounds or friction rubs may be noted with pericardial disease. S_3 and S_4 gallops may be heard with heart failure resulting from the cardiomegaly. Arrhythmias are common with cardiomegaly. Hypertension, as a cause of cardiomegaly, may be present.

2. **Extracardiac.** Examination findings may relate to the underlying causes of cardiomegaly (e.g., autoimmune, infectious, endocrine diseases, and alcoholism). The typical extracardiac findings of heart failure (cough, dyspnea, rales, wheezes, edema, hepatojugular reflux, and jugular venous distension) resulting from the cardiomegaly may be present.

C. Testing.

1. A standard upright posterior–anterior chest X-ray with the 10th rib visible at full inspiration in a nonrotated position without chest deformity is useful for determining the CTR. However, one-fifth of echocardiogram-confirmed cases of cardiomegaly are not seen on chest X-ray.

2. The electrocardiogram (ECG) is almost always abnormal with cardiomegaly, although the changes are often nonspecific. The voltage amplitude is often increased or the axis shifted. Atrial and ventricular arrhythmias are common, with atrial fibrillation occurring in 25% of patients with cardiomyopathy (5). Because lead V_1 is directly over the atria, this lead can best indicate atrial enlargement. A tall P wave in V_1 indicates atrial hypertrophy, while a widened P wave may indicate atrial dilation. As lead V_5 is over the left ventricle, a tall R wave in V_5 indicates left ventricular hypertrophy. There may be ischemic changes noted on the ECG in cardiomegaly as well.

3. Echocardiography is the test of choice for a definitive diagnosis of cardiac enlargement. It can also yield useful information about systolic and diastolic function, wall hypertrophy, ischemic areas, aneurysms, pericardial effusion, and the heart valves (6).

4. Serologic testing primarily identifies systemic causative disorders, and B-type natriuretic peptide (called the CHF peptide in many institutions) increases with ventricular wall stretch. Cardiomegaly caused by congestive heart failure may also result in an elevated serum troponin level (7).

D. Genetics. There are familial dilated as well as obstructive cardiomyopathies and familial right atrial enlargement. Studies have indicated that the presence of certain gene alleles can modify the risk of cardiac hypertrophy (4). Many autoimmune and endocrine causes of cardiomegaly are known to be familial.

IV. DIAGNOSIS

A. Differential diagnosis. It is very important to first distinguish true from factitious cardiomegaly due to suboptimal radiographic technique. Here the most important factor is an adequate inspiration revealing the 10th rib. Otherwise, the heart appears larger and more globular toward the left. Anterior–posterior films and portable chest X-rays, shot closer than the standard upright view, also falsely enlarge the heart. Supine views prevent adequate inspiration. Trunk rotation, scoliosis, and pectus excavatum can also cause apparent cardiomegaly.

B. Clinical manifestations. An enlarged heart is less efficient in providing adequate blood flow to itself and to the body. Therefore, clinical manifestations of cardiomegaly are primarily those of heart failure (e.g., dyspnea, dizziness, and fatigue). Additional symptoms are arrhythmia, angina, and sudden death. Other manifestations are signs and symptoms particular to the specific disease causing the cardiomegaly.

REFERENCES

1. *Stedman's medical dictionary*, 5th ed. Philadelphia, PA: Lippincott Williams & Williams, 2005.
2. Ahlgrim C, Guglin M. Anabolics and cardiomyopathy in a bodybuilder: case report and literature review. *J Card Failure* 2009;15(6):496–500.
3. Schwarz E, Jammula P, Gupta R, et al. A case and review of acromegaly-induced cardiomyopathy and the relationship between growth hormone and heart failure: cause or cure or neither or both? *J Cardiovasc Pharmacol Ther* 2006;11(4):232–244.
4. Lauschke J, Maisch B. Athlete's heart or hypertrophic cardiomyopathy? *Clinic Res Cardiol* 2009;98(2):80–88.
5. Hancock E, Deal B, Mirvis D, et al. AHA/ACCF/HRS recommendations for the standardization and interpretation of the electrocardiogram: part v: electrocardiogram changes associated with cardiac chamber hypertrophy: a scientific statement from the American Heart Association Electrocardiography and Arrhythmias Committee, Council on Clinical Cardiology; The American College of Cardiology Foundation; and The Heart Rhythm Society. Endorsed by The International Society for Computerized Electrocardiology. *J Am Coll Cardiol* 2009;53(11):992–1002.
6. Pewsner D, Juni P, Egger M, et al. Accuracy of electrocardiography in diagnosis of left ventricular hypertrophy in arterial hypertension: systematic review. *BMJ* 2007;335(7622):711.
7. Jungbauer C, Riedlinger J, Buchner S, et al. High-sensitive troponin T in chronic heart failure correlates with severity of symptoms, left ventricular dysfunction and prognosis independently from N-terminal pro-B-type natriuretic peptide. *Clin Chem Lab Med* 2011;49(11):1899–1906.

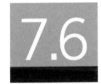

7.6 Congestive Heart Failure
Rebecca Wester

I. BACKGROUND. Heart failure (HF) is defined as "a complex clinical syndrome resulting from any structural or functional cardiac disorder that impairs the ability of the ventricle to fill with or eject blood" (1). The term *heart failure* is preferred over the older term *congestive heart failure* because HF patients may not show evidence of congestion (i.e., fluid overload) at the time of evaluation (1). HF is complex, costly, and deadly. HF is a major public health problem in industrialized nations and is increasing in prevalence and incidence in North America and Western Europe (2). Not unexpectedly, HF-related hospitalization rates have been steadily increasing over the past decade (1). Despite improvements in therapy, the mortality in patients with HF has remained unacceptably high, making early detection of susceptible individuals imperative (3). Approximately 5 million patients have HF, and over 550,000 new patients are diagnosed with HF each year in the United States (1). With the notable exception of lung cancer, HF is as "malignant" as many common types of cancer and is associated with a comparable number of expected life-years lost (4). In 2005, the direct and indirect cost of HF was approximated at $27.9 billion, with $2.9 billion annually spent on HF drug treatment in the United States (1). With improvements in the prognosis of HF, improved survival after acute myocardial infarction, and an aging population, the burden of HF will continue to increase in the years to come.

II. PATHOPHYSIOLOGY

A. Etiology

1. Two interrelated processes, chamber remodeling and left ventricular dysfunction, play critical roles in HF. In patients with HF, approximately 70% have systolic dysfunction, 15% have diastolic dysfunction, and the remaining 15% have both (4). Systolic HF is now referred to as *HF with reduced left ventricular ejection fraction (LVEF)*. Diastolic HF is now referred to as *HF with preserved LVEF* (1). Reduced LVEF (previously systolic HF) is associated with reduced myocardial contractility. Preserved LVEF (previously diastolic HF) is associated with decreased LV filling.

2. Causes of HF differ depending on LV function (reduced or preserved LVEF), left-sided or right-sided, or acute or chronic. In the United States and Western Europe, coronary artery disease and hypertension are the most common causes of both types of LV dysfunction. In 75% of cases, HF has antecedent hypertension (5). The most common cause of right-sided HF is left-sided HF. Other causes of right-sided HF include pulmonary hypertension, cor pulmonale, or dysfunction of right-sided valves (6). Refer to Table 7.6.1 for the common causes of HF.

B. Epidemiology

1. In evaluating patients with HF, it is important to identify not only the underlying cause(s) but also the precipitating factor(s). The OPTIMIZE-HF study identified precipitating factors in patients hospitalized for HF: pneumonia/respiratory condition (15%), ischemia (15%), arrhythmias (14%), uncontrolled hypertension (11%), medication non-adherence (9%), worsening renal function (7%), and diet non-adherence (5%) (6). A total of 61% of these HF patients had one or more factors; 39% did not have an identified precipitating factor (7). Less common precipitating factors are pulmonary embolism, high-output states (i.e., anemia, pregnancy, and thyrotoxicosis), cardiotoxins and medications with HF adverse drug effects (i.e., alcohol, cocaine, antiarrhythmics, calcium channel blockers, nonsteroidal anti-inflammatory drugs, and antineoplastics), and cardiac infections (i.e., myocarditis, endocarditis, and pericarditis).

2. HF is primarily a condition of the elderly (1). The incidence of HF approaches 10 per 1,000 population over age 65 years; and approximately 80% of patients who are hospitalized with HF are over 65 years old (1). In the Framingham Study, the incidence of HF approximately doubled over each successive decade of life (3).

TABLE 7.6.1	Types and Causes of Heart Failure

Heart failure with reduced left ventricular function

Causes include

Ischemic heart disease, hypertension, alcohol toxicity, obesity, valvular disease (e.g., aortic stenosis), or chronic tachydysrhythmia

Heart failure with preserved left ventricular function

Causes include

Transient systolic dysfunction due to acute myocardial ischemia

Left atrial hypertension due to high-output states (e.g., thyrotoxicosis), volume excess, or mitral stenosis

Left ventricular diastolic dysfunction due to hypertension, ischemia, aging, obesity, or sustained tachy-arrhythmias

Miscellaneous disorders such as restrictive cardiomyopathy due to infiltrative diseases (e.g., amyloidosis), constrictive pericarditis and pericardial tamponade, and pure right-sided heart failure

III. EVALUATION

A. History

1. Clinical symptoms occur after hemodynamic changes and are in essence "just the tip of the iceberg" (i.e., a small aspect of something largely hidden) (8). Dyspnea on exertion (DOE), orthopnea, and paroxysmal nocturnal dyspnea (PND) result from underlying pulmonary congestion and are the most specific symptoms of HF. Dyspnea is the most predominant symptom of HF, whereas orthopnea and PND occur in a more advanced stage of HF. Orthopnea can be assessed by asking "Can you breathe comfortably when you lie flat?" PND can be assessed by asking "Do you wake up short of breath after falling asleep?" PND occurs after 2–3 hours of sleep and is relieved with sitting up for 5–30 minutes. Systemic vascular congestion causes peripheral edema, ascites, abdominal pain/fullness, and nausea, whereas low cardiac output causes fatigue and change in mental status. It is not unusual for HF patients to have fatigue, weight gain, worsening exercise tolerance, cough, sleepiness, or decreased mentation. These symptoms are common, but are not present in every HF case. For example, DOE has 66% sensitivity and 52% specificity; orthopnea has 66% sensitivity and 47% specificity (8). HF patients that are sedentary or deconditioned may not have DOE due to their baseline poor exercise tolerance. Older patients with HF often present with atypical symptoms such as dry cough, daytime oliguria with nocturia, or confusion. It is important to assess functional capacity (i.e., the ability to perform activities of daily living, such as bathing, dressing, and ambulation) and desired activities by asking "What are some activities you would like to do but can no longer do?" (1).

2. A detailed family history should be obtained not only to determine whether there is familial predisposition to atherosclerotic disease but also to identify relatives with cardiomyopathy, sudden unexplained death, conduction system disease, and skeletal myopathy. About 30% of cases of idiopathic dilated cardiomyopathy may be familial (1). Noncardiac diseases such as rheumatologic diseases, bacterial or parasitic infection, obesity, amyloidosis, thyroid disorders, or pheochromocytoma can cause HF and are reasonable to consider in select HF patients with a clinical suspicion. Smoking history should be inquired as well (1).

B. Physical examination.

In general, physical examination is more sensitive in detecting acute HF than chronic HF. In mild or moderately severe HF, the patient appears in no distress at rest except feeling uncomfortable when lying flat for more than a few minutes. In severe HF, the pulse pressure may be diminished; and the diastolic arterial pressure may be elevated. Elevated systemic venous pressure may be reflected in the distention of the jugular veins. When this pressure is abnormally high, characteristic abdominojugular reflux is seen. Elevated jugular vein pressure (JVP) is the most specific sign for fluid overload; unfortunately, elevated JVP is present in a minority of dyspneic patients and is difficult to assess in obese patients. The diagnostic value of resting JVD is 70% sensitivity and 42% specificity (8). Third and fourth heart sounds are often audible but are not specific for HF. Other physical findings include pulmonary rales, cardiac edema (which is usually symmetric and dependent on HF, pitting in acute and brawny in chronic HF), hydrothorax, ascites, congestive hepatomegaly, occasional splenomegaly, jaundice, and cardiac cachexia. Pulmonary rales indicate a more acute decompensation, but most patients with chronic HF do not have rales (1). In severe acute HF with hypoperfusion, systolic hypotension may be present with cool, diaphoretic extremities and Cheyne-Stokes respiration. There may be cyanosis in lips and nail beds and sinus tachycardia as well. Initial examination should include the patient's volume status, orthostatic blood pressure changes, weight and height measurements (for body mass index). Weight gain or loss of 3 pounds in 2–3 days usually is due to fluid overload or diuresis. Up to 5 L (11 lb) may accumulate in body tissues before bilateral peripheral edema is seen. Edema can redistribute to dependent areas, such as the sacrum or upper thighs.

C. Testing.

While ordering laboratory tests for patients with HF, it is important to screen for diabetes, kidney disease, anemia, thyrotoxicosis, and liver dysfunction. Initial laboratory evaulation should include complete blood count, urianalysis, electrolytes (including calcium and magnesium), blood urea nitrogen, serum creatitine, fasting blood glucose (and hemoglobin A1C), lipid panel, liver function tests, and thyroid-stimulating hormone (1). Additional tests may be ordered when there is suspicion of certain diseases either causing or precipitating HF, such as cardiac markers in the presence of chest pain (1). Screening for hemochromatosis, sleep-disturbed pattern (i.e., obstructive sleep apnea), or human immunodeficiency virus is reasonable in selected patients (1). Although the sodium and potassium values are usually normal in these patients, hyponatremia and hyperkalemia can be associated with severe HF. Impaired liver function is often associated with hepatic congestion or cardiac cirrhosis.

1. *Echocardiography* is the single most effective diagnostic test in the evaluation of patients with HF. In HF with reduced LVEF, the ejection fraction is less than 40%, whereas a normal ejection fraction could be HF with preserved LVEF. High left ventricular end-diastolic pressure (LVEDP) suggests diastolic dysfunction. The echocardiogram provides information about possible associated pericardial, myocardial, or valvular disease. Reassessment of HF is needed in patients who had a change in clinical status or received treatment that might have had a significant effect on heart function (1).

2. *Electrocardiogram (ECG)* reveals atrial fibrillation in approximately 20–30% patients with HF. ECG may also show evidence of old infarction, left ventricular hypertrophy, left atrial enlargement, arrhythmias other than atrial fibrillation, low voltage, or bundle branch block.

3. *Chest x-ray* typically shows cardiomegaly, with a sensitivity of 97% and specificity of 10% (8). Other x-ray findings of HF include pulmonary vascular redistribution, interstitial and alveolar pulmonary edema, and less often cloud-like appearance with concentration of fluid around the hilum, giving a butterfly or bat wing appearance. Serial chest x-rays are not recommended for routine follow-up (1).

4. *B-type natriuretic peptide (BNP)* is an independent predictor of high LVEDP. Its release is proportional to ventricular volume expansion and pressure overload. A BNP < 100 pg/mL reliably rules out HF diagnosis in the dyspneic patient in the urgent care setting, in whom the clinical diagnosis of HF is uncertain (1, 9).

5. *Cardiac catheterization* with coronary arteriography may be considered in patients with HF, angina, and known or suspected coronary artery disease but without angina, who are candidates for revascularization (1).

6. Magnetic resonance imaging, radionuclide ventriculography, or endomyocardial biopsy is used infrequently for diagnosis in clinical practice. No single noninvasive test can accurately detect HF, and the ability to detect congestion by hemodynamic measurement remains a diagnostic challenge because it usually precedes clincal symptoms (8).

It should be emphasized that HF is not equivalent to cardiomyopathy or to LV dysfunction; these terms describe structural or functional reasons for HF. HF is a clinical syndrome that is characterized by specific symptoms from history (such as dyspnea and fatigue) and by specific signs from examination (such as edema and rales) (1). There is no single diagnostic test for HF because it is for the most part a clinical diagnosis that is based on careful history and physical examination (1, 8).

REFERENCES

1. Hunt SA, Abraham WT, Chin MH, et al. Focused update incorporated into the ACC/AHA 2005 guidelines for the diagnosis and management of heart failure in adults. *Circulation* 2009;119:e391–e479.
2. Cleland JG, Khand A, Clark A. The heart failure epidemic: exactly how big is it? *Eur Heart J* 2001;22:623–626.
3. Ho KK, Pinsky JL, Kannel WB. The epidemiology of heart failure: the Framingham Study. *J Am Coll Cardiol* 1993;22:6A–13A.
4. Stewart S, MacIntyre K, Hole DJ, Capewell S, McMurray JJ. More "malignant" than cancer? Five-year survival following a first admission for heart failure. *Eur J Heart Failure* 2001;3:315–322.
5. Lloyd-Jones D, Adams RJ, Brown TM, et al. Heart diease and stroke statistics-2010 update: a report from the American Heart Association. *Circulation* 2010;121(7):e46–e215.
6. Nohria A, Lewis E, Stevenson LW. Medical management of advanced heart failure. *JAMA* 2002;287:628–640.

7. Fonafrow GC, Abraham WT, Albert NM, et al. Factors identified as precipitating hospital admission for heart failure and clincal outcomes. *Arch Intern Med* 2008;168(8):847–854.
8. Gheorghiade M, Follarth F, Ponikowski P, et al. Assessing and grading congestion in acute heart failure: a scientific statement for the acute heart failure committee of the Heart Failure Association of the European Society of Cardiology and endorsed by the European Society of Intensive Care Medicine. *Eur J Heart Failure* 2010;12:423–433.
9. Battaglia M, Pewser D, Juni P, et al. Accurancy of B-type natriuretic peptide tests to exclude congestive heart failure. *Arch Intern Med* 2006;166:1073–1080.

7.7 Diastolic Heart Murmurs

Douglas J. Inciarte

I. CONCEPT. A diastolic heart murmur occurs during heart muscle relaxation starting with or after S_2 and ending before or after S_1 (*S_2/-murmur-/S_1*). Diastolic murmurs are typically due to the stenosis of the mitral or tricuspid valves or the regurgitation of the aortic or pulmonary valves. The diastolic murmur should more often than not be considered pathological or associated with structural cardiac abnormalities and therefore warrants further evaluation. These murmurs can be classified into four categories:

A. Early diastolic murmur, which starts with S_2 and peaks in the first third of diastole.

B. Mid-diastolic murmur, which starts after S_2 and ends prior to S_1.

C. Late diastolic murmur, which starts in the concluding part of diastole during atrial contraction and persists to S_1.

D. Continuous murmur, which extends from systole into diastole. Such a murmur results from blood flow continuing from a high-pressure to a lower-pressure area (1).

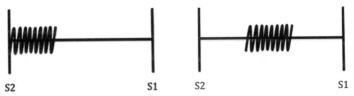

S2   S1   S2   S1

Figure 7.7.1. Early diastolic murmur.
Seen in aortic and pulmonary regurgitation, S3, and left anterior descending stenosis.

Figure 7.7.2. Mid-diastolic murmur.
Seen in mitral and tricuspid stenosis and atrial axiomas.

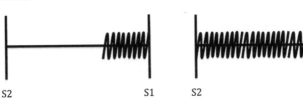

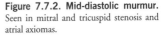

S2   S1   S2   S1

Figure 7.7.3. Late diastolic murmur.
Seen in mitral and tricuspid stenosis, atrial axiomas, left-to-right shunt, complete heart block, and S4.

Figure 7.7.4. Continuous murmur.
Classical for patent ductus arteriosus.

II. PATHOPHYSIOLOGY/EVALUATION/DIAGNOSIS

A. Early diastolic murmur

1. Aortic regurgitation

a. Pathophysiology. Insufficient closing of the aortic valve leaflets, which can be caused by alteration or dilatation of the aortic root and ascending aorta. Aortic regurgitation (AR) causes greater resultant end-diastolic left ventricular volume, resulting in a residual left ventricular dilatation and hypertrophy. Eventually, peripheral signs include increase in the gradient between systolic and diastolic pressure (widened arterial pulse pressure), observable carotid pulse, suprasternal pulsations, rapid rise and fall of pulse ("water-hammer" pulse), flushing pulsations of nail beds (Quincke's pulse), "to-and-fro" murmur from slight stethoscope compression on the femoral artery (Duroziez's murmur), head bob with each pulse (de Musset's sign), and rapid ejection of large stroke volume ("pistol-shot" femoral artery sound) (2, 3).

b. Epidemiology. More common in men than women; more common in adults older than 60 years. If associated with Marfan's syndrome, Ehlers-Danlos syndrome, autosomal recessive or X-linked inheritance, and collagen-vascular diseases, there may be familial predisposition (3).

c. Causes (2–4). Rheumatic heart disease, congenital heart disease (bicuspid aortic valve, prolapsed aortic cusp with ventricular septal defect), collagen-vascular diseases (systemic lupus erythematosus), connective-tissue disease (Marfan's syndrome, Turner's syndrome, pseudoxanthoma elasticum, ankylosing spondylitis, Ehlers-Danlos syndrome, polymyalgia rheumatica), ascending aortic aneurysm, aortitis (syphilis, Takayasu's arteritis, granulomatous aortitis), cystic medial necrosis, Reiter's syndrome, myxomatous aortic valve, calcific changes in aortic valve, anorectic drugs or patients treated with dexfenfluramine or phentermine/fenfluramine, infective endocarditis, aortic dissection, trauma, hypertension, and end-stage renal disease (transient murmur from fluid overload).

d. History. Is there a history of rheumatic fever (RF)? Check for recurrent strep throat, shortness of breath at rest (signs of cardiac decompensation), chest pressure during physical activity, palpitations (symptomatic arrhythmias), lower extremity swelling, trauma (risk of aortic dissection), intravenous drug use, recent dental work (risk of endocarditis), use of fenfluramine/dexfenfluramine (Fen-Phen) or other weight loss drugs, history of lens dislocation/long slender limbs (presence of Marfan's syndrome), sexually transmitted diseases (risk of syphilis), and lax joints (Ehlers-Danlos syndrome) (3).

e. Diagnosis. Decrescendo, "blowing" character, low-intensity, high-pitched diastolic murmur at the left sternal border or over the right second intercostal space while the patient is sitting and leaning forward with breath held in deep expiration, radiating to the cardiac apex, increases with handgrip or squatting; can even present with a musical quality "diastolic whoop." A diastolic rumble at the ventricular apex is known as the *Austin Flint murmur* (1).

f. Presentation. Heart failure symptoms, exertional dyspnea, fatigue, paroxysmal nocturnal dyspnea, pulmonary edema, angina pectoris, atypical chest pain, elevated systolic and decreased diastolic blood pressure (3).

2. Pulmonary regurgitation

a. Pathophysiology. Insufficient closure of the pulmonary valve leaflets.

b. Causes. Usually secondary to pulmonary hypertension. However, pulmonary regurgitation (PR) can also be caused by the idiopathic dilatation of the pulmonary artery, status postsurgery or post-balloon valvuloplasty, right-sided endocarditis, or congenital absence of the pulmonary valve.

c. Diagnosis. Decrescendo, "blowing" character, high-pitched diastolic (Graham Steell) heard best over the left sternal border and left second and third intercostal space (vs. AR, which is heard in the right intercostals). The PR murmur increases with inspiration.

d. Presentation. Right ventricular volume and pressure overload; a significant right ventricular heave, elevated jugular venous pressure (1, 3).

3. **Left anterior descending artery stenosis.** "Dock's murmur" is similar to that of AR and is caused by turbulent flow across the stenotic coronary arteries. Auscultate for murmur at the left second or third intercostal space and the left sternal border (1).

4. **S$_3$ gallop/ventricular gallop.** This can be heard as an early diastolic gallop. In children, it is usually normal; however, in adults, it is typically a sign of heart failure.

B. Mid-diastolic murmur

1. **Mitral stenosis**

   a. **Pathophysiology.** Fibrosis and lack of mobility of the mitral valve leaflets, which cause an impediment in flow from the left atrium to the left ventricle, resulting in increased pressure in the left atrium, pulmonary vasculature, and right side of the heart.

   b. **Epidemiology.** Predominately women.

   c. **Causes.** RF, congenital disease, malignant carcinoid, methysergide therapy, systemic lupus erythematosus, and rheumatoid arthritis.

   d. **History.** Is there a history of RF (most common cause), breathlessness with exertion (most common symptom), palpitations (atrial fibrillation associated with mitral stenosis [MS]), travel history (RF is common in developing countries), and/or migraine medications (methysergide)?

   e. **Diagnosis.** Loud opening snap followed by a low-pitched diastolic rumble heard best at the apex while the patient is lying on the left side; murmur increases with expiration.

   f. **Presentation.** "Mitral facies" (vasoconstriction with resultant pinkish-purple patches on cheeks), heart failure symptoms (exertional dyspnea, edema), atrial fibrillation, chest pain, hoarseness from left atrial enlargement and compression of recurrent laryngeal nerve, and fatigue (4).

2. **Tricuspid stenosis**

   a. **Pathophysiology.** Fibrosis and lack of mobility of the tricuspid valve leaflets with resultant elevation of pressure in the right atrium and jugular veins; more common in mid-diastole when in atrial fibrillation (in normal sinus rhythm, murmur is late diastolic).

   b. **Causes.** Usually in association with MS, RF, carcinoid heart disease, right atrial myxoma (1).

   c. **Diagnosis.** Begins with a tricuspid opening snap and associated with a mid-diastolic rumble best auscultated at the left sternal border; murmur increases with inspiration (Carvallo's sign).

   d. **Presentation.** Can present with atrial fibrillation, right-sided heart failure, hepatomegaly, ascites, dependent edema.

3. **Atrial myxoma.** This is the most common primary heart tumor consisting of a benign gelatinous growth. The growths can cause an obstruction of the mitral and tricuspid valves presenting with chest pain, dyspnea, edema, and syncope. Left atrial myxoma murmur is similar to that of MS (as right atrial myxoma is similar to tricuspid stenosis). Atrial myxoma murmurs can change with alterations of position and also present with the "tumor plop."

4. **Increased flow across the atrioventricular valve.** This is otherwise known as a *flow murmur* (1).

C. Late diastolic murmur

1. **Mitral stenosis.** This murmur becomes a late diastolic murmur when atrial contraction increases the pressure and flow at the end of the diastole.

2. **Tricuspid stenosis.** This late diastolic murmur occurs during sinus rhythm.

3. **Atrial myxoma.** This murmur can also present in late diastole as well as mid-diastole.

4. **Left-to-right shunt**

5. **Complete heart block.** This is a short late murmur called *Rytand's murmur.*

6. **S$_4$/atrial gallop.** This occurs from the resistance of atrial filling after an atrial contraction. It presents as a late diastolic atrial gallop that may be associated with myocardial disease, coronary artery disease, or hypertension and increases sound with deep inspiration (1).

D. Continuous murmur.

This murmur begins in systole, peaks near S$_2$, and continues into all or part of the diastole.

1. **Patent ductus arteriosus.** This continuous machinelike murmur is auscultated best at the left middle and left upper sternal border and second intercostal space with radiation to the back.

2. **Other causes of continuous murmurs.** These include aortopulmonary window, shunts (through an atrial septal defect), arteriovenous fistulas, constriction of systemic/pulmonary arteries, coarctation of the aorta, "mammary soufflé" in pregnancy, venous hum, and pericardial friction rub (1).

III. DIAGNOSTIC EVALUATION

A. The standard test of choice is transthoracic echocardiography. Consider transesophageal for more specific evaluation for endocarditis and to evaluate for vegetations.

B. Other ancillary diagnostic tools to exclude differential diagnosis include electrocardiogram, chest x-ray, cardiac catheterization, blood cultures, complete blood count with differential and erythrocyte sedimentation rate in suspected cases of endocarditis, radionuclide angiography when echocardiography is nonconclusive, aortogram for evaluation of aorta, chest computed tomography (to diagnose dissection), aortic magnetic resonance imaging (to diagnose dissection), exercise testing, tissue testing/DNA testing for genetic abnormalities, and serologic tests for collagen-vascular disease and syphilis (2, 4, 5).

REFERENCES

1. Chatterjee K. *Auscultation of cardiac murmurs. Up To Date:* online 13.2 (www.uptodate.com); updated on April 2005.
2. Cheitlin MD. Surgery for chronic aortic regurgitation: when should it be considered? *Am Fam Physician* 2001;64:1709–1714.
3. Scherger JE, O'Hanlon KM, Jones RC, et al. *Aortic regurgitation. FIRSTConsult* (http://www .firstconsult.com.cuhsl.creighton.edu/?type=med&id=01014202) Updated on Wednesday, June 25, 2005.
4. Cunningham R, Corretti M, Henrich W. *Valvular heart disease in patients with end-stage renal disease. Up to Date:* online 13.2 (www.uptodate.com); updated on April 2005.
5. Ferri FF, Saver DF, Hodgson JM, et al. *Mitral stenosis. FIRSTConsult* (http://www.firstconsult.com. cuhsl.creighton.edu/?type=med&id=01014231) Updated on Friday, May 27, 2005.

7.8 Systolic Heart Murmurs
James E. Hougas, III

Heart murmurs are a common physical examination finding and carry varied amounts of clinical significance. As William James, a pioneering American psychologist and physician, once said: "The art of being wise is the art of knowing what to overlook." The discerning health care provider must be able to tell the difference between murmurs that are clinically insignificant and those that require further workup and management.

I. BACKGROUND. A heart murmur is the description of a heart sound that is different from the primary heart sounds of S1 and S2 and the often-pathologic S3 and S4. The murmur is generally a prolonged sound in comparison to the very short S1–4. Specifically, systolic murmurs occur during the heart's contractile phase (systole) that occurs between S1, the closing of the mitral and tricuspid valves, and S2, the closing of the aortic and pulmonic valves. Diastolic murmurs occur during the heart's relaxation and filling phase (diastole) between S2 and S1. Those murmurs should never be considered innocent and require workup; they are addressed elsewhere in this volume (1).

II. PATHOPHYSIOLOGY. Murmurs are caused by turbulent blood flow in the vasculature, most commonly the heart. They are produced by high blood flow through normal (tachycardia) or abnormal openings (septal defect), forward flow through narrowed or irregular openings into an enlarged chamber or vessel (stenosis), or backward flow through an insufficient valve (regurgitation) (1).

III. EVALUATION

A. History. A thorough and complete history is paramount when evaluating a previously unheard murmur.

1. It is important to note any previous history of valvular disease or congenital heart disease. A social history of intravenous drug use, tobacco abuse, and other high-risk behaviors should be documented. Past medical history of anemia, thyroid disorders, and pregnancy are notably associated with flow murmurs.

2. Review of systems should include any complaints of dyspnea, dyspnea on exertion, diaphoresis, chest pain, palpitations, edema, syncope, exacerbating and relieving factors, as well as a timeline of symptoms and any progression. Other systemic complaints to address include weight loss, fevers and/or chills, new rashes, recent myocardial infarction, and easy fatigability. Family history of early or sudden cardiac deaths may increase the possibility of a genetic disorder such as hypertrophic cardiomyopathy (HCM).

3. Worsening of murmurs over time or the development of symptoms may warrant workup (1, 2).

B. Physical examination

1. Always begin with a review of the vital signs and observation of the patient for signs of distress.

2. The cardiac examination involves auscultation at the four cardiac listening points, palpation of carotid and peripheral pulses, and description of the heart sounds. Murmurs are described by their location, loudness, and timing. It should also be noted if the murmur changes with inspiration, exhalation, Valsalva maneuver, handgrip exercise, or positional change. Right-sided murmurs (pulmonic and tricuspid) will often increase with inspiration and left-sided (aortic and mitral) murmurs increase with expiration. Valsalva maneuver increases the murmur of HCM and mitral valve prolapse (MVP). The handgrip exercise increases the systolic murmurs of mitral regurgitation and ventricular septal defects. Standing decreases all murmurs except for HCM and MVP, while squatting does the reverse.

3. The timing of the murmur can be classified as holosystolic (pansystolic), midsystolic (systolic ejection), early systolic, or mid-to-late systolic. Holosystolic murmurs occur throughout systole. Midsystolic murmurs begin immediately after a usually normal S1. Early systolic murmurs start with and can obscure S1. Mid-to-late systolic murmurs start well after S1. A review of the listening posts and their associated murmurs is found in Table 7.8.1 (1, 3).

4. Murmurs should be graded according to volume and the absence or presence of a palpable thrill (3).
   a. Grade I. Faint and difficult to hear, which is easily missed and requires special effort to hear
   b. Grade II. Soft murmur more easily heard, especially with experience
   c. Grade III. A fairly loud murmur that is not associated with a thrill
   d. Grade IV. A loud murmur that is associated with a thrill
   e. Grade V. A louder murmur with a thrill, but a stethoscope is still required to hear it
   f. Grade VI. A murmur with a thrill that is so loud it can be heard before the stethoscope touches the chest

C. Testing. Midsystolic murmurs that are grade I or II and not associated with symptoms or abnormal electrocardiography (EKG) or chest x-ray (CXR) require no further workup. All other patients should have echocardiography performed. EKG and CXR are not indicated for routine workup of systolic murmurs but may be available due to workup for another clinical situation (e.g., chest pain). Patients with isolated, asymptomatic, grade I or II midsystolic murmurs will likely have a normal EKG and CXR (1).

1. EKG is readily available and inexpensive. It provides useful information about the presence of myocardial ischemia, prior infarct, and arrhythmias and may show ventricular hypertrophy or atrial dilation.

TABLE 7.8.1 Physical Examination Findings of Systolic Heart Murmurs

Systolic murmur	Description	Maneuvers	Location heard
Aortic stenosis	Midsystolic, crescendo–decrescendo	Transmits to carotids, thrill with expiration	Right sternal border, second rib space
Tricuspid regurgitation	Usually early systolic, rarely midsystolic	Increases with inspiration	Lower left sternal border, heard below xiphoid process
Mitral regurgitation	Common, usually early systolic, rarely midsystolic	Handgrip exercise may increase	Apex, radiates to axilla
Mitral valve prolapse	Mid-to-late systolic, may hear click	Increases with standing or Valsalva	Apex, use diaphragm
Pulmonic stenosis	Midsystolic, crescendo–decrescendo	Increases with inspiration, transmits to suprasternal notch	Left sternal border, second to third rib space
Ventricular septal defect	Harsh holosystolic	Radiates to right sternal border, handgrip exercise may increase	Apex to right sternal border
Hypertrophic cardiomyopathy	Harsh midsystolic, ejection murmur	Increases with standing or Valsalva	Aortic area to apex, does not radiate beyond heart

2. Posterioanterior and lateral CXR can provide information about the heart size, vascular calcifications, pulmonary vascular prominence, and pulmonary edema. Signs of heart failure in the face of a new murmur may warrant a more urgent evaluation.

3. Useful laboratory tests may include complete blood count (anemia, infection, red blood cell destruction), thyroid-stimulating hormone (hypothyroidism/hyperthyroidism), blood culture (endocarditis), troponin I creatine kinase (CK)/CK-MB (markers of myocardial damage), and CHF peptide.

4. Transthoracic echocardiography (TTE) is noninvasive and widely available and yields important information by imaging cardiac structures and measuring flow rate and direction through cardiac valves. It can sometimes be limited by the patient's body habitus. TTE is the initial test of choice for the evaluation of murmurs that require workup.

5. Transesophageal echocardiography and cardiac catheterization are also available if the diagnosis is still uncertain after reviewing the TTE. These are invasive, expensive studies and are not appropriate for initial workup of systolic heart murmurs without compelling evidence, such as evidence of acute coronary syndrome.

IV. DIAGNOSIS. A diligent history and physical are often enough to diagnose the root of your patient's systolic heart murmur. When indicated, echocardiography will confirm your clinical suspicion. For additional practice in cardiac auscultation, several web sites have been developed that may be useful for learning to recognize specific murmurs.

A. Virtual Stethoscope. http://sprojects.mmi.mcgill.ca/mvs/mvsteth.htm

B. The Auscultation Assistant. http://www.wilkes.med.ucla.edu/inex.htm

C. Cardiac Auscultation. http://www.egeneralmedical.com/listohearmur.html

REFERENCES

1. Bonow RO, Carabello BA, Chatterjee K, et al. 2008 Focused update incorporated into the ACC/AHA 2006 Guidelines for the Management of Patients with Valvular Heart Disease. *Circulation* 2008;118:e523–e661.
2. Kasper D, Braunwald E, Wilson JD, eds. *Harrison's principals of internal medicine*, 16th ed. New York, NY: McGraw-Hill, 2005.
3. Greenberger N, Hinthorn D. *History taking and physical examination*. St. Louis, MO: Mosby, 1993.

7.9 Hypertension
K. John Burhan

Hypertension (HTN) is a leading cause of morbidity and mortality in the United States. The treatment of HTN is the most common reason for office visits of nonpregnant adults. Estimates suggest that of all individuals with HTN, 34% are receiving adequate therapy, 25% are receiving inadequate therapy, 11% are receiving no therapy, and 30% of individuals with HTN do not know they have the condition (1).

I. **BACKGROUND.** According to *The Seventh Report of the Joint National Committee on Prevention, Detection, Evaluation, and Treatment of High Blood Pressure*, the classification of blood pressure in adults aged 18 years and older is as follows (see Table 7.9.1):

   A. A systolic blood pressure of 120 mmHg or less is considered normal.

   B. A new classification, "prehypertension" is a systolic blood pressure of 120–139 mmHg and/or a diastolic blood pressure of 80–89 mmHg. Prehypertension is not a disease category and individuals who fall into this category *are not* candidates for drug therapy. Patients who fall into this category are identified as being considered at high risk for HTN and should be counseled regarding lifestyle modification to reduce their risk of developing HTN in the future.

   C. Stage 1 HTN is defined as a systolic blood pressure of 140–159 mmHg and/or a diastolic blood pressure of 90–99 mmHg.

   D. Stage 2 HTN is defined as a systolic blood pressure of 160 mmHg or greater based on the average of two or more readings taken at each of two or more visits after initial screening (2).

TABLE 7.9.1	Classification of Blood Pressure in US Adults 18 Years of Age and Older	
Blood pressure classification	**Systolic blood pressure (mmHg)**	**Diastolic blood pressure (mmHg)**
Normal	<120	<80
Prehypertension	120–139	80–89
Stage 1 HTN	140–159	90–99
Stage 2 HTN	≥160	≥100

HTN, hypertension.

Department of Health and Human Service, National Institutes of Health, *The Seventh Report of the Joint National Committee on Prevention, Detection, Evaluation, and Treatment of High Blood Pressure*. www.nhlbi.nih.gov/guidelines/hypertension

II. PATHOPHYSIOLOGY

A. Etiology. The cause of 90–95% of the cases of HTN is not known (1). Patients with no identifiable cause of HTN are said to have primary or essential HTN. Patients with a specific structural organ or gene defect responsible for their HTN are classified as having secondary HTN (3).

B. Epidemiology. Approximately one in three adults in the United States have HTN, and approximately 28% or 59 million of American adults 18 years of age and older have "prehypertension" (1). Approximately 50% of individuals who suffer a first myocardial infarction and two-thirds who undergo a first stroke have a blood pressure higher than 160/95 mmHg. Compared with normotensive individuals, the relative risk of stroke is four times greater for individuals with a systolic blood pressure of 160 mmHg or higher and/or a diastolic blood pressure of 95 mmHg or higher. Individuals at the lower educational and income levels tend to have higher levels of blood pressure.

III. EVALUATION

A. History. After the documentation of HTN is established, a detailed history should reveal information about target end organ damage, the patient's cardiovascular risk status, and secondary causes of HTN. Questions to assess the extent of target organ damage should include any history of acute episodic or progressive visual change or occipital headaches upon arising in the morning that fade in several hours. Review any symptoms consistent with angina pectoris, ischemic heart disease, peripheral vascular disease, congestive heart failure, cerebral vascular disease, retinopathy, and nephropathy (3). Symptoms suggestive of a secondary cause of HTN need to be explored. The patients' age and gender should also be considered. A higher percentage of men than women have HTN until 55 years of age. After 55 years of age, a much higher percentage of women have HTN than men (2). Other important medical history includes previous documentation of HTN by a health-care provider. Part of the health history must address comorbid health conditions such as diabetes mellitus, dyslipidemia, obesity, and family history.

1. **Medication history.** It is important to review current or past antihypertensive medication use. Patients stop antihypertensive therapy for various reasons, including stated reasons such as they were "feeling better" or they "could not afford the medication." It is also necessary to review the herbal and over-the-counter (OTC) therapies the patient currently uses or previously used. Many OTC cough and cold remedies and weight loss pills contain products that can potentially elevate blood pressure. Unfortunately, some OTC herbal therapies may interact with prescription medications, altering the metabolism, serum level, effectiveness, and side effects of many prescription medications and potentially complicating treatment. Potencies of herbal medications can vary dramatically between manufacturers. Therefore, health-care practitioners should have ready access to a guide for herbal medicines that describes their origin, uses, side effects, metabolism, excretion, toxicities, and known potential prescription drug interactions. In addition, many prescription medications may elevate blood pressure.

2. **Social history.** Factors to review include tobacco, caffeine, alcohol, and illicit drug use. A dietary history may illuminate approximate quantities of saturated fats and sodium intake. Time spent in exercise and type of leisure activities should be determined.

B. Physical examination

1. **Blood pressure measurement.** Errors can be minimized by choosing the proper size blood pressure cuff and utilizing a standardized technique. Guidelines for a proper size blood pressure cuff are listed in Table 7.9.2. Patient preparation guidelines to minimize erroneous blood pressure readings are listed in Table 7.9.3. To determine a proper cuff inflation pressure, palpate the radial pulse while inflating the cuff bladder. When the radial pulse is no longer palpable, note this pressure on the manometer and add 30 mmHg to it. Deflate the cuff and wait approximately 30 seconds before attempting cuff reinflation. Place the stethoscope bell lightly over the brachial artery and inflate the cuff rapidly to the above-determined pressure. Deflate it at a rate of about 2–3 mmHg per second. Note the pressure level when at least two consecutive beats are first heard. This level is the systolic pressure. Continue lowering the cuff pressure until the sounds

TABLE 7.9.2	Selecting the Correct Blood Pressure Cuff

- Width of the inflatable bladder of the cuff should be approximately 40% of the upper arm circumference (approximately 12–14 cm in the average adult)
- Length of inflatable bladder should be approximately 80% of upper arm circumference (almost long enough to encircle the arm)
- If aneroid, recalibrate periodically before use

Bickley LS, Szilagyi PG. Beginning the physical examination: general survey and vital signs. In: *Guide to physical examination and history taking,* 8th ed. Philadelphia, PA: Lippincott Williams & Wilkins, 2003:75–78.

become muffled and disappear, again note the pressure on the manometer. Confirm sound disappearance by listening as the pressure falls an additional 20 mmHg. If no further sounds occur, deflate the cuff rapidly to zero. The disappearance point represents the diastolic blood pressure. Measure the blood pressure in each arm (4).

2. **Other important features.** The physical examination should include the eye examination looking for retinal changes consistent with HTN. Palpate the thyroid to evaluate for masses, enlargement, or asymmetry. The cardiovascular examination should include palpation and auscultation of the carotid and femoral pulses, noting symmetry of pulse strength or bruits. Palpate distal extremity pulses and perform a complete cardiac examination, noting any cardiac heave, murmurs, gallops, rubs, jugular venous distension, and intensity of S_1 and S_2 heart sounds. Abdominal examination should evaluate for bruits, pulsatile and nonpulsatile masses, or renal enlargement. A complete pulmonary examination should be performed. Examination of extremities should note edema and changes consistent with peripheral vascular disease. A thorough neurologic and skin examination should be performed.

C. **Testing**

1. Basic laboratory tests, when evaluating a patient with HTN, include uric acid, urinalysis including screening for microalbuminuria, complete blood count, serum creatinine, potassium, calcium, and blood urea nitrogen. A fasting serum glucose and a complete lipoprotein profile should be obtained. The lipoprotein profile should include a total cholesterol, triglyceride, low-density lipoprotein cholesterol, and high-density

TABLE 7.9.3	Preparing to Measure Blood Pressure

- Ideally, ask the patient to avoid smoking or drinking caffeinated beverages for 30 min before the blood pressure is taken and to rest for at least 5 min.
- Check to make sure the examining room is quiet, warm, and comfortable.
- Make sure the arm selected is *free of clothing.* There should be no arteriovenous fistulas for dialysis, scarring from prior brachial artery cutdowns, or signs of lymphedema (seen after axillary node dissection or radiation therapy).
- Palpate the brachial artery to confirm that it has a viable pulse.
- Position the arm so that the brachial artery, at the antecubital crease, is *at heart level*—roughly level with the fourth interspace at its junction with the sternum.
- If the patient is seated, rest the arm on a table a little above the patient's waist; if standing, try to support the patient's arm at the midchest level.

Bickley LS, Szilagyi PG. Beginning the physical examination: general survey and vital signs. In: *Guide to physical examination and history taking,* 8th ed. Philadelphia, PA: Lippincott Williams & Wilkins, 2003:75–78.

TABLE 7.9.4 **Equations for Estimation of GFR from Plasma Creatinine Concentration (P_{cr})**

1. Equation from the Modification of Diet in Renal Disease Study[a]

   Estimated GFR (mL/min/1.73 m^2) = $1.86 \times (P_{cr})^{-1.154} \times (age)^{-0.203}$

   Multiply by 0.742 for women

   Multiply by 1.21 for African Americans

2. Cockcroft-Gault equation

   Estimated creatinine clearance (mL/min) = $\dfrac{(140 - age) \times body\ weight\ (kg)}{72 \times (P_{cr})(mg/dL)}$

   Multiply by 0.85 for women

GFR, glomerular filtration rate.

[a]Kasper DL, Braunwald E, Fauci AS, et al. *Harrison's principles of internal medicine*, 16th ed. Part 8; Chapter 230. McGraw-Hill Companies, 2005.

lipoprotein cholesterol. The estimated glomerular filtration rate (GFR) or creatinine clearance should be calculated using available formulas (see Table 7.9.4). If a secondary cause of HTN is suspected, the appropriate specific laboratory workup should be included.

2. An electrocardiogram may assist with recognizing a previously damaged myocardium, rhythm disturbances, or changes consistent with left ventricular hypertrophy (LVH).

3. Imaging studies may be useful. A chest x-ray may be useful when attempting to evaluate the patient for cardiomegaly, but a limited echocardiogram will give more detailed information about cardiac function and LVH.

D. Genetics. To date, genetic studies have not identified any single gene or combination of genes that appreciably accounts for HTN in the general population.

III. DIAGNOSIS
A. Differential diagnosis
1. Essential HTN
2. Secondary HTN
   a. Renovascular HTN
   i. Stenosis of main renal arteries and/or major branches is responsible for 2–5% of patients with HTN.
   ii. Initial workup involves Doppler ultrasonography with measurement of the intra-renal resistance index.
   iii. This diagnosis includes the subgroups preeclampsia and eclampsia.
   b. Renal parenchymal HTN. Diseases that injure renal parenchymal tissue result in inflammatory and fibrotic changes of small intrarenal vessels, thereby causing decreased profusion and resultant HTN.
   c. Primary aldosteronism. A tumor or bilateral adrenal hyperplasia should be sought.
   d. Cushing's syndrome
   i. Truncal obesity, fatigability, purplish abdominal striae, amenorrhea, hirsutism, edema, glucosuria, moon facies, and buffalo hump
   ii. Most common in the third or fourth decade of life
   iii. Failure to suppress cortisol level with dexamethasone challenge
   e. Pheochromocytoma
   i. Most common in young to mid adult life

    ii. Headaches, palpitations, excessive sweating, impaired glucose tolerance, hypercal-cemia, weight loss, and anxiety

    iii. Twenty-four hour urine collection assayed for vanillylmandelic acid, metaneph-rine, and "free" catecholamines

f. Coarctation of the aorta

    i. Cardiac murmur, possibly heard in the back, over spinous processes, and lateral thorax

    ii. Decreased, delayed, or absent femoral pulses

    iii. Chest x-ray reveals "the three sign" at coarctation sight and notched ribs

g. Hyperparathyroidism

    i. Hypercalcemia

    ii. Renal parenchymal damage due to nephrocalcinosis and renal stones

h. Oral contraceptive medications

i. Malignant HTN (3)

    i. Diastolic blood pressure usually greater than 130 mmHg

    ii. Papilledema, retinal hemorrhages, and exudates

    iii. Possibly vomiting, severe headache, transient visual changes or loss, stupor, coma, oliguria, and cardiac decompensation

j. Obstructive sleep apnea

B. Clinical manifestations. Individuals may have high blood pressure for years and not know it. Sometimes HTN may have subtle symptoms such as epistaxis, hematuria, episodic weakness, dizziness, palpitations, easy fatigability, and impotence. If HTN is part of a disease process, such as secondary HTN, it may be joined by other symptoms of the influencing disease process.

REFERENCES

1. American Heart Association Inc. Accessed at www.americanheart.org, on April 11, 2006.
2. Department of Health and Human Service, National Institutes of Health. The Seventh Report of the Joint National Committee on Prevention, Detection, Evaluation, and Treatment of High Blood Pressure. Accessed at www.nhlbi.nih.gov/guidelines/hypertension, on April 11, 2006.
3. Kasper DL, Braunwald E, Fauci AS, et al. *Harrison's principles of internal medicine*, 16th ed. Part 8; Chapter 230. New York, NY: McGraw-Hill, 2005.
4. Bickley LS, Szilagyi PG. Beginning the physical examination: general survey and vital signs. In: *Guide to physical examination and history taking*, 8th ed. Philadelphia, PA: Lippincott Williams & Wilkins, 2003:75–78.
5. U.S. Preventive Services Task Force. Screening for high blood pressure: reaffirmation recommendation statement. *Am Fam Physician* 2009; 79(12) 1087–1088.

7.10 Palpitations

Naureen Rafiq

I. BACKGROUND. Palpitations are an unpleasant abnormal awareness of the heartbeat. They are usually described as a pounding or racing of the heart.

II. PATHOPHYSIOLOGY

    A. Etiology. Palpitations are a common presenting complaint encountered by the primary care physicians and cardiologists. The list of underlying causes of palpitations is extensive (see Table 7.10.1).

TABLE 7.10.1	Some Causes of Palpitations	

Cardiac	Medications
Arrhythmias	Alcohol
Atrial fibrillation/atrial flutter	Anticholinergics
Multifocal atrial tachycardia	Caffeine
Premature ventricular contractions	Illicit drugs like cocaine
Sick sinus syndrome	Nicotine
Sinus node dysfunction	Sympathomimetics
Sinus tachycardia	Amphetamines
Supraventricular tachycardia	**Endocrine/metabolic**
Ventricular tachycardia	Hyperthyroidism
Wolff-Parkinson-White syndrome	Hypoglycemia
Other cardiac causes	Pheochromocytoma
Cardiac shunts	**Psychiatric**
Cardiomyopathy	Anxiety disorder
Pacemaker	Panic attacks
Valvular heart disease like mitral stenosis	Somatization disorder
	Stress
	Others
	Anemia
	Fever
	Strenuous physical activity

B. Epidemiology. One prospective cohort study of 190 patients showed that 43% had palpitations due to cardiac causes, 31% due to anxiety or panic disorder, and 16% due to an undetermined etiology (1). Remembering that the heart is electrically paced, a good mnemonic to assist in recalling causes of palpitations is E-PACED (Electrolytes, Psychiatric, Anemia, Cardiac, Endocrine, and Drugs) (2).

C. Symptoms. The symptoms can range from just awareness of heart rhythm to chest tightness, shortness of breath, dizziness, light-headedness, or syncope. They can last from a few seconds to prolonged periods of time.

III. EVALUATION. Because patients rarely experience an episode while in the physician's office, the history and physical examination are the most crucial elements of the investigation. Moreover, only occasionally does physical examination provide clues or supporting evidence to affirm a diagnosis, thereby making a thorough and descriptive history assume even greater importance.

    A. History. The history should focus on the age of the patient, detailed description of symptoms, and information such as the circumstances during occurrence, intermittency, duration, and precipitating and resolving factors.

        1. The circumstances during which palpitations occur may indicate an association with anxiety or panic attacks, although one should also keep in mind excess catecholamine during times of stress. Validated screening tools are readily available to assist in identifying patients with such psychiatric illness (3). Occurrence at night while lying down could result from atrial or ventricular premature contractions. Positional changes might indicate atrioventricular nodal tachycardia.

2. Isolated or skipped beats could be premature contractions or benign ectopy.
3. Palpitations precipitated by exercise may be associated with supraventricular arrhythmias or atrial fibrillation. Palpitations terminated by vagal maneuvers point to paroxysmal supraventricular tachycardia.
4. Palpitations described as rapid and regular may indicate paroxysmal supraventricular tachycardia and ventricular tachycardias. Palpitations described as rapid and irregular could imply atrial fibrillation, multifocal atrial tachycardia, and atrial flutter with variable block. Flip-flopping or stopping–starting sensations may be caused by supraventricular or ventricular premature contractions. Palpitations may be sensed as a pounding in the neck. Notably, atrioventricular nodal reentrant tachycardia is associated with a rapid regular pounding in the neck, whereas such a sensation that is less regular and more intermittent may be premature ventricular contractions.
5. The physician should keep in mind that dizziness, presyncope, or syncope accompanying palpitations are factors that help identify patients at risk for fatal results. These symptoms should prompt an investigation for ventricular tachycardias.
6. Age at onset in childhood may suggest supraventricular tachycardia. Symptoms of hyperthyroidism such as heat intolerance should be elicited. Illicit drugs, caffeine, and nicotine habits as well as anemia and metabolic disorders are all important possible associations that should be considered.

B. Physical Examination. The findings of the physical examination may give clues such as a heart murmur, indicating the possibility of valvular disease or cardiomyopathies or the midsystolic click of mitral valve prolapse. A brisk walk down a corridor might reveal a poorly controlled ventricular response and resultant palpitations in a patient with atrial fibrillation and palpitations (1). It is necessary to search for signs of congestive heart failure.

C. Workup

1. Twelve-lead electrocardiography
It is indicated and should be analyzed for short PR interval and delta waves (ventricular pre-excitation), Q waves indicating left ventricular hypertrophy or prior infarction, premature contractions, long QT intervals, heart blocks, or any other abnormality.

2: Laboratory testing
It can usually be limited to investigation of anemia, thyroid function, and electrolyte disturbances (potassium and magnesium). Ambulatory electrocardiography (ECG) can be used for further investigation.

3: Holter monitoring
It should suffice for patients with daily symptoms.

4: Continuous-loop event recorder
It provides a better diagnostic yield (4, 5).

5: Echocardiogram
It can be done to detect any structural abnormality of the heart like valvular heart disease.

IV. DIAGNOSIS. The list of causes of palpitations is extensive (Table 7.10.1). In most cases, the cause is benign. Life-threatening causes are suggested by associated symptoms such as dizziness or syncope. The history is the most important diagnostic tool, and a thorough and descriptive inquiry should be made. The physical examination may provide further clues or supporting evidence. Testing involves 12-lead ECG and a limited laboratory investigation.

REFERENCES

1. Abbott AV. Diagnostic approach to palpitations. *Am Fam Physician* 2005;71:743–750.
2. Weber BE, Kapoor WN. Evaluation and outcomes of patients with palpitations. *Am J Med* 1996;100:138–148.
3. Taylor RB, ed. *The 10-minute diagnosis manual*, 1st ed. Philadelphia, PA: JB Lippincott, 1994.
4. Zimetbaum P, Josephson ME. Evaluation of patients with palpitations. *N Engl J Med* 1998;338:1369–1373.
5. Zimetbaum P, Josephson ME. The evolving role of ambulatory monitoring in general clinical practice. *Ann Intern Med* 1999;130:848–856.

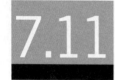

7.11 Pericardial Friction Rub

Stephen L. George

I. BACKGROUND. The pericardium is a sac-like structure consisting of an outer *parietal* layer and an inner *visceral* layer that envelops the heart and root of the great vessels. There is approximately 5–50 mL of ultrafiltrate of plasma between the two layers. It is innervated by the phrenic nerve. It primarily drains into the right pleural space via the thoracic duct. A friction rub is present in 85% of cases of pericarditis and is essentially diagnostic of pericarditis. Patients typically present with acute chest pain and characteristic serial electrocardiographic changes (1–4).

II. PATHOPHYSIOLOGY

A. Etiology of Acute Pericarditis. Acute pericarditis (AP) is generally a benign, self-limited, and readily treatable condition. Inflammation between the two layers can produce a serous, fibrinous, or purulent reaction. A pericardial effusion is not necessarily present. Together, idiopathic and viral (coxsackie virus, echovirus, Epstein-Barr virus, influenza virus, human immunodeficiency virus, hepatitis viruses, varicella, measles, and mumps) etiologies account for 80–90% of cases. Malignancies are the third leading cause at 5%. A specific cause is identified in only about 7% of cases (6, 7). Other etiologies include bacterial (tuberculosis, *Staphylococcus*, *Haemophilus*, *Pneumococcus*, *Salmonella*, *Meningococcus*, and syphilis), fungal (histoplasmosis, blastomycosis, coccidioidomycosis, and aspergillosis), parasitic (echinococcosis, amebiasis, Rickettsia, and Toxoplasma), rheumatoid arthritis, systemic lupus erythematosus, gout, scleroderma (up to 85%), rheumatic fever, sarcoidosis, other inflammatory conditions (Sjögren syndrome, mixed connective tissue disease, Reiter's syndrome, Whipple's disease, familial Mediterranean fever, and serum sickness), uremia, dialysis, hypothyroidism, cholesterol pericarditis, 1–4 days after myocardial infarction, 1–3 days postpericardiotomy, metastatic (breast, lung, lymphoma, melanoma, and leukemia), irradiation, drugs (penicillin, cromolyn sodium, doxorubicin, cyclophosphamide, procainamide, phenytoin, and minoxidil), aortic dissection, cardiac trauma, after cardiac catheterization or pacemaker placement, and hemorrhagic. Infarction-associated pericarditis has diminished significantly with the advent of reperfusion interventions. Dressler's syndrome occurs weeks to months post-acute myocardial infarction (AMI) (1–7).

B. Epidemiology of AP. AP occurs in approximately 0.1% of hospitalized patients and 5% of noncardiac chest pain patients in the emergency department (1, 2, 4) and is more common in males and adults 20–50 years old. Up to 15% of patients may experience recurrence of symptoms within a few months and 25% will eventually have a recurrence (2, 5–7).

III. EVALUATION

A. History

1. Most patients have acute sharp, sternal or left precordial pain. However, they may have a dull, aching, burning, or pressure-type pain. Pain is characteristically referred to the trapezius ridge, worse with inspiration, lying down, swallowing, or body motion and relieved by sitting upright or leaning forward. It may also radiate to the neck, jaw, or arms and is usually not relieved with nitroglycerine (1, 3, 4, 6, 7).

2. There is often a prodrome of fever, malaise, and myalgias. Associated symptoms may include dyspnea (pariticularly with tamponade), weight loss (malignancy), productive cough (with pneumonia and purulent pericarditis) or hemoptysis (tuberculosis). Nonspecific symptoms include hiccups, cough, hoarseness (phrenic nerve), palpitations, nausea, and vomiting (1, 4, 6).

3. Past medical and surgical history may be suggestive of a causal illness or procedure. Examples are recent pericardiotomy, renal failure, rheumatologic diseases, trauma, malignancy, or the use of suspect medications (1–7).

B. Physical Examination. Pericardial friction rub is a creaking leather or scratching high-pitched sound best heard with the diaphragm along the left lower sternal border with the patient leaning forward at end expiration. Most often triphasic (atrial systole, ventricular systole, and early ventricular diastole), but it can be biphasic or monophasic. It can be intermittent and therefore overlooked without serial exams. Beck's triad (muffled heart sounds, JVD, and hypotension) pulsus paradoxus or Kussmaul sign suggest tamponade. With rapid accumulation, tamponade can occur with as little as 200 mL of fluid (1–5).

C. Testing

1. **Laboratory tests.** Clinical circumstances will dictate specifics of testing. The minimum workup should include a complete blood count, erythrocyte sedimentation rate, C-reactive protein, blood urea nitrogen, creatinine, and cardiac enzymes. Elevated cardiac enzymes occur 35–55% of the time due to myopericarditis. Specific rheumatologic testing such as a rheumatoid factor or antinuclear antibody panel may be indicated. For tuberculosis, skin testing and an adenosine deaminase test of pericardial fluid are indicated. Thyroid function tests, streptococcal antigen testing, cytology of pericardial fluid, antibody titers, or pericardial biopsy may be warranted (1, 2, 5, 6).

2. **Electrocardiogram (ECG).** The ECG is indispensable in the diagnosis and management of AP. At first, current injury changes of upwardly concave ST elevation and PR depression is seen in the precordial and limb leads with reciprocal changes in leads V1 and aVR. T waves gradually flatten and then invert. Persistent T wave inversion beyond 3 weeks indicates a chronic fluid accumulation and the need for further testing. Distinct from AMI, there are no Q waves *or reciprocal changes*. Electrical alternans may be seen with an effusion or tamponade. Electrical alternans with tachycardia is relatively specific for tamponade (1, 2, 4, 6, 8).

3. **Imaging studies.** Echocardiography should be performed to assist with the diagnosis, management, and guidance of interventions such as pericardiocentesis. Flask-shaped cardiomegaly on chest radiography requires at least a 200 mL effusion (1, 2, 4, 5).

IV. DIAGNOSIS. The differential diagnosis is extensive, similar to that for chest pain, and is guided by the clinical situation. Salient conditions to consider include acute coronary syndromes, aortic dissection, esophageal rupture, pulmonary embolism, pulmonary infarct, pneumothorax, esophagitis, esophageal spasm, acute gastritis, pneumonia, cholecystitis, and costochondritis (1, 2, 6, 7).

REFERENCES

1. Khandaker MH, Espinosa RE, Nishimura RA, et al. Pericardial disease: diagnosis and management. *Mayo Clin Proc* 2010;85(6):572–593.
2. Tingle LE, Moina D, Calvert CW. Acute pericarditis. *Am Fam Physician* 2007;76:1509–1514.
3. Leal ME. Pericarditis and pericardial effusions. In: Bope ET, Kellerman RD. *Bope and Kellerman: Conn's current therapy 2012*, 1st ed. St. Louis: W.B. Saunders, 2012:458–460.
4. Stehlik J, Benjamin IJ. Pericardial and myocardial disease. In: Andreoli TE, Ivor BJ, Griggs RC, Wing EJ. *Andreoli and Carpenter's Cecil essentials of medicine*, 8th ed. Philadelphia, PA: Saunders Elsevier, 2010:145–148.
5. Delgado GA, Ferri FF, Forunato DJ. *Ferri's clinical advisor 2012*, 1st ed. Philadelphia, PA: Mosby, 2012:768–769.
6. Wu K. Pericarditis. 2011. Accessed at https://www.online.epocrates.com/noFrame/Showpage.do?method=disease&MonographId=243 on May 19, 2012.
7. Massimo I, LeWinter MM. Clinical presentation and diagnostic evaluation of acute pericarditis. 2011. Accessed at http://www.uptodate.com/contents/clinical-presentation-and-diagnostic-evaluation-of-acutepericarditis?source=searchresult&search=pericarditis&selectedTitle=1%7E150 on May 19, 2012.
8. Goldberger A. *Goldberger: clinical electrocardiography: a simplified approach*, 7th ed. Philadelphia, PA: Mosby Elsevier, 2006:139–140.

7.12 Raynaud's Disease

Sandra B. Baumberger

I. BACKGROUND

A. Definition. Raynaud's disease is a vasospastic disorder causing episodic ischemia of the digits of the hands, lasting a varying amount of time. It was named after Maurice Raynaud, who first noted the disorder in 1862. Although the disorder mainly affects the finger and toes, it can also affect the tongue, the nose, the ears, and the nipples (1). Raynaud's disease not associated with any underlying disease is also known as primary Raynaud's disease (PRD). This type of Raynaud's disease tends to be less severe and is more common. Secondary Raynaud's disease (SRD) or Raynaud's phenomenon is often associated with an underlying illness (2).

II. PATHOPHYSIOLOGY.

A. Etiology. Emotional stress and cold seem to be the biggest triggers for attacks. The attacks may last minutes to hours. Classically, the attacks have a three-stage color change. Stage one consists of pallor of the skin, which is sometimes associated with coldness, numbness, and/or paresthesias. The second stage, if present, consists of cyanosis and may include some of the symptoms associated with stage one. Finally, the third stage consists of erythema, which may be associated with throbbing of the digits (3). PRD carries a low risk of progression to an autoimmune disorder, if after 2 years of attacks no other signs or symptoms of autoimmune processes are present. Conversely, Raynaud's can be the presenting sign for scleroderma. It has been proven that those who suffer from PRD or SRD have abnormal blood flow to the digits and abnormal recovery from cold stimulus. In patients with scleroderma, the blood vessels are already narrowed from proliferation of the intimal area. This exacerbates the ischemia caused by the cold stimulus (3).

B. Epidemiology. The prevalence of Raynaud's disease in women ranges from 3% to 20% and in men from 3% to 14%. The prevalence of PRD in the United States is around 5%, while in France it may be as high as 17% (4). PRD usually begins in the second or third decade of life. SRD may begin with the underlying disorder and/or be the presenting sign of an autoimmune disorder. Raynaud's disease is more common in cold climates. It is sometimes associated with certain occupations such as those that require exposure to mechanical vibration on an ongoing basis (5). Other disorders associated with SRD include systemic lupus erythematosus (SLE), rheumatoid arthritis, dermatomyositis, polymyositis, hyperviscosity syndromes, antineoplastic medications, and beta blockers. Vasospastic processes such as vascular headaches, atypical angina, and primary pulmonary hypertension may also be associated with SRD (6).

III. EVALUATION.

A. History and Physical. When interviewing the patient, it is important to determine when the symptoms appear. Patients note that symptoms appear during relative shifts from warm to cold temperatures. Emotional stress is also reported to cause symptoms via the activation of the sympathetic nervous system. Medications used and history of smoking are also important questions to cover during the history (4). Also, questions about the use of machines or tools that produce vibration or other repetitive activities done with the fingers may help determine if the patient has a variant of Raynaud's disease known as hand–arm vibration syndrome (1). The physical exam should focus on a thorough examination of the digits. Inspect the digits carefully for sclerodactyly or digital ulcers and examine the nail fold capillaries for abnormally large capillary loops, alternating with areas without any capillaries. This pattern is suggestive of scleroderma (4). Also inspect for Malar rash, persistent cyanosis, and/or necrotic tissue of the digits.

B. Genetics. Although the exact pathophysiology of PRD and SRD remain unclear, there do seem to be strong genetic influences. Familial analysis and twin studies have confirmed the role of hereditary factors. Pedigree analysis indicates the possibility of an autosomal dominant transmission influenced by sex in some families. At this time, sequencing of candidate genes for genetic mutations remains negative (7).

IV. DIAGNOSIS.

A. Differential Diagnosis. PRD is the most likely diagnosis in a young woman with less severe symptoms and no underlying disease. SRD should be considered in anyone with a known autoimmune disorder such as scleroderma or SLE. Other diagnoses to be considered include thromboangiitis obliterans in a man who smokes, thoracic outlet syndrome, carpal tunnel syndrome related to repetitive use of the hands, acrocyanosis, and cryoglobulinemia, especially associated with hepatitis B or C. Drugs that may induce SRD include but are not limited to beta blockers, oral contraceptives, antineoplastic drugs, ergot alkaloids, cyclosporine, and alfa-interferon (8).

B. Clinical Manifestations. Color changes of the digits when exposed to the cold is the classic presentation. Patients may not undergo all three color changes. Some literature states that pallor followed by cyanosis is the most common pattern, while other sources note that patients who have episodes with cyanosis have more severe disease (1). The most important thing to keep in mind when diagnosing patients with Raynaud's disease is that patients with SRD will almost always have other symptoms of connective tissue disease in addition to the symptoms of Raynaud's disease.

REFERENCES

1. Block, JA. Raynaud's phenomenon. *Lancet* 2001;357:2042–2048.
2. National Heart Lung and Blood Institute. Accessed at www.nhlbi.nih.gov/health/health-topics/topics/raynaud/ on February 23, 2012.
3. National Institute of Arthritis and Musculoskeletal and Skin Diseases. Accessed at www.niams.nih.gov on April 1, 2012.
4. *Clinical manifestations and diagnosis of the Raynaud phenomenon.* Accessed at www.uptodate.com on April 9, 2012.
5. Canada's National Occupational Health and Safety Resource. Accessed at www.ccohs.ca/oshanswers/diseases/raynaud/html on April 11, 2006.
6. *Raynaud's phenomenon,* 2004. Accessed at www.firstconsult.com.
7. Pistorius MA, Planchon B, Schott JJ, Lemarec H. Hereditary and genetic aspects of Raynaud's disease. *J Mal Vasc* 2006;31(1):10–15.
8. *Raynaud's phenomenon,* 2004. Accessed at www.imedicine.com.

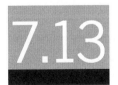

7.13 Tachycardia

Hannah M. Heckart

I. BACKGROUND.
Tachycardia is defined as a condition in which the heart rate is greater than 100 beats/minute for three or more beats. It can be categorized into two main types, supraventricular or ventricular, with the former being further categorized into either wide complex tachycardia or narrow complex tachycardia (1).

II. PATHOPHYSIOLOGY.
In the evaluation of the patient with tachycardia, one needs to discover the etiology of the tachycardia and then identify the specific arrhythmia. Symptoms of tachycardia include chest discomfort, dyspnea, fatigue, light-headedness, presyncope, syncope, and palpitations (2). Conditions to look for in the past medical history may include myocardial

infarction, ventricular hypertrophy, heart failure, valvular heart disease, or congenital abnormalities. Caffeine use, alcohol use, stress, and hypothyroidism can also precipitate tachycardia (1).

III. EVALUATION

A. History. Determine if the patient is hemodynamically stable and if he or she is symptomatic (distressed or unconscious) or asymptomatic (awake and not distressed).

B. Physical Examination. Auscultate the heart, listening for murmurs, rubs, or gallops. Look for jugular venous distention and lower extremity edema, which would indicate heart failure. Listen to the lung fields for crackles. Feel the thyroid for enlargement.

C. Testing

1. **Electrocardiogram (ECG).** Obtain a 12-lead ECG and determine the rate, rhythm, and QRS duration on the rhythm strip (commonly lead II).

2. **Laboratory tests.** Look for hypomagnesemia, hypokalemia, anemia, hyperthyroidism, hypoxemia, illicit drugs, β-type natriuretic peptide, and digitalis toxicity.

IV. DIAGNOSIS

A. Narrow complex tachycardia (QRS < 120 ms)

1. **Sinus tachycardia.** There are numerous reasons for sinus tachycardia in adults: pathologic (anemia, thyrotoxicosis, hypoxemia, hypotension, hypovolemia) or physiologic (anemia, fever). Normal P wave and QRS complexes are seen on the ECG. Therapy consists in treating the underlying cause.

2. **Atrial fibrillation.** Atrial fibrillation is an irregularly irregular rhythm with a variable ventricular rate and no discernable P waves on the ECG. If there is an aberrant conduction from the atria to ventricles or prior bundle branch block, it may be difficult to distinguish atrial fibrillation from atrial flutter as it commonly shifts between fibrillation and flutter.

3. **Atrial flutter.** In atrial flutter, cardiac monitoring shows the classic P wave "sawtooth" appearance with a rate between 180 and 350 beats/minute. The ventricles have a slower rate, demonstrating either 2:1 or 4:1 block with a corresponding ventricular rate of 150 to 75 beats/minute. Atrial flutter is associated with a risk of atrial thromboembolism.

4. **Paroxysmal supraventricular tachycardia (SVT).** Paroxysmal SVT is a rhythm that is most commonly caused by the reentry of the atrial impulse at the atrioventricular (AV) node. Morphology of the rhythm shows a sudden onset with a regular QRS complex and a rate from 140 to 250 beats/minute. P wave may not be apparent because of retrograde atrial depolarization that typically occurs simultaneously with ventricular depolarization. Wolff-Parkinson-White syndrome occurs when there is antegrade conduction via an accessory pathway, producing delta waves (upsloping prior to the QRS complex) and shortened PR intervals.

5. **Multifocal atrial tachycardia (MAT).** MAT is an arrhythmia that may occur in cases of heart failure or chronic obstructive pulmonary disease. MAT exists when there are three different P-wave morphologies unrelated to each other.

B. Wide complex tachycardia (QRS >120 ms)

1. **Ventricular Tachycardia (VT).** There can be much difficulty in distinguishing SVT with an aberrant conduction from VT. If there is any doubt about the origin of a wide-complex tachycardia, the patient should be treated as if the rhythm is VT. These electrocardiogram (EKG) clues can help differentiate between SVT and VT (3).

   a. If an RS complex cannot be identified in any precordial leads, it is VT.

   b. If an RS complex is identified, then an RS interval (the R wave onset to the S wave nadir) of greater than 100 ms strongly suggests a VT.

   c. If the RS interval is less than 100 ms, then there is either a ventricular or a supraventricular origin site of the tachycardia and AV dissociation must be evaluated. However, if AV dissociation is present, it is VT.

   d. If the RS interval is <100 ms and there is no demonstrable AV dissociation, then look for concordance of the precordial QRS complexes (leads V1–V6 all have a similar negative appearance), which would also indicate VT.

2. **Torsade de Pointes (TdP).** A form of polymorphic VT with varying amplitudes of the QRS complex. Particularly seen in patients with a prolonged QT interval. May present in patients with hypokalemia and hypomagnesemia. Medications like erythromycin, phenothiazines, haloperidol, or methadone may cause TdP.

3. **Ventricular fibrillation (VF).** VF is a life-threatening arrhythmia resulting from abnormal ventricular depolarizations that prevent an unified contraction of cardiac muscle. On EKG, VF is characterized by a chaotic irregular appearance without discrete QRS waveforms.

REFERENCES

1. Lilly, L. *Pathophysiology of heart disease*, 4th ed. Baltimore, MD: Lippincott Williams & Wilkins, 2007.
2. Colucci R, Silver M, Shubrook J. Common types of supraventricular tachycardia: diagnosis and management. *Am Fam Physician* 2010;82(8):942–952.
3. Eckardt L, Breithardt G, Kirchhof P. Approach to wide complex tachycardias in patients without structural heart disease. *Heart* 2006;92(5):704–711.

CHAPTER 8

Respiratory Problems

Christopher Bunt

8.1 Cough

Kenji L. Takano

I. **BACKGROUND.** Cough is the most common reason for outpatient clinical visits in the United States (1). It accounts for over 200 million episodes of acute illness per year, and chronic cough is associated with significant morbidity and reduced quality of life (2).

II. **PATHOPHYSIOLOGY.** Cough is a reflex that clears the upper airways of the respiratory tract. It is triggered through sensory activation of afferent fibers in the vagus nerve. This visceral reflex can be controlled by higher cortical centers.

III. **EVALUATION**

A. **History.** A complete history is crucial to determining the etiology.

1. **Cough Characteristics.** In determining the cause for a cough, a distinction from the following should be considered:

a. **Cough Duration:**

i. Acute cough is under 3 weeks in duration

ii. Subacute cough is between 3 and 8 weeks in duration

iii. Chronic cough is over 8 weeks in duration

b. Pediatric versus adult patient

2. **Characteristics of the Cough.** There are specific causes and clinical symptoms associated with acute, subacute, and chronic cough. Special consideration for pediatric causes for chronic cough must also be recognized.

a. Acute cough is most commonly due to self-resolving viral illness, but can be the first sign of potential and serious life-threatening disease (3). A focused history to rule out pneumonia, severe asthma exacerbation, chronic obstructive pulmonary disease (COPD), congestive heart failure (CHF), or pulmonary embolism (PE) should be undertaken and documented. Complaints such as severe pleuritic chest pain and hemoptysis may prompt consideration of PE or positional dyspnea, and bilateral leg swelling may lead to conclusion of CHF. Smoking should be identified and smoking cessation discussed as it can cause chronic bronchitis and bronchogenic cancer. Travel history should also be discussed to consider if patient is possibly exposed to tuberculosis. Immunization history should also be obtained. Discuss medical history of preexisting conditions or environmental or occupational exposure to noxious agents. Once it is established that a non–life threatening diagnosis is likely, the most common causes are viral upper and lower respiratory tract illness, mild exacerbations of asthma or COPD, bronchitis, or environmental exposure.

b. Subacute cough can be considered to be caused by postinfectious versus noninfectious etiologies (3). A history of previous infection with persistence of symptoms may suggest that pneumonia has developed, or that bronchitis has set in. Pertussis should be considered in patients with an inspiratory whooping sound, paroxysmal coughing, or post-tussive emesis. Previous conditions such as asthma, if not treated, can lead to subacute cough. Other etiologies such as gastroesophageal reflux disease (GERD) can also occur; this is suggested by possible gastrointestinal (GI) complaints such as acid reflux or heartburn. Upper airway cough syndrome (UACS) is another condition that can be identified through clinical symptoms in the upper airway such as postnasal drip or sinus symptoms.

   c. Chronic cough has a larger differential diagnosis and includes consideration of medications such as angiotensin converting enzyme inhibitor (ACE-I), environmental influences such as smoking, and persistent asthma (4). GERD can also be the cause for chronic cough and may still be a cause despite a lack of GI symptoms. Usually, patients in this category have been seen previously for their cough and review of previous treatments and treatment response can help guide further diagnostic studies. Chronic cough has many similar etiologies as subacute cough and in many patients is caused by more than one etiology. Neoplasm should always be considered, especially with a smoking history, weight loss, and hemoptysis. Chest radiography is usually indicated in chronic cough evaluation as normal versus abnormal imaging can exclude infectious conditions, neoplasm, and sarcoidosis.

   d. In children, there are some crucial differences in the evaluation of cough (5,6). For instance, aspiration of foreign body should be considered and early chest radiography would be indicated. Spirometry should also be considered early in the evaluation if age appropriate. Children who have cystic fibrosis, tracheoesophageal fistula, or congenital cardiac abnormalities may also present initially with cough, and further history should be obtained if suspected. Children may also be sensitive to environmental irritants such as second-hand smoke. Specific treatment guidelines for pediatric patients should be followed as medication type and starting dosage such as antibiotics may be different from adults. In young children, parents should be discouraged from using over-the-counter cough medications (7).

B. Physical Examination

   1. Focused physical exam. This must include vital signs such as temperature, pulse, respiratory rate, oxygen saturation, and blood pressure. A complete heart and lung examination with bare chest should be performed as well. Ear, nose, sinus, and throat examinations are also essential for the evaluation of cough.

   2. Additional physical exam. Based on clinical history, a cardiac evaluation focused on stigmata of CHF such as jugular venous distention or liver enlargement should be performed. Lymphadenopathy may suggest neoplasm as the cause and evidence of cachexia and wasting can suggest chronic disease, cancer, or human immunodeficiency virus. Clubbing of fingers, barrel chest, or peripheral cyanosis may also indicate COPD if not identified through history.

C. Testing

   1. Clinical laboratory tests. The vast majority of causes for acute non–life threatening cough do not require laboratory testing. If pneumonia is suspected, it would be reasonable to obtain a complete blood count and blood cultures. In an outpatient setting, Gram stain and sputum culture would not likely alter treatment strategy and therefore is unlikely to be practical. If clinical history suggests, a purified protein derivative may be useful if tuberculosis is suspected. Further lab testing can confirm specific diagnosis such as testing for pertussis or cystic fibrosis screening.

   2. Radiologic tests. Chest radiography should be considered if a lower airway cause such as pneumonia is suspected. This would be supported by a patient having a fever, tachypnea, productive sputum, and abnormal physical exam. In children, imaging may detect a foreign body as the cough etiology. As a general rule, patients with a chronic cough should have a chest radiography performed unless they have a specific contraindication such as pregnancy. Appropriate imaging for evaluation of PE should be performed if this is the suspected cause. In a subacute or chronic cough, sinus computed tomography imaging can determine if the cause for the cough is sinusitis.

3. **Pulmonary function tests.** In adults, peak flowmeter measurement with use of a bronchodilator can often identify asthma. In children and adults of chronic cough non-responsive to treatment, spirometry should be performed (5). Children aged 6 and older can reliably perform spirometry (6).

4. **Invasive tests.** Bronchoscopy is useful as a follow-up to abnormal imaging such as a foreign body or neoplasm. For patients with chronic GERD, there is a role in using esophageal pH monitoring or barium esophagography if nonacid GERD is the suspected cause (8).

IV. DIAGNOSIS

A. **Differential Diagnosis.** In general, the acute cough is most likely due to an infectious etiology, specifically viral. Given this, antibiotics are unlikely to be effective unless the condition is bacterial in origin. Life-threatening causes should always be considered when evaluating acute cough such as CHF exacerbation, pneumonia, or PE. Subacute cough can be the result of postinfectious recovery or the persistence of a chronic cause for cough such as asthma, GERD, or COPD. Chronic cough has a much longer differential diagnosis and includes infectious and noninfectious etiologies such as ACE-I use and UACS. UACS should be considered if a nonsmoking, immunocompetent adult has a chronic cough with normal chest x-ray. Often, there is more than one specific disease process that causes chronic coughing. Environmental agents can also cause coughing; unless these are considered and the exposure is reduced, symptoms will persist.

B. **Special Concerns.** Failure to improve despite treatment should prompt a more extensive diagnostic evaluation and possible specialist referral if the etiology is not found or if clinical response is not obtained. In general, patients such as the very young, old, or immunosuppressed warrant close follow-up to ensure clinical recovery.

Disclaimer

The opinions and assertions contained herein are the private views of the author and are not to be construed as official or as reflecting the views of the U.S. Air Force Medical Service, the U.S. Air Force or the Department of Defense at large.

REFERENCES

1. Chun-Ju H, Cherry DK, Beatty PC, et al. National Ambulatory Medical Care Survey: 2007 Summary. *US Department of Health and Human Services, CDC* November 2010: 27.
2. French CL, Irwin RS, Curley FJ, Krikorian CJ. Impact of chronic cough on quality of life. *Arch Intern Med* 1998;158(15):1657–1661.
3. Irwin RS, Baumann MH, Boser DC, et al.; American College of Chest Physicians. Diagnosis and management of cough executive summary: ACCP evidence-based clinical practice guidelines. *Chest* 2006;129(1 suppl):1S–23S.
4. Benich JJ, Carek PJ. Evaluation of the patient with chronic cough. *Am Fam Physician* 2011;84(8): 887–892.
5. Asilsoy S, Bayram E, Agin H, et al. Evaluation of chronic cough in children. *Chest* 2008;134(6): 1122–1128.
6. Custer JW, Rau RE, eds. *The Harriett Lane Handbook*, 18th ed. Philadelphia, PA: Elsevier Mosby, 2009.
7. AAP Practice Guideline: Withdrawal of Cold Medicines, Addressing Parent Concerns 2008. Accessed at http://practice.aap.org/content.aspx?aid=2254 on Feb 20, 2012.
8. Irwin RS. Chronic cough due to gastroesophageal reflux disease: ACCP evidence-based clinical practice guidelines. *Chest* 2006; 129(suppl):805–945.

Cyanosis

Michael J. Gravett

I. BACKGROUND. Cyanosis is a dusky blue discoloration of the skin and mucous membranes caused by an increased quantity of reduced (deoxygenated) hemoglobin or hemoglobin derivatives in these tissues.

II. PATHOPHYSIOLOGY. In general, cyanosis appears when the concentration of reduced hemoglobin in the cutaneous tissues exceeds 4 g/dL (1). This represents systemic arterial oxygen saturations ranging from 60% in a patient with a hemoglobin concentration of 6 g/dL to 88% in a patient with a hemoglobin concentration of 20 g/dL (2). In addition, skin pigmentation and thickness also affect the degree of apparent cyanosis. In darkly pigmented individuals, color changes may not be seen until significantly lower oxygen saturations (1). Cyanosis is categorized as either central or peripheral based on the underlying abnormality.

A. Central cyanosis occurs with systemic arterial oxygen desaturation, in some anatomic shunts, and in certain conditions with abnormal hemoglobin molecules (3). Central cyanosis is characterized by the discoloration of both skin and mucous membranes. It is usually caused by one of the following:

1. Obstruction of oxygen intake (epiglottitis, acute laryngotracheobronchitis, asthma, chronic bronchitis, emphysema, and foreign body aspiration).

2. Decreased oxygen absorption, such as an alveolar capillary block (sarcoidosis, pulmonary fibrosis, pneumonia, pulmonary edema, alveolar proteinosis) or ventilation-perfusion (V/Q) defects from emphysema, pneumoconioses, and sarcoidosis.

3. Decreased lung perfusion (septic shock, cardiogenic shock, pulmonary embolus, pulmonary vascular shunts, and congenital heart disease).

4. Reduced intake of oxygen from altitudes above 8,000 to 13,000 ft (1, 4).

5. A defective hemoglobin molecule that is unable to attach to oxygen (methemoglobinemia, sulfhemoglobinemia, and other hemoglobinopathies). Note that carbon monoxide poisoning causes a cherry red appearance rather than a bluish hue. This is not true cyanosis but is often considered in the same category.

B. Peripheral cyanosis is the result of decreased blood flow and an abnormally high extraction of oxygen from arterial blood. It is caused by reduced cardiac output, cold exposure, and arterial or venous obstruction. In contrast to central cyanosis, the oral mucous membranes are typically spared (2). The following are the most common causes of peripheral cyanosis:

1. Reduced cardiac output from acute myocardial infarction or other causes of heart "pump" failure.

2. Local or regional phenomenon from cold exposure, arterial obstruction from embolus or thrombosis, and venous stasis or obstruction.

3. Generalized cold exposure (Raynaud's disease).

III. EVALUATION

A. History

1. Onset? Is the cyanosis of recent onset or has it been present since birth? A history of cyanosis since birth and "squatting" in childhood suggest congenital heart disease. Chronic cyanosis caused by methemoglobinemia can be congenital or acquired. Other causes of chronic cyanosis include chronic obstructive pulmonary disease (COPD), pulmonary fibrosis, and pulmonary atrioventricular fistula. Acute and subacute cyanosis can be caused by acute myocardial infarction, pneumothorax, pulmonary embolus, pneumonia, or upper airway obstruction.

2. Symptomatic? Asymptomatic patients may have methemoglobinemia (congenital or drug induced) or sulfhemoglobinemia. Exposures to drugs (prescribed and/or illicit)

or environmental factors should be reviewed. Intermittent cyanosis, skin color changes, and pain with cold exposure suggest Raynaud's phenomenon. Symptomatic patients, especially with chest pain and respiratory distress, are more likely to have a cardiac or pulmonary cause of cyanosis.

3. Risk Factors? Does the patient have known risk factors for cardiac or pulmonary disease, including smoking, hyperlipidemia, asthma, drug abuse (especially methamphetamines), severe obesity (sleep apnea), neuromuscular disease, or autoimmune disease? Does the patient have chest pain or intermittent cyanosis with exercise, suggesting angina? Chest pain can be present with acute pulmonary emboli or pneumothorax. Is there a cough and fever suggesting pneumonia? Has the patient had any occupational or environmental exposures that might cause pulmonary problems?

4. Family History or Past Medical History? Is there a family history of abnormal hemoglobin or pulmonary disease? Has the patient suffered an episode of hypotension that could produce adult respiratory distress syndrome (ARDS), such as sepsis or heart failure?

B. Physical Examination

1. **Initial assessment**. Vital signs: tachycardia suggests cardiac arrhythmia, shock, volume depletion, anemia, or fever. An increased or decreased respiratory rate and use of accessory musculature suggest hypoxia. Hypotension can signal vascular collapse.

2. **Additional physical examination**. Stridor suggests upper airway obstruction. Examine the pharynx for evidence of obstruction. If epiglottitis or the presence of a foreign body is suspected, be prepared to intubate the patient. Check the neck for evidence of jugular venous distention. Auscultate the chest for rales suggestive of pulmonary edema, wheezing, and rhonchi consistent with reactive airway disease or absence of breath sounds, suggestive of pneumonia or pneumothorax. Auscultate the heart for murmurs, arrhythmias, and abnormal heart sounds. Feel the pulses in the extremities to assess for arterial embolus or venous thrombosis, especially if cyanosis is localized to one extremity. Examine the abdomen for evidence of intra-abdominal catastrophe or aneurysm. Examine the nails for evidence of clubbing, which is suggestive of chronic pulmonary disease.

C. Testing

1. Pulse oximetry estimates oxygen saturation but does not measure it directly. Direct measurements using arterial blood gases (ABGs) are necessary to assess a patient with cyanosis. Patients with abnormal hemoglobin types have a normal Pao_2 but decreased hemoglobin O_2 saturation. A low Pao_2 is caused by respiratory or cardiac problems in most circumstances.

2. A chest radiograph helps assess heart size and lung parenchyma. Infiltrates suggest pneumonia, ARDS, or pulmonary edema. Exclude pneumothorax. Look for evidence of interstitial lung disease. Pleural effusion can represent infection, malignancy, or pulmonary edema.

3. An electrocardiogram may demonstrate acute myocardial infarction, arrhythmia, or pericardial process. P pulmonale, right ventricular hypertrophy, and right axis shift suggest chronic pulmonary disease.

4. An echocardiogram can help diagnose both diastolic and systolic heart failure, as well as visualize wall motion abnormalities that may be present in acute or prior myocardial infarction. Evidence of pulmonary hypertension can also be seen on echocardiogram.

5. Chest computed tomography (CT) may identify pulmonary emboli and provide more information than chest x-ray in a variety of cardiac and pulmonary diseases.

6. V/Q scanning may also demonstrate pulmonary embolus. It can be helpful in cases where a CT scan is contraindicated such as in patients with renal disease or contrast allergy.

7. Pulmonary artery catheterization and pressure measurements can help distinguish cardiac causes from pulmonary etiologies.

8. Pulmonary function testing can also be a useful adjunct for diagnosis.

IV. DIAGNOSIS

A. Focused history, physical examination, and diagnostic testing usually reveal the cause of cyanosis. Response to supplemental O_2 can also help pinpoint the cause of cyanosis (4). Decreased oxygenation secondary to mild-to-moderate V/Q mismatches caused by pneumonia, pulmonary embolus, and asthma may be reversible with supplemental oxygen. Severe V/Q mismatch caused by intrapulmonary shunting from severe pulmonary edema or ARDS may be refractory to supplemental O_2. Moderate V/Q mismatch associated with ventilatory failure COPD may respond to supplemental O_2, but be aware of increasing CO_2 levels. ABGs directly measure Pao_2 and O_2 saturation. Abnormal hemoglobin types are also measured and they can help guide therapy. Hypoxia with an elevated CO_2 suggests COPD or asthma, whereas hypoxia with a normal or decreased CO_2 suggests pneumonia, ARDS, pulmonary edema, pulmonary emboli, or interstitial lung disease (5).

B. Once the cause of the cyanosis is determined, the objective is to treat the underlying process. Causes of pseudocyanosis include argyria or bismuth poisoning (slate blue-gray coloring of mucous membranes), hemochromatosis (brownish color), or polycythemia (ruddy red color). For peripheral cyanosis caused by decreased cardiac output, correct the causes of hypovolemia (e.g., dehydration, shock, heart failure).

Disclaimer

The opinions and assertions contained herein are the private views of the author and are not to be construed as official or as reflecting the views of the U.S. Air Force Medical Service, the U.S. Air Force or the Department of Defense at large.

REFERENCES

1. Longo DL, Fauci AS, Kasper DL, et al., eds. *Harrison's Principles of Internal Medicine*, 18th ed. New York, NY: McGraw-Hill; 2012:Vol. 1:287–291.
2. Fathman L, ed. *Evidence-Based Physical Diagnosis*, Philadelphia, PA: Saunders, 2001:90–95.
3. Alvero R, Ferri FF, Borkan JM, et al., eds. *Ferri's Clinical Advisor 2012: 5 Books in 1*, 1st ed. Philadelphia, PA: Mosby, 2012:1136–1137.
4. Woodley M, Whelan A. *Manual of medical therapeutics,* Boston, MA: Little, Brown and Company, 1993:179–181.
5. Khan MG. *Cardiac and pulmonary management,* Philadelphia, PA: Lea & Febiger, 1993:818–825.

8.3 Hemoptysis

Sean P. Wherry

I. BACKGROUND. Hemoptysis is the expectoration of blood or blood-tinged sputum originating from the lower respiratory tract, encompassing the lung parenchyma, bronchioles, and trachea.

II. PATHOPHYSIOLOGY. Hemoptysis is often an anxiety-provoking symptom, creating fear more often than being life-threatening. With that being said, cases of massive hemoptysis, defined in the literature as the expectoration of ≥600 mL/24 h, can indeed be life-threatening, and impaired oxygenation can occur with as little as 400 mL of blood in the alveolar space (1).

A. Etiology and Epidemiology

a. Infection. According to the American Thoracic Society, there are greater than 100 possible causes of hemoptysis (2). By far the most common etiology is infection, accounting for 60–70% of cases presenting to a primary care setting (3). Resulting from its prevalence in Third World countries, tuberculosis (TB) remains the most common infectious etiology worldwide (4). Within the United States, viral bronchitis and bacterial pneumonia have surpassed TB as the primary cause (3). It is thought that pulmonary infections are responsible for superficial mucosal inflammation and rupture of blood vessels, resulting in blood-tinged sputum.

   b. Neoplasm. Neoplastic disease is responsible for 19–20% of hemoptysis cases (2). Bronchogenic carcinomas comprise 90% of these cases, with metastatic disease (renal, colon, and breast) accounting for the rest (1, 3). Neoplastic causes should be considered in patients over the age of 40 years with a history of smoking.

   c. Pulmonary Venous Hypertension. Conditions that result in elevated pulmonary artery pressures are known to cause hemoptysis. These include congestive heart failure, severe mitral stenosis, pulmonary embolism, and pulmonary arterial hypertension (2, 3).

   d. Idiopathic. Idiopathic hemoptysis is a diagnosis of exclusion occurring in 7–34% of patients (3). Typically, these patients do well and do not have any long-term sequela. Despite this, patients over the age of 40 years with a history of smoking should undergo close follow-up, as there is evidence for increased incidence of lung cancer (3).

III. EVALUATION. The initial evaluation of patients with hemoptysis is similar regardless of the rate of bleeding. Despite this, the mortality from a massive bleed decreases with expeditious evaluation (2). Regardless of the rate, the initial step in the evaluation is to differentiate whether the patient truly has hemoptysis versus bleeding from another source, e.g., hematemesis or pseudohemoptysis (bleeding originating in the naso/oropharynx).

   A. History. Close attention should be paid to the nature of the hemoptysis and its associated symptoms to include the presence of a productive cough, documented fevers, and increased dyspnea. Even though it is often exaggerated by the patient, an attempt should be made to assess the volume of expectorant. Frothy, bright red/pink, or clotted appearance is more likely to be associated with true hemoptysis, whereas dark brown/black, coffee ground appearance is likely to be gastric in origin. Likewise, the presence of nausea and emesis, a history of gastric or hepatic disease, or a history of epistaxis decrease the likelihood of a pulmonary source. If a pulmonary source is suspected, a thorough review of systems and review of the patient's past medical history will often be enlightening as to the etiology of the hemoptysis. A history of anticoagulant use, breast/colon/renal cancer, calf tenderness/swelling, pleuritic chest pain, cardiac disease/heart failure, orthopnea, recent travel, hematuria, unintentional weight gain/loss, chronic obstructive pulmonary disease, and smoking may assist in the diagnosis and management of hemoptysis (3).

   B. Physical Exam. Vital signs should include heart rate, blood pressure, temperature, respiratory rate, and oxygen saturation. Any signs of shock, hypovolemia, hypoxia, or respiratory failure should be identified and acted upon immediately. A thorough ENT exam should be performed. The presence of saddle nose with rhinitis and a septal perforation may be seen with Wegener's granulomatosis. The presence of oral or genital ulcers should raise the concern for Behçet's disease (4). The pulmonary exam should note the work of breathing, any chest wall abnormalities, as well as the presence of stridor, rales, wheezes, or decreased breath sounds. A cardiac exam should be done with particular attention paid to the presence of murmurs, an S4 heart sound, and jugular venous distention. An exam of the patient's extremities should note the presence of edema, clubbing of the digits, or cyanosis. Cervical, axillary, and inguinal lymph nodes should be assessed for lymphadenopathy.

   C. Diagnostic Evaluation

   a. Labs. The severity of the patient's symptoms, the patient's comorbidities, and the associated symptoms will dictate what laboratory tests will be appropriate. In all patients with signs of respiratory distress, an arterial blood gas should be obtained (1). In most patients, routine blood work to include a complete blood count, renal function panel, coagulation profile, electrolytes, and urinalysis should be performed (1, 2). Sputum should be analyzed and cultured for the presence of bacteria (Gram stain, potassium hydroxide, acid fast). Sputum cytology should be performed in all smokers older than 40 years and in any patient where there is concern for neoplasm (4).

b. **Imaging.** Following a thorough history and physical, all patients presenting with hemoptysis should obtain a chest radiograph to evaluate lung parenchyma, heart, and pulmonary vasculature (1–5). Evidence of cavitary lesions, tumors, infiltrates, and atelectasis may be demonstrated and aid in diagnosis and management (4); 20–40% of chest radiographs are interpreted as normal (1). In stable patients with a normal chest radiograph who have no risk factors for neoplasm and do not have recurrent episodes of hemoptysis, no further evaluation is needed, and a course of observation is warranted. In patients with abnormal chest radiographs, recurrent symptoms, or risk factors for neoplasm, a high-resolution computed tomography should be performed (3).

c. **Bronchoscopy.** Bronchoscopy may be performed in patients in whom there is a strong concern for neoplasm (3). Advantages include direct visualization of the endobronchial processes to include site of bleeding, and it allows for immediate intervention to control bleeding. Rigid bronchoscopy is recommended for massive hemoptysis requiring immediate intervention. This is due to its greater suctioning capabilities and its ability to maintain a patent airway. It does, however, require general anesthesia and often fails to visualize the upper lobes (4). Fiber-optic bronchoscopy is often reserved for mild hemoptysis typically 24–48 hours after presentation (3), can be done at the bedside, and may reach more peripheral lesions (4).

Disclaimer

The opinions and assertions contained herein are the private views of the author and are not to be construed as official or as reflecting the views of the U.S. Air Force Medical Service, the U.S. Air Force or the Department of Defense at large.

REFERENCES

1. Corder R. Hemoptysis. *Emerg Med Clin N Am* 2003;21:421–435.
2. Lenner R, Schilero G, Lesser M. Hemoptysis: diagnosis and management. *Comp Ther* 2002;28(1):7–14.
3. Bidwell JL, Pachner RW. Hemoptysis: diagnosis and management. *Am Fam Physician* 2005;72(7):1253–1260.
4. Jean-Baptiste E. Clinical assessment and management of massive hemoptysis. *Crit Care Med* 2000;28(5):1642–1647.
5. Marshall TJ, Flower CDR, Jackson JE. The role of radiology in the investigation and management of patients with haemoptysis. *Clin Radiol* 1996;51:391–400.

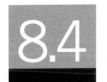

8.4 Pleural Effusion

Kenisha R. Heath

I. **BACKGROUND.** Pleural effusions represent an imbalance between the formation and removal of pleural fluid and are characterized by an excessive accumulation of fluid in the pleural space (1). There are many medical conditions that may cause pleural effusions, but the most common causes in adults are congestive heart failure, infection, pulmonary embolism, and malignancy (2).

II. **PATHOPHYSIOLOGY.** Causative mechanisms for pleural effusion include an increased hydrostatic pressure in the microvascular circulation such as in congestive heart failure, a decreased oncotic pressure in the microvascular circulation which may be secondary to hypoalbuminemia, and increased negative pressure in the pleural space suggestive of atelectasis. Other common mechanisms include separation of the pleural spaces from a trapped lung, increased permeability of the microvascular circulation due to inflammatory mediators from infectious processes, impaired lymphatic drainage from the pleural surface due to blockage by tumor or fibrosis, and movement of ascitic fluid from the peritoneal space through diaphragmatic lymphatics (1).

III. EVALUATION

A. History

1. **Pulmonary**. Symptoms experienced by the patient are largely dependent upon the amount of accumulated fluid in the pleural space. With significant fluid accumulation, patients may report pleuritic pain, dyspnea, and a nonproductive cough. With minimal fluid accumulation, patients may remain asymptomatic.

2. **Associated Symptoms**. Patients may also experience fever in the presence of infection; hemoptysis in the presence of pulmonary embolism and lung cancer; or weight loss in the presence of malignancy, tuberculosis, or infection (2).

3. **Past Medical History**. Patients with a recent history of abdominal surgery may experience postoperative pleural effusion or effusion secondary to pulmonary embolism. Pleural effusion secondary to malignancy should be excluded (2). Congestive heart failure should be considered in patients with multiple cardiac risk factors.

4. **Family History**. Consideration of family history of malignancy, heart disease, and infectious diseases should be discussed.

5. **Social History**. Patients with a history of alcohol abuse, misuse, or pancreatic disease may have pleural fluid accumulation secondary to a pancreatic effusion. Chronic and prolonged exposure to asbestos may cause effusion secondary to mesothelioma or benign asbestos pleural effusion (2).

B. Physical Exam

1. **Focused Pulmonary Exam**. The patient's respiratory rate, respiratory effort, and breath sounds should be thoroughly evaluated. Possible findings on exam suggestive of pleural effusion may include dullness to percussion, decreased or absent breath sounds, and reduced tactile fremitus. Presence or absence of the findings may be dependent upon the severity of the effusion.

2. **Additional Physical Exam**. The presence of a heart murmur and cardiomegaly on imaging suggests possible heart failure, whereas ascites may suggest the presence of hepatic hydrothorax. Consider pulmonary embolism in patients exhibiting swelling of a lower extremity and pericarditis in those with the presence of a pericardial friction rub (2).

C. Testing

1. **Radiography**. Anteroposterior (AP) and lateral chest radiographs should be completed when concern for pleural effusion exists. In the upright position, free pleural fluid will flow beneath the lung, causing the following on imaging: blunting of the costophrenic angle, lateral displacement of the dome of the diaphragm, and elevation of the hemithorax (1). Views of the lateral decubitus are helpful in viewing smaller effusions, as typically only effusions of 200 mL or larger are seen on the AP view (3).

2. **Ultrasound**. The use of ultrasonography is helpful in identifying small effusions undetectable by radiograph. It is also helpful in differentiating between solid and liquid components. Additionally, an ultrasound may be used to guide thoracentesis for small or loculated effusions (1).

3. **Computed Tomography (CT)**. CT is used in cases where plain radiography and ultrasound are unsuccessful in identifying anatomy. It is helpful for detecting small effusions as well as differentiating pleural fluid from pleural thickening (2).

4. **Thoracentesis**. Thoracentesis should be performed in cases where the cause of effusion is not known following history and physical exam. Not all effusions, however, will require a thoracentesis.

   a. **Relative contraindications**. Thoracentesis should not be performed in several circumstances: patients with obvious heart failure, effusions that are too small to be aspirated safely, patients who have recently underwent thoracic or abdominal surgery (1), and patients with severe chronic obstructive pulmonary disease or bilateral lung or pleural involvement (4).

   b. **Transudate or exudate?** Pleural fluid should be evaluated for protein, lactate dehydrogenase (LDH), pH, Gram stain, acid fast bacilli (AFB) stain, cytology, and microbiologic culture (4). Evaluation of the fluid obtained will assist in determining if the

TABLE 8.4.1	Light's Criteria		
	Pleural fluid protein/serum protein	Pleural fluid LDH/serum LDH	Pleural fluid LDH/upper limit normal serum LDH
Exudate	>0.5	>0.6	>2/3
Transudate	≤0.5	≤0.6	≤2/3

LDH, lactate dehydrogenase.

effusion is transudative, due to an imbalance in hydrostatic and oncotic forces, or exudative, due to increased permeability of the pleural surfaces and blood vessels or impaired lymphatic drainage of the pleural space (3). Transudative effusions are commonly caused by congestive heart failure and cirrhosis. They require no further workup and usually respond to treatment of the causative condition. Exudative effusions, however, have many more possible causes to include malignancy and infection and require more investigation.

Light's criteria is a reliable tool for differentiating between exudative and transudative effusions. This tool compares the LDH and protein levels of serum and pleural fluid (3). The presence of at least one of the following three criteria would classify the fluid as an exudates:

1. Pleural fluid protein/serum protein ratio greater than 0.5
2. Pleural fluid LDH/serum LDH ratio greater than 0.6.
3. Pleural fluid/LDH greater than two-thirds the upper limit of the laboratory's normal serum LDH (Table 8.4.1).

c. Other measures have been used to identify exudative pleural effusions and include pleural fluid cholesterol, triglycerides, glucose, and albumin (3).

IV. **DIAGNOSIS.** Pleural effusion analysis is an essential component to diagnosis.

   A. If the pleural fluid is found to be transudative, the causative condition is commonly congestive heart failure, hypoalbuminemia, atelectasis, or nephrotic syndrome (3). Using clinical clues from the H&P is now required.

   B. Typical causes of exudative effusion are pneumonia and other infections, malignancy, tuberculosis, pulmonary embolism, lung entrapment, and connective tissue diseases. Exudative effusions, however, have a vast number of causes and thus further investigation is warranted with glucose level, cell count, pH level, amylase, and triglycerides. Thoracoscopy, bronchoscopy, repeat thoracentesis, or pleural biopsy may also be helpful.

   C. In the majority of cases, a diagnosis can be determined based on the patient's exam and thoracentesis results, but in a small number of cases, no diagnosis is ever established (5). When no diagnosis is made, the patient should be closely monitored and pulmonary consultation should be obtained.

REFERENCES

1. Yataco JC, Dweik RA. Pleural effusions: evaluation and management. *Cleveland Clin J Med* 2005;72:854–872.
2. Porcel JM, Light RW. Diagnostic approach to pleural effusion in adults. *Am Fam Physician* 2006;73(7):1211–1220.
3. Heffner JE. *Diagnostic evaluation of a pleural effusion in adults: initial testing.* Accessed at http://www.uptodate.com/contents/diagnostic-evaluation-of-a-pleuraleffusion-in-adults-initial-testing on June 2012.
4. Medford A, Maskell N. Pleural effusion. *Postgrad Med J* 2005;81:702–710.
5. Rodriquez-Panadero F, Janssen J.P, Astoul P. Thoracoscopy: general overview and place in the diagnosis and management of pleural effusion. *Eur Resp J* 2006;28,2:409–422.

Pleuritic Pain

Lisa B. Norton

I. BACKGROUND. Pleuritic chest pain is pain that is referable to the parietal pleura, lining the inner wall of the thoracic cavity. The character of the pain is typically described as sharp, burning, or catching but may be perceived as dull (1). It is most appropriate to consider "pleuritic pain" a descriptor of the source rather than character of the pain. "Pleurisy" is often used synonymously with pleuritic pain.

II. PATHOPHYSIOLOGY

A. Etiology. The parietal pleura is the primary source of respiratory pain and lines the inner chest wall, superior surface of the diaphragm, and lateral boundaries of the mediastinum. It is innervated by somatic intercostal nerves inside the chest wall and along the lateral portions of the diaphragm. Inflammation involving these areas results in localized chest pain. The parietal pleura at the central portion of the diaphragm is innervated by the phrenic nerve, and inflammation in this region is frequently referable to the ipsilateral shoulder or neck. The visceral pleura, or pleura pulmonalis, represents a layer of mesothelial tissue that is insensate and covers the entire surface of the lung (1–3).

B. Epidemiology. Determining that chest pain is of a pleural origin, rather than from cardiac or pulmonary vasculature sources, is an important initial distinction. The incidence of primary care evaluations for chest pain varies from 1% to 3% (4). In an emergency setting in Belgium, a cardiovascular etiology for chest pain was found 18% of the time and a noncardiac etiology was found 30% of the time (5). In contrast, the same study and two others from the United States and Switzerland found the incidence of a cardiovascular cause of chest pain in the outpatient primary care setting to be 13–16% and a noncardiac etiology to be present 68–80% of the time (5–7).

III. EVALUATION

A. History

1. **History of Present Illness**. The history alone rarely leads to a definitive etiology of pleuritic chest pain (4, 8). The primary value of the history during an evaluation is to describe the temporal course and to identify markers that increase the likelihood that a life-threatening condition is present (8). Acute (minutes to hours) processes of concern include myocardial infarction, pulmonary embolism, pneumothorax, and trauma. Subacute (hours to days) processes include pneumonia, parapneumonic infections, and some inflammatory processes such as pericarditis. Chronic (days to weeks) presentations may be associated with malignancy or connective tissues diseases such as rheumatoid arthritis or systemic lupus erythematosus.

2. **Review of Systems.** The review of systems should be used to generate a differential diagnosis and establish pretest probabilities for possible etiologies prior to ordering diagnostic tests. Typical angina symptoms may lead to consideration of acute coronary syndrome (9); exertional dyspnea may suggest congestive heart failure (10); a Wells score of >2 increases the likelihood of pulmonary embolism (11); and a sudden, ripping or tearing pain in the chest or back should suggest dissecting aortic aneurysm (4).

3. **Past Medical History.** Its greatest value is in refining the initial differential diagnosis that was generated based upon the description of symptoms provided by the patient.

B. Physical Examination.
The negative and positive predictive values for most exam findings in pleuritic pain are low (4). A pleural friction rub may be heard in as many as 4% of patients with either pulmonary embolism or pneumonia (8, 12). Myocardial infarction may cause diaphoresis, an S3 gallop, or evidence of new valvular dysfunction. Pneumonia, pleural effusion, or pneumothorax all may be associated with a focal area of decreased breath

sounds. Pneumonia can be associated with egophony on examination, whereas pleural effusion is not. Pneumothorax may cause tympany with percussion, while pleural effusion and pneumonia do not.

C. Testing

1. A posteroanterior and lateral chest radiograph should be obtained in all patients being evaluated for pleuritic chest pain. This may quickly identify, or suggest, life-threatening conditions such as pneumothorax or thoracic aortic aneurysm. However, the study is imperfect for all causes of chest pain. Other studies to consider include electrocardiogram, chest computed tomography, cardiac enzymes, rheumatologic serology studies, or lung ultrasound. In one study of various diagnostic tests in the bedside evaluation of pleuritic chest pain in the emergency department with an apparently normal chest radiograph, the lung ultrasound was found to have better positive predictive value (94.12%), negative predictive value (98.21%), and area under the curve of receiver operator curve (0.967) for pain etiology versus the D-dimer or C- reactive Protein (CRP) blood studies (13).

D. Genetics.
Most common causes of pleuritic chest pain are not directly related to identified genetic abnormalities, although this area of research is evolving rapidly. Notable exceptions include hypercoagulable states (caused either directly by a genetic abnormality or indirectly due to a genetically related condition such as some cancers).

IV. DIAGNOSIS

A. Differential Diagnosis.
The differential diagnosis of what clinically appears to be a pleuritic chest pain syndrome is quite broad. Viral infection, due to the Coxsackie B virus in particular, is among the most common causes of pleuritic chest pain (8). Some of the conditions, such as myocardial infarction, in the differential diagnosis are not truly causes of inflammation of the parietal pleura, but are included in the differential because of similarity in presentation. Commonly considered causes of a pleuritic chest pain syndrome include (4) acute coronary syndrome, pulmonary embolism, aortic dissection, pneumonia, lung cancer, pneumothorax, chest wall syndrome, costochondritis, trauma, fibromyalgia (14), odynophagia, gastroesophageal reflux disease, and psychogenic chest pain. The latter is always a diagnosis of exclusion (Table 8.5.1).

Disclaimer

The opinions and assertions contained herein are the private views of the author and are not to be construed as official or as reflecting the views of the U.S. Air Force Medical Service, the U.S. Air Force or the Department of Defense at large.

TABLE 8.5.1	Differential Diagnosis of Pleuritic Pain

- Acute coronary syndrome
- Pulmonary embolism
- Pneumothorax
- Pneumonia
- Pleural effusion
- Empyema
- Aortic dissection
- Pericarditis
- Costochondritis
- Neoplasm
- Fibromyalgia
- Other known cause: infection, autoimmune disorder, or medications

REFERENCES

1. Brims FJH, Davies HE, Lee YC. Respiratory chest pain: diagnosis and treatment. *Med Clin N Am* 2010;94:217–232.
2. English JC, Leslie KO. Pathology of the pleura. *Clin Chest Med* 2006;27:157–180.
3. Cagle PT, Allen TC. Pathology of the pleura: what the pulmonologists need to know. *Respirology* 2011;16:430–438.
4. Yelland M, Cayley WE, Vach W. An algorithm for the diagnosis and management of chest pain in primary care. *Med Clin N Am* 2010;94:349–374.
5. Buntinx F, Knockaert D, Bruyninckx R, et al. Chest pain in general practice or in the hospital emergency department: is it the same? *Fam Pract* 2001;18(6):586–589.
6. Ruigomez A, Rodriguez LA, Wallander MA, et al. Chest pain in general practice: incidence, comorbidity and mortality. *Fam Pract* 2006;23(2):167–174.
7. Nilsson S, Scheike M, Engblom D, et al. Chest pain and ischaemic heart disease in primary care. *Br J Gen Pract* 2003;53:378–382.
8. Kass SM, Williams PM, Reamy BV. Pleurisy. *Am Fam Physician* 2007;75:1357–1364.
9. Gibbons RJ, Balady GJ, Bricker JT, et al. ACC/AHA 2002 guideline update for exercise testing: summary article: a report of the American College of Cardiology/American Heart Association Task Force on Practice Guidelines (Committee to Update the 1997 Exercise Testing Guidelines). *Circulation* 2002;106:1883–1892.
10. Davie AP, Caruana FL, Sutherland GER, et al. Assessing diagnosis in heart failure: which features are any use? *QJM* 1997;90:335–339.
11. Wells PS, Anderson DR, Rodger M, et al. Derivation of a simple clinical model to categorize patients probability of pulmonary embolism: increasing the models utility with the SimpliRED D-dimer. *Thromb Haemost* 2000;83:416–420.
12. Miniati M, Prediletto R, Formichi B, et al. Accuracy of clinical assessment in the diagnosis of pulmonary embolism. *Am J Respir Crit Care Med* 1999;159:864–871.
13. Volpicelli G, Cardinale L, Berchialla P, et al. A comparison of different diagnostic tests in the bedside evaluation of pleuritic pain in the ED. *Am J Emerg Med* 2012;30:317–324.
14. Almansa C, Wang B, Achem SR. Noncardiac chest pain and fibromyalgia. *Med Clin N Am* 2010;94:275–289.

8.6 Pneumothorax

Carlton J. Covey

I. BACKGROUND. Pneumothorax occurs when air collects between the lung and the chest wall (the pleural space), due to a disruption in either the visceral or parietal pleura. The clinical manifestations can be asymptomatic, mild, or life-threatening, necessitating immediate intervention.

II. PATHOPHYSIOLOGY. Pneumothorax can be classified into two major categories—spontaneous and nonspontaneous. Spontaneous pneumothoraces occur without any obvious precipitating cause and are further subclassified as primary or secondary. Nonspontaneous pneumothoraces are traumatic and can be either iatrogenic or noniatrogenic.

A. Spontaneous Pneumothorax

1. Primary spontaneous pneumothorax (PSP) occurs in previously healthy individuals without a history of lung disease. It is found more frequently in tall, slender young adults (age 20–30 years) and is uncommon in those older than 40 years (1, 2). PSP is often caused by a rupture of alveolar apical blebs or bullae. Cigarette smoking increases the possibility of PSP in a dose-dependent fashion. Light smokers (1–12 cigarettes a day) have a seven times higher lifetime relative risk, while heavy smokers (>22 cigarettes per day) have greater than 100 times increased risk (1). The estimated annual incidence

of PSP is 7.4–18 cases per 100,000 men and 1.2–6 cases per 100,000 women (3). Patients who have had a PSP have an approximate 30% rate of recurrence. However, the consensus remains that these patients should not undergo definitive preventive treatment (1, 4).

2. Secondary spontaneous pneumothorax (SSP) occurs as a complication in individuals with underlying pulmonary disease and therefore can be a much more serious entity. A multitude of lung disorders have been described as etiologies for SSP, but chronic obstructive pulmonary disease (COPD) is by far the most commonly associated condition (5). SSP can also be seen in individuals with pulmonary infections, particularly *Pneumocystis carinii* pneumonia and tuberculosis, as well as with primary lung neoplasms or metastatic tumors. The incidence is similar to that of PSP, with an estimated 15,000 cases per year in the United States (1). Patients who have had an SSP have an approximately 40–80% rate of recurrence. This high recurrence rate, and the increased clinical severity of a pneumothorax in this subset of patients, has led to the consensus that these patients should receive immediate definitive therapy for recurrence prevention, even after the first episode (1, 4).

B. Traumatic Pneumothorax

1. Iatrogenic pneumothorax is more common than PSP and SSP combined and, by definition, occurs as a complication of medical procedures (6). The leading cause of iatrogenic pneumothorax is transthoracic needle biopsy, but it can also occur during other procedures such as central venous catheter placement, thoracentesis and bronchoscopy, or as a complication of mechanical ventilation.

2. **Penetrating and Blunt Trauma.** Penetrating trauma, such as a stab wound, allows air to enter through the chest wall wound. Pneumothorax can also be a result of blunt trauma (e.g., when a rib fracture pierces the visceral pleura). However, the majority of nonpenetrating trauma and resultant pneumothorax lack a preceding rib fracture (1). The decelerating force of blunt chest trauma and subsequent thoracic compression leads to an increase in alveolar pressure that can cause a pneumothorax.

III. EVALUATION

A. History

1. **Spontaneous Pneumothorax.** Sudden ipsilateral chest pain or discomfort, most often pleuritic, is the most common symptom. In PSP, symptom onset is usually at rest, and patients often do not immediately seek medical attention (2). Dypsnea may be present but is often mild in PSP. In patients with underlying lung disease (SSP) who have impaired pulmonary reserve, symptoms are generally more severe and dyspnea is the most prominent clinical feature.

2. **Traumatic Pneumothorax.** The symptoms are preceded by a medical procedure or a traumatic event and are similar to those seen in spontaneous pneumothorax. In cases of iatrogenic pneumothorax, symptoms may not occur for 24 hours or more after the diagnostic or therapeutic procedure (2). Any mechanically ventilated patient with acute deterioration should always be evaluated for pneumothorax and is more likely in ventilated patients with acute respiratory distress syndrome, aspiration pneumonia, COPD, or interstitial lung disease (1, 2).

B. Physical Examination.
Vital signs can be normal with small pneumothoraces, but tachycardia is the most common sign of spontaneous pneumothorax (3). In larger pneumothoraces, or in patients with SSP, significant tachypnea, cyanosis, and hypoxemia can occur and deterioration can be rapid and fatal. These symptoms can also be accompanied by hypotension in patients with tension pneumothorax, a life-threatening medical emergency. During chest and lung examinations, patients may be found to have unilateral enlargement of the chest cavity, loss of tactile fremitus, hyperresonance to percussion, and decreased, or absent, breath sounds on the affected side (1, 5).

C. Testing

1. Chest x-ray is paramount in the diagnosis, with visualization of the visceral pleural line and the absence of lung markings distal to this line. The radiographical pleural line is defined by air density on either side of the line and should be sharp and well demarcated.

This is best seen on an upright inspiratory posteroanterior film (7). There is no value of adding additional expiratory films and this is not recommended for diagnosis. Lateral decubitus films (with the affected side up) may be helpful when the diagnosis is in question or in critically ill patients who cannot sit upright (1, 7).

2. Arterial blood gas typically reveals hypoxia and occasionally hypocarbia secondary to hyperventilation (1). The hypoxia is due to both the creation of low ventilation-perfusion ratios and absent ventilation (creating a shunt) in affected areas of the lung.

3. Computed tomography (CT) can be useful when the chest x-ray is not diagnostic, but is not routinely recommended for patients with a first-time pneumothorax (4). In patients with SSP, the radiographic appearance of the pneumothorax can be altered by the underlying lung abnormalities, making the chest x-ray more difficult to interpret. These complicated patients may need a CT scan for diagnosis. Utilization of CT can also be important when diagnosing traumatic pneumothoraces as up to 40% are not detected by chest x-ray alone (8). More recently, bedside ultrasound has been utilized to diagnose pneumothoraces, especially in the emergency department setting. Unfortunately, there is a high rate of false-positive scans, especially in patients with underlying COPD, and most patients will require a confirmatory CT scan (8).

IV. DIAGNOSIS
A. Differential Diagnosis
1. The differential diagnosis of pleuritic chest pain and dyspnea includes other life-threatening conditions such as myocardial infarction, COPD exacerbation, aortic dissection, pericarditis, pneumonia, and pulmonary embolism (9). PSP can be diagnosed by the clinical history and physical examination in tall, thin patients who have had acute onset of chest pain and mild dyspnea and confirmed with a chest radiograph visualizing the visceral pleural line.

2. SSP can be more complicated to diagnose. Although the symptoms are more prominent, the signs on physical examination are often subtle, especially in patients with COPD who tend to have decreased breath sounds and decreased tactile fremitus, because of their underlying disease. As previously addressed, radiographic evaluation can also be more difficult. Because of the lack of interstitial markings in the emphysematous lung, little difference is seen in the appearance proximal and distal to the visceral line.

B. Clinical Manifestations
1. Symptoms of a pneumothorax can range from being mild to life-threatening. Most healthy individuals never seek care for their PSP. A high index of suspicion for a spontaneous pneumothorax should be kept for young, tall, slender males with acute-onset chest pain occurring at rest. Patients with pleuritic chest pain and dyspnea after a diagnostic or therapeutic procedure, and all patients with significant blunt trauma to the chest, should be evaluated for pneumothorax, including all patients with rib or scapula fractures. All patients with underlying lung conditions, especially COPD, have an increased risk of spontaneous pneumothorax and usually present with more significant clinical symptoms.

2. Tension pneumothorax is a rare but life-threatening entity that occurs when a condition exists that allows air into, but not out of, the pleural space. As pressure in the pleural space exceeds the atmospheric pressure, the ipsilateral lung, mediastinum, and contralateral lung are compressed. The diagnosis of tension pneumothorax must be made clinically and appropriate treatment rendered promptly. Diagnosis should never be delayed for radiographic confirmation. The diagnosis can be confirmed by treatment: insert a large bore needle (14–16 G) through the second anterior intercostal space at the clavicular midline. A rush of air and rapid improvement of symptoms confirms the diagnosis (1).

Disclaimer
The opinions and assertions contained herein are the private views of the author and are not to be construed as official or as reflecting the views of the U.S. Air Force Medical Service, the U.S. Air Force or the Department of Defense at large.

REFERENCES

1. Light RW, Lee YC. Pneumothorax, chylothorax, hemothorax, and fibrothorax. In: *Murray and Nadel's textbook of respiratory medicine,* 5th ed. Philadelphia, PA: Saunders, 2010:1764–1778.
2. Baumann MH, Noppen M. Pneumothorax. *Respirology* 2004;9:157–164.
3. Sahn SA, Heffner JE. Spontaneous pneumothorax. *N Engl J Med* 2000;342:868–874.
4. Baumann MH, Strange C, Heffner JE, et al. Management of spontaneous pneumothorax: an American College of Chest Physicians Delphi consensus statement. *Chest* 2001;119:590–602.
5. Noppen M. Spontaneous pneumothorax: epidemiology, pathophysiology and cause. *Eur Respir Rev* 2010;19:217–219.
6. Gordon CE, Feller-Kopman D, Balk EM, Smetana GW. Pneumothorax following thoracentesis. *Arch Intern Med* 2010;170(4):332–339.
7. O'Connor AR, Morgan WE. Radiologic review of pneumothorax. *BMJ* 2005;330:1493–1497.
8. Rowen KR, Kirkpatrick AW, Liu D, et al. Traumatic pneumothorax detection with thoracic US: correlation with chest radiography and CT-initial experience. *Radiology* 2002;225:210–214.
9. Kass SM, Williams PM, Reamy BV. Pleurisy. *Am Fam Physician* 2007;75:1357–1364.

8.7 Shortness of Breath

David K. Gordon II

I. BACKGROUND. Shortness of breath, or dyspnea, is defined as "a subjective experience of breathing discomfort that is comprised of qualitatively distinct sensations that vary in intensity. The experience derives from interactions among multiple physiologic, psychological, social, and environmental factors and may induce secondary physiologic and behavioral responses" (1).

Given the potential for patient distress when experiencing dyspnea, it is common for dyspneic patients to present to the emergency department (ED) or acute care clinic. In 2009, dyspnea was the chief complaint in 2.7% of the more than 136 million ED visits in the United States. Dyspnea-related complaints such as cough and chest pain accounted for 8.8% of ED visits in 2009 (2).

II. PATHOPHYSIOLOGY. The respiratory system is responsible for maintaining appropriate gas exchange and acid–base regulation within the body. Factors that impair oxygenation or cause acidemia, whether they originate in the heart, lungs, or elsewhere, can lead to the sensation of breathing difficulty or shortness of breath.

Dyspnea can be the primary manifestation of various life-threatening conditions (Table 8.7.1), but the vast majority of patients who experience dyspnea have one of the following five chronic conditions (3, 4):
- Asthma
- Chronic obstructive pulmonary disease (COPD)
- Interstitial lung disease
- Myocardial dysfunction
- Obesity/deconditioning

The most common diagnoses for elderly patients (age >65 years) who present to the ED with shortness of breath and the signs of respiratory distress (respiratory rate > 25, Spo_2 < 93%) are (5)
- Decompensated heart failure
- Pneumonia
- COPD
- Pulmonary embolism
- Asthma

III. EVALUATION. Cardiac disease remains the leading cause of death in the United States. Shortness of breath is one of the hallmark symptoms, and occasionally the only symptom, of

TABLE 8.7.1   Life-Threatening Causes of Dyspnea

Upper airway

- Tracheal foreign objects
- Angioedema
- Anaphylaxis
- Infections of the pharynx and neck
- Airway trauma

Pulmonary/lower airway

- Pulmonary embolism
- Chronic obstructive pulmonary disease
- Asthma
- Pneumothorax/hemothorax and pneumomediastinum
- Pulmonary infection
- Noncardiogenic pulmonary edema
- Direct pulmonary injury
- Acute Respiratory Distress Syndrome
- Pulmonary hemorrhage

Cardiac

- Acute coronary syndrome
- Acute decompensated heart failure
- Flash pulmonary edema
- High-output heart failure
- Cardiomyopathy
- Cardiac arrhythmia
- Valvular dysfunction
- Cardiac tamponade

Neurologic

- Stroke
- Neuromuscular disease

Toxic and metabolic

- Poisoning, e.g., salicylates and carbon monoxide
- Toxin-related metabolic acidosis
- Diabetic ketoacidosis
- Sepsis
- Anemia
- Acute chest syndrome

myocardial infarction and angina (6). As such, heart disease must remain on the top of the differential diagnosis when beginning the workup of a patient with dyspnea.

A. History. Knowing how to differentiate between respiratory system causes of dyspnea and cardiovascular system causes of dyspnea is essential for accurate diagnosis. Health-care providers should approach the evaluation of dyspneic patients in much the same way that they approach the evaluation of pain, by asking the patient to use descriptive words to explain their shortness of breath. Several causes of dyspnea have been found to have common terms used in the description of the patients' symptoms:

- COPD patients report an increased "effort to breathe," a sensation of "unsatisfying breaths," and a feeling that they "cannot get a deep breath" (7).
- Heart failure patients commonly report feelings of "air hunger" and "suffocation" (8).
- Cardiovascular deconditioning is commonly associated with "heavy breathing" (9).
- Bronchospasm is frequently described as chest tightness.
- Interstitial disease often corresponds to rapid, shallow breathing.

Other historical questions should also be asked such as past medical history, prescribed medication compliance, symptom duration, allergens or toxin exposure, preceding events, recent onset of cough or fever, recent surgical history or immobilization that could increase the risk of pulmonary embolism, or recent trauma.

B. Physical Examination. The physical examination begins with your first observation of the patient and within the first minute you should be able to assess the patient for signs of significant respiratory distress.

- Signs of impending respiratory arrest
  o Cyanosis
  o Decreased ability to sustain respiratory effort
  o Depressed mental status
- Signs of severe respiratory distress
  o Chest retractions
  o Use of accessory muscles to maintain respiratory effort
  o Extreme diaphoresis
  o Staccato, disjointed speech
  o Nervousness, anxiety
  o Refusal to lie supine
  o Altered mental status

If the patient is deemed to be stable after the quick initial assessment, the examiner continues with a more detailed and thorough examination with the aim of determining whether the patient's dyspnea is due to a respiratory or cardiac disease. Begin with a review of the vital signs—specifically the respiratory rate and pulse oximetry reading. Next, proceed with an examination of the face and neck where you should look for nasal flaring, postnasal drip, pharyngeal inflammation/infection, foreign bodies, tracheal deviation, and jugular venous distension.

Moving down to the chest, observe for symmetric chest rise and fall, retractions, accessory muscle use, tripod seated position, general shape of the chest/thorax (e.g., barrel-shaped chest commonly seen in COPD). Listen for abnormal breath sounds:

- Inspiratory stridor—obstruction above the vocal cords (e.g., epiglottitis, foreign body).
- Expiratory stridor—obstruction below the vocal cords (e.g., croup, bacterial tracheitis, foreign body).
- Wheezing—obstruction below the trachea (e.g., asthma, anaphylaxis, foreign body in bronchus).
- Crackles (rales)—fluid accumulation in the interalveolar space (e.g., pneumonia, acute decompensated heart failure [ADHF]).
- Decreased breath sounds—any source that prevents air entry into the lung (e.g., pneumothorax, tension pneumothorax, hemothorax).

There are several possible findings in the heart exam that can reveal the etiology of the patient's dyspnea. An abnormal rhythm, such as atrial fibrillation in a heart failure patient, may cause dyspnea. Cardiac tamponade produces muffled or distant heart sounds and the impaired function of the heart with this condition leads to a systemic decrease in oxygen delivery and resultant dyspnea. S3 and S4 heart sounds are suggestive of left ventricular dysfunction. Jugular venous distension can be seen in patients with ADHF and cardiac tamponade.

Next, the examiner should perform an abdominal exam to assess for an intraab-dominal mass that may be compressing the diaphragm and decreasing the intrathoracic space and total lung volume or compressing the inferior vena cava and decreasing blood return to the heart. Finally, a close inspection of the patient's skin and extremities should be performed looking for discoloration suggestive of poor perfusion or hypoxia and peripheral edema suggesting ADHF.

C. Testing

1. A chest x-ray (CXR) and pulse oximetry are useful in evaluating a variety of cardiac and pulmonary causes of dyspnea. Cardiomegaly, pleural effusion, and cephalization of blood vessels are indicative of acute heart failure. Pulmonary infiltration is diagnostic of pneumonia and a pneumothorax can be identified as an area of increased lucency, typically at the lung apices, on CXR. COPD and asthma are identified by increased lung volumes and flattening of the diaphragm. All of these conditions will result in a decreased pulse oximetry reading.

2. An electrocardiogram (ECG) is necessary to assess for cardiac ischemia/infarction, cardiomegaly, pulmonary embolism, cardiac arrhythmia, and pericardial tamponade. It should be noted that a normal ECG upon initial presentation does not rule out myocardial infarction. A normal initial ECG is found in nearly 20% of patients subsequently diagnosed with myocardial infarction and only 33% of initial ECGs are diagnostic (10). Echocardiography should be considered in dyspneic patients with cardiomegaly on CXR to further assess for left ventricular heart failure.

3. Pulmonary function tests (PFTs) should be performed in a stable patient in whom lung disease is suspected as part of an evaluation for restrictive and obstructive lung disease. If the initial PFTs are normal and the suspicion still remains high that lung disease is present, a methacholine challenge test can be performed to help identify asthma in patients who have intermittent dyspnea symptoms.

4. A variety of other tests should also be considered in order to accurately identify the source of the patient's dyspnea symptoms:
   - Blood tests:
     o Elevated cardiac biomarkers indicate cardiac ischemia or infarction.
     o An elevated brain natriuretic peptide is helpful in confirming suspected ADHF.
     o A positive D-dimer is useful if the patient's pretest probability of pulmonary embolism is high.
     o A complete blood count will identify anemia as well as possible sepsis and subsequent ARDS.
   - Imaging:
     o Chest computed tomography (CT) and ventilation-perfusion (VQ) scan can be used to identify pulmonary embolism, pneumonia, malignancy, and pulmonary edema.
   - Other:
     o Negative inspiratory pressure and forced vital capacity measurements are helpful bedside tests in dyspneic patients suspected of having neuromuscular disorders such as myasthenia gravis or Guillain-Barré syndrome. Electomyogram and nerve conduction studies should be performed to confirm a diagnosis of a neuromuscular disorder.

IV. DIAGNOSIS. The underlying disease causing the patient's dyspnea can be identified 70% of the time using the clinical evaluation, CXR, and pulse oximetry (11). If the disease is not identified using these three modalities, the examiner must proceed with a systematic evaluation, focusing primarily on the pulmonary and cardiac systems.

A. 75% of dyspnea cases are caused by pulmonary disease (3). CXR and pulse oximetry should be followed by PFTs and chest CT/VQ scan if indicated by the historical and exam findings.

B. If a pulmonary etiology has been ruled out or if the history and physical are more indicative of a cardiac etiology, a cardiac workup should be initiated immediately. A CXR, pulse oximetry, ECG, and cardiac biomarkers should all be performed. Once immediate life-threatening causes have been ruled out, the examiner should proceed with echocardiogram and arrhythmia evaluation as indicated by history, physical, and study findings.

Disclaimer
The opinions and assertions contained herein are the private views of the author and are not to be construed as official or as reflecting the views of the U.S. Air Force Medical Service, the U.S. Air Force or the Department of Defense at large.

REFERENCES

1. Dyspnea. Mechanisms, assessment, and management: a consensus statement. American Thoracic Society. Am *J Respir Crit Care Med* 1999;159:321.
2. American College of Emergency Physicians. Accessed at http://www.acep.org/uploadedFiles/ACEP/newsroom/NewsMediaResources/StatisticsData/2009%20NHAMCS_ED_Factsheet_ED.pdf on July 17, 2012.
3. Pratter MR, Curley FJ, Dubois J, Irwin RS. Cause and evaluation of chronic dyspnea in a pulmonary disease clinic. *Arch intern Med* 1989;149:2277.
4. Martinez FJ, Stanopoulos I, Acero R, et al. Graded comprehensive cardiopulmonary exercise testing in the evaluation of dyspnea unexplained by routing evaluation. *Chest* 1994;105:168.
5. Ray P, Birolleau S, Lefort Y, et al. Acute respiratory failure in the elderly: etiology, emergency diagnosis, and prognosis. *Crit Care* 2006;10:R82.
6. Cook DG, Shaper AG. Breathlessness, lung function and the risk of heart attack. *Eur Heart J* 1988;9:1215.
7. O'Donnell DE, Bertley JC, Chau LK, Webb KA. Qualitative aspects of exertional breathlessness in chronic airflow limitation: pathophysiologic mechanisms. *Am J Respir Crit Care Med* 1997;155:109.
8. Simon PM, Schwartzstein RM, Weiss JW, et al. Distinguishable types of dyspnea in patients with shortness of breath. *Am Rev Respir Dis* 1990;142:1009.
9. Mahler DA, Harver A, Lentine T, et al. Descriptors of breathlessness in cardiorespiratory diseases. *Am J Respir Crit Care Med* 1996;154:1357.
10. UpToDate: Accessed at http://www.uptodate.com/contents/evaluation-of-the-adult-with-dyspnea-in-the-emergency-department on July 17, 2012.
11. Mulrow CD, Lucey CR, Farnett LE. Discriminating causes of dyspnea through clinical examination. *J Gen Intern Med* 1993;8:383–392.

Stridor
Dillon J. Savard

I. **BACKGROUND.** Stridor is a harsh, noisy breath sound produced by turbulent air flow created by partial airway obstruction. Though most commonly found in early childhood, stridor may present at any age (1, 2).

II. **PATHOPHYSIOLOGY.** Stridor is usually inspiratory, indicating an obstruction at or above the larynx. Biphasic stridor can occur with obstruction at or below the larynx in the upper trachea and suggests a fixed obstruction. Expiratory stridor suggests obstruction in the distal trachea or mainstem bronchi. The vocal cords are likely involved when hoarseness or aphonia is present (1, 2).

III. **EVALUATION.** Stabilize the patient first. Some patients with stridor are in respiratory distress and require immediate emergency intervention.
   A. History
      1. To rapidly narrow the differential diagnosis (Table 8.8.1), first identify whether or not the patient is febrile and if the stridor is acute (new), persistent, or recurrent. Also ask about recent upper respiratory infection (URI) symptoms and positioning or activities that relieve or exacerbate the symptoms. Further inquire about feeding difficulties, failure

TABLE 8.8.1	Common Causes of Stridor

Congenital[a]	Inflammatory
Laryngomalacia[b]	Laryngotracheobronchitis (croup)
Laryngeal cysts and webs	Epiglottitis, bacterial tracheitis
Laryngeal hemangiomas	Retropharyngeal abscess
Tumors	Allergic edema
Subglottic stenosis[c]	Diphtheria, tetanus
Vocal cord paralysis[c]	
Micrognathia	**Noninflammatory**
Vascular ring	Foreign body
Ectopic thyroid	Gastroesophageal reflux disease
Cri du chat	Hysterical stridor
Macroglossia	Trauma

[a]More common in children younger than 6 months of age.

[b]Also found in older children or adults with neuromuscular disorders.

[c]Commonly congenital but may be iatrogenic.

to thrive, choking or gagging, voice changes, immunocompromised state, history of intubations, neck or thoracic surgery, neuromuscular disorder, prematurity, or congenital syndromes. Congenital causes of stridor commonly present prior to 6 months of age. A child older than 6 months of age with stridor lasting hours to days usually has viral croup or foreign body aspiration, although if the child is toxic appearing, consider epiglottitis or an abscess. Any history of smoking or alcohol abuse should raise suspicion for cancer in adults (2–4).

   a. Viral laryngotracheitis (croup) accounts for 90% of childhood cases of stridor. A typical history is a nontoxic febrile child younger than 6 years of age with a 2–3 day history of URI and barking cough with inspiratory stridor.

   b. Laryngomalacia is the most common cause of stridor in infants. It presents with intermittent inspiratory stridor worse when supine and feeding difficulties within the first 2 weeks of life and usually resolves spontaneously in about 9 months. Gastroesophageal reflux and neuromuscular disorders frequently accompany laryngomalacia (2, 4, 5).

   c. Epiglottitis and bacterial tracheitis are life-threatening infections that are typically associated with high fevers, rapid progression, drooling, voice changes, and marked odynophagia in a toxic-appearing patient (4, 5).

   d. An afebrile history of acute choking or gagging suggests aspiration or ingestion of a foreign body.

B. Physical Examination

   1. Focused physical examination

   a. Include temperature, respiratory rate, heart rate, work of breathing and emphasize general appearance. Also examine the neck, palate, tonsils, jaw, tongue size, lungs, ears, and nose (fog on a mirror assesses patency).

   b. Signs of respiratory distress may be present, including dyspnea, tachypnea, chest retractions, or nasal flaring. Degree of retractions may be a better indicator of severity than the stridor, as stridor can become quieter as the obstruction gets worse. Cyanosis is an ominous sign.

2. Additional physical examination
   a. A toxic-appearing child with high fever, drooling, severe respiratory distress, and a preference for sitting and leaning forward with head in a "sniffing" position suggests epiglottitis or pharyngeal abscess.
   b. Look for features of known syndromes, which may suggest particular sources of airway obstruction. Examples: micrognathia (Pierre Robin), macroglossia (Beckwith-Wiedemann), or cutaneous hemangiomas (subglottic hemangiomas) (4, 5).

C. Testing
1. If epiglottitis or bacterial tracheitis is strongly suspected, or if the patient is unstable, then further testing is not indicated prior to starting treatment. When further testing is needed, endoscopy is the gold standard, but x-ray images may provide limited diagnostic information. Chest or head/neck x-rays may show a foreign body or signs of one, such as relative oligemia, mediastinal shift, or air trapping. Croup can be diagnosed on clinical grounds, though a "steeple sign" may be present on posterior–anterior x-ray imaging of the neck. Abscess is suggested by the presence of a retropharyngeal or retrotracheal space (3, 4, 6, 7).
2. Computed tomography and magnetic resonance imaging of the neck may help in the search for causes of persistent chronic stridor, though they are insensitive for identifying airway stenosis. Vocal cord ultrasound is used when vocal cord paralysis is suspected (4).
3. Respiratory virus antibody panels or direct fluorescence antibody testing can be done. A complete blood count can be useful in the acutely ill patient (bacterial infection being more likely to have leukocytosis with neutrophil predominance). Arterial blood gas measurement will reveal acid–base status. Carbon dioxide levels may be high in partial airway obstruction despite reassuring pulse oximetry in a patient being given supplemental oxygen (3, 4).

IV. DIAGNOSIS.
In making the diagnosis of stridor, three basic patterns exist: acute febrile, acute nonfebrile, and chronic.

A. Acute Stridor
1. Laryngotracheobronchitis (croup) accounts for 90% of cases of stridor in children. Generally, this diagnosis is made on clinical grounds (acute onset in a mildly febrile child). It is due to a viral infection; most commonly parainfluenza virus but could be respiratory syncytial virus, rhinovirus, adenovirus, or influenza virus. The entire illness usually abates in 5 days. Hospitalization, unlike with epiglottitis, is rarely needed (3, 5).
2. Laryngomalacia can be confidently suspected in the right clinical setting (chronic, afebrile, less than 6 months old) and confirmed by endoscopy.
3. Epiglottitis is a medical emergency. A patient with epiglottitis classically appears as a toxic young child with fever, respiratory distress, sore throat, or drooling. *Haemophilus influenzae* was the most common cause of stridor (and epiglottitis) prior to the Hib vaccine. Now streptococcus, staphylococcus, and viral agents are more likely causes. A muffled voice suggests retropharyngeal abscess.
4. Foreign body aspiration can present acutely with symptoms similar to epiglottitis, but without fever. Foreign body aspiration is common in 1- to 2-year-old children, although it does occur in adults and can even be a cause of chronic stridor (3).
5. Acute allergic reaction can also cause stridor. The history should herald a possible offending noninfectious agent, and although respiratory collapse may be eminent, the patient is afebrile.
6. Trauma causing acute stridor is readily identified by history.

B. Chronic stridor.
Causes of chronic stridor typically occur in early childhood. Laryngeal papillomas, tumors, and subglottic stenosis are typically congenital, whereas foreign body aspiration and hysterical stridor can occur at any age. Laryngomalacia and laryngeal lesions are caused by webs, hemangiomas, and cysts; they are usually identified early in life (5).

Disclaimer

REFERENCES

1. Marx JA, Hockberger RS, Walls RM, eds. *Rosen's emergency medicine,* 7th ed. Philadelphia, PA: Mosby, 2009:2104–2105.
2. Rakel RE, Rakel DP, eds. *Textbook of family medicine,* 8th ed. Philadelphia, PA: WB Saunders, 2011:334–336.
3. Long SS, Pickering LK, Prober CG, eds. *Principles and practice of pediatric infectious diseases revised reprint,* 3rd ed. Philadelphia, PA: Churchill Livingstone, 2009:172–177.
4. Flint PW, Haughey BH, Lund VJ, et al., eds. *Cummings otolaryngology—head and neck surgery,* 5th ed. Philadelphia, PA: Mosby, 2010:2866–2868, 2896–2901.
5. Kliegman RM, Stanton BF, St. Geme III JW, Schor NF, Behrman RE, eds. *Nelson textbook of pediatrics,* 19th ed. Philadelphia, PA: WB Saunders, 2011:283, 314, 1450–1451, 1445–1446, 1445. e3–1445.e4.
6. Barratt GE, Koopmann CF Jr, Coulthard SW. Retropharyngeal abscess—a ten-year experience. *Laryngoscope* 1984;94:455.
7. Stankiewicz JA, Bowes AK. Croup and epiglottitis: a radiologic study. *Laryngoscope* 1985;95:1159.

8.9 Wheezing

Katrina N. Wherry

I. BACKGROUND. Wheezing is one of the most common respiratory complaints to present to primary care physicians. Up to 25% of children under the age of 5 years present to their primary care manager with a wheezing illness (1).

II. PATHOPHYSIOLOGY AND ETIOLOGY. Expiratory wheezing is the sound heard on auscultation when air is rapidly passed through smaller, narrowed airways. Younger children and infants have smaller airways than adults and thus have more frequent wheezing symptoms (2).

A. Wheezing in Infants. The most common cause for wheezing in this age group is infectious lower respiratory tract illnesses, e.g., respiratory syncytial virus and coronavirus. Edema in the smaller airways caused by the infection results in airway constriction, which can then lead to small airway collapse and air trapping. If this process leads to wheezing in a child less than 2 years, it is called bronchiolitis (1). Another common cause of wheezing in infants is asthma. Many infants with recurrent wheezing and lower respiratory tract illnesses are very likely to have asthma, even without evidence of ectopic disease and despite their young age (3). Some common risk factors for asthma are second-hand smoke exposure, male sex, and unclean living conditions. A third common cause (but often unrecognized) of recurrent wheezing in infants is inhalation/aspiration of food and liquids, which is usually associated with gastroesophageal reflux disease (GERD). A classic related symptom is coughing while feeding; however, this may extinguish as the cough reflex is diminished from repeated larynx stimulation by foreign substances (1). Some of the more uncommon and rare causes of wheezing in infants are listed in Table 8.9.1.

B. Wheezing in Children. The most common cause of recurrent wheezing in children is asthma, and the prevalence is highly linked to elevated serum immunoglobulin E (IgE) levels. As with infants, children with asthma have decreased lung function compared with those without asthma, and second-hand smoke exposure increases the risk of developing a wheeze (3). Likewise, another common cause of recurrent wheeze is repeated aspiration of foods and liquids associated with GERD. An isolated, sudden episode of localized wheezing in children may be due to foreign body inhalation. More common than aspiration, a swallowed foreign body, if stuck in the esophagus, may cause a wheeze by compression of the trachea (1). Single episodes of wheezing in children can also be caused by infections, with viruses being the most common pathogens (e.g., respiratory syncytial and parainfluenza viruses) (Table 8.9.1).

TABLE 8.9.1	Uncommon and Rare Causes of Wheezing by Age Group (1, 5)
Infants and Children	**Adults**
Infectious pertussis and tuberculosis	Pulmonary embolism
Bronchopulmonary dysplasia	Benign and malignant tumors causing obstruction
Cystic fibrosis	Eosinophilic pulmonary infiltration
Congestive heart failure	Vocal cord dysfunction
Congenital vascular anomalies	
Mediastinal masses	
Bronchiolitis obliterans	
Immune deficiency	
Tracheobronchial anomalies	

C. **Wheezing in Adults.** Asthma is one of the most common causes of wheezing in adults, with a prevalence of 10–12% in developed countries (4). While the majority of adults with asthma are diagnosed in early childhood, asthma can develop in adulthood without a history of recurrent wheeze in childhood (4). The prevalence of asthma in adults is also highly linked to elevated serum IgE levels (1). Chronic obstructive pulmonary disease (COPD) is another cause of recurrent wheezing in adults who typically have a significant smoking history. These patients will usually have other symptoms associated with wheezing, such as cough, exertional dyspnea, and sputum production (4). Episodic wheezing in adults can also be secondary to congestive heart failure (CHF) and pulmonary embolism (5). See Table 8.9.1 for more diagnoses.

III. **EVALUATION.** Given that asthma is a common cause of wheezing in all age groups, the initial evaluation of a wheezing patient should aim to exclude other diagnoses that can cause wheezing (1).
A. **Clinical History**
   a. **Onset.** If within the first few weeks of life, consider a congenital cause of wheezing. If it started suddenly, foreign body aspiration may be more likely (1, 2).
   b. **Timing and Pattern.** If the wheezing is episodic and recurrent, asthma may be more likely. If the wheezing occurs during a certain time of the year, then infectious causes or asthma that is triggered by certain environmental allergens may be more likely (1, 2).
   c. **Associated Symptoms.** If there are cough and sputum production, fever, and upper respiratory symptoms, then consider infectious causes and COPD. In an infant and child, cough during feeding may be associated with aspiration and reflux. If there is poor weight gain in the child or infant, then consider GERD and cystic fibrosis (CF) (2, 6).
   d. **Family and Social History.** If there is a family history of the atopic triad, asthma, eczema, and environmental allergies, then asthma may be more likely. If the patient has a significant smoking history, or a parent smokes, consider asthma and COPD. Although most patients with CF do not have a family history of the disease, recurrent infections causing wheezing may be secondary to CF (6).
B. **Physical Examination.** Inspect the newborn for persistent cyanosis, as this can be associated with congenital anomalies. Inspect the adult and child for clubbing in the setting of recurrent wheezing episodes, as this can be associated with CF. Palpate the chest of the infant and child for a localized vibration consistent with wheezing in the setting of foreign body aspiration. Dullness to percussion can be consistent with consolidation caused by significant infection. Wheezes can be heard on auscultation, and their location should be noted

as localized wheezes are more consistent with foreign body aspiration. Other breath sounds should also be noted: crackles can be present in infection or CHF, and stridor can be heard in viral infections that also affect the upper airways (6).

   C. Testing. The decision to order a test will depend on the differential diagnosis being considered after a careful history and physical is performed. For suspected asthma or COPD, spirometry should be performed. Generally, patients older than 5 years will be able to follow the necessary steps to perform spirometry. Infants may be tested by their response to treatment with an inhaled beta agonist (1, 5). Chest x-ray findings may support infectious causes of wheezing or rare causes such as masses or congenital malformations. A swallow study may help identify patients with frequent aspiration or GERD, swallowed foreign objects, or anatomic abnormalities. Bronchoscopy should be considered if other testing does not help narrow the differential diagnosis (6). If CF is considered, genetic and sweat chloride testing should be performed. When pertussis or tuberculosis is considered, testing for antibodies to pertussis and purified protein derivative skin testing should be performed (1).

IV. DIAGNOSIS. The differential diagnosis will be created after a careful history is taken and will be supported by physical exam findings and testing. One of the most common causes of wheezing in all age groups is asthma, and an effort should be made to exclude the other causes of wheezing especially in infants, where many other conditions (some rare) can produce similar symptoms to asthma (1).

Disclaimer

The opinions and assertions contained herein are the private views of the author and are not to be construed as official or as reflecting the views of the U.S. Air Force Medical Service, the U.S. Air Force or the Department of Defense at large.

REFERENCES

1. Martinati LC, Boner AL. Clinical diagnosis of wheezing in childhood. *Allergy* 1995;50:701–710.
2. Weiss LN. The diagnosis of wheezing in children. *Am Fam Physician* 2008;77(8):1109–1114.
3. Martinez FD, Wright AL, Taussig LM, et al.; Group Health Medical Associates. Asthma and wheezing in the first six years of life. *N Engl J Med* 1995;332:133–138.
4. Fauci AS, Braunwald E, Kasper DK, et al., eds. *Harrison's principles of internal medicine*, 17th ed. New York, NY: McGraw Hill Medical, 2008. Accessed at http://accessmedicine.com/resourceTOC.aspx?resourceID=4 on May 1, 2012.
5. Summary report 2007 National Asthma Education and Prevention Program expert panel report 3: Guidelines for the diagnosis and management of asthma. Accessed at http://www.nhlbi.nih.gov/guidelines/asthma/asthsumm.pdf on May 1, 2012.
6. Finder JD. Understanding airway disease in infants. *Curr Probl Pediatr* 1999;29:65–81.

CHAPTER 9

Gastrointestinal Problems

Richard Fruehling

9.1 Abdominal Pain

Zachary W. Meyer and Richard Fruehling

I. **BACKGROUND.** Abdominal pain is a common complaint and comprises up to 10% of total visits to the emergency department. The etiology may be quite varied resulting from extra-abdominal pathology or intra-abdominal sources. Physical findings are variable and sometimes misleading, where life-threatening conditions may evolve from seemingly benign presentations.

II. **PATHOPHYSIOLOGY.** The common reasons for intra-abdominal pain that causes concern are presented in Table 9.1.1 (1). Selected causes of severe intra-abdominal pain are listed in Table 9.1.2. Causes of extra-abdominal pain are listed in Box 9.1.

TABLE 9.1.1	Common Causes of Abdominal Pain	
Diagnosis	**Etiology**	**Epidemiology**
Gastric, esophageal, or duodenal inflammation	Gastric hypersecretion, breakdown of mucoprotective barriers, infection, exogenous source	All age groups. Gastroenteritis may be seasonal, with travel history and affected family
		See peptic ulcer disease
Acute appendicitis	Appendiceal lumen obstruction leads to swelling, ischemia, infection, and perforation	Adolescence to young adulthood
		Higher perforation rate in children, women, and elderly
		Mortality rate of 0.1% (2–6% with perforation)
Biliary tract disease	Passage of gallstones causes biliary colic	Peak age of 35–60 y
		Rare in patients <20 y of age
	Impaction of a stone in cystic duct or common duct causes cholecystitis or cholangitis	Female-to-male ratio of 3:1
		Risk factors: multiparity, obesity, alcohol intake, birth control pills
Ureteral colic	Family history, dehydration, urinary tract infections, gout, certain medications	Average age of 30-40 y, primarily in men, less common in children

(Continued)

TABLE 9.1.1 Common Causes of Abdominal Pain *(Continued)*

Diagnosis	Etiology	Epidemiology
Diverticulitis	Diverticular infection or inflammation or perforation	Incidence increases with advancing age; male > female
	May develop peritonitis, fistulas, or abscesses	Recurrences are common
		Called "left-sided appendicitis"
Peptic ulcer	Sometimes associated with *Helicobacter pylori* infection	Occurs in all age groups; peaks at the age of 50 y
	Risk factors include nonsteroidal anti-inflammatory drug use, tobacco and alcohol use	Men affected twice as much as women. Severe bleeding or perforation is rare

Bengiamin RN, Budhram GR, King KE, Wightman JM. Abdominal pain. In: Marx JA, ed. *Rosen's emergency medicine: concepts and clinical practice*, 7th ed. Philadelphia, PA: Mosby, 2010: 160–194.

III. EVALUATION
A. History
1. The history should include the following: **P**alliative/alleviating factors, **Q**uality of pain, **R**adiation or referred pain pattern, **S**everity, and **T**ime of onset/temporal relationships. The character of pain is particularly helpful (e.g., colicky, steady, sharp, burning, tearing, and gnawing). The associated symptoms should be identified (e.g., dysuria, hematuria, melena, hematochezia, change in bowel habits, diarrhea, vomiting). The exact sequence of symptoms may be especially helpful; for example, in acute appendicitis, generalized pain and anorexia typically precede point tenderness.
2. A thorough gynecologic history should be performed in all women with abdominal pain, and pregnancy (including ectopic pregnancy) should be considered.
3. Small bowel obstruction in patients with prior abdominal surgery should be considered. Alarming symptoms generally involve escalating symptoms, fever, profound illness, and extremes of age.

TABLE 9.1.2 Selected Life-threatening Causes of Abdominal Pain

Diagnosis	Etiology	Epidemiology
Ruptured or leaking aortic aneurysm	Exact etiology undetermined. Contributing factors: atherosclerosis, genetic predisposition, connective tissue disease, infection	More frequent in men Risk factors: hypertension, diabetes mellitus, smoking, chronic obstructive pulmonary disease, coronary artery disease (CAD)
Acute pancreatitis	Alcohol, gallstones, hypertriglyceridemia, hypercalcemia, post endoscopic retrograde cholangiopancreatography (post-ERCP)	Peak age in adulthood, rare in childhood More frequent in males
Mesenteric ischemia	Often multifactorial, including transient hypotension in the presence of atherosclerosis. Occlusion occurs in 65% of cases (75% embolic)	Most common in elderly people with cardiovascular disease, congestive heart failure (CHF), diabetes mellitus, sepsis, dehydration Mortality 70%

BOX 9.1	Important Extra-Abdominal Causes of Abdominal Pain

Thoracic: myocardial infarction/unstable angina, pneumonia, PE, pericarditis, herniated disk

Genitourinary: testicular torsion

Abdominal Wall: muscle spasm, muscle hematoma, herpes zoster

Infections: streptococcal pharyngitis (often in children), mononucleosis, Rocky Mountain spotted fever

Systemic: diabetic ketoacidosis, alcoholic ketoacidosis, uremia, sickle cell disease, porphyria, systemic lupus erythematosus, vasculitis, glaucoma, hyperthyroidism

Toxic: methanol poisoning, heavy metal toxicity, scorpion bite, snake bite, black widow spider bite

Bengiamin RN, Budhram GR, King KE, Wightman JM. Abdominal pain. In: Marx JA, ed. *Rosen's emergency medicine: concepts and clinical practice*, 7th ed. Philadelphia, PA: Mosby, 2010: 160–194.

B. Physical Examination

1. Analysis of the general appearance of the patient is especially helpful. Patients with colicky (hollow viscus obstruction) pain often writhe about, seeking a comfortable position. Peritonitis causes patients to be still and jarring the bed or heel tap may exacerbate the pain. Check complete vital signs for evidence of sepsis/shock; identify fever, tachycardia, or hypotension.
2. Inspect the abdomen for distension, pulsations, or ecchymosis (Grey Turner's or Cullen's sign).
3. Auscultate for the presence of bowel sounds or bruits suggestive of aneurysms. Bowel sounds are sometimes absent in appendicitis.
4. Palpation begins distal to areas of pain and should be gentle. Guarding and rigidity should be noted. Masses and organomegaly should be assessed. Murphy's sign may help identify gallbladder pathology. The iliopsoas and obturator signs may indicate appendicitis. Genital examination is important to exclude hernia and a rectal examination may help identify a retrocecal appendicitis.

C. Testing

1. **Laboratory Evaluation.** It is necessary to obtain a serum human chorionic gonadotropin from any patient who could potentially be pregnant. Electrolytes can rule out metabolic abnormalities such as hypercalcemia. A complete blood count should be considered in infectious etiologies and for the purpose of monitoring hematocrit stability and platelet count. Elevated liver tests can identify hepatocellular or obstructive biliary disease. Elevated amylase may be found in pancreatitis, salivary disease, mesenteric ischemia, and fallopian pathology. Lipase is very specific to the pancreas. Urinalysis is useful to exclude urinary tract infections. Hematuria is found in 90% of renal stones. Pyuria can be present when an inflammatory mass (e.g., appendicitis) is close to the urinary tract (2).
2. **Imaging.** Plain film acute abdominal series (upright and supine) identify free air and abnormal gas patterns. Plain films may identify calcifications associated with renal stones (85%), biliary lithiasis (15%), and pneumonia as an extra-abdominal cause for pain. Ultrasound is useful to rule out ectopic pregnancy, appendicitis, biliary tract disease, abdominal aortic aneurysm, and hydroureter. Computed tomography (CT) scan has largely replaced other modalities, because it provides a quick accurate imaging modality to detect appendicitis, urolithiasis, cholecystitis, diverticulitis, and pancreatitis. In elderly patients with abdominal pain, CT scan alters the initial diagnosis in 45% of cases and affects admission decisions in 26% of cases (3).

IV. DIAGNOSIS

A. **Differential Diagnosis.** This is usually broad and needs frequent reconsideration. If a treatment modality is unsuccessful, the working diagnosis must be questioned and the

TABLE 9.1.3	Types of Abdominal Pain
Visceral pain	Results from stretching unmyelinated nerve fibers surrounding an organ; may be "crampy, dull, or achy," can be either steady or intermittent. This type of pain is often ill-defined and diffuse. Examples include appendicitis, cholecystitis, bowel obstruction, and renal colic. Foregut structures often refer to the epigastrium (stomach, duodenum, pancreatic-biliary tree), and midgut structures (small bowel, ascending colon) refer to periumbilical area. Hindgut structures (descending colon) often refer to the suprapubic area or the back
Somatic pain	Arises from pain fibers in parietal peritoneum; usually sharper, localized, and more constant; may develop after visceral pain. Usually, it represents peritoneal inflammation from various sources (bleeding, chemical irritation, infectious causes) and most often causes great concern. Patients prefer immobility
Referred pain	Defined as pain felt at a distance from the diseased organ. Diaphragmatic irritation often radiates to shoulders, and ureteral colic often radiates to groin. Referred pain is often localized to the developmental dermatome and can be misleading in localizing the source. However, it is usually perceived on the same side as the involved organ (4)

differential expanded. Serial examination and close follow-up are needed if the diagnosis is in question.

B. Clinical Manifestations. Patterns associated with the different types of abdominal pain are presented in Table 9.1.3. Multiple causes necessitate a broad differential diagnosis. Numerous diagnostic modalities exist, including physical examination, laboratory studies, and ancillary studies.

REFERENCES

1. Bengiamin RN, Budhram GR, King KE, Wightman JM. Abdominal pain. In: Marx JA, ed. *Rosen's emergency medicine: concepts and clinical practice,* 7th ed. Philadelphia, PA: Mosby, 2010:159–169.
2. Kamin RA, Nowicki TA, Courtney DS, et al. Pearls and pitfalls in the emergency department evaluation of abdominal pain. *Emerg Med Clin North Am* 2003;21:61–72.
3. Esses D, Birnbaum A, Bijur P, et al. Ability of CT to alter decision making in elderly patients with acute abdominal pain. *Am J Emerg Med* 2004;22:270–272.
4. O'Brien MC. Chapter 74. Acute abdominal pain. In: Tintinalli JE, ed. *Tintinalli's emergency medicine,* 7th ed. New York, NY: McGraw-Hill, 2011.

9.2 Ascites
Manoj Kumar and Milton (Pete) Johnson

I. BACKGROUND. Ascites involves an accumulation of fluid in the peritoneal cavity. It is known as the most common major complication of cirrhosis. About 50% of patients with compensated cirrhosis develop ascites in 10 years (1). The 1- and 5-year mortality among patients with ascites due to cirrhosis is approximately 15% and 44%, respectively (2). Spontaneous bacterial peritonitis and hepatorenal syndrome are known complications of ascites, contributing to significant morbidity and mortality, with a median survival of 25 years. Patients with ascites are commonly referred for liver transplantation as the later improves the survival rate by approximately 40% in this population (3).

II. PATHOPHYSIOLOGY. The widely accepted theory for ascites formation is peripheral arterial vasodilatation hypothesis in cirrhosis patients. Portal hypertension (PH) in advanced stages of cirrhosis causes increased sinusoidal pressure, which subsequently triggers vasodilatation in splanchnic and peripheral arterial system mediated by nitric oxide. This vasodilatation activates renin–angiotensin system, sympathetic nervous system, and antidiuretic hormone to maintain fluid homeostasis (4). These factors activate salt and fluid retention and interrupt the balance among the Starling forces. Thus, the fluid with the greater pressure displaces into the tissues and then "weep" from the surface of the liver and collects in the peritoneal cavity in the form of ascites. Elevated levels of epinephrine and norepinephrine along with hypoalbuminemia also contribute to ascites formation in chronic liver disease patients. Hypoalbuminemia contributes by decreasing plasma oncotic pressure and favors the extravasation of fluid from the plasma to the peritoneal cavity. The low arterial pressure and reduced systemic vascular resistance induce renal vasoconstriction and renal hypoperfusion and thus eventually trigger renal injury. The renal system then loses its ability to clear free water and eventually develop dilutional hyponatremia and hepatorenal syndrome.

III. EVALUATION

A. History. The history should cover questions about risk factors for liver disease. History of alcoholism, transfusions, tattoos, HIV, and other risk factors for infectious hepatitis is relevant. Other pertinent past medical history could be of cancers (leukemia, lymphomas), heart failure, renal disease, and tuberculosis. In patients with no clear etiology of cirrhosis, lifetime body weight, diabetes, and hyperlipidemia should be evaluated to include nonalcoholic steatohepatitis in the differential diagnosis.

B. Physical Examination. Patients with full and distended abdomen should have their flanks examined by percussion method. If flank dullness is significantly appreciated then, shifting dullness should be tested. The presence of shifting dullness has sensitivity and specificity of greater than 80% and 50%, respectively, in the diagnosis of ascites, and its presence usually indicates at least 1500 cc of fluid in the peritoneal cavity (5). In obese patients with liver disease, distinguishing ascites from obesity by physical examination can frequently be a challenge and abdominal ultrasound may be required. Signs of PH and liver failure include collateral veins over the abdominal wall, jaundice, palmar erythema, spider angiomas, etc.

C. Testing. Once ascites is confirmed, diagnostic abdominal paracentesis should be done in all patients. Bleeding is sufficiently uncommon and thus administration of fresh frozen plasma or platelets is not recommended (6). Besides new-onset ascites, other indications for abdominal paracentesis include ascites with fever, abdominal pain, tenderness, hypotension, ileus, acidosis, azotemia, hypothermia, or encephalopathy and tense ascites. Cell count, differential count, ascitic fluid total protein, and serum–ascites albumin gradient should be checked as routine tests on ascitic fluid. If infection of the fluid is suspected, bedside culture in blood culture bottles should be performed and then empiric antibiotic coverage should be initiated and continued until infection is ruled out by routine laboratory investigation of the fluid. Total serum CA125 is not helpful in the differential diagnosis of ascites of any type (6). pH, lactate, cholesterol, fibronectin, and glycosaminoglycans testing is not helpful (7). The significance and interpretation of the laboratory findings from the ascitic fluid are described in Tables 9.2.1 and 9.2.2.

IV. DIAGNOSIS.

A. Differential Diagnosis. The differential diagnosis of ascites is listed in Table 9.2.3. Some rare causes of ascites include trauma to lymphatics or ureters, chlamydia, coccidioides, gonococcus induced, nephrotic syndrome, serositis, hypothyroidism, acquired immunodeficiency syndrome, Fitz-Hugh-Curtis syndrome, and peritoneal mesothelioma.

B. Clinical manifestation. The general symptoms include nausea, anorexia, heart burn, dyspnea, abdominal distension, orthopnea, weight gain, and pedal edema. Patients can also present with signs of spontaneous bacterial peritonitis and hepatic

TABLE 9.2.1	Paracentesis Fluid Findings and Their Significance	

Characteristic	Specific findings	Significance
Appearance	Clear	Cirrhosis
	Turbid/cloudy	Infection
	Opalescent	Elevated triglyceride concentration
	Milky	Traumatic tap, malignancy
	Pink/bloody	Patient with jaundice, ruptured gallbladder,
	Brown	duodenal ulcer
Cell count and differential	Polymorphonuclear leukocytes count >250	Spontaneous bacterial peritonitis
Serum to ascites albumin gradient (serum albumin–ascites albumin) (g/dL)	>1.1	**Portal hypertension**: cirrhosis, alcoholic hepatitis, compression from large liver metastases, portal vein thrombosis, Budd-Chiari syndrome, cardiac ascites, acute fatty liver of pregnancy, myxedema, mixed ascites
	<1.1	**No portal hypertension**: peritoneal carcinomatosis (most common), tuberculosis, pancreatic or biliary ascites, bowel infarction or obstruction, nephritic syndrome

encephalopathy. Those with esophageal varices may present with signs of variceal hemorrhage. Hepatosplenomegaly, umbilical hernia, and scrotal edema are frequently seen as well. Masses or lymphadenopathy suggest underlying malignancy. Distended neck veins, cardiomegaly, S3 on auscultation support cardiac cause of ascites. Nephrotic syndrome can present in the form of anasarca.

TABLE 9.2.2	Clinical Association of Paracentesis Fluid Results

Characteristic	Association
Amylase	Elevated in small bowel or pancreatic injury
LDH	In uncomplicated ascites, LDH is fewer than half the serum values. Peritonitis > SBP > serum LDH
Glucose concentration	Mildly depressed in carcinomatosis and SBP. In bowel perforation or late SBP, the glucose level may be as low as 0
Cytology	This is of benefit when carcinomatosis is present. This test requires the release of malignant cells into the ascitic fluid, sensitivity 67% of all malignancy-related cases
Renal panel	Assess for hepatorenal syndrome

LDH, lactate dehydrogenase; SBP, spontaneous bacterial peritonitis.

(Continued)

TABLE 9.2.3	Differential Diagnosis of Ascites *(Continued)*
Cause	**Comment**
Cirrhosis	Etiology in ~80% of ascites (3)
Alcoholic hepatitis	
Carcinomatosis	Two-thirds of malignancy-related ascites
Metastases	One-third of malignancy-related ascites
Congestive heart failure	History of heart failure or severe lung disease
Tuberculosis	Cause in ~1% of ascites (3)
Hepatitis B and C	Leads to cirrhosis
Pancreatic disease	Ascites amylase is five times the serum values
Wilson's disease	Effects range from liver test abnormalities to hepatic failure
Hemochromatosis	Iron deposition causes cirrhosis
Constrictive pericarditis	Leads to hepatic congestion
Mixed ascites	~5% (cirrhosis + another etiology)

REFERENCES

1. Gines P, Quintero E, Arroyo V, et al. Compensated cirrhosis: natural history and prognostic factors. *Hepatology* 1987;7:12–18.
2. Planas R, Montoliu S, Balleste B, et al. Natural history of patients hospitalized for management of cirrhotic ascites. *Clin Gastroenterol Hepatol* 2006;4:1385–1394.
3. Gines P, Cardenas A, Arroyo V, et al. Current concepts: management of cirrhosis and ascites. *N Engl J Med* 2004;350:1646–1654.
4. Schrier RW, Arroyo V, et al. Peripheral arterial vasodilation hypothesis: a proposal for the initiation of renal sodium and water retention in cirrhosis. *Hepatology* 1988;8:1151–1157.
5. Cattau EL Jr, Benjamin SB, Knuff TE, Castell DO. The accuracy of the physical exam in the diagnosis of suspected ascites. *JAMA* 1982;247:1164–1166.
6. Runyon BA, AASLD Practice Guidelines Committee. Management of adult patients with ascites due to cirrhosis: an update. *Hepatology* 2009;49(6):2087.
7. Haubrich WS, Schaffner F, Brek J, et al. *Bockus gastroenterology,* 5th ed. Philadelphia, PA: WB Saunders, 1994:2009.

9.3 Constipation
Timothy McAuliff and Richard Fruehling

I. **BACKGROUND.** Constipation is a common gastrointestinal complaint among the general population. The definition varies from patient to patient, being described as stools that are too hard, too small, too difficult, or too infrequent (1). To clarify and offer an objective diagnosis for the clinician, an international panel in 2006 developed a consensus definition called The Rome-III criteria (2) (see Table 9.3.1).

II. **PATHOPHYSIOLOGY.** The colon and rectum are responsible for both digestive and excretive functions, including continued mixing of the output of the ileum, further processing of undigested carbohydrate (including digestion and absorption), absorption of water to create

TABLE 9.3.1	**Rome-III Criteria for the Diagnosis of Functional Constipation**

Adults

- Two or more of the following symptoms are present for at least 3 months, with onset at least 6 months prior to diagnosis.

  o Straining during at least 25% of defecations.

  o Lumpy or hard stools in at least 25% of defecations.

  o Sensation of incomplete evacuation for at least 25% of defecations.

  o Sensation of blockage or obstruction in anus or rectum for at least 25% of defecations.

  o Use of manual maneuvers (e.g., digital expression of stool, pelvic floor support) to facilitate at least 25% of defecations.

  o Fewer than three defecations per week

- Loose stools are rarely present without the use of laxatives.

- Symptoms do not meet the criteria for irritable bowel syndrome

Infants and young children

- Two or more weeks of one of the following symptoms:

  o Hard stools (pebblelike = scybalous) in most bowel movements

  o LESS THAN three FIRM stools per week

- Symptoms not explained by a metabolic, endocrine, or anatomic cause

Adapted with permission from Longstreth GF, Thompson WG, Chey WD, et al. Functional Bowel Disorders. *Gastroenterology* 2006;130:1480–1491.

semisolid or solid stool, and ultimately evacuation of stool from the body. These processes are coordinated through a variety of neurotransmitters, a parasympathetic neural plexus, and a variety of other voluntary and involuntary mechanisms.

A. Etiology. Changes in the texture of the stool, the peristaltic function or internal diameter of the colon, or the expulsive function of the rectum and pelvic floor can lead to constipation (3, 4). Risk factors are numerous and more common causes include a low-fiber diet, inactivity, and medications (5) (see Table 9.3.2).

B. Epidemiology. Prevalence rates range between 2% and 28% and it is a more common complaint among women and the elderly (6).

TABLE 9.3.2	**Causes of Constipation (Rated by the Likelihood of Being a Cause of Constipation)**	
Functional (common)	**Medications (less common)**	
Low-fiber diet	Antacids	Clonidine
Sedentary lifestyle	Anticholinergics	Diuretics
Dehydration	Antidepressants	Sinemet
Slow transit time	Calcium channel blockers	Narcotics
Outlet delay	Cholestyramine	Sympathomimetics

(Continued)

TABLE 9.3.2 | Causes of Constipation (Rated by the Likelihood of Being a Cause of Constipation) *(Continued)*

Functional (common)	Medications (less common)	
Irritable bowel syndrome	Nonsteroidal anti-inflammatory drugs	Psychotropics
Inflammatory bowel disease		
Excessive milk intake		
Stool withholding		
Structural (less common)	**Neurogenic (rare)**	**Endocrine/metabolic (rare)**
Anal fissures	Cerebrovascular events	Diabetes mellitus
Hemorrhoids	Multiple sclerosis	Hypercalcemia
Colonic strictures	Parkinson's disease	Hyperparathyroidism
Diverticulitis	Hirschsprung's disease	Hypokalemia
Ischemia	Spinal cord tumors or abnormalities	Hypothyroidism
Radiation colitis	Cerebral palsy	Uremia
Adenocarcinoma	Chagas disease	Celiac disease
Imperforate anus	Botulism	Cystic fibrosis
Pelvic masses	Down syndrome	Pregnancy
	Prune belly syndrome	
Psychogenic (less common)	**Connective tissue (rare)**	
Anxiety	Amyloidosis	
Depression	Scleroderma	
Somatization	Systemic lupus erythematosus	

III. EVALUATION (see Figure 9.3.1)

A. **History and Physical Examination.** Initially, the patient should be screened for alarming features that require more extensive testwork (hematochezia, >10 lb weight loss, obstipation, family history of colon cancer). If these are absent, then evaluate via history and physical (including rectal exam with hemoccult) to distinguish idiopathic constipation from secondary causes. (Table 9.3.3 presents findings in the history and physical examination that aid in distinguishing idiopathic or functional causes from secondary causes.) If a secondary cause is found, treat the underlying cause. If no cause is found on initial clinic visit, treat the patient empirically with a trail of fiber, increased physical activity, and constipation medications. If the patient fails conservative management, then further diagnostic testing is warranted (7).

Note: Obstipation (lack of flatus) may be indicative of a bowel obstruction, which requires immediate surgical evaluation.

B. **Testing.** Laboratory tests include serum chemistries (including calcium and glucose), complete blood count (for anemia), and thyroid function tests. Abdominal x-ray may show fecal retention. Colon transit time may be measured using a "pill camera" or radiopaque marker study. Anorectal or colonic manometry may provide information about colonic tone and motility (8). Colonoscopy is indicated when any of the following are present: anemia, rectal bleeding, hemoccult positive stools, obstructive symptoms, new onset of constipation, unintended weight loss, a change in stool caliber, or if the patient is older than 50 years and is due for colon cancer screening (9).

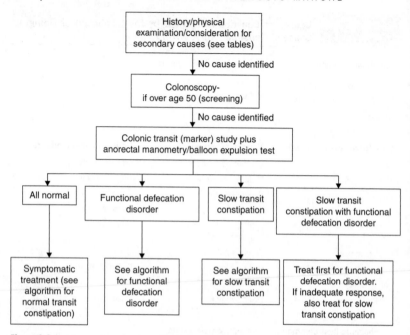

Figure 9.3.1. Diagnostic approach to chronic constipation unresponsive to conservative therapy.

Courtesy of Arnold Wald, MD. 2012 UpToDate "Etiology and evaluation of chronic constipation in adults"

TABLE 9.3.3	History and Physical Examination Findings	
Component	**Finding**	**Condition suggested**
	History	
Age at onset	Childhood onset	Congenital causes
Duration	Acute onset	Correctable causes
	Longer duration	Functional cause
The most troubling symptom	Straining	Pelvic floor dysfunction
	Need for manual maneuvers for evacuation	
	Cramping/bloating between bowel movements	Irritable bowel syndrome
Medication history		See the list of common offenders in Table 9.3.2
	Physical examination	
Digital rectal examination	Tender puborectalis	Puborectalis spasm
	Inability to expel rectal finger	Pelvic floor dysfunction

(Continued)

TABLE 9.3.3 History and Physical Examination Findings *(Continued)*

Component	Finding	Condition suggested
	Rectal mass, anal stricture	Obstruction
	Anal fissure	Cause or effect?
	Impacted stool	Slow transit constipation
Simulated defecation	Laxity of anal verge	Neurogenic causes
Perineal function during simulated expulsion and retention	Low activity	Pelvic floor dysfunction
Vaginal examination (women)	Observe for rectocele	Pelvic relaxation
Neurologic examination	Other focal neurologic deficits	Neurogenic causes
Abdominal examination	Masses, scars	Causes of obstruction

IV. DIAGNOSIS

A. Differential Diagnosis. A differential diagnosis of functional constipation is presented in Table 9.3.2.

REFERENCES

1. Stewart WF, Liberman JN, Sandler RS, et al. Epidemiology of constipation (EPOC) study in the United States: relation of clinical subtypes to sociodemographic features. *Am J Gastroenterol* 1999;94:3530.
2. Longstreth GF, Thompson WG, Chey WD, et al. Functional bowel disorders. *Gastroenterology* 2006;130:1480–1491.
3. Arce DA, Ermocilla CA, Costa H. Evaluation of constipation. *Am Fam Physician* 2002;65:2283–2290.
4. Faigel DO. A clinical approach to constipation. *Clin Cornerstone* 2002;4(4):11–21.
5. Leung FW. Etiologic factors of chronic constipation: review of the scientific evidence. *Dig Dis Sci* 2007;52(2):313–316.
6. Satish-Rao SC. Constipation: evaluation and treatment. *Gastroenterol Clin North Am* 2003;32:659–683.
7. Barnett JL, Hasler WL, Camilleri M. American Gastroenterological Association medical position statement on anorectal testing techniques. American Gastroenterological Association. *Gastroenterology* 1999;116:732.
8. Rao SS, Singh S. Clinical utility of colonic and anorectal manometry in chronic constipation. *J Clin Gastroenterol* 2010;44:597.
9. Qureshi W, Adler DG, Davila RE, et al. ASGE guideline: guideline on the use of endoscopy in the management of constipation. *Gastrointest Endosc* 2005;62:199.

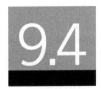

9.4 Diarrhea
Safana Anna Makhdoom and Robert C. Messbarger

I. BACKGROUND. Clinically, the most useful definition of diarrhea is the most vague and patient-centric, that is, frequent, loose stools. Diarrhea can also be defined as daily stools cumulatively weighing over 200 g in teenagers and adults and weighing over 10 g/kg/d for infants and young children (1, 2). Another way to characterize diarrhea is as a definite increase in frequency and decrease in consistency of stools, relative to said individual's baseline. The last definition is more clinically useful in children.

These stools are often watery, excessive, and can be uncontrolled. Diarrhea can be associated with fever, abdominal cramping, painful defecation, mucousy stools, and/or bloody stools. Additionally, the duration of diarrhea is of significant clinical importance. Acute diarrhea is of less than 14 days duration, while diarrhea beyond 30 days' duration is termed chronic; persistent diarrhea is diarrhea lasting beyond 14 days (3).

In selected clinical settings (e.g., impoverished or immunocompromised patients), this ailment can be life threatening.

II. PATHOPHYSIOLOGY
A. Etiology

1. Acute diarrhea can be infectious or noninfectious. By and large, most acute diarrhea in the developed world and developing world is infectious. The pathogenic organisms can be bacteria, protozoa, and/or viruses. Noninfectious causes include food allergies, drugs, and/or adverse drug effects, and other disease states including inflammatory bowel disease, thyrotoxicosis, and carcinoid syndrome.

   For pediatric patients, acute diarrhea is also commonly due to infectious gastroenteritis. However, other etiologies in the pediatric population include other infections (e.g., acute otitis media, urinary tract infection); life-threatening conditions (e.g., intussusception; toxic megacolon, appendicitis; hemolytic uremic syndrome); overfeeding; starvation stools; antibiotic associated diarrhea (AAD). More rare etiologies can include endocrinologic pathologies, anatomic abnormalities, and genetic disorders (e.g., congenital adrenal hyperplasia; blind loop syndrome; cystic fibrosis).

   Large-volume stools result from a small bowel pathology, while smaller volume, bloody, and painful stools may be more likely to derive from distal, colonic pathology.

2. Chronic diarrhea is categorized as one of four types: fatty, inflammatory, secretory, or osmotic.

   a. Fatty diarrhea contains excess stool fat, shown either by direct measurement or Sudan staining.

   b. Inflammatory diarrhea may contain mucous, blood, and/or fecal leukocytes in the stool.

   c. Secretory diarrhea is watery and has a low osmotic gap of <50 mOsm/kg (normal: 290 mOsm/kg).

   d. Osmotic diarrhea is also watery but has an osmotic gap of over 125 mOsm/kg.

B. Epidemiology

1. The epidemiology of diarrhea in the United States has not been well studied, in contrast to the developing countries. It is well established that acute diarrhea is the leading cause of childhood death worldwide. In the US population, viruses are likely the most common cause, with bacterial infection producing most of the severe cases. However, most studies show that less than 10% of stool cultures will show a bacterial agent. In the United States, acute diarrhea rarely requires a significant diagnostic evaluation and usually no more than symptomatic oral rehydration* and reassurance.

2. Chronic diarrhea is a worldwide childhood problem, with infection being the most common cause. In adults in developed countries, chronic diarrhea is most frequently because of irritable bowel syndrome, inflammatory bowel disease, and malabsorption syndromes. In developed countries, the common causes of chronic diarrhea in children include malabsorption or maldigestion (2). Two common causes are chronic nonspecific diarrhea and celiac disease.

III. EVALUATION.
Most patients with acute diarrhea experience a mild, self-limited illness and no laboratory testing is necessary. The challenge of the initial evaluation is to distinguish these patients from the more serious disorders. "Red flags" associated with severe illness include hypovolemia; bloody diarrhea; fever; more than five unformed stools in 24 hours;

severe abdominal pain; antibiotic use or hospitalization; or diarrhea in an infant, geriatric, or immunocompromised patient (4).

Chronic diarrhea with the above "red flags" or with weight loss, systemic symptoms (fevers, anorexia), abdominal masses, or other signs pointing to a malignancy should be worked up beyond a physical exam.

Pediatric patients with acute diarrhea, if afebrile or febrile, and nonbloody stools usually have viral enteritis, which do not usually require extensive lab workup. The afebrile or febrile child with bloody diarrhea is most worrisome because of the possibility of bacterial enteritis (usually febrile), HUS, intussusception or pseudomembranous colitis (the latter three listed are usually afebrile), all of which warrant further evaluation.

Persistent or chronic diarrhea in the pediatric patient can warrant further evaluation. Severe abdominal pain, dehydration, abdominal masses all may warrant further evaluation.

A. History. Evaluation of acute diarrhea begins with a history of the onset, duration, pattern (time of day; relation to dietary intake; urgency) and characteristics (bloody; malodorous; floating; greasy) of the stools. Patients should be questioned regarding occupation (e.g., exposure to raw meat at work), travel (e.g., Mexico; mountains in the United States), sexual practices (risk of human immunodeficiency virus and possible immunocompromise), pets, and hobbies that could signal exposure to potential pathogens. Other key points include inquiries regarding fevers, medication use (e.g., metformin), a dietary history, and a complete past medical history (to determine risk of nosocomial infection or immunocompromised status).

A concern of chronic diarrhea should thoroughly explore the onset, duration, pattern, and characteristics of the stools. Major findings include significant weight loss, diarrhea for longer than 1 year, nocturnal diarrhea, and straining with stool. Other questions should focus on social and epidemiologic history (travel, foods, sexual practices, living conditions, water sources), family history (e.g., inflammatory bowel disease), associated symptoms (e.g., fever, fecal incontinence, abdominal pain, mouth ulcers, joint pains), and aggravating or palliative factors (diet, stress, medication). A detailed medical history evaluates for iatrogenic causes (e.g., medication; total parenteral nutrition in past; bowel resection; cholecystectomy; or other surgeries), immunocompromised state, and possible psychiatric pathology (e.g., laxative abuse; anorexia nervosa). A thorough review of systems provides evidence of systemic processes that can cause diarrhea such as diabetes mellitus, hyperthyroidism, rheumatologic disease, and tumors.

In pediatric patients, in addition to the above questions, inquire about formula use, recent feeding changes, appearance of stools, appearance of infant ("well" vs. "toxic"), recent medications or hospitalizations, attendance at daycare, and exposure to sick contacts.

B. Physical Examination. Examination should focus on signs of hypovolemia (e.g., dry mucous membranes, orthostatic hypotension). Observation of fever or peritoneal signs can indicate an invasive source (Shigella, Campylobacter) (3, 5). Abdominal signs (masses, ascites, liver changes), anorectal signs (loss of tone, fissures, fistulas), lymphadenopathy, mouth ulcers, rashes, and thyroid changes can provide diagnostic clues (6).

In pediatric patients, abdominal masses can indicate intussusception. Toxic-appearing infants or children may be suffering from toxic megacolon, pseudomembranous colitis, or intussusception. In children having purpuric rashes, consider HUS as a diagnosis. Peritoneal signs may signal an appendiceal pathology.

C. Testing. See Figures 9.4.1 and 9.4. 2 for evaluation of acute and chronic diarrhea.

Threshold for imaging (e.g., ultrasound [U/S] or contrast enema for intussusception; U/S or computed tomography for appendiceal pathology) for a pediatric patient with bloody or febrile diarrhea should be lower, especially in a difficult to console child.

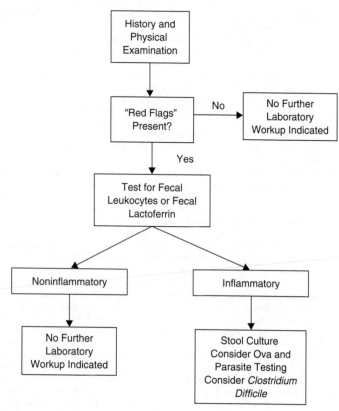

Figure 9.4.1. Laboratory evaluation of acute diarrhea. (Adapted from Thielman NM, Guerrant RL. Clinical practice. Acute infectious diarrhea. *N Engl JMed* 2004;350:38.)

IV. DIAGNOSIS

A. Differential Diagnosis. See Table 9.4.1 for a differential diagnosis of diarrhea.

B. Clinical Manifestations

1. Acute diarrhea features a few well-described patterns. Traveler's diarrhea commonly begins 3–10 days after arrival in a foreign location where the patient is exposed to food or water contaminated with enterotoxigenic *E. coli*, Salmonella, or Campylobacter, among other bacteria. Diarrhea that develops within 6 hours of food ingestion is commonly because of a preformed bacterial toxin (*Staphylococcus aureus*). Symptoms that begin after more than 8 hours suggest either a bacterial (*Clostridium perfringens* at 8–16 hours) or viral infection (3). Febrile diarrhea is suggestive of invasive bacteria, enteric viruses, or a cytotoxic organism. If diarrhea occurs in the setting of a recent course of antibiotic therapy or recent hospitalization, *Clostridium difficile* toxin should be considered. *C. difficile* is being seen in those without recent hospitalizations or recent antibiotic use and the threshold for testing for stool *C. difficile* toxin should also be lower.

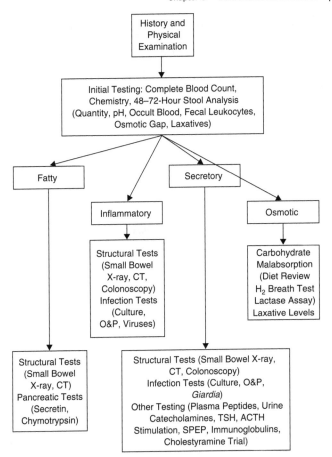

Figure 9.4.2. Laboratory evaluation of chronic diarrhea. ACTH, adrenocorticotropic hormone; CT, computed tomography; O&P, ova and parasites; SPEP, serum protein electrophoresis; TSH, thyroid-stimulating hormone. (Adapted from Fine KD, Schiller LR. AGA technical review on the evaluation and management of chronic diarrhea. *Gastroenterology* 1999;116:1464.)

2. Chronic diarrhea has a myriad possible underlying etiologies. However, crampy abdominal pain with bowel habits varying between diarrhea and constipation is common in irritable bowel syndrome. Diarrhea with abdominal pain, weight loss, and fever is a hallmark of inflammatory bowel disease. Finally, malabsorption classically presents with weight loss and voluminous, fatty, malodorous stools. Flatulence is seen more commonly with carbohydrate malabsorption, while pancreatic exocrine insufficiency can present with pale stools.

*Note: Oral rehydration therapy solution can be made at home with 0.25 teaspoons each of sodium chloride and sodium bicarbonate mixed in 1 L of water. To this, add 4 tablespoons of table sugar (3).

TABLE 9.4.1 Differential Diagnosis of Acute and Chronic Diarrhea

Acute diarrhea

Infectious

Bacteria (*Salmonella, Campylobacter, Shigella, Escherichia coli*)

Virus (rotavirus, norovirus)

Protozoa (*Cryptosporidium, Giardia, Entamoeba histolytica*)

Noninfectious

Food intolerance

Medications

Inflammatory bowel disease

Carcinoid

Thyroid disease

Chronic diarrhea

Fatty

Intestinal malabsorption

Maldigestion

Inflammatory

Inflammatory bowel disease

Infection

Ischemia

Neoplasia

Secretory

Medications

Motility disorder

Neoplasia

Inflammatory bowel disease

Toxin

Osmotic

Carbohydrate malabsorption

Ingestion of magnesium, sulfates, or phosphates

REFERENCES

1. Feldman M, Friedman L, Brandt L (eds.) (2010). *Sleisenger and Fordtran's gastrointestinal and liver disease: pathophysiology/diagnosis/management*, 9th ed. Chapter 15: Diarrhea. Accessed online at MDConsult.com.
2. Kellermayer R, Shulman RJ. *Approach to the causes of chronic diarrhea in children.* Accessed at UpToDate.com (http://www.uptodate.com/contents/overview-of-the-causes-of-chronic-diarrhea-in-children?source=see_link) on May 5, 2012.
3. Wanke CA (2011). Approach to the adult with acute diarrhea in developed countries. Retrieved from UpToDate.com
4. Thielman NM, Guerrant RL. Clinical practice. Acute infectious diarrhea. N Engl J Med 2004;350:38.
5. DuPont HL. Guidelines on acute infectious diarrhea in adults. The practice parameters committee of the American college of gastroenterology. Am J Gastroenterol 1997;92:1962.
6. Schiller LR. Chronic diarrhea. Gastroenterology 2004;127:287.

9.5 Dysphagia

Susan M. Newman and Richard Fruehling

I. BACKGROUND. Dysphagia is defined as difficulty in swallowing. This is a common complaint in primary care practices, especially in aging persons. Up to 10% of adults older than 60 years, 25% of hospitalized patients, and 30–40% of nursing home patients experience swallowing problems; 7% of Americans will experience dysphagia in their lifetime.

II. PATHOPHYSIOLOGY. Organic swallowing problems occur at two primary sites: in the oropharynx at the initiation of the swallow reflex or in the esophagus with propulsion of food. Dysfunctional transfer of the food past the upper esophageal sphincter into the esophagus causes oropharyngeal dysphagia symptoms, and disordered peristalsis or conditions that obstruct the flow of a food bolus through the esophagus cause esophageal dysphagia symptoms. Mechanical obstruction or neuromuscular motility disorders occur in both the oropharynx and the esophagus. Common causes of oropharyngeal and esophageal dysphagia are listed in Table 9.5.1 (1).

TABLE 9.5.1	Differential Diagnosis of Dysphagia

Oropharyngeal dysphagia

Neuromuscular disease (diseases of the central nervous system)

   Cerebrovascular accident

   Parkinson's disease

   Brain stem tumors

   Degenerative diseases

   Amyotrophic lateral sclerosis

   Multiple sclerosis

   Huntington's disease

   Postinfectious

   Poliomyelitis

   Syphilis

   Peripheral nervous system

   Peripheral neuropathy

   Motor end-plate dysfunction

   Myasthenia gravis

   Skeletal muscle disease (myopathies)

   Polymyositis

   Dermatomyositis

   Muscular dystrophy (myotonic dystrophy, oculopharyngeal dystrophy)

   Cricopharyngeal (upper esophageal sphincter), achalasia

Obstructive lesions

Tumors

Inflammatory masses

(Continued)

TABLE 9.5.1	Differential Diagnosis of Dysphagia *(Continued)*

Trauma/surgical resection
Zenker's diverticulum
Esophageal webs
Extrinsic structural lesions
Anterior mediastinal masses
Cervical spondylosis

Esophageal dysphagia

Neuromuscular disorders

Achalasia

Spastic motor disorders

   Diffuse esophageal spasm

   Hypertensive lower esophageal sphincter

   Nutcracker esophagus

Scleroderma

Obstructive lesions

Intrinsic structural lesions

   Tumors

   Strictures

   Peptic

   Radiation-induced

   Chemical-induced

   Medication-induced

   Lower esophageal rings (Schatzki's ring)

   Esophageal webs

   Foreign bodies

Extrinsic structural lesions

   Vascular compression

   Enlarged aorta or left atrium

   Aberrant vessels

   Mediastinal masses

   Lymphadenopathy

   Substernal thyroid

From Castell DO. Approach to the patient with dysphagia. In: Yamada T, ed. *Textbook of gastroenterology*, 2nd ed. Philadelphia, PA: Lippincott Williams & Wilkins, 1995.

III. EVALUATION. Choosing the best study depends on many factors including age, acuity of onset, comorbidities, and availability of testing modalities in the community.

    A. History. A careful history identifies 80–85% of causes by differentiating whether the dysphagia is oropharyngeal or esophageal in location and whether it is obstructive or neuromuscular in nature. The onset, severity, and duration of dysphagia combined with questions about associated symptoms can help narrow the differential diagnosis (see Table 9.5.2) (3). Alcohol and tobacco consumption histories provide important information. It is also

TABLE 9.5.2	Associated Symptoms and Possible Causes of Dysphagia

Condition	Diagnoses to consider
Progressive dysphagia	Neuromuscular dysphagia
Sudden dysphagia	Obstructive dysphagia, esophagitis
Difficulty in initiating swallow	Oropharyngeal dysphagia
Food "sticks" after swallow	Esophageal dysphagia
Cough	
Early in swallow	Neuromuscular dysphagia
Late in swallow	Obstructive dysphagia
Weight loss	
In the elderly	Carcinoma
With regurgitation	Achalasia
Progressive symptoms	
Heartburn	Peptic stricture, scleroderma
Intermittent symptoms	Rings and webs, diffuse esophageal spasm, nutcracker esophagus
Pain with dysphagia	Esophagitis
	Postradiation
	Infectious: herpes simplex virus, monilia
	Pill induced
Pain made worse by	
Solid food only	Obstructive dysphagia
Solids and liquids	Neuromuscular dysphagia
Regurgitation of old food	Zenker's diverticulum
Weakness and dysphagia	Cerebrovascular accidents, muscular dystrophies, myasthenia gravis, multiple sclerosis
Halitosis	Zenker's diverticulum
Dysphagia relieved with repeated swallows	Achalasia
Dysphagia made worse with cold foods	Neuromuscular motility disorders

From Johnson A. Deglutition. In: Scott-Brown WG, Kerr AG, eds. *Scott-Brown's otolaryngology*, 6th ed. Boston, MA: Butterworth-Heinemann, 1997.

important to obtain a thorough past medical history to evaluate for gastroesophageal reflux disease, cancer or radiation, immunocompromised states, and other medical problems associated with dysphagia such as scleroderma. Medications can cause direct esophageal injury, dysmotility, decreased lower esophageal sphincter tone with reflux, or xerostomia with subsequent dysphagia (see Table 9.5.3) (4).

  B. Physical Examination. Examination should focus on the head, eyes, ears, nose, and throat (HEENT), neck, and neurologic systems. A pulmonary exam is also important to evaluate for aspiration, a possible complication of dysphagia. However, physical exam typically provides limited information unless the patient has experienced an obvious cerebrovascular accident. Gag reflexes are also of little use because this is absent in up to 13% of nondysphagic patients.

  C. Testing. Few screening laboratory tests are indicated in the evaluation of dysphagia unless history or clinical examination findings dictate otherwise. Imaging studies are often required for

TABLE 9.5.3	Medications Associated with Dysphagia

Medications that can cause direct esophageal mucosal injury

Doxycycline (Vibramycin)

Tetracycline

Clindamycin (Cleocin)

Trimethoprim–sulfamethoxazole (Bactrim, Septra)

Nonsteroidal anti-inflammatory drugs

Alendronate (Fosamax)

Zidovudine (Retrovir)

Ascorbic acid

Potassium chloride tablets (Slow-K)[a]

Theophylline

Quinidine gluconate

Ferrous sulfate

Medications, hormones, and foods associated with reduced lower esophageal sphincter tone and reflux

Butylscopolamine

Theophylline

Nitrates

Calcium antagonists

Alcohol, fat, chocolate

Medications associated with xerostomia

Anticholinergics: atropine, scopolamine (Transderm Scop)

α-Adrenergic blockers

Angiotensin-converting enzyme inhibitors

Angiotensin II receptor blockers

Antiarrhythmics

Disopyramide (Norpace)

Mexiletine (Mexitil)

Ipratropium bromide (Atrovent)

Antihistamines

Diuretics

Opiates

Antipsychotics

[a]Especially the slow-release formulation.

From Boyce HW. Drug-induced esophageal damage: diseases of medical progress. [Editorial] *Gastrointest Endosc* 1998;47:547–550; Stoschus B, Allescher HD. Drug-induced dysphagia. *Dysphagia* 1993;8:154–159.

definitive diagnosis. According to the American College of Radiologist Appropriateness Criteria for dysphagia, an X-ray biphasic esophagram is usually appropriate for evaluation of unexplained oropharyngeal or substernal dysphagia. Videoradiography is also commonly done. In addition, manometry and endoscopy (nasopharyngeal laryngoscopy or upper gastrointestinal endoscopy) should be considered depending on various clinical factors, but is generally not advisable prior to barium studies. Endoscopy is more sensitive (92% vs. 54%) and more specific (100% vs. 91%) than double-contrast upper gastrointestinal radiography and also generally allows for biopsy of lesions or therapeutic maneuvers such as dilation, but is also more expensive and invasive.

IV. DIAGNOSIS

A. **Differential Diagnosis.** The diagnosis of dysphagia centers on the answers to two questions: is the dysphagia oropharyngeal or esophageal in location? Is it neuromuscular or obstructive in nature (Table 9.5.1)? Patients with oropharyngeal dysphagia present with difficulty in initiating swallowing and have associated coughing, choking, or nasal regurgitation. Speech quality may have a nasal tone. Oropharyngeal dysphagia is associated with stroke, Parkinson's disease, or other long-term neuromuscular disorders. Local structural lesions are less common. Esophageal dysphagia often causes the sensation of food sticking in the throat or chest. Motility disorders and mechanical obstructions are common. Several medications have been associated with direct esophageal mucosal injury, whereas others can decrease lower esophageal sphincter pressures and cause reflux (Table 9.5.3) (4, 5).

B. **Clinical Manifestations.** Patients with neuromuscular dysphagia experience gradually progressive difficulty in swallowing solid food and liquids. Cold foods often aggravate the problem. Patients may succeed in passing the food bolus by repeated swallowing, by performing the Valsalva maneuver, or by making a positional change. They are more likely to experience pain when swallowing than patients with simple obstruction. Achalasia, scleroderma, and diffuse esophageal spasm are the most common causes of neuromuscular motility disorders. Obstructive pathology is typically associated with dysphagia of solid food but not liquids. Patients may be able to force food through the esophagus by performing a Valsalva maneuver, or they may regurgitate undigested food. Rapidly progressing dysphagia of a few months' duration suggests esophageal carcinoma. Weight loss is more predictive of a mechanical obstructive lesion. Peptic stricture, carcinoma, and Schatzki's ring are the predominant obstructive lesions.

REFERENCES

1. ACR Appropriateness Criteria® dysphagia. 1998 (revised 2010). NGC:007921.
2. Castell DO. Approach to the patient with dysphagia. In: Yamada T, ed. *Textbook of gastroenterology*, 2nd ed. Philadelphia, PA: Lippincott Williams & Wilkins, 1995.
3. Johnson A. Deglutition. In: Scott-Brown WG, Kerr AG, eds. *Scott-Brown's otolaryngology*, 6th ed. Boston, MA: Butterworth-Heinemann, 1997.
4. Koch WM. Swallowing disorder. Diagnosis and therapy. *Med Clin North Am* 1993;77:571.
5. Boyce HW. Drug-induced esophageal damage: diseases of medical progress [Editorial]. *Gastrointest Endosc* 1998;47:547–550.
6. Stoschus B, Allescher HD. Drug-induced dysphagia. *Dysphagia* 1993;8:154–159.

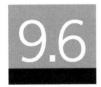

9.6 Epigastric Distress

Daniela Cardozo and Milton (Pete) Johnson

I. **BACKGROUND.** Epigastric discomfort was a term initially used to describe an alteration in the digestion of food; however, it can be caused by a wide array of conditions occurring in multiple organs across the gastrointestinal, cardiovascular, and pulmonary systems. Serious causes, such as gastric, esophageal, bowel, and pancreatic cancers, are rare but must also be considered. Common reported symptoms are bloating and early satiety; nevertheless, overlapping symptoms make initial diagnosis difficult, and in many patients a definite cause is not established. Pulmonary, cardiac, and vascular causes of epigastric discomfort are previewed in other chapters.

II. PATHOPHYSIOLOGY

A. Etiology. Up to 25% of the cases of epigastric discomfort are caused by peptic ulcer disease; the most common cause encountered by primary care physicians is idiopathic, referred also as functional dyspepsia. Gastroesophageal reflux disease (GERD) should be suspected when regurgitation and heartburn are primary complains. Esophagitis can be related to GERD but also can be caused by hypersecretory conditions. Esophagitis and gastritis can also be primarily inflammatory conditions, related to medications such as nonsteroidal anti-inflammatory drugs and toxins such as alcohol. Most peptic ulcer diseases are related to *Helicobacter pylori* infection. Gallstones, formed by supersaturation of bile, cause pain by obstructing the cystic duct. Obstruction of the cystic duct by gallstones can cause cholecystitis, an acute inflammatory condition.

B. Epidemiology. Epigastric discomfort and dyspepsia occur in 25% of the population each year, but most affected persons do not seek medical care. Patients at increased risk for gallstones include the elderly, the obese (especially those who try a rapid weight loss), the pregnant, and those on medications such as fibrates, estrogens, and contraceptives. Also at increased risk for gallstones are certain ethnicities, those with maternal family history, the female gender, and those with metabolic diseases such as diabetes, cirrhosis, and hypertriglyceridemia.

III. EVALUATION.
Typical history, physical examination, and laboratory findings associated with common causes of epigastric distress are listed in Table 9.6.1.

A. Genetics. Most causes of epigastric discomfort result from environmental factors, but some, such as cholelithiasis, exhibit hereditary components. Colonic and esophageal malignancies arise in certain inherited disorders. Hereditary pancreatitis is caused by a mutation in the cationic trypsinogen gene.

TABLE 9.6.1	Typical Historical, Physical Examination, and Laboratory Findings for Gastrointestinal Etiologies of Epigastric Discomfort		
	History	**Physical examination**	**Laboratory tests**
GERD	Heartburn, regurgitation, sour belches, pain radiating to throat, pain worsened by lying supine, chronic cough, hoarseness, beneficial trial of treatment with proton pump inhibitors	Dental erosions, examination often normal	Usually normal
PUD	Personal or family history of PUD, smoking history, nonsteroidal anti-inflammatory drug use, pain reduced by the intake of meals	Hypotension or tachycardia (GI bleeding), melena	Positive *Helicobacter pylori* antibody testing, positive urea breath test, stool *H. pylori* testing, heme-positive stools
GI malignancy	Dysphagia, weight loss, continuous pain, anorexia, protracted vomiting, age >50 y, smoking or alcohol history, family history	Weight loss, palpable mass, Virchow's nodes, hypotension or tachycardia (GI bleeding), melena, acanthosis nigricans, brittle nails, cheilosis, conjunctival pallor	Anemia, heme-positive stools
Pancreatitis	Abrupt-onset pain, stabbing, severe, and radiating to back; history of alcohol use	Diffuse, severe pain	Elevated amylase, lipase

(Continued)

TABLE 9.6.1	Typical Historical, Physical Examination, and Laboratory Findings for Gastrointestinal Etiologies of Epigastric Discomfort *(Continued)*

	History	Physical examination	Laboratory tests
Cholelithiasis	Rapid-onset pain, increasing in intensity, <3 h duration, radiation to scapula or right shoulder, sweating, vomiting, pain brought on by meals, more common at night, genetic component	No palpable mass	Usually normal
Cholecystitis	>3 h duration of pain, shifts from epigastrium to right upper quadrant, acholic stools, dark urine	Palpable mass (30–40%), fever, jaundice (15%), positive Murphy's sign	Leukocytosis (with left shift), elevated sedimentation rate, elevated bilirubin, elevated aminotransferases, elevated alkaline phosphatase, elevated amylase
Irritable bowel	Constipation and/or diarrhea, pain relieved by defecation	Normal	Normal

GERD, gastroesophageal reflux disease; GI, gastrointestinal; PUD, peptic ulcer disease.

From Bazaldua OV, Schneider FD. Evaluation and management of dyspepsia. *Am Fam Physician* 1999;60:1773–1788; Dyspepsia and GERD Practice Guideline. Institute for Clinical Systems Improvement (ICSI); 2004 Jul; Marshall BJ. Gastritis and peptic ulcer disease. In: Rakel RE, ed. *Conn's current therapy*, 57th ed. Elsevier, 2005:600–603; Ahmad M, et al. Differential diagnosis of gallstone induced complications. *South Med J* 2000;93:261–264.

IV. DIAGNOSIS
A. Clinical Approach.
1. The patient's history, a thorough physical exam along with limited laboratory workup, helps initially to put into evidence the most common causes of epigastric discomfort. Complete blood count and a comprehensive metabolic panel can be ordered depending on the clinical presentation. These provide information regarding the presence of alarm signs and might mandate further invasive testing. Recommendations made by American Gastroenterological Association (AGA) suggest the test and treatment approach that consists in a simple trial of treatment with a double-dosed proton pump inhibitor, such as omeprazole in young patients less than 55 years of age without alarm symptoms for 4–8 weeks along with *H. pylori* testing with stool antigen or 13c urea breath test and treating accordingly if positive. If symptoms remit, further workup may not be necessary. If symptoms do not remit, then an upper endoscopy is warranted. Patients 55 years or older and the presence of alarm symptoms irrespective of age should prompt the clinician to proceed with more invasive diagnostic workup, specifically upper gastrointestinal endoscopy.
2. The biliary colic of gallstones consists of epigastric or right upper quadrant pain of rapid onset that increases in intensity over a 15-minute interval and lasts as long as 3 hours, usually without any palpable mass. Pain may radiate to the interscapular region or to the right shoulder. Associated sweating and vomiting are common. Attacks of biliary colic are often brought on by eating, which stimulate contraction of gallbladder, especially a fatty meal. Fever, tachycardia and a positive Murphy's sign are usually absent.

TABLE 9.6.2	Medications Associated with Epigastric Discomfort

Acarbose

Bisphosphonates

Iron supplements

Nonsteroidal anti-inflammatory drugs

Oral antibiotics

Potassium supplements

Systemic corticosteroids

Acute cholecystitis causes epigastric or right upper quadrant tenderness or mass and fever. The pain typically lasts longer than 3 hours and, over time, shifts from the epigastrium to the right upper quadrant. In the elderly, localized tenderness may be the only presenting sign. The gallbladder is palpable 30–40% of the time, and jaundice is seen in about 15% of patients with acute cholecystitis. Leukocytosis and left shift in complete blood count are usually present in cholecystitis. Elevation of serum alkaline phosphatase and total bilirubin is not a prominent feature of cholecystitis. If present, it could potentially represent more serious condition such as cholangitis, choledocolithiasis or Mirizzi syndrome. Physical examination often cannot provide information about the source of inflammation and pain, and that is the reason why it is mandatory to obtain an ultrasound immediately when the aforementioned laboratory results are present (2).

3. Malignancies that cause epigastric discomfort are rare. Symptoms of gastric and esophageal cancers are similar to those of other causes of epigastric distress. Alarm symptoms such as progressive dysphagia, unexplained iron deficiency anemia, unintended weight loss, history of gastrointestinal bleeding, odynophagia, lymphadenopathy, jaundice, persistent emesis, or hematemesis can differentiate patients with a more serious disease. Numerous medications induce nonulcer dyspepsia (see Table 9.6.2). Costly diagnostic studies can be avoided by identifying medication-associated dyspepsia.

4. Irritable bowel syndrome is generally associated with chronic complex abdominal pain and with abnormal bowel habits. There is significant overlap with functional dyspepsia.

5. It must be mentioned that the pain of ischemic heart disease may originate in the epigastrium and must be ruled out. Metabolic disorders are a rare cause of epigastric discomfort, but a complete differential should include malabsorption syndromes, collagen vascular disorders, Zollinger-Edison syndrome, and Crohn's disease.

B. Differential Diagnosis. The differential diagnosis of gastrointestinal causes of epigastric discomfort is presented in Table 9.6.3.

TABLE 9.6.3	Differential Diagnosis of Gastrointestinal Causes of Epigastric Discomfort

Esophagus

Esophagitis

Gastroesophageal reflux disease

Medications

Lung

Pneumonia

Pulmonary embolism

Pneumothorax

(Continued)

TABLE 9.6.3	Differential Diagnosis of Gastrointestinal Causes of Epigastric Discomfort *(Continued)*

Pancreas

Pancreatitis

Heart

Cardiac ischemia

Pericarditis

Stomach

Gastritis

Peptic ulcer disease

Bleeding

Gastroparesis

Medications

Gallbladder

Cholelithiasis

Cholecystitis

Bowel

Irritable bowel syndrome

Bleeding

REFERENCES

1. Bazaldua OV, Schneider FD. Evaluation and management of dyspepsia. *Am Fam Physician* 1999; 60:1773–1788.
2. Ahmed A, Cheung RC, Keeffe EB. Management of gallstones and their complications. *Am Fam Physician* 2000; 61:1673–1680, 1687–1688.
3. Singer AJ, McCracken G, Henry MC, et al. Correlation among clinical, laboratory, and hepatobiliary scanning findings in patients with suspected acute cholecystitis. Ann Emerg Med 1996; 28:267.
4. Thompson W, Longstreth, Drossman D. Functional bowel disorders and functional abdominal pain. Gut 1999; 45 Suppl 2: 1143
5. Klauser AG, Schindlbeck NE, Müller-Lissner SA. Symptoms in gastro-oesophageal reflux disease. Lancet 1990; 335:205.

Upper Gastrointestinal Bleeding

9.7

Lindsey M. Mosel and Milton (Pete) Johnson

I. BACKGROUND. Upper gastrointestinal (GI) bleeding, defined as bleeding proximal to the ligament of Treitz, is responsible for 400,000 hospital admissions in the United States, with a mortality rate of 13%. It is seen twice as commonly in men than in women, and the prevelance is noted to increase with age (1). Bleeding can be either acute or chronic, and the source can be overt or occult. The patient may be either hemodynamically stable or unstable on presentation.

TABLE 9.7.1	Common Causes of Gastrointestinal Bleeding and Diagnostic Clues

Cause	Diagnostic clue
Peptic ulcer (55%)	Nonsteroidal anti-inflammatory drug use, *Helicobacter pylori* infection, stress
Esophagogastric varices (14%)	Ethanol use, umbilical or rectal varices, palmar erythema, ascites, spider hemangiomas
Arteriovenous malformations (6%)	History of previous episodes
Mallory-Weiss tears (5%)	Vomiting prior to hematemesis, ethanol use, occurs in young men
Tumors (4%)	Ethanol use, smoking, smoked foods, gastroesophageal reflux disease, Barrett's esophagus, weight loss

From Jutabha RJ, Jensen DM. Approach to the patient with upper gastrointestinal bleeding. UpToDate June 2005.

II. PATHOPHYSIOLOGY. Bleeding from the upper GI tract usually results when disruption occurs between the protective barriers to the vasculature and the harsh environment of the digestive tract. The most common causes (as percentages) are listed in Table 9.7.1.

III. EVALUATION. The key to successful evaluation and diagnosis is a systematic approach with emphasis on the overall hemodynamic status of the patient (see Figure 9.7.1).

    A. History. Clinical history accurately points to the source of bleeding in only 40% of cases (3). Hematemesis and melena are the most common presentations of acute upper GI bleeding. Other historical features include abdominal pain, coffee-ground emesis, dysphagia, black tarry stools, bright red blood per rectum, hematemesis, or chest pain. It is important to ask about a prior history of bleeding as 60% rebleed from the same site (3). History of other comorbid diseases (peptic ulcer disease, pancreatitis, cirrhosis, and cancer) may point to an etiology as well as a review of medication use (i.e., clopidogrel, coumadin, nonsteroidal anti-inflammatory drugs, aspirin, SSRIs, or corticosteroids) (1). A history of alcohol or drug use is also improtant to elucidate. Particular attention must be given to the patient's cardiopulmonary status because this affects urgency and degree of resuscitative efforts. Table 9.7.1 lists other diagnostic clues to common causes, and Table 9.7.2 lists the less common causes.

    B. Physical Examination

        1. Vital Signs. The single most important aspect of the initial physical examination is determining the patient's hemodynamic stability. Unstable patients should be managed as trauma patients. A nasogastric (NG) tube is often placed at presentation to help confirm the diagnosis. After ensuring hemodynamic stability, the initial physical examination should eliminate a nasal or oropharyngeal source of bleeding.

        2. Skin Examination. Ecchymoses, petechiae, and varices should be noted. Conjunctival pallor is a sign of chronic anemia. Numerous mucosal telangiectasias can point to an underlying vascular abnormality.

        3. Abdominal Examination. Look for stigmata of chronic liver disease (hepatosplenomegaly, spider angiomata, ascites, palmar erythema, caput medusae, gynecomastia, and testicular atrophy).

        4. Rectal Examination. Rectal varices, hemorrhoids, and fissures should be noted and hemeoccult testing done.

    C. Testing. Basic laboratory studies should include a complete blood count (CBC), with particular attention to the hematocrit, coagulation studies (prothrombin time [PT]) and partial thromboplastin time [PTT]), liver function tests (LFTs), serum chemistries (blood urea nitrogen is elevated disproportionate to creatinine in patients with GI blood loss),

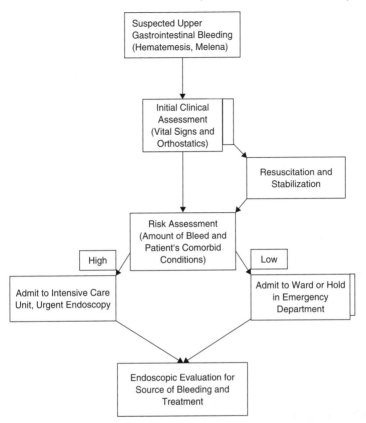

Figure 9.7.1. Approach to upper gastrointestinal bleeding. (Modified from Eisen GM, Dominitz JA, Faigel DO. An annotated algorithmic approach to upper gastrointestinal bleeding. *Gastrointest Endosc* 2001;53:853–858.) (2)

TABLE 9.7.2	Uncommon Causes of Upper Gastrointestinal Bleeding
Cause	**Diagnostic clue**
Dieulafoy's lesion	Congenital lesion usually diagnosed during endoscopy
Gastric antral vascular ectasia	Associated with cirrhosis and elderly women
Hemobilia	Usually associated with recent biliary tree injury
Aortoenteric fistulas	Primary cases associated with AAA, secondary cases with fistulas from AAA repairs; may present with back pain and fever

AAA, abdominal aortic aneurysm.

From Jutabha RJ, Jensen DM. Approach to the patient with upper gastrointestinal bleeding. UpToDate June 2005 (4).

electrocardiogram (ECG), and NG aspirate analysis. Initially, the hematocrit is a poor indicator of blood loss; however, serial hematocrits can be useful in assessing ongoing blood loss. The CBC indices, particularly an elevated red cell distribution width and low mean corpuscular volume, point toward a chronic bleed. A prolonged PT or PTT suggests an underlying coagulopathy. Elevated LFTs suggest underlying liver disease. An ECG is important, especially in elderly patients, to search for evidence of cardiac ischemia. If the aspirate is bright red, or "coffee ground" in appearance, an upper GI source of bleeding is likely. Additionally, NG lavage removes blood and helps with the performance of endoscopy. In cases in which no source can be identified, lower endoscopy should be considered in the search for a lower GI bleed.

IV. DIAGNOSIS. The differential diagnosis of an upper GI bleed should include bleeding from the upper airways or pharynx that is swallowed and regurgitated and lower GI bleeding that may be manifested as melanic stools due to delay in transit through the colon. Endoscopy is typically preformed within 24 hours (1). In most cases, diagnosis can be confirmed and the source localized and treated. In rare cases in which upper endoscopy is unable to adequately identify the source of GI bleeding, specialized nuclear medicine and angiographic studies can be used. Colonoscopy would also be considered.

REFERENCES

1. Wilkins T, Khan N, Nabh A, Schade R. Diagnosis and management of upper gastrointestinal bleeding. *Am Fam Phys* 2012;469–476.
2. Eisen GM, Dominitz JA, Faigel DO. An annotated algorithmic approach to upper gastrointestinal bleeding. *Gastrointest Endosc* 2001;53:853–858.
3. McGuirk TD, Coyle WJ. Upper gastrointestinal tract bleeding. *Emerg Med Clin North Am* 1996;14:523–545.
4. Laine L. Acute and chronic gastrointestinal bleeding. In: Feldman M, Sleisinger MH, Scharschmidt BF, eds. *Gastrointestinal and liver disease: pathophysiology, diagnosis, and management*. Philadelphia, PA: WB Saunders, 1998:198–218.

9.8 Hepatitis

Manoj Kumar and Milton (Pete) Johnson

I. BACKGROUND. Hepatitis involves inflammation of the liver resulting from infectious or non-infectious causes. Among infections, viral hepatitis accounts for 50% of acute hepatitis in the United States but bacterial, fungal, and parasitic etiology can also be responsible.

II. PATHOPHYSIOLOGY. Hepatitis involves hepatocellular injury and subsequent necrosis. Injury can be acute or chronic. Progressive damage of liver parenchyma causes fibrosis, which eventually causes cirrhosis and portal hypertension with loss of hepatic function. Once 80–90% of hepatic function is affected, liver failure ensues with a mortality of 70–95%.

A. Etiology. Multiple viruses can cause hepatitis. Hepatitis A is most common for acute hepatitis and hepatitis B (HBV) and hepatitis C mostly result in chronic infection. Hepatitis D virus can occur as coinfection or superinfection in persons with established HBV infection especially in intravenous drug users. Hepatitis E is mostly seen in endemic areas in underdeveloped nations. Clinically, it presents similar to hepatitis A. During pregnancy, hepatitis E infection can lead to fulminant hepatic failure.

1. Drug-induced liver injury (DILI) is the most common cause for liver transplantation. The exposure could be acute or chronic. Most common drug culprit is acetaminophen. Other offenders are antibiotics (augmentin is most common), medications for central nervous system, musculoskeletal, and gastrointestinal system. Antiretroviral agents (especially protease inhibitors) and lipid lowering agents are other offenders. Alcohol causes hepatitis either due to its direct long-term effect or due to its effect on the metabolism of other drugs. Few herbal and dietary supplements can also be responsible for DILI.

2. Fatty liver disease aka hepatic steatosis involves lipid droplets accumulation within hepatocytes. In alcoholics, it leads to alcoholic hepatitis and finally to alcoholic cirrhosis. Nonalcoholic fatty liver disease results from insulin resistance. It follows a spectrum of disease from hepatic steatosis to nonalcoholic steatohepatitis and eventually leads to cirrhosis and even liver failure.

3. Autoimmune hepatitis is four times more common in females. α1-antitrypsin (A1AT) deficiency disease affects the lung as well as liver. Unlike lungs, in liver, A1AT accumulates within the hepatocytes due to a failure in its export into the circulation and causes hepatitis. Hereditary hemochromatosis (HFE gene on chromosome 6) is characterized by excess iron deposition in the liver and several other organs. Hepatic iron overload can also occur due to excess iron supplement, multiple frequent transfusions, or hematopoietic disorders. Wilson's disease (ATP7B gene, on chromosome 13) involves defect of intrahepatic copper metabolism resulting in excess copper deposition in the liver and other organs. These patients have normal copper absorption from proximal bowel, but their capability of biliary copper excretion is severely decreased leading to its accumulation in the hepatocytes which causes hepatitis due to free radical injury. Deficiency of ceruloplasmin is not a cause of Wilson's disease. Ischemia in the presence of hypovolemic shock or hypoxemia can also cause hepatitis.

B. Epidemiology. In 2009, a total of 1,987 acute symptomatic cases of hepatitis A, 3,371 of hepatitis B, and 781 cases of hepatitis C were reported in the United States (1). An incidence rate of 0.6 (lowest ever) cases per 100,000 population of hepatitis A, 0.1–4.6 for hepatitis B, and 0.3 for hepatitis C was recorded (2, 3). There are approximately 800,00–1.4 million people living with chronic hepatitis B and 2.7–3.9 million with chronic hepatitis C. About 5% of all acute cases of hepatitis B and 60–85% of hepatitis C develop into chronic infection. Many cases present just with asymptomatic elevations in their liver-associated enzymes. Fatty liver disease is considered the most common cause of mild liver-associated enzyme elevation mostly seen in obese patients.

III. EVALUATION

A. History. Risk factors should be identified while obtaining the history from hepatitis patients. If acute hepatitis is suspected, the history of recent drug intake as well as risk factors for viral hepatitis should be obtained. History of alcohol is very important in any form of liver injury including hepatitis. History of travel to endemic areas, ingestion of shell fish, children in day care centers, and institutionalization are other important components especially if hepatitis A is suspected. History of sexual promiscuity, intravenous drug use, blood transfusions should be elicited if hepatitis B or C is suspected. History containing exposures to hepatotoxins and family history of A1AT deficiency, hereditary hemochromatosis, or Wilson's disease are other useful components while obtaining history (4, 5).

B. Physical Examination. Physical examination helps in identifying the severity and sometimes the cause of hepatitis. Low-grade fevers, jaundice, and signs of dehydration are some of the common features of acute hepatitis. Liver can be diffusely enlarged, firm, and tender with a smooth edge. Nodules or mass-like appearance can also be encountered. In early chronic hepatitis, the liver may or may not be tender and other constitutional signs may be masked. During advanced chronic disease, new signs may appear. Liver can be hard, nodular along with the signs of liver failure (e.g., alopecia, palmar erythema, gynecomastia, testicular atrophy, and spider angioma). Ascites can be seen in patients who have portal hypertension secondary to cirrhosis. Signs of iron overload like hyperpigmentation in hereditary hemochromatosis and Kayser-Fleischer ring encircling the iris in Wilson's disease are important findings.

C. Testing

1. While ordering the lab test, the clinician should be mindful of various causes of hepatitis. Most of the time the basic labs (serum alanine and aspartate aminotransferases, alkaline phosphatase, γ-glutamyl transpeptidase, serum albumin, bilirubin levels) provide great information about the severity and possible mechanism of the liver injury. Tables 9.8.1 and 9.8.2 show commonly used tests and their clinical significance. Specific tests (e.g., serum antigen, antibody test, iron studies, quantitative tissue copper analysis) are used to identify the type of viral hepatitis as well as other causes of hepatitis.

TABLE 9.8.1	Common Laboratory Tests for Evaluating Liver Disease	
Test	**Implication**	**Notes**
ALT and AST	Hepatocellular injury or necrosis	ALT is more specific than AST for liver injury; AST/ALT $\geq$ 2 in alcoholic liver disease. Improvement in ALT level (longer half-life) lags behind AST
Bilirubin (conjugated/ unconjugated)	Hepatobiliary disease	Conjugated hyperbilirubinemia patients have dark urine (hyperbilirubinuria) and light colored stool
GGT	Hepatobiliary disease	Increased by alcohol ingestion or medications; used to confirm hepatic origin of alkaline phosphatase
Alkaline phosphatase	Cholestatic disease	Not liver specific (also in placenta and bone); used to rule out cholestasis
Prothrombin time and albumin	Marker of hepatic synthesis function	Short-term and long-term indicators; not specific

ALT, alanine aminotransferase; AST, aspartate aminotransferase; GGT, γ-glutamyl transpeptidase.

From Goldman L, Ausiello D, eds. *Cecil textbook of medicine*, 22nd ed. Philadelphia, PA: Saunders, 2003; Green RM, Flamm S. AGA technical review on the evaluation of liver chemistry tests. *Gastroenterology* 2002;123:1367–1384. http://www2.us.elsevierhealth.com/inst/serve?action= searchDB&searchDBfor=art&artType=abs&id=agast 1231367&nav=abs&special=hilite&query= [all_fields](liver+chemistry+tests,).

TABLE 9.8.2	Diagnostic Tests for Suspected Hepatitis
Hepatitis A	Anti-HAV IgM
Hepatitis B	Hepatitis B surface antigen, antihepatitis B core IgM
Hepatitis C	Anti-HCV antibody (ELISA or RIBA), HCV RNA
Non alcoholic fatty liver disease (NAFLD)	Ultrasound of liver, liver biopsy
Alcoholic liver disease	Liver biopsy, improvement with alcohol abstinence
A1AT deficiency	Serum A1AT activity, A1AT phenotyping or genotyping, liver biopsy
Autoimmune hepatitis	First exclude other causes of hepatitis, antinuclear, antismooth muscle, liver–kidney microsomal antibodies, soluble liver antigen antibody, IgG, liver biopsy
Iron overload	Serum ferritin and transferrin saturation, HFE gene test, liver biopsy
Wilson's disease	Serum ceruloplasmin, 24-h urine copper, slit lamp examination for Kayser Fleisher rings, liver biopsy, and quantitative tissue copper analysis

A1AT, α_1-antitrypsin; ELISA, enzyme-linked immunosorbent assay; HAV, hepatitis A virus; HCV, hepatitis C virus; Ig, immunoglobulin; RIBA, recombinant immunoblot assay.

From Goldman L, Ausiello D, eds. *Cecil textbook of medicine*, 22nd ed. Philadelphia, PA: Saunders, 2003; Green RM, Flamm S. AGA technical review on the evaluation of liver chemistry tests. *Gastroenterology* 2002;123:1367–1384. http://www2.us.elsevierhealth.com/inst/serve?action= searchDB&searchDBfor=art&artType=abs&id=agast 1231367&nav=abs&special=hilite&query= [all_fields](liver+chemistry+tests,).

2. Ultrasound and computed tomography scan of biliary tract and liver is helpful in biliary tract obstruction or fatty liver disease. Genetic testing is done in hereditary hemochromatosis, Wilson's disease, or A1AT deficiency. Liver biopsy plays an important role in diagnostic confirmation as well as to evaluate the severity of the disease.

IV. DIAGNOSIS

A. **Differential Diagnosis.** Table 9.8.3 represents the differential diagnosis of hepatitis.

B. **Clinical Manifestations**

1. **Acute Hepatitis.** It may manifest as completely asymptomatic (like in hepatitis C) or with symptoms such as flu-like illness, lethargy, jaundice, fever, nausea, vomiting, anorexia, etc., as in acute hepatitis A or B. Approximately 1% cases of acute hepatitis A or B may develop into fulminant hepatic failure. Acute hepatitis C as the cause of fulminant failure remains controversial. The acute viral hepatitis follows a classic pattern of four phases, which is described in Table 9.8.4.

2. **Chronic Hepatitis.** Hepatitis with a sustained elevation in aminotransferases (>3 months) is described as chronic hepatitis. The symptoms of chronic hepatitis are either mild or may be absent. They can present with nonspecific signs of fatigue, weight loss, insomnia, and malaise. In advanced stages, patients may present with upper or lower GI bleeding due to variceal bleed. Endocrinologic abnormalities like hypogonadism, hypothyroidism (in hereditary hemochromatosis), and arthropathies can also be encountered. In very advanced cases, patients can show signs of encephalopathy, ascites, and anasarca (due to liver function abnormality). Generalized bleeding can also occur due to thrombocytopenia secondary to hypersplenism from portal hypertension or coagulopathic liver disease. Since prognosis is poor in advanced liver disease secondary to chronic hepatitis, serial clinical and laboratory checkups and follow-ups play a crucial role in the management of patients once they get diagnosed with hepatitis (4).

TABLE 9.8.3	Differential Diagnosis of Hepatitis
Biliary tract obstruction	Conditions such as choledocholithiasis, neoplasm, pancreatitis, primary sclerosis cholangitis
	SURGICAL CAUSES MUST BE EXCLUDED EARLY
Liver infiltration	Granulomatous liver disease: immunologic and hypersensitivity disorders; fungal, mycobacterial, parasitic, other infections; inflammatory bowel disease; lymphoma; primary biliary cirrhosis; drug, foreign body, toxic reactions; rheumatic diseases; sarcoidosis; infiltrating malignancy
Other infections	Bacterial: ehrlichiosis, gonococcal perihepatitis, Legionnaires' disease, leptospirosis, listeriosis, Lyme disease, pyogenic abscess, Q-fever, Rocky Mountain spotted fever, salmonellosis, secondary syphilis, tularemia
	Fungal: candidiasis
	Parasitic: amebic abscess, babesiasis, malaria, toxoplasmosis
	Viral: adenovirus, cytomegalovirus, Epstein-Barr virus, herpes simplex virus
Pregnancy	Acute fatty liver of pregnancy, HELLP syndrome, hyperemesis gravidarum

HELLP, hemolysis, elevated liver enzymes, and low platelet count.

From Goldman L, Ausiello D, eds. *Cecil textbook of medicine,* 22nd ed. Philadelphia, PA: Saunders, 2003; Green RM, Flamm S. AGA technical review on the evaluation of liver chemistry tests. *Gastroenterology* 2002;123:1367–1384. http://www2.us.elsevierhealth.com/inst/serve?action= searchDB&searchDBfor=art&artType=abs&id=agast 1231367&nav=abs&special=hilite&query= [all_fields](liver+chemistry+tests,).

TABLE 9.8.4	Phases of "Classic" Acute Hepatitis		
Phase	**Symptoms**	**Findings**	**Duration**
Preicteric/ prodromal	Anorexia, nausea, fatigue, malaise, vague right upper quadrant pain	Greater than tenfold elevation of ALT and AST	2 weeks after exposure till appearance of jaundice
Icteric	Worsening of preicteric symptoms, dark urine, jaundice	Jaundice, liver tenderness, hyperbilirubinemia	Begins 1–2 weeks after prodromal phase and lasts 2–6 weeks
Convalescent/ recovery	Gradual resolution	Gradual resolution	6–8 weeks after exposure until full recovery of liver function and injury

ALT, alanine aminotransferase; AST, aspartate aminotransferase.

From Goldman L, Ausiello D, eds. *Cecil textbook of medicine*, 22nd ed. Philadelphia, PA: Saunders, 2003.

REFERENCES

1. Surveillance Data for Acute Viral Hepatitis—United States, 2009, CDC. Accessed at http://www.cdc .gov/hepatitis/Statistics/2009Surveillance/index.htm#
2. Recommendations for identification and public health management of persons with chronic hepatitis B virus infection. *MMWR* 2008;57(No. RR-8).
3. Armstrong GL et al. The prevalence of hepatitis C virus infection in the United States, 1999 through 2002. *Ann Int Med* 2006;144:705–714.
4. Goldman L, Ausiello D, eds. *Cecil textbook of medicine*, 22nd ed. Philadelphia, PA: Saunders, 2003.
5. Mersy DJ. Recognition of alcohol and substance abuse. *Am Fam Physician* 2003;67:1529–1532. Accessed at http://www.aafp.org/afp/20030401/1529.html

9.9 Hepatomegaly
Zoilo O. Lansang and John C. Huscher

I. **BACKGROUND.** Hepatomegaly is a physical finding associated with hepatobiliary disease. It is not specific or sensitive to one cause and defining it can be enigmatic because of the highly variable liver size that makes establishment of what constitutes normal somewhat difficult. The normal adult liver has a midclavicular range of 8–12 cm for men and 6–10 cm for women, with most studies defining hepatomegaly as a liver span greater than 15 cm in the midclavicular line (1).

II. **PATHOPHYSIOLOGY**

A. **Etiology.** Liver enlargement can have multiple pathophysiologic pathways. Enlargement occurs in the early hepatic inflammatory response to viral pathogens, toxic substances, and other stimulants and is then followed by scarring and shrinking in chronic conditions. Fatty infiltration causes enlargement in obesity and metabolic syndrome. Vascular congestion results in liver swelling in acute and chronic heart diseases as well as in conditions of decreased vascular outflow. Focally enlarging lesions such as vascular cysts, infectious cysts, and cancerous growths also occur. Abnormal deposition of amyloid, lipids, or iron can also result in liver enlargement. Common causes are listed in Table 9.9.1.

TABLE 9.9.1	**Common Causes of Hepatomegaly**

Infective

- *Glandular fever* (infectious mononucleosis) caused by the Epstein-Barr virus (EBV).
- *Hepatitis* (not all hepatitis viruses cause hepatomegaly)
- *Liver abscess* (pyogenic and amoebic abscess)
- *Malaria*
- *Amoeba* infections
- *Hydatid cyst*
- *Leptospirosis*
- *Actinomycosis*

Neoplastic

- Metastatic tumors (most common)
- *Hemangiomas*
- *Hepatocellular carcinoma*
- *Myeloma*
- *Leukemia*
- *Lymphoma*
- *Carcinoma*

Cirrhotic

- Portal
- Biliary
- Cardio
- *Hemochromatosis*

Metabolic

- *Fatty infiltration*
- *Amyloidosis*
- *Gaucher's disease*
- *Niemann Pick disease*
- *Von Gierke disease (glycogen storage disease type 1)*
- *Glycogen storage disease types III, VI and IX*

Drugs and toxins

- *Alcoholism*
- *Poisoning*

Congenital

- *Hemolytic anemia*
- Riedel's lobe is an extended, tongue-like, right lobe of the liver
- *Polycystic disease*
- *Cori's disease*

Others

- *Hunter syndrome*
- *Zellweger's syndrome*

(Continued)

TABLE 9.9.1	Common Causes of Hepatomegaly *(Continued)*

- *Carnitine palmitoyltransferase I deficiency*
- *Right ventricular failure*
- Granulomatous: *Sarcoidosis*
- *Glycogen storage disease type II*

B. Epidemiology. The incidence of hepatomegaly has not been studied in any large population group. However, a recent summary article of multiple studies found that a palpable liver margin had a likelihood ratio of 2.5 (confidence interval [CI], 2.2–2.8) for hepatomegaly and a nonpalpable liver margin had a negative likelihood ratio of 0.45 (CI, 0.38–0.52) (2).

III. EVALUATION

A. History

1. Risk Factors. See Table 9.9.2
2. Symptoms associated with liver disease. See Table 9.9.3

B. Physical Examination. Examination of the liver is difficult given its irregular shape and its location within the abdomen.

1. It is typical to use one of the two directions for palpation of the right upper quadrant: palpate from below using the fingertips to palpate superiorly or from above with the fingertips hooked over the lower rib. Either method is facilitated by the patient's deep inspiration. Palpation must include the midline to identify an enlarged left lobe of the liver. On palpation, note the liver position, the extent of its palpation below the costal margin, and its texture and consistency. Palpate for the lower edge and percuss for the upper margin. These two points give the highest accuracy in estimating liver size (3). If the margin is not palpated but hepatomegaly is suspected, attempt direct percussion of both margins. The "scratch method" (gently stoking or scratching the skin surface in a parallel plane while listening with the stethoscope for change in sound and intensity of frequency) has been used to identify margins; however, a recent study comparing ultrasound to the results of the scratch test found that this test was unreliable and inaccurate (4).

2. Auscultation of the right upper quadrant has poor clinical utility. Other physical examination findings consistent with liver disease include jaundice, vascular spiders, palmar erythema, gynecomastia, ascites, splenomegaly, testicular atrophy, peripheral edema, Dupuytren's contracture, parotid enlargement, and encephalopathy. Although none of these physical examination signs are pathognomonic for hepatobiliary disease, their presence prompts further diagnostic tests for hepatic disease.

C. Testing. Diagnostic tests should include computed tomography (CT) scan of the right upper quadrant and initial laboratory tests (complete blood count, serum blood tests [CHEM-7]), liver enzyme tests (aspartate aminotransferase, alanine aminotransferase, γ-glutamyl transpeptidase, and alkaline phosphatase), and true liver function tests (albumin, prothrombin time, partial thromboplastin time, and bilirubin). If liver enzymes are elevated,

TABLE 9.9.2	Risk Factors for Liver Disease	
Acupuncture	Alcoholism	Bisexuality
Blood product transfusion	Dietary supplements	Family history of liver disease
Gallstones	Gastrointestinal bleeding	Irritable bowel disease
Sexually transmitted disease	Male homosexuality	International travel
Tattoos		

TABLE 9.9.3	Symptoms of Liver Disease		
Abdominal pain	Pruritus	Nausea	Loss of appetite
Confusion	Arthralgias	Rashes	Night sweats
Fatigue	Diarrhea	Chills	Sleep disturbance
Gastric bleeding	Fever	Easy bruisability	Vomiting
Myalgia	Heavy menses	Frequent epistaxis	

TABLE 9.9.4	Specific Tests to Evaluate hepatomegaly
Suggested diagnosis	**Test**
Autoimmune hepatitis	Smooth muscle antibody, anti–liver–kidney microsomal antibody
Biliary cirrhosis	Antimitochondrial antibody
Hemochromatosis	Ferritin
Wilson's disease	Ceruloplasmin
Hepatocellular cancer	α-Fetoprotein
α_1-Antitrypsin deficiency	Enzyme assay of the same

proceed with hepatitis serology. Ultrasound can be used when CT scan is contraindicated or not available. Further testing used to elucidate the differential diagnosis is listed in Table 9.9.4.

IV. DIAGNOSIS

A. **Differential Diagnosis.** This can be approached on the basis of the findings of the physical examination.

1. Smooth nontender liver. Suspect fatty infiltration, congestive heart failure (CHF), portal cirrhosis, lymphoma, portal obstruction, hepatic vein thrombosis, lymphocystic leukemia, amyloidosis, schistosomiasis, or kala-azar.

2. Smooth tender liver. Suspect early CHF, acute hepatitis, amoebic abscess, or hepatic abscess.

3. Nodular liver. Suspect late portal cirrhosis, tertiary syphilis, hydatid cyst, or metastatic carcinoma.

4. Very hard nodular liver. This nearly always indicates metastatic carcinoma.

B. **Clinical Manifestations.** The clinical manifestations of hepatomegaly, although somewhat ill defined, should prompt a thorough evaluation and workup. Appropriate diagnostic tests generally provide a quick and accurate diagnosis. New therapies for chronic liver diseases make early diagnosis critical for obtaining good results.

REFERENCES

1. Unal B, Bilgili Y, Kocacikli E, et al. Simple evaluation of liver size on erect abdominal plain radiography. *Clin Radiol* 2004;59:1132–1135.
2. Seupaul RA, Collins R. Physical examination of the liver. *Ann Emerg Med* 2005;45:553–555.
3. Naylor CD. Physical examination of the liver. *JAMA* 1994;27:1859–1865.
4. Tucker WN, Saab S, Leland SR, et al. The scratch test is unreliable for determining the liver edge. *J Clin Gastroenterol* 1997;25:410–414.

9.10 Jaundice

Vijaya Subramanian and John C. Huscher

I. **BACKGROUND.** Jaundice refers to a yellowish discoloration of the skin, sclerae, and mucous membranes caused by the deposition of bile pigments. Normal serum bilirubin in children and adults is less than 1 mg/dL. Typically, physical examination is unable to detect elevations of bilirubin until the serum level exceeds 2.0–3.0 mg/dL.

II. **PATHOPHYSIOLOGY**

    A. Etiology. Bilirubin is formed primarily through the metabolic breakdown of heme rings, predominantly from the catabolism of red blood cells. Dysfunction of any of the phases of bilirubin metabolism (prehepatic, intrahepatic, or posthepatic) can lead to jaundice. Normally, 96% of plasma bilirubin is unconjugated (indirect). When the plasma elevation is caused predominantly by unconjugated bilirubin, the defect is likely to be the result of overproduction, impaired hepatic uptake, or abnormalities in conjugation. When the plasma elevation includes a substantial contribution from conjugated (direct) bilirubin, then hepatocellular disease, defective canalicular excretion, and biliary obstruction are the more likely causes.

    B. Epidemiology. Among adults presenting with jaundice, serious underlying disease is common. In one study, 20% of patients with jaundice had pancreatic or biliary carcinoma, 13% experienced gallstone disease, and 10% suffered from alcoholic cirrhosis (1). Jaundice rarely represents a medical emergency but can present as massive hemolysis, kernicterus, ascending cholangitis, and fulminant hepatic failure.

III. **EVALUATION**

    A. History

        1. A careful history gives multiple clues to the etiology of jaundice. Sudden onset is consistent with viral hepatitis, acute biliary obstruction, trauma, or toxin-mediated fulminant liver failure. More gradual onset is indicative of chronic liver disease (including alcoholic cirrhosis) or malignancy. A lifelong history suggests an inherited metabolic or hemolytic cause. Acholic stools, dark urine, and right upper quadrant (RUQ) pain, especially following a fatty meal, should suggest cholestasis or cholelithiasis. A history of fever or prior biliary surgery, especially if RUQ pain is present, points to cholangitis. Charcot's triad of cholangitis includes fever, RUQ pain, and jaundice. In the presence of a history of anorexia, malaise, or myalgias, a viral etiology should be considered. Typically, pruritus or weight loss is associated with noninfectious etiologies such as primary biliary cirrhosis in which pruritus is commonly the initial symptom (2). Numerous medications can induce hepatocellular injury or cholestasis (see Table 9.10.1).

        2. Blood transfusions, intravenous drug use, sexual contacts, travel to endemic regions, or ingestion of contaminated foods can also expose patients to viral-related hepatocellular injury. Past medical history and surgical history, prior episodes of jaundice, and a history of a rheumatologic disease or inflammatory bowel disease should be examined. Family history may reveal an inherited defect in bilirubin conjugation or transport, Wilson's disease, α1-antitrypsin deficiency, or hemochromatoses.

    B. Physical Examination. In addition to icterus, examination findings of ascites, splenomegaly, spider angiomas, caput medusa, gynecomastia, testicular atrophy, palmar erythema, or Dupuytren's contracture suggest chronic liver disease and portal hypertension. An abdominal examination to assess liver size and tenderness is important. Altered consciousness and asterixis point toward liver failure. Kayser-Fleischer rings are seen in Wilson's disease, and Courvoisier's sign (a painless palpable gallbladder) is suggestive of pancreatic cancer.

    C. Testing

        1. Initial laboratory testing for a jaundiced patient includes a complete blood count (CBC) and peripheral smear, a fractionated serum bilirubin (total and direct), and a urinalysis.

TABLE 9.10.1	Medications Associated with the Development of Jaundice
Alcohol	Antibiotics
Diuretics	Diuretics
Acetaminophen	Oral hypoglycemics
Cholesterol-lowering agents	Inhaled anesthetics
Anticonvulsants	Chemotherapy agents
Sex hormones	Nonsteroidal anti-inflammatory drugs
Psychotropic medications	Herbal compounds

Additional testing should include aspartate aminotransferase/alanine aminotransferase (AST/ALT), γ-glutamyl transpeptidase, and alkaline phosphatase. Pure liver function should be evaluated by obtaining an albumin and a prothrombin time.

2. Further laboratory testing and imaging are predicated on obtaining the initial results and may include serologic testing for viral hepatitis, autoimmune markers (antimitochondrial antibodies: primary biliary cirrhosis, or anti-smooth muscle antibodies and antimicrosomal antibodies: autoimmune hepatitis), serum iron, transferrin and ferritin (hemochromatosis), ceruloplasmin (Wilson's disease), and α1-antitrypsin activity (α_1-antitrypsin deficiency). Ultrasound and computed tomography (CT) can help distinguish obstructive disease from hepatocellular disease (3).

IV. DIAGNOSIS. Historical features corroborated by physical examination and laboratory studies should distinguish obstructive causes from nonobstructive causes, differentiate acutely presenting conditions from more chronic diseases, and discriminate unconjugated and conjugated sources of bilirubin (see Table 9.10.2). Dubin-Johnson and Rotor's syndrome are inherited disorders that affect transportation of conjugated bilirubin.

A CBC is useful in detecting hemolysis, which is indicated by the presence of schistocytes and increased reticulocytes on the smear. Results of the patient's aminotransferases further refine the differential diagnosis. Hepatocellular injury is distinguished from cholestasis by substantial

TABLE 9.10.2	Differential Diagnosis of Jaundice	
Disorders of unconjugated hyperbilirubinemia		
Overproduction	**Impaired uptake**	**Impaired conjugation**
Intravascular hemolysis	Congestive heart failure	Crigler-Najjar syndrome, types I and II
Extravascular hemolysis	Cirrhosis	Advanced cirrhosis
Dyserythropoiesis	Gilbert's disease	Wilson's disease
Extravasation of blood into tissues	Medication—rifampin, probenecid	Antibiotics, ethinyl estradiol
		Neonates
Disorders of conjugated hyperbilirubinemia		
Extrahepatic cholestasis	**Intrahepatic cholestasis**	**Hepatocellular injury**
Sclerosing cholangitis	Viral hepatitis	See Table 9.10.1
Choledocholithiasis	Alcoholic hepatitis	
Pancreatitis	Nonalcoholic steatohepatitis	
Tumors	Biliary cirrhosis	
AIDS cholangiopathy	Toxins	

(Continued)

TABLE 9.10.2	Differential Diagnosis of Jaundice *(Continued)*
Disorders of unconjugated hyperbilirubinemia	
Strictures	Infiltrating diseases
Parasitic infections	Total parenteral nutrition
	Pregnancy
	End-stage hepatic disease

AIDS, acquired immunodeficiency syndrome.

elevations in the aminotransferases (AST/ALT). A ratio of AST/ALT of >2.0 suggests alcoholic liver disease. Infectious causes of hepatitis cause greater elevations of ALT than AST. Levels greater than 10,000 U/L usually occur with acute injury to the liver (e.g., acetaminophen or ischemia). Normal aminotransferases argue against hepatocellular injury and increase the likelihood that hemolysis or a disorder of bilirubin processing exists. However, this can be misleading in chronic liver disease when there is little liver parenchyma left for being injured. Alkaline phosphatase and gamma glutamyltransferase are markers for cholestasis. Ultrasound is the most sensitive imaging technique for detecting biliary stones. CT scan provides more information about liver and pancreatic parenchymal disease. Further imaging may be done by a gastroenterologist or interventional radiologist such as endoscopic retrograde cholangiopancreatography and percutaneous transhepatic cholangiography in case of extrahepatic obstruction (4).

REFERENCES

1. Reisman Y, Gips GH, Lavelle SM, et al. Clinical presentation of (subclinical) jaundice. *Hepatogastroenterology* 1996;43:1190.
2. Leuschner U. Primary biliary cirrhosis-presentation and diagnosis. *Clin Liver Dis* 2003;7:741.
3. Namita Roy Chowdury, Jayan Roy Chowdury, Diagnostic approach to the patient with jaundice or asymptomatic hyperbilirubinemia. Accessed at http://www.uptodate.com/contents/diagnostic-approach-to-the-patient-with-jaundice-or-asymptomatic-hyperbilirubinemia?source=search_result&search=jaundice&selectedTitle=1~150.
4. Sean PR, Rebecca K. Jaundice in the adult patient. *Am Fam Physician* 2004;69(2):299–304.

9.11 Rectal Bleeding

Nirmal Bastola and Robert C. Messbarger

I. BACKGROUND. Rectal bleeding is a common problem primary care physicians are faced with in the outpatient and emergency department setting. The spectrum of rectal bleeding can range from mild to severe: bright red blood per rectum, which can present as blood on the toilet paper, a small amount of blood in the toilet bowl, or fresh blood on the stool. This mostly tends to be chronic intermittent bleeding. Many patients with mild rectal bleeding do not seek health care for this problem (1). Acute massive rectal bleeding with hematochezia or melena can be life threatening (2).

II. PATHOPHYSIOLOGY. Rectal bleeding is typically a sign of local mucosal or vascular disease, but it can also signify proximal intestinal disease in the small or large bowel. Scant or minimal rectal bleeding is a common problem present in up to 15% of the population. Constipation traumatizes local venous and mucosal tissues. Pregnancy can inhibit venous blood flow in the pelvis and lead to hemorrhoid formation. Bleeding from sources proximal to ligament of Treitz tends to produce stools that are black and tarry because of metabolism of heme.

III. EVALUATION

A. Initial Evaluation. The initial evaluation should determine the acuity and hemodynamic stability of the patient and establish the origin of the bleeding as upper or lower gastrointestinal (GI) tract in nature. Potential hemodynamic compromise warrants volume resuscitation with two large-bore intravenous lines, preferably in an intensive care setting involving a gastroenterologist on the team. If rectal bleeding is minimal or has stopped, and the patient is stable, evaluation can occur in the outpatient setting (3–5, 9).

B. History and Differential Diagnosis (2). By far, the most common anorectal bleeding source is hemorrhoidal disease. Risks of hemorrhoids increase with advancing age, pregnancy, prolonged sitting or standing, chronic diarrhea, or constipation. Associated complaints from hemorrhoids include anal pruritus, pain, and prolapse. Other anorectal sources of minimal bleeding include anal fissures, polyps, proctitis, rectal ulcers, and cancer (4). It is also necessary to take the history of any use of blood thinners.

1. Upper GI tract

Peptic ulcer disease: Use of aspirin, nonsteroidal anti-inflammatory drugs, or tobacco

Esophageal varices: Alcohol abuse; jaundice; signs of portal hypertension, including ascites, palmar erythema, spider angiomata, hepatomegaly, splenomegaly, and rectal varices

Mallory-Weiss tear: Bleeding preceded by vomiting, retching, or seizures

Gastric cancer: Left supraclavicular adenopathy; palpable mass; abdominal pain; weight loss; cachexia

2. Lower GI tract

Diverticular disease: Age >60 years; painless bleeding; possible recent constipation

Arteriovenous malformations: Age >60 years; painless bleeding; chronic renal failure

Colonic neoplasms: Age >50 years; abdominal pain; weight loss; muscle wasting; protein calorie malnutrition; right-sided colon cancer may be associated with palpable right-sided abdominal mass; hepatomegaly; liver nodules; history of adenomatous polyps or long-standing ulcerative colitis; prior exposure to ionized radiation; family history of familial polyposis coli or cancer family syndrome (6).

3. Inflammatory bowel disease

Ulcerative colitis: starts in younger patients (20–40 years of age); usually involves the rectum; associated with diarrhea mixed with blood and mucus

Crohn's disease: starts in younger patients (20–40 years of age); perianal, peritoneal, and/or abdominal wall fistulas may be associated

Radiation colitis: History of radiation treatment to abdomen and/or pelvis

Hemorrhoids: Perianal mass may be painful (external hemorrhoid) or painless (internal hemorrhoid); commonly starts in younger patients; associated with constipation, pregnancy, or postpartum period

Anal fissures: More common in patients with history of constipation; associated with severe sharp pain occurring with straining on defecation; pain resolves within an hour after defecation; commonly starts at 20–40 years of age

Colon tuberculosis: History of pulmonary tuberculosis or past exposure to tuberculosis

Aortoduodenal fistula: History of abdominal aortic aneurysm surgically repaired with synthetic vascular graft placement

C. Workup

1. Initial laboratory tests to assess hemodynamic stability and clotting ability are complete blood count to assess for anemia, type and screen, stool hemoccult test, serum blood urea nitrogen and creatinine, and coagulation panel (9).

2. Imaging studies can be directed at the most likely source of bleeding. Younger patients with intermittent mild rectal bleeding can be evaluated with anoscopy or flexible sigmoidoscopy. Persons older than 50 years of age with painless bleeding are assumed to have colon cancer until proved otherwise by colonoscopy, even if the rectal examination is abnormal.

IV. DIAGNOSTIC PROCEDURES

A. Chronic Intermittent Rectal bleeding. Colonoscopy is the diagnostic tool of choice in a hemodynamically stable patient with a suspected lower GI source of bleeding (2, 7). **Double-contrast barium enema with sigmoidoscopy** may be an alternative in patients who have a relative contraindication to colonoscopy. Some physicians may consider a limited evaluation of the anorectosigmoid area with sigmoidoscopy in patients younger than 40 years because only 5% of colorectal cancer cases occur in this population (8). In addition, the most common cause of rectal bleeding in patients younger than 30 years is anal pathology such as hemorrhoids or fissures, which can be diagnosed with **anoscopy** (9). In cases where the source of bleeding cannot be confirmed, or if bleeding and anemia continue, a colonoscopy should be performed for complete evaluation of the large bowel (10). Small bowel sources of GI bleeding are uncommon, accounting for only 2–10% of all cases. Because of its location, evaluation is technically difficult. For these reasons, therefore, evaluation of the small bowel is less commonly indicated (11, 12). However, when endoscopy is nondiagnostic, the small bowel should be evaluated. Obscure GI bleeding is the recurrent blood loss without an identifiable source of bleeding even after esophagogastroduodenoscopy (EGD) and colonoscopy. When evaluation of the small bowel is considered necessary, several procedures can be employed including barium-contrast upper GI series with small bowel follow through (SBFT), capsule endoscopy, angiography (requires blood loss at a rate of 1 mL/min), technetium radiolabeled RBC scan (requires blood loss at a rate of 0.1 mL/min), and push enteroscopy (13).

B. Acute Massive Rectal Bleeding. Acute massive rectal bleeding frequently arises from an upper GI source. The diagnostic workup begins with an **EGD**. If the patient is not experiencing hematemesis and endoscopy is not immediately available, a nasogastric tube may be placed for gastric lavage while awaiting endoscopy. If no blood is returned and bile is identified, an upper GI source is much less likely, and the workup can focus on the large bowel. **Colonoscopy** is one of two diagnostic tools of choice used to evaluate acute lower GI bleeding. Colonoscopy may be performed urgently or electively, depending on the patient's hemodynamic status and risk stratification criteria (2, 7, 11, 14, 15).

REFERENCES

1. Talley NJ, Jones M. Self-reported rectal bleeding in a United States community: prevalence, risk factors, and health care seeking. Am J Gastroenterol 1998;93:2179–2183.
2. Maltz C. Acute gastrointestinal bleeding. Best Pract Med 2003;16:1–19. Accessed online March 11, 2005.
3. Bounds B, Friedman L. Lower gastrointestinal bleeding. Gastroenterol Clin 2003;32:1107–1125.
4. Gopal D. Diseases of the rectum and anus: a clinical approach to common disorders. Clin Cornerstone 2002;4:34–48.
5. Peter D, Dougherty J. Evaluation of the patient with gastrointestinal bleeding: an evidence based approach. Emerg Med Clin North Am 1999;17:239–261.
6. Manning LL, Dimmitt, Dimmitt SG, Wilson GR. Diagnosis of gastrointestinal bleeding in adults. Am Fam Physician 2005;71(7):1339–1346.
7. Eisen GM, Dominitz JA, Faigel DO, et al. An annotated algorithmic approach to acute lower gastrointestinal bleeding. Gastrointest Endosc. 2001;53:859–863.
8. Steele GD Jr. The National Cancer Data Base report on colorectal cancer. Cancer 1994;74:1979–1989.
9. Lewis JD, Brown A, Localio AR, Schwartz JS. Initial evaluation of rectal bleeding in young persons: a cost-effectiveness analysis. *Ann Intern Med* 2002;136:99–110.
10. Fine KD, Nelson AC, Ellington RT, Mossburg A. Comparison of the color of fecal blood with the anatomical location of gastrointestinal bleeding lesions: potential misdiagnosis using only flexible sigmoidoscopy for bright red blood per rectum. *Am J Gastroenterol* 1999;94:3202–3210.
11. Fallah MA, Prakash C, Edmundowicz S. Acute gastrointestinal bleeding. *Med Clin North Am* 2000;84:1183–1208.
12. Ell C, Remke S, May A, Helou L, Henrich R, Mayer G. The first prospective controlled trial comparing wireless capsule endoscopy with push enteroscopy in chronic gastrointestinal bleeding. Endoscopy 2002;34:685–689.
13. Zuckerman GR, Prakash C, Askin MP, Lewis BS. AGA technical review on the evaluation and management of occult and obscure gastrointestinal bleeding. Gastroenterology 2000;118:201–221.
14. Wilcox CM, Clark WS. Causes and outcome of upper and lower gastrointestinal bleeding: the Grady Hospital experience. South Med J 1999;92:44–50.
15. Zuccaro G Jr. Management of the adult patient with acute lower gastrointestinal bleeding. American College of Gastroenterology. Practice Parameters Committee. *Am J Gastroenterol* 1998;93:1202–1208.

9.12 Steatorrhea

Monica Sarawagi and Milton (Pete) Johnson

I. BACKGROUND. Steatorrhea results from fat malabsorption. It is quantitatively defined as the presence of more than 7 g of fat in the stool during a 24-hour period while the patient is on a diet containing no more than 100 g of fat per day. It manifests as a history of greasy, foul smelling stools that leave an oily residue in the toilet bowl, increased flatulence, and weight loss. Normally more than 90% of daily dietary fat is absorbed into the general circulation, but any defects in the processes can reduce this uptake and lead to fatty diarrhea.

II. PATHOPHYSIOLOGY. This can result from defects in any of the three phases required for proper digestion and absorption of fat.

A. Luminal Phase. This phase includes substrate (fat) hydrolysis by the help of digestive enzyme, followed by fat solubilization in the presence of bile salts.

B. Mucosal Phase. This can be also called as absorptive phase where mucosal uptake and reesterification occur. This phase is defective in celiac disease where changes occur in the mucosal structure.

C. Postabsorptive process. During this phase, the chylomicrons are formed and transported to the lymphatic system.

1. Etiology. Chronic pancreatitis is the most common cause of steatorrhea, which results from ethanol abuse. It causes steatorrhea due to pancreatic lipase deficiency. Steatorrhea is evident only when more than 90% of pancreatic exocrine insufficiency occurs (2). Other causes are cystic fibrosis and pancreatic duct obstruction. Cirrhosis and biliary obstruction may cause mild form of steatorrhea due to deficiency of intraluminal bile acid concentration. Similar pathology can be seen in bacterial overgrowth in the small intestine which may deconjugate bile acids and alter micelle formation, thus impairing fat digestion. Bacterial overgrowth can be seen in stasis from a blind loop, small bowel diverticulum, or dysmotility, which is very common in the elderly.

Mucosal malabsorption can result from a variety of enteropathies, the most common being celiac disease. Celiac disease is characterized by villous atrophy and crypt hyperplasia in the proximal small bowel; these mucosal changes can cause fatty diarrhea. Other causes of fat malabsorption due to mucosal changes are tropical sprue, mycobacterium avium intracellulare infection of the intestinal mucosa, and AIDS. Abetalipoproteinemia is a very rare defect of chylomicron formation and fat malabsorption seen commonly in children. Giardiasis is a protozoal infection that also causes fat malabsorption. Other miscellaneous causes are neomycin, colchicine, and cholestyramine consumption. Amyloidosis and chronic small bowel ischemia can also be considered as causes of steatorrhea (1).

Postmucosal malabsorption of fat can result from a very rare condition called intestinal lymphangiectasia or acquired lymphatic obstruction secondary to trauma, cardiac disease causing congestion of the mucosal lining. In these conditions, there is fat malabsorption and enteric losses of protein and there is associated lymphocytopenia. It is seen that carbohydrate and amino acid absorption are preserved.

2. Epidemiology. The incidence and prevalence of steatorrhea are difficult to estimate because this condition arises from an array of diverse underlying conditions that are difficult to amass into an overall figure. These other conditions are nonreportable illnesses or surgical procedures performed for other reasons and so are not readily tabulated in the literature.

III. EVALUATION

A. History. A careful history often provides clues to probable diagnoses and guides the clinician to do tests that are most likely to provide a definitive diagnosis or helps to narrow down the differential diagnosis for steatorrhea. Abdominal pain in the epigastric region will be seen in patients with chronic pancreatitis. Jaundice will be seen in cholestasis. Cramping, abdominal pain, bloating, and flatulence in addition to steatorrhea will be seen in celiac disease and giardiasis.

B. Physical Examination. Physical findings associated with steatorrhea are limited. A thorough examination of the abdomen to exclude palpable masses should be undertaken along with a search for signs of alcoholic liver disease. There might be evidence of lack of subcutaneous fat, temporal wasting, signs suggestive of end-stage cirrhosis like palmar erythema and telangiectasias. Other findings noted can be skin jaundice suggesting biliary obstruction.

C. Testing. The role of laboratory and radiologic investigation is

1. Confirmation of steatorrhea.
2. Determination of the type of steatorrhea.
3. Assessment for conditions that cause fat malabsorption.

Patients with suspected steatorrhea can be tested for fecal fat presence by any of these methods:

   a. Sudden stain of a random sample of homogenized stool.

   b. Steatocrit is a quantitative measure of fat as a proportion of a whole centrifuged homogenized stool sample. A spot acid steatocrit level (normal less than 10%) has been reported as having a sensitivity of 100% and a specificity of 95% when compared with 72-hour quantitative fat analysis.

   c. The gold standard for diagnosis remains the quantitative determination of fecal fat from stool samples collected over 72 hours while the patient ingests a diet with a limited fat content. Once true steatorrhea is demonstrated, further testing helps determine the underlying disorder.

   d. Measurement of fecal elastase-1 is a simple noninvasive test for pancreatic exocrine insufficiency (3).

   e. The D-xylose test measures the absorptive capacity of the proximal small bowel mucosa (4). D-xylose does not require pancreatic exocrine function to be absorbed. Disorders of the intestinal mucosa that impede absorption lead to low levels of the sugar in both serum and urine samples. Inadequate renal function, dehydration, or hypothyroidism can also depress urine levels, so determinations of serum thyroid-stimulating hormone, blood urea nitrogen, and creatinine are warranted. Bacterial overgrowth of the small intestine can also produce an abnormal D-xylose test. An abnormal D-xylose test should prompt referral for small intestine biopsy to search for evidence of mucosal diseases including gluten enteropathy, Whipple's disease, giardiasis, tropical sprue, or intestinal lymphoma. Some of these entities may also be diagnosed by their characteristic appearance on an upper gastrointestinal series. A normal D-xylose test indicates proper mucosal function and so the problem is usually the digestion of fats within the intestinal lumen. The most frequent etiology is pancreatic insufficiency (see Table 9.12.1). A secretin test may be required to measure pancreatic function. A therapeutic trial of pancreatic enzymes with improvement in symptoms is considered presumptive proof of the diagnosis. The bile

TABLE 9.12.1	Causes of Pancreatic Exocrine Insufficiency
Alcohol-induced liver diseases	Cystic fibrosis
Chronic pancreatitis	Zollinger-Ellison syndrome
Hypertriglyceridemia	Gastrectomy
Cancer of the pancreas	Vagotomy
Resection of the pancreas	Hemochromatosis
Blockage of the pancreatic duct	Shwachman-Diamond syndrome
Traumatic pancreatitis	Trypsinogen deficiency
Hereditary pancreatitis	α_1-Antitrypsin deficiency
Enterokinase deficiency	Somatostatinoma
Graft vs. host disease	

salt breath test, a nuclear medicine study, measures bile acid absorption. Because the terminal ileum is also the site of vitamin B12 absorption, the Schilling test may also be utilized to search for disorders of absorption. Disorders of the terminal ileum (Crohn's disease, granulomatous ileitis, and prior ileal resection) result in poor absorption of bile salts, which then pass into the colon where bacteria deconjugate them. Poor reabsorption depletes the supply of bile salts, resulting in maldigestion of fats. Noninvasive testing for small bowel bacterial overgrowth (SBBO) is available by the c-xylose breath test, the bile acid breath test, or the breath hydrogen test (6). A therapeutic trial of oral tetracycline with resolution of steatorrhea is presumptive confirmation of bacterial overgrowth, avoiding a more costly testing. The upper small intestine is normally bacteriologically sterile except for contaminants from the mouth and upper respiratory tract. Aspiration of fluid through an endoscope or a small intestine tube placed under fluoroscopic guidance that yields a bacterial colony count greater than 100,000/mL is diagnostic of SBBO. Abdominal computed tomography (CT) scan with oral and IV contrast can be done to look for small bowel lymphoma, Crohn disease, or pancreatic abnormalities. Alternatively, ultrasound of the pancreas can be helpful to look for any structural abnormality of the pancreas in the absence of CT scan.

D. Genetics. Genetics plays little role in this disorder with the exception of those conditions with familial tendencies such as cystic fibrosis, gluten enteropathy, and acanthocytosis. In approximately 25% of cases, Zollinger-Ellison syndrome occurs in association with a genetic syndrome, multiple endocrine neoplasia type 1 (5).

IV. DIAGNOSIS

A. Differential diagnosis. The following conditions can be considered as some of the common causes of steatorrhea:

o Chronic pancreatitis
o Bacterial overgrowth syndrome
o Ileal disease
o Celiac disease
o Intestinal lymphangiectasia
o Graves disease
o Lipase inhibitors, for example, tetrahydrolipstatin (orlistat).

The degree of steatorrhea can lend clues to the source. Mild steatorrhea can occur with any disorder that causes rapid transit of intestinal contents, because the shortened exposure of the fats prevents proper absorption. The explosive urgent diarrhea of irritable bowel syndrome can mimic steatorrhea, but the fecal fat content does not usually meet the criteria for true steatorrhea. The proper workup of this symptom frequently requires specialized testing and procedures, necessitating consultation with a gastroenterologist if initial history and the more readily available tests fail to reveal its source.

Treatment

Patients with steatorrhea may or may not present with diarrhea; dietary restriction of fat plays a important role in controlling episodes of diarrhea. Initial fat intake can be restricted to 50 g/d and then gradually increased until diarrhea appears. Maximum allowed quantity is usually not more than 100 g/d distributed equally among four meals. For patients with pancreatic insufficiency, pancreatic extract containing 30,000–50,000 units of lipase can be given. This dose of lipase is distributed throughout each of four daily meals.

REFERENCES

1. Gruy-Kapral C, Little KH, Fordtran JS, et al. Conjugated bile acid replacement therapy for shortbowel syndrome. *Gastroenterology* 1999;116:15.
2. Grigg AP, Angus PW, Hoyt R, et al. The incidence, pathogenesis and natural history of steatorrhea after bone marrow transplantation. *Bone Marrow Transplant* 2003;31(8):701–703.
3. Beharry S, Ellis L, Corey M, et al. How useful is fecal pancreatic elastase 1 as a marker of exocrine pancreatic disease? *J Pediatr* 2002;141(1):84–90.
4. Craig RM, Ehrenpreis ED. D-xylose testing. *J Clin Gastroenterol* 1999;29(2):143–150.
5. Domínguez-Muñoz JE. Pancreatic exocrine insufficiency: diagnosis and treatment. *J Gastroenterol Hepatol* 2011;26(Suppl. 2):12–16.
6. Ziegler TR, Cole CR. Small bowel bacterial overgrowth in adults: a potential contributor to intestinal failure. *Curr Gastroenterol Rep* 2007;9(6):463–467.

CHAPTER 10

Renal and Urologic Problems
David M. Quillen

10.1 Dysuria
David M. Quillen and Daniel Rubin

I. BACKGROUND. Dysuria is defined as "painful urination." Acute dysuria is a frequent problem seen in ambulatory practices, accounting for >3 million office visits a year. The most common diagnosis given for patients with dysuria is a urinary tract infection (UTI). The estimated cost of traditional management of acute UTIs approaches $1 billion per year in the United States. Although a UTI is the most common cause of dysuria symptoms, many other causes need to be accurately diagnosed. The differential diagnosis for patients with dysuria can be separated into broad categories. With a few notable exceptions, the differential diagnoses for men and women are similar, although the incidences are greatly different and change with age (1, 2).

II. PATHOPHYSIOLOGY
    A. Causes of dysuria—female (3)
        1. Infectious
            a. Cystitis, lower UTI, with or without pyelonephritis
            b. Urethritis caused by a sexually transmitted disease (STD): *Chlamydia*, *Neisseria gonorrhoeae*, herpes simplex virus (HSV)
            c. Vulvovaginitis—bacterial vaginosis, trichomoniasis, yeast, genital HSV
        2. Noninfectious—trauma, irritant, allergy, atrophy, sexual abuse
    B. Causes of dysuria—male (4)
        1. Infectious
            a. Urethritis caused by *Chlamydia*, *N. gonorrhoeae*, yeast (uncircumcised → balanitis), HSV
            b. Cystitis (if culture positive, possible anatomic abnormality, further workup indicated)
            c. Prostatitis, acute more common than chronic (5)
        2. Noninfectious
            a. Penile lesions, trauma, sexual abuse
            b. Benign prostatic hypertrophy (BPH) particularly in older men (1). Infection can be evident but is primarily an obstructive process

III. EVALUATION
    A. History. A good general history is critical and can help direct further questions. Careful questioning about other associated symptoms and risk factors is the key to sorting out the diagnosis.
        1. Internal Dysuria versus External Dysuria
            a. Internal dysuria is where the discomfort seems to be centered inside the body and begins before or with the initiation of voiding.
                i. Inflammation of the bladder or urethra
            b. External dysuria is when the discomfort appears after voiding has initiated.
                ii. Vaginitis, vulvar inflammation, or external penile lesions
        2. Other important history items
            a. New sex partner → STD cause

b. Diaphragm usage → bladder infection
c. Gradual onset → urethritis and external causes
d. Suprapubic pain, costovertebral angle tenderness, fever, and flank pain → pyelonephritis
e. Older men → questioning about BPH
B. Physical Examination. The examination is essential in narrowing the diagnosis.
  1. Rule out pyelonephritis
    a. Fever
    b. Flank tenderness
    c. Suprapubic tenderness
  2. Genital examination
    a. Speculum examination in women
    b. Foreskin retraction in uncircumcised men
    c. Prostate examination
  3. Collection of samples for testing
    a. HSV lesions
    b. Discharge—yeast, bacterial vaginosis, gonorrhea, and trichomoniasis
    c. Trauma
C. Testing
  1. Urine analysis dipstick test—nitrates and leukoesterase (urea-fixing bacteria and leukocytes)
  2. Direct microscopic examination of the urine can detect the following:
    a. Leukocytes, bacteria, and blood
    b. Pyuria (defined as white blood cell count $>10/mm^3$ of urine)
  3. Urine culture: takes up to 48 hours

IV. DIAGNOSIS. Given the many causes of dysuria, an accurate diagnosis can be difficult without a thorough approach to each patient. Because most causes have other associated symptoms and findings, a diagnosis can usually be made with a carefully taken history, a focused physical examination, and appropriate laboratory tests. Separating an uncomplicated UTI or STD from the more serious pyelonephritis and other possible diagnoses is the challenge in these patients.

REFERENCES

1. Bremnor JD, Sadovsky R. Evaluation of dysuria in adults. *Am Fam Physician* 2002;65(8):1589–1596.
2. Johnson JR, Stamm WE. Diagnosis and treatment of acute urinary tract infections. *Infect Dis Clin North Am* 1987;4(1):773–791.
3. Kurowiski K. The woman with dysuria. *Am Fam Physician* 1998;57(9):2155–2164, 2169–2170.
4. Ainsworth JG, Weaver T, Murphy S, et al. General practitioners' immediate management of men presenting with urethral symptoms. *Genitourin Med* 1996;72(6):427–430.
5. Roberts RO, Lieber MM, Rhodes R, et al. Prevalence of a physician-assigned diagnosis of prostatitis: the Olmsted County study of urinary symptoms and health status among men. *Urology* 1998;51(4):578–584.

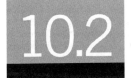

Hematuria
Ku-Lang Chang and Siegfried Schmidt

I. BACKGROUND. Hematuria, defined as "blood in the urine," is frequently an outpatient complaint. It can manifest as gross (macroscopic) hematuria with obvious reddish discoloration, greater than 50 red blood cells/high power field (400×), or microscopic hematuria detected with a dipstick followed by a microscopic examination. Although there is existing controversy pertaining to what constitutes microhematuria, the American Urological Association defines significant microscopic hematuria as three or more red blood cells/high power field from two of three properly collected urine specimens (1).

II. PATHOPHYSIOLOGY

A. Etiology. The list of the potential causes of hematuria is lengthy and includes diseases of the urinary tract, as well as nonurologic causes. Some of these are life threatening (e.g., renal and bladder cancer), whereas others are insignificant (e.g., exercise-induced hematuria, bladder polyps, and renal cysts). It is important to note that hematuria in an adult is more often urologic than renal in origin. The extent of the workup should be determined by considering factors such as the likelihood of coexisting illnesses, potential complications from procedures, and the cost to the patient. Benign causes such as menstruation, infection, and trauma should always be excluded before further evaluation and referral to urology or nephrology is initiated.

B. Epidemiology. Overall prevalence varies greatly (0.1–13%) and depends on many variables (e.g., the number of screening tests performed and the type of population studied). However, screening of the general population for microscopic hematuria is not recommended. The decision to check for hematuria should depend on various risk factors for significant underlying disease and remains a physician's judgment call. Risk factors of significant urological disease include age > 40 years, cigarette smoking (past or present, including second-hand smoke), history of urinary tract infections, history of hematuria, exposure to various drugs (analgesics, anti-inflammatory drugs, cyclophosphamide, and human immunodeficiency virus therapy), exposure to occupational hazards (benzenes, 2-naphthylamine, aromatic amines, and aniline dyes), and pelvic radiation. In many cases of microhematuria, no cause can be found despite a complete evaluation.

III. EVALUATION

A. History. A thorough history is of utmost importance.

1. General questions should cover the type of hematuria (macro/gross/microscopic) and the relationship between urination and the timing of hematuria. The three-container method assists in separating the micturition into three portions—initial, middle, and final portions. Anatomically, initial hematuria usually originates from anterior urethral disease, and final hematuria results from disease of the bladder neck, posterior urethra, or prostate. Hematuria throughout the micturition suggests pathology more proximal. Worm-like clots suggest a location above the bladder neck. Urine color should be questioned, which can be affected by the following: phenazopyridine (orange), nitrofurantoin (brown), rifampin (yellow-orange), l-dopa, methyldopa, and metronidazole (reddish-brown), phenolphthalein in laxatives, red beet and rhubarb consumption, food coloring, and vegetable dyes (red).

2. Associated symptoms can hint at various particular problems; for example, a recent sore throat, fever, chills, and flu-like symptoms may be the first signs of immunoglobulin A nephropathy or postinfectious glomerulonephritis. Urinary frequency, urgency, dysuria, fever, and chills point to an infectious process. Diminished urine flow and abdominal or flank pain radiating into the groin can indicate the presence of urinary tract obstruction. Vaginal discharge or bowel movement changes may hint at a nonurinary tract cause such as a foreign body (especially in children). A rash, joint pain, photosensitivity, flu-like symptoms, and Raynaud's phenomenon point to a collagen vascular disease.

3. Past medical history should also include travel history. If the patient has traveled to areas where bilharzia (*Schistosoma haematobium*) is endemic, parasitic infestation is highly probable. Furthermore, if the history includes the use of analgesics, especially anti-inflammatory drugs, renal papillary necrosis should be considered. Past exposure to cyclophosphamide may cause chemical cystitis, because past exposure to antibiotics (e.g., penicillin and cephalosporins) may cause interstitial nephritis. Of special note is that the mere use of oral anticoagulants does not cause hematuria. To the contrary, these patients may in fact present earlier in their disease process and should be evaluated promptly (2).

4. Family history may lead to suspicion of polycystic kidney disease, sickle cell trait and disease, nephrolithiasis, various glomerular diseases, tuberculosis, and benign familial

hematuria. The combination of renal failure, deafness, and hematuria suggests Alport's hereditary nephritis.

B. Physical Examination. Examination should focus on signs of systemic disease (e.g., fever, rash, lymphadenopathy, joint swelling, and abdominal or pelvic mass) and underlying medical or renal disease (e.g., hypertension, peripheral and generalized edema). Multiple telangiectasias and mucous membrane lesions indicate hereditary hemorrhagic telangiectasia (Rendu-Osler-Weber disease). The finding of an abdominal mass may indicate Wilms' tumor in children and abdominal cancer and aneurysm in adults. On rectal and genitourinary examination, one can find signs of prostatitis, prostate hypertrophy, prostate cancer, vaginal and urethral changes, and pelvic masses.

C. Testing

1. Laboratory testing initially begins with examining a freshly voided, clean catch urine sample by a dipstick. It is important to confirm hematuria by a microscopic examination of the urine sediment. This sediment is obtained by centrifugation of a fixed volume of urine (5 mL) for 5 minutes at 3,000 rotations/min. Afterward, the supernatant is poured off, and the remaining sediment is resuspended in the centrifuge tube by gently tapping the bottom of the tube. A pipette is used to sample the residual fluid and transfer it to a glass slide, and a cover slip is applied to the slide for microscopic evaluation (3). The specimen is examined under high magnification (400×) to determine cell type and distinct morphologic features. Results are recorded as the number of red blood cells per high-power field. If a patient is asymptomatic and has no particular risk factors, two additional urine analyses should be obtained. If one of them is abnormal, it is necessary to proceed with further workup. For those asymptomatic patients with one to two red blood cells/high-power field and risk factors for significant underlying disease, consider full urologic evaluation (1). When the dipstick testing is positive for blood, but urine microscopy reveals no red blood cells, hemoglobinuria or myoglobinuria should be considered. The use of a benzidine dipstick allows the differentiation of these discolorations from those of hematuria and myoglobinuria. As a next step, a urine culture can be obtained to rule out an infection. The urine could also be sent for cytology to assess for abnormal cells.

2. Blood tests include a renal panel and a complete blood count with differential, sedimentation rate, prothrombin time, and partial thromboplastin time. Any further evaluation is highly dependent on the suspected cause. Further blood tests may include serum complement titer (significant if low), antistreptolysin-O titer (significant if high), antinuclear antibody and extended panels with anti-deoxyribonuclease B titer (significant if high), and hemoglobin electrophoresis.

3. A tuberculin skin test or chest x-ray can be done to detect tuberculosis. Upper urinary tract workup such as intravenous pyelogram (limited sensitivity for small renal lesions), abdominal and pelvic ultrasound (limited ability to detect solid tumors that are less than 3 cm), computed tomography (high sensitivity for renal calculi and small lesions), or magnetic resonance imaging (high cost and not widely supported in the literature) (3) may detect benign conditions such as urolithiasis, obstructive uropathy, renal cysts, parenchymal abnormalities, and nonurinary tract lesions, as well as malignancies of various anatomic areas. Abnormalities of the urethra and bladder maybe found using cystoscopy. Biopsies of various areas, as well as invasive vascular studies, may be necessary. At any time during an evaluation, it remains within the physician's judgment to refer the patient to a subspecialist.

IV. DIAGNOSIS. The keys to the diagnosis of hematuria are the clinical history and the physical examination. Laboratory and imaging studies only aid to confirm or rule out initial suspicions. The goal is to diagnose a variety of serious illnesses, including malignancies and renal parenchymal diseases. In general, the degree of hematuria is of little diagnostic or prognostic value (4). As little as 1 mL of blood can cause a visible color change. In addition, a variety of drugs, foods, and food coloring can discolor the urine. Also, it is necessary to remember that transient hematuria, especially in a young individual, is quite common and rarely indicative of significant pathology (5). When present in patients older than 40 years, however, transient hematuria warrants a comprehensive evaluation to rule out malignancy. Similarly, a diagnostic workup should be performed when persistent hematuria is found in patients of any age. A summary of the best practice policy recommendations by the American Urologic Association can be obtained from the article "Asymptomatic Microscopic Hematuria in Adults (1)." It contains an excellent flowchart of the workup of asymptomatic microscopic hematuria plus a strategy to identify patients with significant disease, while minimizing cost and morbidity associated with unnecessary tests.

Repeat evaluations are indicated for those patients with a negative evaluation and in whom a malignancy is suspected (mainly older adults). A reasonable time frame appears to be 3–6 months for less invasive tests and 1–5 years for more invasive tests (6, 7).

Other clinical manifestations should also be considered. Until otherwise proven, painless gross hematuria in the absence of infection in elderly men is caused by malignancy, just as hematuria associated with "sterile" pyuria is caused by genitourinary tuberculosis or interstitial nephritis. Finally, other medical problems such as prostate hypertrophy, diabetes mellitus (nephrosclerosis), nephrolithiasis, trauma (including vigorous masturbation), previous urinary tract malignancies with recurrence, and sickle cell disease (papillary necrosis) may cause hematuria.

REFERENCES

1. Grossfeld GD, Wolf JS Jr, Litwan MS, et al. Asymptomatic microscopic hematuria in adults: summary of the AUA best practice policy recommendations. *Am Fam Physician* 2001;63(6):1145–1154.
2. Yun EJ, Meng MV, Carroll PR. Evaluation of the patient with hematuria. *Med Clin North Am* 2004;88(2):329–343.
3. McDonald MM, Swagerty D, Wetzel L. Assessment of microscopic hematuria in adults. *Am Fam Physician* 2006;73(10):1748–1754.
4. Thaller TR, Wang LP. Evaluation of asymptomatic microscopic hematuria in adults. *Am Fam Physician* 1999;64(4):1143–1152, 1154.
5. Murakami S, Igarashi T, Hara S, Shimazaki J. Strategies for asymptomatic microscopic hematuria: a prospective study of 1,034 patients. *J Urol* 1990;144(1):99–101.
6. Messing EM, Young TB, Hunt VB, et al. Hematuria home screening: repeat testing results. *J Urol* 1995;154(1):57–61.
7. Loo R, Whittaker J, Rabrenivich V. National practice recommendations for hematuria: how to evaluate in the absence of strong evidence? *Perm J* 2009;13(1):37–46, PMCID: 3034463.

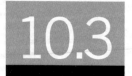

10.3 Erectile Dysfunction

Louis Kuritzky and Michel B. Diab

I. BACKGROUND. Erectile dysfunction (ED), previously commonly labeled "impotence," defined as the consistent inability to get or maintain an erection sufficient for intercourse, is in essence a patient-defined diagnosis (1,2). The role of the clinician is to confirm ED, rule out correctable secondary causes, and expeditiously restore sexual function. To encourage hopefulness, clinicians would do well to explain at the outset that essentially 100% of men can have restoration of sexual function using currently available treatments.

II. PATHOPHYSIOLOGY. The most recent large epidemiologic survey of American men found some degree of impotence in 52% of men older than 40 years of age. Most organic ED is on a vascular basis. Because integrity of the endothelium is necessary to provide adequate penile engorgement, disorders that cause endothelial dysfunction are predictably associated with ED. Diabetes, smoking, hypertension, dyslipidemia, and peripheral vascular disease are all associated with impaired endothelial function and may hence induce or contribute to ED. Whether the correction of these pathogenic vasculopathic factors improves erectile function in men with ED remains to be determined. Studies that have looked at global implementation of cardiovascular risk factor reduction (i.e., weight loss, blood pressure control, lipid control, diet modulation, smoking cessation, and exercise in combination) have shown improvements in erectile function, although it is difficult to ascertain—due to the combination of interventions—which specific intervention(s) can be confirmed to be efficacious.

III. EVALUATION
A. History
1. Although written questionnaires may elicit sexual dysfunction, most patients prefer to communicate such issues in the privacy of verbal communication with their primary care provider. Initial inquiry can simply be "Are you sexually active?" For sexual dysfunction evaluation, gender orientation is not relevant to diagnosis or therapy, so that whether the patient is homosexual, heterosexual, or bisexual has no distinct bearing on the diagnostic or therapeutic direction. For individuals who are not sexually active, the next inquiry should be to determine whether this is a matter of choice or due to an obstacle that prevents sexual activity (e.g., lack of partner, impotence, and physical disorder).
2. For individuals who are sexually active, a series of follow-up questions uncovers most relevant psychosexual pathology. You could begin with "How would you rate your sex life on a scale of 1 to 10?" If the response is 10, sexual dysfunction is decidedly unlikely. However, most individuals respond "Oh, about a 7." You can follow with, "What would have to be different to change your sex life from a 7 to a 10?" This forced-choice inquiry often produces responses that directly indicate problematic underlying issues such as "Well, if I could just get a good erection" or "If my erection could last >30 seconds." Inquiry about libido is a crucial diagnostic point for testosterone deficiency. Men who present with good libido only have a remote possibility of having testosterone deficiency. Although testosterone enhances response of nitric oxide synthase, and hence can augment the response to erectogenic stimuli, testosterone is not necessary to have erections. Most experts suggest routine measurement of testosterone, nonetheless.
3. A medication history should be taken. Most medication-induced ED is evident by the temporal relationship between the onset of ED and medication initiation. On the other hand, agents such as thiazides may produce ED after months of use. Similarly, some antidepressants may produce sexual dysfunction early or after weeks of therapy. Relationship of medications to ED can often be clarified by a drug holiday.

B. Physical Examination.
Although physical examination is usually not enlightening, there is general agreement that the genitals should be examined for evidence of overt testicular atrophy and the penis for Peyronie's disease. Peyronie's disease produces palpable plaques in the corpora cavernosa that can lead to angulation upon erection, pain, or both. Treatment is surgical. A rectal examination to document rectal sensation as well as tone can be complemented by the bulbocavernosus reflex. This reflex is elicited by briskly squeezing the glans penis in one hand while a single digit from the other is in the rectum. A normal examination, indicating an intact reflex arc, is manifest as a rectal contraction in response to the glans squeeze. Prostate examination is pertinent at this point, in the event testosterone therapy is required.

C. Testing.
Reasonable screening tests for ED include plasma glucose, lipid profile (seeking vasculopathic risk factors), total morning testosterone, and a urinalysis. If total morning testosterone is low, luteinizing hormone (LH) and follicle-stimulating hormone (FSH) levels should be measured, because an increase in these indicates gonadal failure, for which testosterone replacement is indicated; a normal or decreased LH/FSH indicates potential hypothalamic or pituitary insufficiency, necessitating central nervous system (CNS) imaging to rule out a mass lesion. Recently, expert consensus guidance has suggested that because some midlife males do not respond with a vigorous LH or FSH elevation to testicular failure, only men with distinctively low testosterone levels (<150 ng/dL) and nonelevated LH/FSH require CNS imaging.

Similarly, testosterone may be suppressed by an elevated prolactin, whether induced by a CNS lesion, hypothyroidism, medications, or other factors. A low (or low-normal) total testosterone should be repeated and confirmed; equivocal total morning testosterone levels should be further clarified by means of measuring the free testosterone, sex hormone binding globulin or both.

IV. DIAGNOSIS

A. Differential Diagnosis. ED is broadly divided into psychogenic and organic categories, although there is often a substantial degree of overlap. Men who report sudden, complete loss of sexual function, or "circumstantial" ED: (i) good function with one partner, but not another; (ii) good erections with masturbation but not with a partner; (iii) good morning erections, but not with a partner, are much more likely to have psychogenic ED. Because organic ED generally leads to psychological consequences, many patients suffer a combination of psychogenic and organic ED.

B. Clinical Manifestations

1. Psychogenic ED may reflect depression, relationship conflict, performance anxiety, or partner-directed hostility. The history is definitive in most cases. Sudden complete loss of function, situation or partner variability, along with maintenance of morning or masturbatory erections, is typical. Occasionally, patients with dysfunctions other than ED seek advice; for instance, mistaking premature ejaculation for ED. In such cases, corrective education combined with appropriate attention to the alternate diagnosis is the logical next step.

2. Organic sexual dysfunction is characterized by incremental loss of erectile function. In middle age, men with organic ED note reduced erectile turgidity, increasing requirement for tactile stimulation to produce an erection, and a lengthening refractory period (i.e., the amount of time required after ejaculation before the male is receptive to restimulation and erection). Such stepwise loss of sexual function corroborates organicity.

3. In primary care, as many as 98% of patients have no correctable cause of impotence discerned after appropriate history and physical examination. This is not to say that hypertension, diabetes, and dyslipidemia are not remediable, but rather that correction of such risk factors has not been confirmed to ameliorate ED. Additionally, the presence of such additional risk factors need not delay the immediate provision of highly effective oral agents (PDES inhibitor [phosphodiesterase type 5 inhibitors]), Tadalafil 5 mg daily (3), vacuum constriction devices, or intra-corporeal injection, any of which may be provided in the primary care setting. However, before providing *any* tool which can restore sexual function, clinicians should be confident that the patient's cardiovascular status is sufficient that vigorous physical activity—sexual activity, exercise, or work exertion—is safe. In general, an adult who can tolerate 4 mets of activity (brisk walking) can safely engage in other vigorous activities such as sexual activity. Patients who fail to respond to the standard treatment tools should be referred (4).

REFERENCES

1. Kuritzky L. Primary care issues in the management of erectile dysfunction. In: Seftel AD, ed. *Male and female sexual dysfunction*. Edinburgh: Mosby, 2004:1–15.
2. Kuritzky L, Ahmed O, Kosch S. Management of impotence in primary care. *Comp Ther* 1998;24(3):137–146.
3. Egerdie RB, Auerbach S, Roehrborn CG, et al. Tadalafil 2.5 mgor 5 mg administration once a daily for 12 weeks in men with both erectile dysfunction and symptoms of benign prostatic hyperplasia: results of a randomized, placebo-controlled, double blind study. *J Sex Med* 2012:9:271–281.
4 Gupta BP, Murad HM, Clifton MM, Prokop L, Nehra A, Kopecky SL. The effect of lifestyle modification and cardiovascular risk factor reduction on erectile dysfunction a systematic review and meta-analysis. *Arch Intern Med* 2011;171(20):1797–1803. doi:10.1001/archintemmed.2011.440

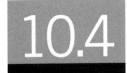

Urinary Incontinence
Richard Rathe and David M. Quillen

I. **BACKGROUND.** Urinary incontinence (UI) is defined by the International Continence Society as the "complaint of involuntary loss of urine." Rates of UI increase with age and are as high as 34% in women and 11% in men (1). It is a major cause of social withdrawal and loss of independent living. Patients are often too embarrassed to discuss this problem, even with their physician. Some even view it as a natural part of aging, but this is not the case. UI is a symptom, not a disease. Understanding the types of disorders that cause incontinence is the key to correct diagnosis and effective treatment (2–5).

A. **Definition.** UI is the involuntary loss of urine.

B. **Classification.** The classification of UI is presented in Table 10.4.1.

C. **UI can be acute or chronic.**
   1. Acute causes include
      a. infection
      b. medications
      c. delirium
      d. exacerbation of systemic diseases (e.g., diabetes mellitus, diabetes insipidus, congestive heart failure, or stroke)

TABLE 10.4.1   Types of Incontinence

Type	Definition	Mechanism	Disorders
Urge	Inability to delay voiding once the urge occurs	Detrusor hyperactivity	Idiopathic (common in the elderly)
			Genitourinary conditions (cystitis, stones)
Stress	Loss of urine with increased abdominal pressure	Sphincter failure	Weak or injured pelvic muscles
			Sphincter weakness
Overflow	Partial retention of urine behind an obstruction	Outlet obstruction	Obstruction (prostate, cystocele)
		Loss of innervation	Neuropathic (diabetes, nerve injury)
Functionality	Inability to get to the toilet	Physical or cognitive impairment	Dementia or delirium
			Physical limitations (lack of mobility)
			Psychological or behavioral causes
Mixed	Any combination of the above		

    2. Chronic conditions that are associated with UI fall into two categories:
      a. local
        i. pelvic floor weakness following childbirth
        ii. bladder tumor or deformity
        iii. tumors
        iv. obstruction by an enlarged prostate or cystocele
        v. postsurgic
      b. systemic
        i. menopause
        ii. neuropathy (diabetes, alcoholism)
        iii. dementia
        iv. depression
        v. stroke
        vi. tumor
        vii. Parkinson's disease

  D. The DRIP mnemonic is often cited as a way to remember the reversible (and curable) causes of UI:
    1. D: Delirium and drugs
    2. R: Restricted mobility and retention
    3. I: Infection, inflammation, and (fecal) impaction
    4. P: Polyuria from uncontrolled diabetes and other conditions

II. EVALUATION

  A. History
    1. Voiding History. It is important to fully characterize the patient's problem by taking a detailed history, including the duration of the symptoms, timing of voluntary or involuntary voiding, amounts voided involuntarily, and the relationship to voluntary voiding. Focus on the following areas:
      a. Need for pads or diapers (measure of severity)
      b. Loss of urine with coughing or laughing (suggests stress type)
      c. Inability to hold urine after having the urge to urinate (suggests urge type)
      d. Pain or discomfort (suggests infection or inflammation)
      e. Inability to fully empty bladder (suggests obstruction)
      f. Decreased urinary stream (suggests obstruction)
      g. What impact does UI have on the patient's life?
      h. What does the patient think is going on?
    2. Major Medical Problems.
      a. Does the patient have any known condition that is associated with UI?
        i. Diabetes
        ii. Heart failure
        iii. Menopause
        iv. Neurologic problems
      b. Does the patient have other genitourinary symptoms? In female patients, be sure to take a detailed obstetric history.
    3. Medication History. Since medications are a major cause of incontinence, a thorough medication history is essential. Offending agents include
      a. Diuretics
      b. Older antidepressants
      c. Antihypertensives
      d. Narcotics
      e. Alcohol
    4. Special Concern. Central and nephrogenic diabetes insipidus can present with UI because of increased urine output (many liters per day). These patients frequently have

a concomitant polydipsia that closely matches their water loss. Consider this diagnosis when the patient gives a history of voiding large volumes of urine.

B. Physical Examination. The physical examination is often normal in cases of UI. Focus efforts in an attempt to uncover the underlying cause(s):

1. **General.** Is the patient physically capable of getting to the toilet?
2. **Mental Status.** Can the patient understand and act on the urge to void?
3. **Neurologic**, including the anal reflex; focal signs suggest a neurologic cause.
4. **Abdominal Examination.** Is the bladder distended?
5. **Rectal or Prostate.** Does the patient have a fecal impaction or an enlarged prostate?
6. **Pelvic Examination.** Look for atrophic vaginitis, uterine prolapse, or a pelvic mass.

C. Testing

1. **Voiding Journal.** A voiding journal is a good way to get additional information about the patient's problem. Have the patient record the time and approximate amount of each voiding, and whether they were wet or dry.
2. **Urinalysis.** Be cautious when interpreting the urine analysis; in the absence of other symptoms, bacteriuria is seldom the primary cause of UI. Treat cystitis or urethritis when the rest of the clinical picture confirms them. Unexplained, persistent microhematuria requires investigation.
3. **Postvoiding Urine Volume.** The patient should be catheterized immediately after voiding. In general, the postvoid urine volume should be less than 50 mL. Volumes in the range of 100–200 mL may suggest impaired bladder contractility or obstruction. Volumes greater than 200 mL strongly suggest obstruction.
4. **Blood Urea Nitrogen, Creatinine, and Glucose** are simple blood tests that help rule out underlying renal disease and diabetes.
5. **Special tests** are available via urologic consultation to further delineate the cause of UI. These include cystoscopy, cystometry, and other voiding studies. Up to two-thirds of patients can be successfully treated without urologic referral.

III. DIAGNOSIS. The clinical history is the most important factor leading to the correct diagnosis and successful treatment of UI. However, it is an imperfect tool at best. In one review, clinical history had a sensitivity and specificity for stress incontinence of 0.90 and 0.50, respectively. For detrusor instability, the figures were 0.74 and 0.55, respectively (2).

The task becomes even more problematic when considering the reluctance of patients to talk about their symptoms and the tendency for UI to be of a mixed type. Response to therapy (or lack thereof) often drives the practical management of this condition. Lack of response to multiple trials of therapy is a good indication for consulting a urologist. Remember that your initial assessment will often be incorrect, so keep an open mind and consider all possible diagnoses. Finally, recall that UI frequently involves more than one causal factor. For example, many elderly people have a functional component (can't get to the toilet quickly) in addition to one of the other types.

REFERENCES

1. Fong E, Nitti VW. Urinary incontinence. *Prim Care* 2010;37(3):599–612, ix.
2. Jensen JR, Nielsen FR, Ostergard DR. The role of patient history in the diagnosis of urinary incontinence. *Obstet Gynecol* 1994;83(5):904–910.
3. Finding Out about Incontinence. AAFP patient information handout. *Am Fam Physician* 1998;57(11):2688–2690.
4. Goode PS, Burgio KL. Pharmacologic treatment of lower urinary tract dysfunction in geriatric patients. *Am J Med Sci* 1997;314(4):262–267.
5. Weiss BD. Diagnostic evaluation of urinary incontinence in geriatric patients. *Am Fam Physician* 1998;57(11):2665–2687.

10.5 Nocturia
Umar Ghaffar

I. BACKGROUND. Nocturia is defined as the need for an individual to wake up one or more times from sleep during the night to void. The prevalence of nocturia increases with age, ranging from 4% in children aged 7–15 years to approximately 70% in patients >60 years of age. Although the prevalence of nocturia does increase with age, it would be difficult to conclude that nocturia is a normal part of aging, because it is not universally present in all older adults. The clinical significance of nocturia has been increasingly recognized because of its association with reduced quality of life and increased morbidity and mortality (1–3).

II. PATHOPHYSIOLOGY. The pathophysiology of nocturia is complex and multifactorial. A number of conditions can result in alteration of more than one regulatory pathway controlling normal voiding. The underlying pathophysiology may depend on some conditions being purely mechanical and for others may involve complex neurohormonal mechanisms. Atrial natriuretic peptide (ANP) and vasopressin appear to be two of the known hormones associated with pathophysiology of some conditions resulting in nocturia.

A. The etiology of nocturia can be divided into four main categories:
   1. Diurnal Polyuria. A continuous overproduction of urine, not limited only to sleep hours, with a 24-hour urine output of more than 40 mL/kg. Diurnal polyuria may be related to either **free water diuresis** or to **osmotic diuresis**.
      a. Free water diuresis.
         i. Diabetes insipidus (DI): Defect in production of arginine vasopressin (AVP; central DI) or impaired response to AVP, medications, hereditary (nephrogenic DI)
         ii. Gestational DI
         iii. Primary polydipsia
      b. Osmotic dieresis
         i. Diabetes mellitus
         ii. Medications
               Sorbitol and mannitol
               Diuretics (multiple mechanisms)
               Lithium
               Calcium channel blockers (variable affect)
               Selective serotonin re-uptake inhibitor (SSRI)
         iii. AVP suppression caused by low calcium and potassium
   2. Nocturnal Polyuria. This is defined as an increase in nighttime urine production with a corresponding decrease in daytime urine production, resulting in a normal 24-hour urine production
      a. Nocturnal Polyuria Syndrome. This is thought to be caused by a lack of normal diurnal variation in the production of urine and lack of nocturnal AVP level increase, which occurs normally.
      b. Edema-Forming States. CHF, chronic kidney disease (CKD), hypoalbulinemia, chronic liver disease, venous insufficiency, enhanced ANP release resulting from a redistribution and mobilization of fluid and solute at night.
      c. Obstructive Sleep Apnea (OSA). AVP production through hypoxic-induced vasoconstriction.
      d. Alzheimer Disease. Loss of circadian AVP release.
      e. Medications. Tetracycline AVP inhibition.
      f. Behavioral. Excessive late night fluid intake, late evening diuretic usage.
   3. Reduced Bladder Capacity. This includes
      a. Overactive bladder, e.g., detrusor over- or underactivity

    b. Reduced bladder capacity due to benign prostatic hypertrophy, bladder cancer, neurogenic bladder, tuberculosis, interstitial cystitis

    c. Others, e.g., infection, stones, pelvic floor laxity

    d. Medications, e.g., SSRIs

    e. Fecal impaction

    f. Obstetric or gynecologic disease

  4. Mixed Nocturia. A significant number of nocturia patients may have more than one etiology for their symptoms, and therefore a thorough history taking is crucial.

    a. History. A comprehensive history should be elicited to obtain information regarding any of the above-mentioned conditions that would contribute toward nocturia.

      i. History of: Lower urinary tract symptoms (e.g., urgency, hesitancy, straining, and feeling of incomplete bladder evacuation) that may suggest bladder storage/capacity-related issues.

      ii. History of: Symptoms related to conditions resulting in diurnal polyuria, e.g., diabetes mellitus, DI, CKD.

      iii. Conditions causing edema-forming state (CHF, chronic liver disease (CLD), hypoalbulinemia)

      iv. Underlying neurologic disorders (prior cerebrovascular accident (CVA), Alzheimer's spinal cord injuries)

      v. Attention should be paid to daily fluid intake schedule, baseline voiding pattern and changes therein, severity of nocturia, sleep pattern, and quality

      vi. Use of frequently used medications such as diuretics, SSRIs, tetracycline, and calcium channel blockers as well as their time of dosing should be sought.

III. EVALUATION

  A. Physical Exam. *A thorough system-wise approach is warranted*:

    1. General vitals: include body weight (obesity contributing to OSA) and orthostatic blood pressure (possibly indicating autonomic dysfunction).

    2. Cardiopulmonary exam: Should focus on clues to CHF, OSA, and edema-forming states.

    3. Abdominal exam: bladder distention, prostate enlargement, ascites, rectal exam for sphincter laxity, tumors, impaction, and signs of spinal cord damage, each pointing toward a specific etiology.

    4. Neurologic exam: general appearance and visual field testing to evaluate for pituitary or endocrine dysfunction.

  B. Testing

    1. Labs including

      a. Urinalysis by dipstick

      b. Urine culture

      c. Selected cases: microscopy may identify a urologic cause

      d. Elevated PSA may point toward a prostatic etiology

      e. Blood urea nitrogen (BUN), creatinine, and electrolytes can help in evaluating for renal disease as well as hypercalcemia

      f. Serum glucose and osmolality and urine electrolytes and water deprivation tests can identify diabetes mellitus or DI

      g. Liver function tests (LFTs) and albumin can be obtained for liver function

    2. Postvoid residual volume measurement can help distinguish bladder outlet obstruction or neurogenic bladder.

    3. Urodynamic studies although very helpful require interpretation by specialists.

IV. DIAGNOSIS. The key to diagnosis of the etiology of nocturia in a given patients is:

  A. Obtaining a thorough history and physical exam.

  B. Identifying other medical conditions and an accurate medication history will often give a strong clue toward the underlying pathology.

  C. Identifying the pattern of normal baseline voiding.

  D. Identifying the pattern of fluid intake, frequency and severity of nocturia.

  E. Appropriate diagnostic testing.

  F. Referral to a urological specialist may, however, be required in some cases for further evaluation with urodynamic studies and cystoscopy.

REFERENCES

1. Boongird S, Shah N, Nolin TD, Unruh ML. Nocturia and aging: diagnosis and treatment. *Adv Chronic Kidney Dis* 2010;17(4):e27–e40.
2. Jin MH, Moon du G. Practical management of nocturia in urology. *Indian J Urol* 2008;24(3): 289–294.
3. Pressman MR, Figueroa WG, Kendrick-Mohamed J, Greenspon LW, Peterson DD. Nocturia. A rarely recognized symptom of sleep apnea and other occult sleep disorders. *Arch Intern Med* 1996;156(5):545–550.

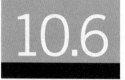

10.6 Oliguria and Anuria

Deepa J. Borde and George P. Samraj

I. BACKGROUND

A. Oliguria is defined as urine volume less than 400 mL/d or less than 0.5 mL/kg/h over a 6-hour period in adults and children and less than 1 mL/kg/h in infants (1, 2). While anuria is defined as the total absence of urine, in the clinical setting, a patient with a urine output of less than 50–100 mL/24 h is considered to be anuric. The presence of oliguria signifies a renal insult that has led to a marked decrease in the glomerular filtration rate (GFR), causing increased urea and creatinine levels and subsequent water and sodium retention. While oliguria is typically one of the earliest manifestations of acute kidney injury (AKI), it often occurs before changes in serum creatinine. However, not all patients with AKI demonstrate oliguria.

B. Patients presenting to the office setting with acute oliguria should be hospitalized due to the risk of developing potentially fatal complications such as hyperkalemia (manifested by weakness or paralysis and electrocardiogram changes), fluid overload, metabolic acidosis, and pericarditis (1). Fortunately, the prognosis of oliguria that develops outside the hospital is typically good if treated early as it is typically due to one cause (3): dehydration. Hospital-acquired oliguria and AKI, however, carry a worse prognosis because the cause is often multifactorial leading to more severe and permanent renal injury (4).

II. PATHOPHYSIOLOGY

A. **Oliguria.** The cause of oliguria is (1) prerenal, (2) renal (intrinsic), or (3) postrenal (see Table 10.6.1).

1. **Prerenal** causes are due to renal hypoperfusion resulting in a decrease in GFR. Often, renal function recovers with prompt treatment of the underlying cause (5).

2. **Renal** disorders are characterized by structural damage to the kidney parenchyma itself and are categorized based on the location of injury. The most common cause of renal AKI is acute tubular necrosis, which is typically due to ischemia or nephrotoxins.

3. **Postrenal** disorders are a result of obstruction in the urinary tract anywhere from the renal pelvis down to the urethra. In order to develop oliguria, however, upper tract obstruction must be bilateral or occur in patients with a solitary kidney. The absence of oliguria does not rule out partial or intermittent obstruction; these patients often have normal or even elevated urine output (6). In children, congenital ureteral or urethral strictures or valves predominate as a cause of obstruction while malignancy, benign prostatic hypertrophy, and calculi are the most common causes of obstructive uropathy in adults (5).

B. Anuria is most commonly a result of complete bilateral urinary tract obstruction or shock. Other more rare causes of anuria include hemolytic uremic syndrome, bilateral renal cortical necrosis, bilateral renal arterial or venous obstruction, and rapidly

TABLE 10.6.1	Causes of Acute Oliguria

Prerenal	Renal	Postrenal
Hypovolemia	Acute GN	Upper tract obstruction
Hemorrhage	Postinfectious GN	Intrinsic
GI loss (including nasogastric suction)	Endocarditis-associated GN	Nephrolithiasis
Diuretics	Systemic vasculitis	Papillary necrosis
Glucosuria	Rapidly progressive GN	Blood clots
Cutaneous loss (burns or sweat)	Membranoproliferative GN	Malignancy
Third spacing (burns, peritonitis, pancreatitis, trauma)	Mesangial proliferative GN	Extrinsic
	IgA nephropathy	Retroperitoneal fibrosis
		Malignancy
Decreased effective blood volume	Acute interstitial nephritis	Endometriosis
Sepsis	Drug-induced (penicillins, cephalosporins, sulfonamides, rifampin, phenytoin, furosemide, PPIs, and NSAIDs)	AAA
Congestive heart failure		Lower tract obstruction
Cirrhosis		Bladder
Nephrotic syndrome	Pyelonephritis	Neurogenic bladder
Vasodilatory drugs	Malignancy	TCC
Anaphylaxis		Blood clots
Anesthetic drugs		Bladder calculus
		Prostate
		Prostate cancer
		BPH
		Urethra
		Stricture
		Phimosis
		Urethral valves
		Urinary catheter
		Obstructed
		Kinked
		Misplaced
Decreased cardiac output	Acute tubular necrosis	
Myocardial infarction	Ischemic (sustained prerenal injury)	
Pulmonary embolus	Nephrotoxic (aminoglycosides, radiocontrast media, hemolysis, rhabdomyolysis, amphotericin, cisplatin, ifosfamide, acetaminophen)	
Cardiac tamponade		
Mechanical ventilation		
Impaired renal perfusion	Acute vascular disease	
ACE inhibitors	Bilateral renal artery stenosis, thrombosis, embolism, or dissecting aneurysm	
NSAIDs		
Intrarenal vasoconstriction	Atheroembolic disease	
Hypercalcemia	HELLP syndrome	
Hepatorenal	Malignant hypertension	
	TTP	
	Hemolytic uremic syndrome	

(Continued)

TABLE 10.6.1	Causes of Acute Oliguria *(Continued)*	
Prerenal	**Renal**	**Postrenal**
	Acute intratubular obstruction	
	Paraprotein (multiple myeloma)	
	Crystalline (ethylene glycol ingestion, tumor lysis, acyclovir, methotrexate)	

AAA, abdominal aortic aneurysm; ACE, angiotensin-converting enzyme; BPH, benign prostatic hypertrophy; GI, gastrointestinal; GN, glomerulonephritis; HELLP, hemolysis, elevated liver enzymes, and low platelets; IgA, immunoglobulin A; NSAIDs, nonsteroidal anti-inflammatory drugs; PPI, proton pump inhibitor; TCC, transitional cell carcinoma; TTP, thrombotic thrombocytopenic purpura.

progressive glomerulonephritis (7). In patients with an indwelling catheter prior to the development of anuria, catheter blockage, kinks, and malposition must be ruled out prior to initiating an extensive workup.

III. EVALUATION

  A. **History.** Patients with oliguria may or may not report decreased urine output, but may report other symptoms that can help to discern the cause of their illness.

   1. Does the patient report symptoms of dehydration or bleeding that would lead to prerenal causes of AKI? Nausea and vomiting may be present, either as a result of gastrointestinal illness or as symptoms of uremia. Other uremic symptoms include anorexia, fatigue, confusion, pruritus, and even seizures. Diarrhea, bleeding, dyspnea, lower extremity edema, or diuretic use may indicate a prerenal cause of oliguria.

   2. Does the patient report symptoms of voiding dysfunction or pelvic or retroperitoneal disease pointing to an obstructive cause of oliguria?

   3. Does the patient have a history of recent travel, occupational hazards, or new medications, specifically antibiotics or over-the-counter nonsteroidal anti-inflammatory drug use that could lead to a renal cause of AKI? Does the patient have any recent exposure to radiocontrast agents, episodes of prolonged hypotension, or angiographic studies involving the aorta?

  B. **Physical Examination.** After review of the patient's vital signs, including orthostatics where indicated, the patient should be evaluated for physical signs of volume depletion or fluid overload. A thorough abdominal exam should be performed to evaluate for bladder distension and renal artery bruits and consideration should be given to performing a pelvic exam if a pelvic mass is suspected or rectal exam if the history indicates prostate enlargement. A careful skin exam may reveal purpura consistent with vasculitis, livedo reticularis indicating atheroembolic disease, or rash consistent with interstitial nephritis.

  C. **Laboratory Tests**

   1. **Urinalysis** is typically normal in prerenal causes of oliguria, but hyaline and fine granular casts may be present in the urine sediment and the specific gravity may be elevated. In renal causes, on the other hand, examination of the urine sediment is quite useful, often revealing brown granular casts and tubular epithelial cells in patients with acute tubular necrosis and dysmorphic red blood cells and red cell casts in those with glomerulonephritis. White blood cells or casts and eosinophils are present in the urine sediment in patients with interstitial nephritis, and crystalluria or proteinuria in those with intratubular obstruction.

   2. **Urinary Indices**. Table 10.6.2 outlines the use of urinary indices to differentiate prerenal, renal, and postrenal etiologies of oliguria. In prerenal AKI, the kidneys respond

Table 10.6.2	Initial Laboratory Testing for Oliguria		
	Prerenal	Renal	Postrenal
Serum BUN:creatinine	>20:1	<20:1	>20:1
Fractional excretion sodium (%)	<1	>1	Variable
Urine sodium (mmol/L)	<20	>40	>20
Fractional excretion urea (%)	<35	<60	

BUN, blood urea nitrogen.

to hypoperfusion by retaining sodium in order to retain water. Thus, the fractional excretion of sodium (FENa) in prerenal causes of oliguria is typically less than 1%. There are two main instances of prerenal AKI in which compensatory sodium reabsorption is impaired leading to a FENa that is greater than 1%: diuretic therapy and chronic kidney disease patients who develop a prerenal state. In patients on diuretic therapy, the fractional excretion of urea is a more useful measure, typically being less than 35% (8). There are two renal causes of AKI in which the FENa is less than 1%: contrast nephropathy and pigment nephropathy (due to rhabdomyolysis or hemolysis).

   D. **Diagnostic Testing.** An indwelling urinary catheter is useful as a diagnostic tool, for accurate urine volume measurement, and also for treatment in cases of lower urinary tract obstruction. Patients suspected of having obstructive uropathy should have a bladder scan or urinary catheter placement after voiding to obtain measurement of postvoid residual (PVR). A PVR of greater than 100 mL is indicative of bladder outlet obstruction. Upper tract obstruction may be evaluated with renal ultrasound or renal protocol computed tomography. A careful intravenous fluid trial can be used as a diagnostic tool in patients suspected of having prerenal AKI. Renal causes of oliguria are in rare instances diagnosed by renal biopsy.

IV. **DIAGNOSIS.** Early recognition of oliguria and, more importantly, anuria is critical because it affords the clinician an opportunity to diagnose AKI at an earlier stage, thereby facilitating prompt treatment and prevention of permanent renal dysfunction (9). Hospitalization is usually necessary to treat the life-threatening complications of AKI. A thorough history and physical exam, evaluation of the serum blood urea nitrogen to creatinine ratio, the urine sediment, FENa, and renal ultrasound often lead to an accurate diagnosis.

REFERENCES

1. Klahr S, Miller SB. Acute oliguria. *N Engl J Med* 1998;338:671–675.
2. Behrman RE, Kliegman RM, eds. *Nelson essentials of pediatrics*, 4th ed. Philadelphia, PA: WB Saunders, 2002.
3. Feest TG, Round A, Hamad S. Incidence of severe acute renal failure in adults: results of a community based study. *BMJ* 1993;306:481–483.
4. Elasy TA, Anderson RJ. Changing demography of acute renal failure. *Semin Dial* 1996;9:438–443.
5. Khalil P, Murthy P, Palevsky PM. The patient with acute kidney injury. *Prim Care Clin Office Pract* 2008;35:239–264.
6. Klahr S. Pathophysiology of obstructive nephropathy. *Kidney Int* 1983;23:414–426.
7. Rose BD. *Pathophysiology of renal disease*, 2nd ed. New York, NY: McGraw-Hill, 1987.
8. Carvounis CP, Nisar S, Guro-Razuman S. Significance of the fractional excretion of urea in the differential diagnosis of acute renal failure. *Kidney Int* 2002;62:2223–2229.
9. Macedo E, Malhotra R, Bouchard J, Wynn SK, Mehta RL. Oliguria is an early predictor of higher mortality in critically ill patients. *Kidney Int* 2011;80:760–767.

10.7 Priapism

David B. Feller

I. BACKGROUND. Priapism is defined as a persistent, often painful, penile erection not associated with sexual stimulation. No time course is specifically defined, but priapism is usually diagnosed when the erection lasts greater than 4 hours. Although relatively uncommon (incidence 1.5 per 100,000 person-years and 2.9 per 100,000 person-years for men aged 40 years and older) (1), priapism often represents a urologic emergency (2).

II. PATHOPHYSIOLOGY

A. Etiology. Two types of priapism (low flow or veno-occlusive and high flow or arterial) have been described based on the underlying precipitating event (3). Arterial priapism usually occurs after injury to the cavernous artery from perineal or direct penile trauma. This injury then leads to uncontrolled high arterial inflow within the corpora cavernosa. Veno-occlusive priapism is characterized by inadequate outflow and is far and away the most common. Distinction between the two is imperative since ultimate treatment varies significantly.

B. Epidemiology. A history of penile or perineal trauma almost always precedes arterial priapism and is the most important historic information that distinguishes between the two types of priapism. The injury may be related to direct trauma to the penis or pelvic region (2) or with less severe trauma such as with penile body piercing (4) or penile tattooing (5). Studies have suggested that up to 41% of patients who present with priapism (veno-occlusive) have taken some type of psychotropic medication, usually neuroleptics, trazodone, and alpha-blockers such as prazosin (6). Priapism has been commonly reported (1–17%) after intracavernous injection with prostaglandins for the treatment of erectile dysfunction. Other drug- or substance-induced causes include the phosphodiesterase-5 inhibitors such as sildenafil citrate, testosterone, heparin, warfarin, cocaine, tacrolimus, and even scorpion toxin (3). Patients with any history of malignancy, especially genitourinary or pelvic carcinoma and new-onset priapism, should be evaluated for penile metastasis. In a recent review, 20–50% of cases with penile metastases initially presented with priapism (7).

The most common cause of priapism in children is sickle cell disease. It has been reported that over 60% of all sickle cell disease children eventually develop priapism (8).

III. EVALUATION

A. History and Physical. Specific questions may help identify the type of priapism, cause, and urgency of treatment. Always inquire how long the priapism has been present. Have they had "stuttering" symptoms (priapism lasting less than 4 hours that resolves spontaneously but then recurs)? How much pain does the patient experience? Moderate to severe, persistent pain is characteristic of veno-occlusive priapism and results from tissue ischemia. Pain is generally much more mild or transient with arterial priapism. Is there a history of penile or perineal trauma? Trauma more commonly precedes arterial priapism. Does the patient take any medications that may predispose to priapism? Is there any history of malignancy? Is there any history of sickle cell disease or any other vaso-occlusive disease?

The physical should include a thorough genitourinary exam to look for trauma or malignancy. The corpora cavernosa but not the corpora spongiosum is involved with priapism, and therefore, the glans will remain flaccid while the shaft is erect and tender. The examination should also include palpation for inguinal lymphadenopathy (genitourinary (GU) malignancy) and an abdominal exam (abdominal or GU malignancy and trauma).

B. Laboratory Tests. In most instances, the history and physical exam will determine the cause of priapism. A complete blood count and sickle cell screen may be useful, looking for malignancy and sickle cell disease, respectively. Coagulation studies are also recommended (in case aspiration is contemplated for treatment). Blood gas measurement from a cavernosal sample may be useful if differentiation between low- and high-flow priapism is difficult (2).

In most cases, further diagnostic testing is not needed. If objective studies are needed, color duplex ultrasonography is the method of choice followed by penile scintigraphy and magnetic resonance imaging. If pelvic malignancy is suspected, computed tomography is generally the next step. If trauma preceded priapism, arteriography may be indicated.

C. Genetics. Sickle cell anemia, an autosomal recessive disorder, is associated with a high incidence of priapism (over 40% of adults and over 60% of children).

IV. DIAGNOSIS

A. Differential Diagnosis. The key to determining the cause of priapism is the clinical history. Examination will reveal an erect, usually tender penis with flaccid glans. Early distinction between arterial and veno-occlusive priapism should be done, with the former often associated with trauma and less painful or painless erections. If the penis is only partially erect, ischemic priapism is less likely. Evaluation of priapism is aimed at determining how long it has been present, since permanent damage may occur within as little as 4 hours, and at determining the cause. The most common causes are due to psychotropic medications or medications for erectile dysfunction. Less common causes include trauma, sickle cell disease, and pelvic malignancy.

B. Clinical Manifestations. Priapism is considered a urologic emergency and should be managed aggressively. Without prompt recognition and treatment, priapism may result in urinary retention, cavernosa fibrosis, impotence, or even gangrene. Treatment within 4–6 hours of onset has been shown to decrease morbidity, the need for invasive procedures, and impotence (6).

REFERENCES

1. Eland IA, van der Lei J, Strickler BH, Sturkenboom MJ. Incidence of priapism in the general population. *Urology* 2001;57:970–972.
2. Burnett AL, Bivalacqua TJ. Priapism: new concepts in medical and surgical management. *Urol Clin North Am* 2011;38:185–194.
3. Huang YC, Harraz AM, Shindel AW. Evaluation and management of priapism: 2009 update. *Nat Rev Urol* 2009;6:262–271.
4. Holbrook J, Minocha J, Laumann A. Body piercing: complications and prevention of health risks. *Am J Clin Dermatol* 2012;13(1):1–17.
5. Zargooshi J, Rahmanian E, Motaee H, et al. Nonischemic priapism following penile tattooing. *J Sex Med* 2012;9(3):844–848.
6. Thompson JW Jr, Ware MR, Blashfield RK. Psychotropic medication and priapism: a comprehensive review. *J Clin Psych* 1990;51:430–433.
7. Lin, Yu-H, Kim J, Stein N, et al. Malignant priapism secondary to metastatic prostatic cancer: a case report and review of the literature. *Rev Urol* 2011;13(2):90–94.
8. Morrison BF, Burnett AL. Priapism in hematological and coagulative disorders: an update. *Urology* 2011;8:223–230.

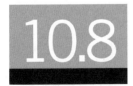

10.8 Scrotal Mass
Ernestine M. Lee and Eddie Needham

I. BACKGROUND. The term scrotal mass is general and includes discrete masses such as carcinomas as well as general swelling. Scrotal masses can be benign, anatomic, infectious, or malignant in origin. The clinical significance can range from entirely benign to emergent requiring immediate surgical treatment. The differential diagnosis of scrotal masses can be classified on the basis of anatomy: skin, spermatic cord, epididymis, and testis. Skin lesions include sebaceous cysts, cellulitis to include Fournier's disease (necrotizing fasciitis of the perineum and scrotum), and squamous cell carcinoma. Lesions of the spermatic cord include indirect inguinal hernia,

234 | TAYLOR'S DIFFERENTIAL DIAGNOSIS MANUAL

varicocele, hematocele, torsion of the appendix testis, and hydrocele. Epididymal swelling could represent epididymitis or spermatocele. Testicular masses include hydrocele, carcinomas, varicocele, testicular torsion, and orchitis (1).

II. PATHOPHYSIOLOGY. During the evaluation of any scrotal mass, the primary goal is to determine whether immediate referral is indicated, as in the case of testicular torsion, Fournier's disease, and hernias that are incarcerated or strangulated (2). Torsion is a surgical emergency. Testicular salvage is 90% when detorsion is performed within 6 hours of symptom onset (1).

III. EVALUATION
  A. History
    1. **Trauma**. Only 10% of patients presenting with testicular torsion report antecedent trauma (1). Hematoceles are more frequently associated with direct trauma (2).
    2. **Pain.** Acute pain (<24 h) is more likely to be associated with torsion, orchitis, epididymitis, hematocele, incarcerated or strangulated hernias, or Fournier's disease (1–3). More indolent pain is associated with non-incarcerated or strangulated hernias, hydroceles, skin infection depending on cause, and tumors. In some cases, masses are painless as is the case with some tumors, varicoceles, and some hydroceles (2).
    3. **Patient Age.** Scrotal masses of a variety of pathology can occur throughout the life span. Varicoceles occur in 15% of the male population (3). The most common cause of acute mass in children up to age 13 years is torsion of the appendix testis (4). Testicular tumors are the most common malignant tumors encountered in men aged 25 to 35 years (1).
    4. **Gastrointestinal Symptoms**. Patients with torsion, epididymo-orchitis, and some cases of epididymitis may also complain of nausea. Emesis may be present with torsion (1).
    5. **Symptoms of Infection**. Fever can accompany cellulitis, Fournier's disease, epididymitis, and orchitis. Patients with Fournier's disease will often exhibit signs of systemic infection such as hypotension, vomiting, and lethargy (1, 2). A history of penile discharge is often found in patients with epididymitis. In up to 80% of patients with mumps, orchitis symptoms are first observed within 8 days of involvement of the salivary gland (5). Tuberculosis and syphilis can also cause orchitis.
    6. **Sexual History**. Risk factors for sexually transmitted illnesses increase the possibility of epididymitis. Traumatic intercourse may lead to hematocele.
    7. **Other Symptoms**. Weight loss, poor appetite, night sweats, and fever may herald metastatic cancer. A mass that changes size may suggest communicating hydrocele.
  B. Physical Examination
    1. **Exam Position.** The standing position may accentuate a varicocele or hydrocele, especially if accompanied by the Valsalva maneuver. Prehn's sign, in which gentle elevation of the affected testicle relieves pain, suggests epididymitis.
    2. **Palpation**. The testes are slightly oblong in shape. Asking the patient to demonstrate the mass can be quite beneficial. A varicocele, most frequently located on the left, feels like a cord of worms and lies between the testicle and the inguinal canal. A spermatocele lies as a firm nodule in the spermatic cord. A hydrocele can be a diffuse unilateral scrotal enlargement. Testicular torsion is quite painful to palpation.
    3. **Neurologic Exam.** The cremasteric reflex is performed by gently stroking the medial thigh. Normally, the ipsilateral testicle will rise perhaps 5–10 mm toward the inguinal canal. With testicular torsion, the cremasteric reflex may be absent.
    4. **Transillumination**. Holding a light against the skin of the scrotum will demonstrate transillumination with a hydrocele. The scrotal sac will appear red as the light diffuses through the fluid.
    5. **General Exam.** The left testicle tends to rest slightly lower and more posterior in most men. The epididymis is generally located on the superomedial pole. The testicular appendix is not palpable in most men but can become painful, enlarged, and dark with torsion and strangulation (Blue dot sign). With metastatic disease, regional and generalized lymphadenopathy may be present.

C. Testing
  1. **Imaging**. For suspected acute torsion, Doppler ultrasound is frequently the easiest and most readily available modality. The waveforms will demonstrate decreased or absent blood flow to the affected testis. Sensitivity for torsion is 86–88% and specificity is 90–100. Urology consultation should be considered at the time of ordering Doppler ultrasound so as not to delay surgical treatment and preserve the testis.
  2. **Laboratories**. If testicular cancer is suspected, consider tumor markers: human chorionic gonadotropin, AFP (alfa-fetoprotein).

IV. DIAGNOSIS. Testicular torsion is the most emergent scrotal mass. The diagnosis is usually straightforward given the level of pain and the acuity. Incarcerated hernias may likewise have an urgent presentation. The non-testicular inguinal mass suggests this diagnosis. Many benign scrotal masses present over weeks to months and can be diagnosed with the history, physical exam, and ultrasound. Infectious causes of scrotal masses have a subacute course.

REFERENCES

1. Tiemstra JD, Kapoor S. Evaluation of scrotal masses. *Am Fam Physician* 2008;78:1165–1170.
2. Davis JE, Silverman M. Scrotal emergencies. *Emerg Med Clin North Am* 2011;29:469–484.
3. Montgomery JS, Bloom DA. The diagnosis and management of scrotal masses. *Med Clin North Am* 2011:95;235–244.
4. Lewis AG, Bukowski TP, Jarvis PD. Evaluation of acute scrotum in the emergency department. *J Pediatr Surg* 1995;6:637–646.
5. Beard CM, Benson RC Jr, Kelalis PP, Elveback LR, Kurland LT. The incidence and outcome of mumps orchitis in Rochester, Minnesota, 1935 to 1974. *Mayo Clin Proc* 1977;52:3–7.

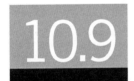

10.9 Scrotal Pain

George P. Samraj

I. BACKGROUND
  A. Definition. Scrotal pain can be acute, intermittent, or chronic. Chronic scrotal pain is pain lasting over 3 months. Scrotal pain is a common problem in adults and the incidence is unknown. Scrotal pain can result from pathology within the scrotum, trauma to the scrotum, scrotal sac, or extra-scrotal pathology, referred pain from intra-abdominal pathology, or systemic diseases. Scrotal and testicular problems may range from benign to malignant and debilitating conditions. Most common causes of scrotal pain are due to benign conditions like epididymitis, varicocele (postvasectomy is a common reason) (1), hydrocele, spermatocele, polyarteritis nodosa, and epididymal or testicular cysts. With the exception of trauma or torsion of testis, scrotal pain in an adult rarely requires emergent surgical intervention. Testicular torsion is common in child and adolescent population (1 in 4,000 males younger than 25 years) and requires urgent intervention (2). The risk of testicular torsion includes malformations, increase in testicular volume, testicular tumor, testicles with horizontal lie, a history of cryptorchidism, and a long spermatic cord. Trauma is a less common cause of torsion. The testis may be salvaged if appropriately treated in time (90% < 6 hours and 50% in 12 hours and <10% at 24 hours) (3).

II. PATHOPHYSIOLOGY
  A. Etiology
  1. **Intrascrotal Pathology**. Testicular torsion (torsion of testicular appendage), spermatic cord torsion (intravaginal, extravaginal, acute, or intermittent), epididymitis, orchitis, vasculitis (e.g., Henoch-Schönlein purpura), varicocele, spermatocele, and primary or metastatic testicular tumor.

2. **Pathology of the Scrotal Sac.** Infections, early Fournier gangrene, trauma, animal or insect bites, cysts and idiopathic scrotal edema, and sexual abuse.

3. **Extrascrotal Pathology**. Direct/indirect hernia, incarcerated hernia, hydrocele (communicating hydrocele or encysted hydrocele with or without torsion or associated with acute abdominal pathology, e.g., appendicitis, peritonitis, splenic rupture), associated urinary tract infection (UTI), prostatitis, and sexually transmitted disease (STD).

4. **Pain Referred from Intra-abdominal Pathology or Systemic Disease**. renal colic, mononucleosis, Coxsackie B virus, Buerger's disease, and polyarteritis nodosa.

B. **Epidemiology**
   1. **Intrascrotal Pathology**
      a. Testicular torsion: Torsion can occur at any age, but is uncommon in adults. In pediatric patients, appendix testis torsion is more common (40–60%) than spermatic cord torsion (20–30%) (4). Peak age of testicular torsion is 12–16 years and most (86–93%) occur after age 10 years. Intrascrotal pathology is the most common cause of scrotal pain in the first year of life (often misdiagnosed as colic or intra-abdominal disorder).
      b. Epididymitis: Epididymitis is the most common cause of acute scrotal pain in adults. Epididymitis in children can be due to infectious or noninfectious causes. If it occurs in prepuberty, suspect urogenital anomaly or dysfunction.
      c. Orchitis: Orchitis is usually due to extension of epididymitis. Approximately 20% of postpubertal mumps infection produces mumps orchitis. Approximately 70% of cases are unilateral. This is less common since the mumps vaccine (5).
      d. Varicocele: It is an abnormal dilatation of the pampiniform plexus veins due to increased pressure secondary to the venous backflow associated with incompetent valves in the spermatic vein. This is common in adults and adolescents. It is uncommon in prepubertal children. Intra-abdominal lesion obstructing venous drainage may present with acute rupture or thrombosis.
      e. Testicular tumor: This can be primary or secondary. Testicular cancer accounts for 1% of all male cancers, and it is the leading cause of cancer among men aged between 15 and 35 years. Most cancers are germ cell in origin and few (4%) are sex cord-stromal tumors.
      f. Spermatocele (epididymal cyst): This is a benign cystic collection of fluid which arises from the epididymis, common after vasectomy, not seen in prepuberty, and very rare in adolescents.
   2. **Extrascrotal Pathology**
      a. Direct/indirect hernia, incarcerated hernia. This is equally prevalent in adults and children.
      b. Hydrocele: Primarily in neonates. Often resolves spontaneously in the first year. If it persists beyond the second year, surgical consultation may be required. Occurs in adults, but not common.
      c. Prostatitis/UTI/STD. UTI should be considered in young children. If the patient has UTI, further evaluation of urinary tract for reflux or congenital anomalies needs to be done. If STD is diagnosed, sexual abuse should be considered in children. STD is common in adolescents and adults.

C. **Scrotal Trauma**
   1. Significant damage to a testicle from trauma, in any age group, is rare. Scrotal trauma with straddle injury, bicycle handle bars injury, and sports injury is common. Scrotal pain due to trauma is generally self-evident or self-reported. Traumatic damage in prepuberty is rare due to small testicles. Testicular pain lasting more than an hour after a traumatic injury is evaluated for testicular rupture or hematoma.

III. EVALUATION
A. **History**
   1. A comprehensive history is essential for the evaluation of scrotal pain. The patient's age, onset, severity of the pain, and sexual history are essential for diagnosis. The speed of worsening symptoms and signs, associated symptoms like fever, nausea, vomiting, urinary symptoms, and history of urethral discharge are noted. Conditions affecting the

scrotum may be secondary to abdominal pathology. Epididymitis usually occurs in one testis and progressively gets worse over days to weeks, whereas testicular torsion is sudden and abrupt in onset. Histories of previous episodes were noted in many patients with torsion. Time of onset of symptoms of torsion is immensely useful in managing torsion and the outcome.

2. History of trauma needs to be elicited. Torsion of testicular appendage has less intense pain than testicular torsion. Epididymitis can be abrupt or insidious in onset. Fever and voiding symptoms may be present with epididymitis.

B. Physical

1. A comprehensive physical examination is essential for the diagnosis of scrotal diseases. A focused exam should include observation and examination of the abdomen, scrotum, genital organs, and prostate when indicated. Typical examination includes inspection, palpation, and transillumination of the scrotum when indicated. Scrotum is noted for swelling, color change, ulcers, or evidence of trauma or asymmetry. In small children, observation for irritability, restlessness, and crying is helpful in diagnosing severe conditions. Any neonate or small child with abdominal pain should be observed for scrotal conditions. Testicular numbers and locations should be noted to rule out cryptorchidism. The scrotum is examined for evidence of trauma, unilateral or bilateral swelling, infection, or masses. Discoloration is usually due to trauma, but can be seen with torsion and epididymitis. The cremasteric reflex is the most sensitive physical finding for testicular torsion. The specificity of this test varies with age group. If cremasteric reflex is present on the painful side, testicular torsion may be ruled out in most cases. In order for the absence of a cremasteric reflex to be a reliable indicator, its presence must be demonstrated on the nonpainful side. Other useful findings of torsion include Prehn's sign (elevation of testis increases pain for torsion and reduced pain in epididymitis), elevation of scrotum on the affected side, abnormal testicular lie, and abnormal and exquisitely tender testis. Unilateral swelling without skin changes indicates hernia or hydrocele. Palpation of the scrotum is performed for the assessment of edema, infections, or other skin conditions. Transillumination of the scrotum may differentiate a hydrocele from hematocele. Focal tenderness at the upper pole of testis and "blue dot sign" (necrotic appendix seen through the scrotal skin) may be present in torsion of appendix. However, this sign is also observed in torsion of the testis (6).

C. Laboratory Tests. Very few laboratory tests are indicated in the evaluation of scrotal pain.

1. Urinalysis (UA): It is performed to rule out bacteriuria or pyuria. Usually positive UA is helpful in differentiating epididymitis from testicular or appendiceal torsion. However, pyuria may be present with torsion and may create diagnostic confusion.

2. Complete blood count (CBC) and comprehensive metabolic panel (CMP): Leukocytosis is a nonspecific finding. More commonly, it is elevated in epididymitis and in late stages (after 24 hours) of testicular or appendiceal torsion. Occasionally, a CMP may be beneficial in identifying the causes of scrotal swelling (e.g., hypoproteinemia or liver or kidney failure).

D. Imaging

1. Color Doppler ultrasound examination (CDUS): CDUS is the first-line modality for the diagnosis of torsion after history and physical. CDUS provides a definitive diagnosis of testicular torsion in 91.7% of cases. However, it is less reliable (63–90% sensitive) in spermatic cord torsion. The findings of torsion in CDUS include reduced or absent Doppler waveforms, parenchymal heterogeneity, and/or altered echotexture compared with the contralateral testis. High-resolution ultrasonography may improve the diagnostic accuracy when available.

2. Nuclear Scan: It measures testicular perfusion with high sensitivity and specificity in testicular torsion. However, the process is often too slow to be used universally in determining the need for surgical intervention in a narrow therapeutic window. Primary uses are evaluation in trauma, with asymptomatic masses, and when elective surgical exploration is contraindicated and Doppler studies are equivocal.

3. Magnetic Resonance Imaging (MRI): MRI provides good anatomic data, but it is not useful in the acute setting to evaluate for blood flow. It is highly valuable in assessing cryptorchidism or abdominal pathology contributing to scrotal pain.

4. Surgical exploration must always be considered whenever the history and/or physical examination is consistent with testicular torsion or when the data do not completely rule it out. The opportunity to salvage the testis is in the first 6 hours from the onset of symptoms.

IV. DIAGNOSIS

A. Differential Diagnosis. Most critical is testicular torsion due to a short window of opportunity to salvage the testis. Other etiologies (appendiceal torsion, epididymitis, trauma, hernia/hydrocele, infections, bites, and tumor and edema of scrotum) have larger window of opportunity. All tests should be directed toward excluding testicular torsion initially, as rapidly as possible. The age of the patient and time of onset of symptoms and time lapsed are the most important clinical information necessary for diagnosis. Severe unilateral pain of less than 6 hours worsened by elevation of the scrotum in an adolescent is testicular torsion until proven otherwise. Every neonate with abdominal symptoms must have a scrotal examination as part of the workup. CDUS is the diagnostic modality of choice for the evaluation of acute scrotal pain. Surgical exploration of acute scrotum of less than 6 hours duration is required unless torsion is excluded.

REFERENCES

1. Wampler SM, Llanes M. Common scrotal and testicular problems primary care: *Clin Office Pract* 2010;37(3):613–626.
2. Espy PG, Koo HP. Torsion of the testicle. In: Graham SD, Glenn JF, Keane TE, eds. *Glenn's urologic surgery*, 6th ed. Philadelphia, PA: Lippincott Williams & Wilkins, 2004:513–517.
3. Ringdahl E, Teague L. Testicular torsion. *Am Fam Physician* 2006;74(10):1739–1743.
4. Barthold JS. *Abnormalities of the testis and scrotum and their surgical management*, 10th ed. Wein: Campbell-Walsh Urology Saunders, 2011:3557–3596.
5. Turgut AT, Bhatt S, Dogra VS. The acute pediatric scrotum. *Ultrasound Clin* 2006;1(3):93–107.
6. David JE, Yale SH, Goldman IL. Urology. *Scrotal Pain Clin Med Res* 2003;1(2):159–160.

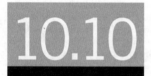

10.10 Urethral Discharge

George P. Samraj

I. BACKGROUND. Urethral discharge (UD) is a common symptom, with etiology varying from various sexually transmitted infections to cancer. UD may be profuse or scanty, clear, yellowish or white, purulent, mucopurulent or serous, brown, green or bloody, watery or frank pus. UD may be an acute or chronic condition and patients may or may not have symptoms. Urethritis is defined as the presence of urethral inflammation and leukorrhea.

II. PATHOPHYSIOLOGY. UD is the presenting sign of many disorders and can be classified as follows:

A. Sexually Transmitted Diseases

1. Gonococcal (GC) infection is more common in men than in women. The Centers for Disease Control and Prevention reported about 700,000 new infections in the United States in 2009, with a rate of 122–116.2/100,000 population/year. It is 20 times more common in young patients from large cities and the African American population (1). In some studies, gonococcus is coinfected with chlamydia (up to 60%).

2. Non-gonococcal (NGC) infection is the most common sexually transmitted disease (STD) in the United States, with 2.8 million new cases occurring annually (1). As many as 85% of women with chlamydial infections and 40% of infected men are asymptomatic.

NGU has a variable incubation period ranging from 2 to 35 days (50% of patients will present with symptoms in 4 days).

3. *Chlamydia trachomatis* (15–40% of NGC)
4. *Mycoplasma genitalium* (15–25% of NGC)
5. *Ureaplasma urealyticum*
6. *M. hominis*

B. Other Organisms Linked to UD

1. **Bacteria**. *Gardnerella vaginalis*, *Escherichia coli*, tuberculosis, *Corynebacterium genitalium*, bacterioides, mycoplasmas, anaerobes.
2. **Viruses**. Herpes simplex virus (up to 60% of men with primary herpes will have NGU), adenoviruses, cytomegalovirus, human papillomavirus, and others.
3. **Protozoal**. *Trichomonas vaginalis*. About 5 million cases occur annually in the United States.
4. **Fungal**. Candida species.

C. Non-sexually Transmitted Diseases

1. **Infections**. Cystitis, prostatitis
2. **Anatomic and Congenital Abnormalities**. Urethral stricture, phimosis
3. **Iatrogenic**. Catheterization, instrumentation, and other procedures
4. Chemical irritation from douches, lubricants, and other chemicals
5. Tumors, malignant lesions, and new growths
6. **Foreign Bodies**. Common in children, teenagers
7. **Substance Abuse**. Chronic use of amphetamines or other stimulants produces a serous discharge. Caffeine and alcohol are also implicated in UD

D. Miscellaneous Factors Linked to UD

1. Sexual practices, masturbation, oral sex, etc.
2. **Unknown**. No organisms may be found in up to one-third of patients

III. EVALUATION

A. History

1. A comprehensive medical history is essential for the evaluation of UD. It should include questions about
   a. dysuria
   b. UD
   c. itching at the urethra
   d. hematuria
   e. rectal symptoms
   f. contact with infectious agents
   g. testicular pain
   h. low back pain and constitutional symptoms
2. The characteristic of UD is characterized in relation to color (purulent, mucoid, or bloody), quantity, odor, consistency, frequency, past history, or any previous treatment and relationship to urination.
   a. Profuse, thick yellow to grayish UD 3–7 days after sexual exposure is characteristic of GC.
   b. Clear to white scanty or mucopurulent UD (23–55%) developing gradually at least a week after exposure with waxing and waning in intensity is suggestive of chlamydial infection.
   c. Mucoid, scant watery discharge developing over a period of 2–3 weeks is common with NGC UD.
   d. A bloody discharge is suggestive of urethral carcinoma.
   e. Dysuria with scanty discharge is a presentation of chlamydial infection.
   f. Sexual history should include sexual orientation, past sexual history, sexual behaviors, condom usage, number of sexual partners, recent sexual contacts, and the orifices used for sexual contacts.
   g. Consistent usage of condoms prevents sexually transmitted urethritis.
   h. Oral sex increases UD due to infections from oral flora.

B. Physical Examination

1. A focused physical examination includes the vital signs and urologic and rectal examination. In men, the examination is best performed at least 2 hours after micturition or preferably before passing the first urine. In males, the examination should include examination of the penis, perimeatal region for evidence of erythema, urethral meatus, scrotum, testicles, epididymis, prostate, and perianal and the inguinal region for lymph nodes. Stains present on the patient's underwear may indicate the characteristics of the discharge, particularly in a patient who has urinated shortly before examination. Recent micturition can eliminate much inflammatory discharge. Sometimes, it may be necessary to examine the patient in the morning before voiding to enhance the diagnosis. In females, a complete gynourologic examination should be performed. A complete examination of the abdomen may be indicated to rule out intra-abdominal pathology like masses, inflammation, obstruction, and distention of organs. Additional physical examination should include examination of skin and other systems as needed. If a GC infection is suspected, it may be essential to check the patient's joints, skin, throat, eye, and other organs.

C. Laboratory Testing

1. Proper collection and handling of UD specimens is essential for the diagnosis. When the discharge is not spontaneous, the urethra should be gently stripped. This is best accomplished by grasping the penis firmly between the thumb and forefinger, with the thumb pressing on the ventral surface. The examiner's hand is then moved distally, compressing the urethra. This maneuver may express small amount of discharge. UD for testing preferably should be collected without contamination by the various bacteria present in the urethral meatus. The urethral meatus can be gently spread and UD collected by gently inserting (2–4 cm into the urethra) calcium alginate urogenital swab (cotton swabs are uncomfortable due to the large size and may interfere with the culture) by rotating for 3–6 seconds. UD should be collected 1–4 hours (preferably 4 hours) after urination. Pharyngeal swabs may be collected when clinically indicated. The specimen should be directly placed into the culture medium. The same swab may be used for a Gram stain (2, 3).

2. Gram Stain and Culture: The presence of polymorphs with intracellular diplococci is diagnostic of GC. Polymorphs without the intracellular diplococci are suggestive of NGC. Few or no polymorphs are suggestive of other etiologies. Gram stain is quite accurate for men, but it is not very sensitive for women (50%), where cultures of the throat, rectum, and sometimes conjunctivae are required to establish the diagnosis (2–4).

3. Wet preparation of the UD is done to establish the diagnosis of trichomonas, candida, and some viral and bacterial infections (bacterial vaginosis—clue cells, viral inclusions, etc.).

IV. DIAGNOSIS

A. Urethritis is confirmed with one of the three finding in an appropriate clinical setting.

1. Presence of purulent or mucopurulent discharge

2. More than 4 (5) white blood cells (WBCs) per high-power field in the oil immersion (1000×) microscopy of the Gram stain (85% of men with confirmed urethritis will have >4 polymorphs/field whereas in 15% it may be absent) of the discharge

3. Presence of leukocyte esterase in the first voided urine or the presence of >10 WBCs per high-power field (400×) in the sediment of the spun urine

B. Urine analysis and urine cultures are essential for the diagnosis of urinary infections. Collection of a urine specimen as described by Stamey (6) with four sterile containers (before and after prostatic massage) is sometimes useful to identify the site of infection in men. Another approach is to test the first 10 mL of urine sample by either microscopy or "dipstick" testing for the presence of leukocyte esterase for chlamydial and GC infections in asymptomatic men. Microscopy and culture of urine from the first voided sample (morning specimen) and urethral swab culture are valuable in diagnosing trichomonas vaginalis. Many centers now use nucleic acid–based tests (nucleic acid amplification assay test [NAATs], nucleic acid hybridization test [probe test], nucleic acid genetic transformation test) due to the simplicity, high sensitivity, and specificity when compared with the difficulties encountered with traditional culture test (low sensitivity and storage problems). NAATs are more popular and use various techniques (performed using polymerase chain reaction [PCR], ligase chain reaction, or strand displacement amplification of DNA) to identify an infection. These tests can be performed from UD or 20–40 mL (more volume can interfere with the test) of first voided first catch initial stream of urine. Female patients should not cleanse labial and urethral region before collection of the first stream urine. Some centers prefer a urine specimen for its simplicity and increased detection rate, especially with scanty UD (4). PCR testing is performed for the diagnosis of *U. urealyticum* infections.

C. Blood studies like complete blood count, chemistry profile, rapid plasma reagin (RPR), human immunodeficiency virus, and immunologic studies may be required.

D. Diagnostic imaging with an urethrogram or pelvic, vaginal, and rectal ultrasound studies may be indicated in some clinical conditions.

E. Examination under anesthesia for children and elderly patients is sometimes necessary in the evaluation of UD.

F. Anoscopy is appropriate for patients who have anal intercourse or for those with anal and rectal symptoms.

G. Cysto-urethroscopy and laparoscopy may also be useful in certain conditions (7).

V. SPECIAL CONCERNS

A. *Neisseria gonorrhea* and *C. trachomatis* infections are reportable to State Health Departments and a specific diagnosis is essential. The partner management is not permitted in all the states in the United States. Occasionally, urethral swab collection may stimulate the vagus. UD secondary to STD involves many psychosocial and medicolegal implications for the patient, his or her partner, their families, and society. Sexual partners should be traced, tested, and treated. In children with UD, sexual abuse should be suspected. Pregnant women with GC infection or chlamydia may infect the infant at birth (ophthalmia neonatorum).

VI. COMPLICATIONS FOLLOWING UD AND URETHRITIS. Some of the complications following UD are post-GC urethritis, pelvic inflammatory disease (PID) in women, infertility, perihepatitis, chronic pelvic pain, adhesions of the intra-abdominal organs, obstructions in gastrointestinal and genitourinary tracts, chronic urethritis, periurethral abscess, fistula, prostatitis, epididymitis, orchitis, urethral syndrome, psychosexual problems, and Reiter's syndrome.

REFERENCES

1. Workowski KA, Berman S. Centers for Disease Control and Prevention (CDC). Sexually transmitted diseases treatment guidelines, 2010. *MMWR Recomm Rep.* 2010;59(RR-12):1–110.
2. Gerber GS, Brendler CB. *Evaluation of the urologic patient: history, physical examination, and urinalysis.* 10th ed. Wein: Campbell-Walsh Urology W.B. Saunders, 2011,Vol I, chapter 3.
3. Lyon CJ. Urethritis. *Clin Fam Pract* 2005;7(1):31–41.
4. Koeijers JJ, Kessels AG, Nys S, et al. Evaluation of the nitrite and leukocyte esterase activity tests for the diagnosis of acute symptomatic urinary tract infection in men. *Clin Infect Dis* 2007;45:894.
5. McCormack WM. Urethritis. In: Mandell GL, Bennett JE, Dolin R, eds. *Principles and practice of infectious diseases,* 7th ed. Philadelphia, PA: Elsevier Churchill Livingstone, 2009:chap 106, 1485–1494.
6. Meares EM, Stamey TA. Bacteriologic localization patterns in bacterial prostatitis and urethritis. *Invest Urol* 1968;5:492–518.
7. Cohen MS. Approach to the patient with a sexually transmitted disease. In: Goldman L, Ausiello D, eds. *Cecil medicine,* 24th ed. Philadelphia, PA: Saunders Elsevier, 2011:chap 293.

CHAPTER 11

Problems Related to the Female Reproductive System

Sanjeev Sharma

11.1 Amenorrhea

Sumit Singhal and Sanjeev Sharma

I. BACKGROUND. Amenorrhea is a clinical term used to describe the absence of menstruation in women in the reproductive age group. It has many potential causes.

II. PATHOPHYSIOLOGY. Amenorrhea is usually divided into primary and secondary forms.

A. Primary Amenorrhea. It is defined as the absence of menses by age 15 or 16 years if normal growth and secondary sexual features are present and at age 13 years if no secondary sexual features are present. If regular cyclic pelvic pain is present without bleeding, specific evaluation for outflow obstruction might be considered at age 13 years or younger (1,2).

B. Secondary Amenorrhea. It is defined as the absence of menstruation for more than three cycles in women who had reasonably regular cycles in the past or 6 months in women who previously had menses.

The etiology of primary and secondary amenorrhea can be divided into four types:

1. Hypothalamus/pituitary (25%). Ovaries do not respond to hypothalamic–pituitary stimulation. This may be due to congenital gonadotropin-releasing hormone (GnRH) deficiency (when associated with anosmia it is Kallmann syndrome), functional hypothalamic amenorrhea (abnormal hypothalamic GnRH secretion), pituitary diseases (such as infiltrative diseases and tumors), or hyperprolactenemia.

2. Ovarian (50%). These are primary ovarian failure due to gonadal dysgenesis (Turner's syndrome), testicular feminizing syndrome, polycystic ovary syndrome (PCOS), autoimmune oophoritis, and chemo- or radiation therapy.

3. Outflow tract abnormalities (20%). Müllerian agenesis (absence of uterus, fallopian tubes, or uterus) and imperforate hymen.

4. Other rare causes (5%). Receptor abnormalities and enzyme deficiencies such as complete androgen insensitivity syndrome, and 5α-reductase deficiency.

Etiology of secondary amenorrhea:

The commonest cause of secondary amenorrhea is pregnancy. Other causes in decreasing order of frequency are ovarian (40%), hypothalamic (35%), pituitary (19%), uterine/outflow tract (9%), and others (1%).

1. Hypothalamic. Functional hypothalamic amenorrhea (decreased GnRH secretion of unknown etiology; risk factors include weight loss nutritional deficiency, and exercise), infiltrative diseases (lymphoma and sarcoidosis), or systemic illnesses.

2. Pituitary. Tumors (prolactinoma, adrenocorticotropic hormone–secreting tumors, and adenomas), acromegaly, Sheehan's syndrome, head irradiation, infiltrative diseases such as hemochromatosis, and hyperprolactinemia.

3. Ovarian. Primary ovarian insufficiency or premature ovarian failure (depletion of oocytes before 40 years of age) and PCOS.
4. Uterine/outflow tract obstruction. Asherman's syndrome.
5. Others including thyroid dysfunction.

III. EVALUATION

A. **History.** Medical history should include a detailed menstrual and obstetric history, past medical and surgical history, social history, medications, and risk factors for amenorrhea. The menstrual and obstetric history should include the date of last menstrual period if known, frequency and duration of menses, contraceptive use, number of pregnancies, parity, miscarriages, and elective abortions. Other symptoms including cold or heat intolerance, voice changes, excessive hair, weight loss or gain, exercise intensity, headaches, visual field defects, dyspareunia, and signs of estrogen deficiency (hot flashes, vaginal dryness, and poor sleep) should be sought.

B. **Physical Examination.** Complete physical examination, including height, weight, and BMI, and complete pelvic examination are required. Assessment of mood, nutritional status, and oral cavity (dental exam for bulimia) is also important.

Acne, hirsutism, acanthosis nigricans, a buffalo hump, the presence and distribution of pubic/axillary hair, easy bruisability, goiter, webbed neck, and galactorrhea are features that can point toward a diagnosis.

Amenorrhea with hirsutism may suggest PCOS or an androgen-secreting tumor of the ovary or adrenals (3).

C. **Diagnosis.** The first step in diagnosis is to rule out pregnancy by performing serum or urine β-human chorionic gonadotropin testing. Other laboratory tests include thyroid-stimulating hormone, serum prolactin, follicle-stimulating hormone (FSH) (high levels indicate ovarian failure), estradiol (low levels with low FSH indicate hypothalamic hypogonadism), and total testosterone and dehydroepiandrosterone-sulfate (high levels may indicate androgen secreting tumors).

Progesterone challenge: Medroxyprogesterone acetate 10 mg/day for 10 days is given. Withdrawal bleeding indicates adequate estrogen levels for endometrial proliferation, in addition to the absence of outflow tract abnormalities.

If the progesterone challenge fails, the endometrium can be primed with oral unconjugated estrogens 0.625 mg/day for 35 days, and addition of a progestin (medroxyprogesterone acetate 10 mg/day) from days 26 to 35. An absence of bleeding is a strong indicator of Asherman's syndrome. Further imaging including hysterosalpingogram and hysteroscopy for lysis of adhesions may be required.

Other tests that may be considered, if indicated, are genetic testing for karyotyping to check for chromosomal abnormalities, such as Turner's syndrome, and bone density scans for patients at risk for osteoporosis.

REFERENCES

1. Up-to-date. *Etiology, diagnosis, and treatment of secondary amenorrhea.* Accessed at www.utdol.com, 2011.
2. First Consult. *Amenorrhea.* Accessed at www.firstconsult.com.
3. E-medicine. *Amenorrhea.* Accessed at www.emedicine.com.

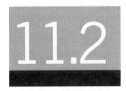

11.2 Breast Mass

Shailendra K. Saxena and Mikayla L. Spangler

I. **BACKGROUND.** A palpable breast mass is a common reason for women to seek an appointment with their primary care physician. Evaluation of a breast mass requires a thorough and systematic approach to ensure that cancers of the breast are not missed or are diagnosed and treated at an early stage. A family physician is in an ideal position to evaluate, treat, or refer to a specialist based on an appropriate evaluation of the breast mass. Although breast self-examination has not been shown to improve survival, it is a useful technique since many patients do detect their own breast masses and bring it to the attention of their health care providers.

A. **Epidemiology.** The vast majority of breast masses are benign. However, one in eight women will develop invasive breast cancer in her lifetime (1). Although the majority of breast cancers are diagnosed in women older than 50 years of age, one third of them are in younger women (2).

II. **EVALUATION AND RISK.** The evaluation of a breast mass should begin with a complete history and physical examination. It is important to identify patient risks for breast cancer (Table 11.2.1). However, physicians should be aware that most women with breast cancer do not have any identifiable risk factors.

In addition to obtaining the information from the table above, a thorough history regarding the mass itself should begin with the following questions:

1. How did you discover the breast mass?
2. Did you notice any changes in the breast mass after it was first noted?
3. Is the mass painful? If painful, is there any cyclic variation to the pain? Cyclic pain and rapid fluctuations in the size of the breast mass may suggest a benign cystic lesion that may be due to fibrocystic changes in the breast.

A. **Physical Examination.** In premenopausal women, the breast examination should optimally be done 7 to 9 days after the onset of menses. Examination should also include examination of the neck, chest wall, and axillae.

1. Inspection: Both breasts should be inspected for asymmetry, abnormal contour, skin changes, including skin retraction, rashes, ulceration, erythema, and peau d'orange. The nipples should be inspected for lesions, retraction, inversion, or discharge.
2. Palpation: Both breasts should be palpated for consistency, abnormal thickening, or mass. If a mass is felt, determine whether it is tender or not. A cancerous lesion is classically hard and immovable with ill-defined borders. Conversely, a round, rubbery, discrete, mobile non-tender mass is more suggestive of a benign fibroadenoma (Table 11.2.2). Palpation of regional lymph nodes in cervical, supraclavicular, infraclavicular, and axillary areas should also be performed. The location of any abnormality should be described and the "clock system" can be used to document localization (3).

B. **Further Tests.** History and careful physical examination are the key elements in evaluation of a patient with a breast mass. However, most patients require further analysis which may include attempted needle aspiration, ultrasound, mammogram, and/or biopsy of the breast mass.

1. Ultrasonography is an important tool to evaluate whether a mass is solid or cystic in nature. It can also be used to guide for biopsies or to aspirate fluid if the mass is cystic.
2. Mammography is not routinely ordered in women under the age of 30. However, it is often used as a first diagnostic test in a woman over the age of 30 with a new breast complaint.
3. A breast mass that is not definitively classified as benign on imaging requires a biopsy to exclude breast cancer.
   i. Fine needle aspiration biopsy (FNAB): FNAB has been used for several years to evaluate masses of the breast. The procedure can be easily and quickly performed. The results can be obtained immediately to expedite early discussion about diagnosis and treatment. However, FNAB cytology cannot distinguish between in situ and invasive breast cancer.
   ii. Core needle biopsy (CNB): This procedure requires a larger gauge needle and provides a histologic material for evaluation of a breast mass. It also can distinguish between in situ and invasive breast cancer. In most centers, CNB is usually performed in conjunction with ultrasound or stereotactic mammography. The stereotactic table allows mammographic guidance for CNB.
   iii. Open excisional biopsy: Where CNB is non-diagnostic and there is a suspicion of breast cancer, excision of the entire lesion is recommended. Patients may also prefer this approach as the entire mass is removed, even if it is benign.
4. Triple test for a solid mass: The triple test includes assessment of the breast mass by physical examination, mammographic findings, and cytologic results through FNAB.

TABLE 11.2.1	Risk Factors for Breast Cancer (3)

Non-modifiable	**Modifiable**
Age (>50 y)	Alcohol consumption (>1 alcoholic beverage/day)
Atypical hyperplasia	Hormone replacement therapy
Chest wall radiation	Oral contraceptive use
Early menarche (prior to age 12)	Obesity
Late menopause (after age 50)	Parity (nulliparous or first child after age 35)
Race (whites have greatest risk)	Smoking
Sex (females at greatest risk)	
Diethylstilbestrol exposure in utero	
Previous personal history of breast cancer, endometrial cancer, or fibrocystic disease	
Family history of breast or ovarian cancer*	

* The family history should also include all other cancers in the immediate family

TABLE 11.2.2	Differential Diagnosis of Benign Breast Masses (3)

Fibrocystic breast disease
Fibroadenoma of the breast
Breast abscess
Galactocele
Hematoma

Testing for the BRCA gene has been used to evaluate the risk of breast cancer. Recently, the United States Preventive Services Task Force (USPSTF) has supported testing for the BRCA gene in women with a suspicious family history. Grade B recommendation indicating benefits of testing outweigh the harms (5).

Combining the results of these three tests together, a sensitivity of 97% to 100% and a specificity of 98% to 100% can be obtained. Inconclusive results may still require an excisional biopsy (5).

5. Emerging technology for breast mass evaluation: Vacuum-assisted biopsy and magnetic resonance imaging–guided breast biopsy are new technologies that have been used to evaluate breast masses.

REFERENCES

1. American Cancer Society. *Cancer facts and figures 2003*. Accessed at http://www.cancer.org/downloads/STT/CAFF2003PWSecured.pdf on August 7, 2012.
2. National Cancer Institute. *SEER 1973-2001 public-use data*. Accessed at http://seer.cancer.gov/publicdata/ on August 7, 2012.
3. Marcia K, Files J, Pruthi S. Reducing the risk of breast cancer: a personalized approach. *J Fam Pract* 2012;61:340–347.
4. Santen RJ, Mansel R. Benign breast disorders. *N Engl J Med* 2005;353:275–278.
5. National Cancer Institute Conference. The uniform approach to breast fine-needle aspiration biopsy (editorial opinion). *Am J Surg* 1997;174(4):371–385.

11.3

Chronic Pelvic Pain

Jayashree Paknikar

I. BACKGROUND. Chronic pelvic pain is defined as episodic or continuous pain that persists for 6 months or longer and is sufficiently severe to have a significant impact on a woman's lifestyle, day-to-day functioning, or relationships.

II. PATHOPHYSIOLOGY (1). Any anatomic structure in the abdomen or pelvis can contribute to the etiology of chronic pelvic pain. It is helpful to attempt to categorize the pain as either gynecologic or nongynecologic when seeking a specific diagnosis. Gynecologic conditions that cause chronic pelvic pain include endometriosis, gynecologic malignancies, and pelvic inflammatory disease. In addition, nongynecologic conditions that can cause chronic pelvic pain are cystitis, inflammatory bowel disease, pelvic floor myalgia, and somatization disorder (1). Therefore, a comprehensive and detailed multisystem evaluation is warranted when evaluating chronic pelvic pain.

III. EVALUATION

    A. History

        1. Components of an appropriate medical history are as follows (2):

            a. Onset, duration, and pattern of the pain

            b. Location, intensity, character, and radiation of the pain

            c. Aggravating or relieving factors

            d. Relationship of the pain to sexual activity or menstruation

            e. Review of urinary, musculoskeletal, and gastrointestinal systems

            f. Medication history (e.g., use of birth control pills and over-the-counter medications)

            g. Systemic symptoms, such as fatigue and anorexia

            h. Past obstetric, gynecologic, and general surgical histories

            i. A questionnaire developed by the International Pelvic Pain Society and available at www.pelvicpain.org may be helpful in the initial evaluation (3)

        2. Women with a history of pelvic inflammatory disease are at high risk for developing chronic pelvic pain. An individual suffering with multiple symptoms that might include intestinal, sexual, urinary, musculoskeletal, and systemic symptoms may be suffering from a psychiatric disorder (e.g., depression and somatization). Specific questions should explore the possibility of a current or remote history of sexual abuse.

        3. Dyspareunia is often a feature of chronic pelvic pain (Chapter 11.5). Cyclic pain that is related to menstruation often, but not always, indicates a gynecologic problem. Pain referred to the anterior thighs is associated with irregular uterine bleeding, or new-onset dysmenorrhea may have a uterine or ovarian cause. Urethral tenderness, dysuria, frequency, or bladder pain suggests interstitial cystitis or a urethral problem (Chapter 10.1). Pain on defecation, melena, bloody stools, or abdominal pain with alternating diarrhea and constipation suggests myofascial pelvic floor problems, irritable bowel syndrome, or inflammatory bowel disease.

    B. Physical Examination

        1. The general appearance of the patient should be noted. Does the patient appear to be chronically ill, which may suggest a pelvic malignancy or an inflammatory bowel disorder? Does the patient appear anxious or stressed?

            a. Can the patient point to the pain with one finger? If so, this can indicate that the pain may have a discrete source, such as abdominal wall pain.

            b. An examination of the lower back, sacral area, and coccyx, including a neurologic examination of the lower extremities, is important. A herniated disk, exaggerated lumbar lordosis, and spondylolisthesis can all cause pelvic pain due to neuropathic or myofascial pathology.

TABLE 11.3.1	Etiology of Chronic Pelvic Pain			
Gynecologic	**Urinary**	**Gastrointestinal**	**Neurologic /Musculoskeletal**	**Psychological**
• Endometriosis • Chronic pelvic inflammatory disease • Pelvic adhesions • Pelvic congestion • Adenomyosis	• Urinary intestinal cysts • Recurrent urinary tract infection • Chronic urethral syndrome • Radiation cystitis	• Irritable bowel syndrome • Inflammatory bowel disease • Diverticulitis • Chronic intermittent bowel obstruction • Chronic constipation • Celiac disease	• Fibromyalgia • Posture • Osteitis pubis • Coccygodynia • Neuralgia • Herniated nucleus pulposus • Neoplasia • Neuropathic pain • Abdominal epilepsy • Abdominal migraine	• Somatization • Sexual abuse • Depression • Substance abuse • Sleep disorders

    c. Examine the abdomen, with attention to surgical scars, distention, or palpable tenderness, particularly in the epigastrium, flank, back, or bladder.

   2. A thorough and careful pelvic examination with a wet mount and cultures is the most important part of the evaluation.

C. Testing (4). If no obvious cause is apparent from the examination, it is reasonable to obtain a complete blood count, urinalysis, sedimentation rate, and serum chemistry profile. If the patient is of childbearing age, a pregnancy test can be considered. A pelvic ultrasound is often helpful, especially if the pelvic examination is inconclusive. Magnetic resonance imaging exam may be useful, particularly when diagnosing adenomyosis. Laparoscopy may be helpful, though is often noncontributory if less invasive testing is negative. A multidisciplinary approach using medical, psychological, environmental, and nutritional disciplines may be helpful in reducing symptoms.

IV. DIAGNOSIS. Chronic pelvic pain has an extensive differential diagnosis (3) (see Table 11.3.1). While gastrointestinal, gynecologic, neuromusculoskeletal, and psychiatric conditions can all cause chronic pelvic pain, a thorough gynecologic history and pelvic examination are the cornerstones of the diagnostic assessment. A few laboratory tests are helpful. A pelvic ultrasound is often useful. A team approach, coordinated by a trusted family physician, can bring much relief to patients who suffer from this frustrating clinical problem.

REFERENCES

1. American College of Obstetricians and Gynecologists. Chronic pelvic pain. ACOG practice bulletin No. 51. *Obstet Gynecol* 2004;103(3):589–605.
2. Gunter J. Chronic pelvic pain: an integrated approach to diagnosis and treatment. *Obstet Gynecol Surv* 2003;58(9):615–623.
3. Howard, F. *Evaluation of chronic pelvic pain in women. UpToDate.* Accessed at www.upto date.com on March 13, 2012.
4. Chan PD, Winkle CR, eds. *Gynecology and obstetrics, 1999–2000.* Laguna Hills, CA: Current Clinical Strategies Publishers, 1999:23–25.

11.4 Dysmenorrhea

Sanjeev Sharma

I. BACKGROUND. Dysmenorrhea can be defined as recurrent, crampy pain experienced during or immediately before menstruation. This is the most common gynecologic symptom reported by women (1).

II. PATHOPHYSIOLOGY (1, 2). Dysmenorrhea can be divided into two broad categories, primary and secondary. Primary dysmenorrhea is the most common form seen in women with no identifiable pelvic pathology. It is usually caused by myometrial activity augmented by prostaglandins resulting in uterine ischemia causing pain. The prevalence of primary dysmenorrhea is highest in younger women, affecting up to 90% of women at some point in their lives. Risk factors include early menarche, heavy menstrual flow, nulliparity, cigarette smoking, disruption of close relationships, depression, anxiety, obesity, and a family history of alcoholism. There is controversy about the association of dysmenorrhea with obesity, alcohol, physical activity, pregnancy history, and dietary factors.

Less commonly, secondary dysmenorrhea is encountered. By definition, secondary dysmenorrhea is associated with some form of pelvic pathology. Common causes of secondary dysmenorrhea include endometriosis, uterine myomas, chronic pelvic inflammatory disease, pelvic adhesions, and obstructive malformations of the genital tract. A pelvic mass can sometimes present with secondary dysmenorrhea.

III. EVALUATION (1–3).

A. History

The diagnosis of primary dysmenorrhea is made clinically, while secondary dysmenorrhea should be considered in the differential diagnosis if symptoms are atypical, or escalating discomfort appears after several years of a stable pattern of menstrual symptoms.

Primary dysmenorrhea usually starts at the onset of ovulatory menstrual cycles, which may be several years after menarche. Symptoms are typically colicky lower abdominal pain starting just before, at the time or a few hours after the start of bleeding. Pain recurs during every menstrual period. It may be associated with diarrhea, nausea and vomiting, fatigue, dizziness, or lightheadedness.

Whenever a patient presents with menstrual pain a detailed menstrual history should be obtained. Menstrual history should focus on the onset of menarche, the time between menarche and onset of symptoms, recurrence of symptoms, duration and quantity of bleeding, characteristics of the pain, including radiation, degree of disability, and any other associated symptoms.

Additionally, a history of sexually transmitted infections, dyspareunia, contraception, infertility, pelvic surgery, family history of endometriosis, the types of therapy tried, and the presence of other medical or psychiatric conditions should be sought.

An atypical history, including pelvic pain beginning at menarche, an atypical pattern or progressive worsening of the pain, or a history of a pelvic infection should alert the physician to the possibility of secondary dysmenorrhea.

In younger women, secondary dysmenorrhea that is sufficiently severe to affect daily functioning or relationships suggests endometriosis. This condition affects as many as 19% of women. Deep dyspareunia and sacral backache with menses are common symptoms. Premenstrual tenesmus or diarrhea correlates with endometriosis of the rectosigmoid area, whereas cyclic hematuria or dysuria may indicate bladder endometriosis.

B. Physical Examination. A thorough physical examination is essential to rule out any pelvic pathology. A detailed pelvic examination, with attention to areas of tenderness, fullness, nodules, or irregularity, is important. In addition, an assessment of the spine, abdomen, and bladder is important. For adolescent patients who present with dysmenorrhea but have never been sexually active, pelvic examination is rarely necessary. However, examination of the external genitalia to exclude outlet abnormalities is important.

IV. DIAGNOSIS (1–5). Primary dysmenorrhea is primarily a clinical diagnosis, and routine laboratory and imaging is usually not required. However, a wet mount, cervical cultures, pregnancy test, urinalysis, and transabdominal or transvaginal ultrasound examination may be very helpful in the appropriate setting to rule out other pathology. Magnetic resonance imaging may be helpful in making a diagnosis of adenomyosis.

A definitive diagnosis of endometriosis can be made by laparoscopy while hysteroscopic examination can help diagnose endometrial polyps and submucosal leiomyomas which may contribute to symptoms.

REFERENCES

1. Lefebvre G, Pinsonneault O, Antao V, Black A. Primary dysmenorrhea consensus guideline. *J Obstet Gynaecol Can* 2005;27(12):1117–1146. Accessed at http://www.ncbi.nlm.nih.gov/pubmed/16524531#.
2. Jamieson DJ, Steege JF. The prevalence of dysmenorrhea, dyspareunia, pelvic pain and irritable syndrome in primary care practices. *Obstet Gynecol* 1996;87:55–58.
3. Apgar BS. Dysmenorrhea and dysfunctional uterine bleeding. *Prim Care* 1997;24(1):161–179.
4. Proctor ML, Farquhar CM. Dysmenorrhoea. *Clin Evid Concise* 2005;14:573–576.
5. Chan PD, Winkle CR. *Gynecology and obstetrics 1999–2000*. Laguna Hills, CA: Current Clinical Strategies Publishers, 1999:25–26.

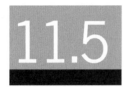

11.5 Dyspareunia
Shailendra K. Saxena and Mikayla L. Spangler

I. BACKGROUND. Dyspareunia is defined as pain experienced during sexual intercourse. The term is most often used in connection with female sexual dysfunction. However, it is important to understand that a small proportion of males also suffer from dyspareunia.

II. EPIDEMIOLOGY. The World Health Organization reviewed 54 studies that included 35,973 women and found the prevalence of dyspareunia to be between 8% and 22% (1). In contrast, it is estimated that only 5% of men suffer from pain associated with sexual intercourse (1). The low incidence of dyspareunia in men may be due to social stigma or low reporting. Dyspareunia may be defined as primary, beginning with first intercourse, or secondary, occurring after previous pain-free intercourse.

A. **Diagnosis and Evaluation.** Many patients are embarrassed by discussions about sexual concerns or dyspareunia. It is important to begin the evaluation of dyspareunia by asking open-ended questions. An important goal in the history is to assess the relative contributions of physical, social, and psychological factors leading to the symptoms that the patient is experiencing. Superficial dyspareunia in females is often related to vulvodynia, vaginitis, urethritis, or inadequate lubrication. Conversely, deep dyspareunia may be related to a pelvic pathology, such as endometriosis or pelvic inflammatory disease (PID). It is often difficult to distinguish vaginismus (muscular spasm of the outer third of the vagina preventing penetration) from other pathologies on the basis of history alone. Premenopausal women are more likely to suffer from vulvodynia and endometriosis, while postmenopausal women tend to have symptoms secondary to urogenital atrophy.

B. **Physical Examination.** Patients may have significant anxiety regarding examination, and care should be taken to minimize this anxiety and any associated discomfort. It may be helpful to have a support person in the examination room and to use a pediatric speculum during the pelvic examination in female patients. The external genitalia, perineum, perianal areas, and skin of the groin should be evaluated thoroughly. After careful evaluation of the external genitalia for tenderness, application of topical lidocaine may help with speculum insertion. Careful evaluation of the vaginal epithelium may reveal pallor or atrophy related to estrogen insufficiency. Female patients will often require bimanual and rectovaginal examinations with careful attention to areas of discomfort. Detection of urethral or vaginal discharge should prompt careful evaluation for infection.

C. **Common Causes of Dyspareunia in Women.** Infections are a common cause of dyspareunia in women. This may include vulvovaginitis due to candidiasis or trichomoniasis, and PID. Other common causes include vulvodynia, vaginismus, insufficient vaginal lubrication, and endometriosis. Less common, but important causes include interstitial cystitis, urethral diverticula, adnexal lesions, and pelvic adhesions. These may be detected by cystoscopy, ultrasound, or laparoscopy, as indicated.

D. **Common Causes of Dyspareunia in Men.** Male dyspareunia is less likely to have an infectious etiology (2). The most frequent causes include chronic prostatitis/chronic pelvic pain, phimosis, and Peyronie's disease.

REFERENCES

1. Lathe P, Latthe M, Say L. WHO systemic review of prevalence of chronic pelvic pain: a neglected reproductive health morbidity. *BMC Public Health* 2006;6:177–182.
2. Luzzi G, Law L. A guide to sexual pain in men. *Practitioner* 2005;249:73–77.

11.6 Menorrhagia
Jayashree Paknikar

I. **BACKGROUND.** Menorrhagia is defined as menstrual blood loss greater than 80 ml (1), which occurs at regular intervals (≥21 to 35 days) or lasts ≥7 days in duration. Assessing the volume of blood loss has limited utility, however. It fails to differentiate among etiologies, direct a diagnostic strategy, or indicate prognosis (1). Practically, it is difficult to quantify the amount of blood loss. Menorrhagia is diagnosed when a woman subjectively reports that menstrual bleeding is heavier or longer than is typical for her.

II. **PATHOPHYSIOLOGY**

A. **Etiology (Table 11.6.1) (2).** The etiology varies considerably with the patient's age, history, and physical findings. Pregnancy and its complications among women in their reproductive years must always be excluded; if "missed," it may be life threatening. Bleeding as a side effect of hormonal contraceptives, intrauterine devices, contraceptive implants, and other medications is common. Other frequent causes are anovulation, uterine fibroids, polyps, endometriosis, adenomyosis, coagulation disorders, endocrinopathies, malignancy, pelvic inflammatory disease (PID), and liver or kidney disease (2).

B. **Epidemiology (1).** Menorrhagia is common. In women aged 30 to 49 years of age, it represents 5% of gynecologic visits (1). Once referred to a gynecologist, women have an increased risk of operative interventions, including hysterectomy. Menorrhagia accounts for two thirds of all hysterectomies; no pathology is identified in at least 50% of these.

TABLE 11.6.1	Overview of Diagnosis
1. Source of bleeding	Vaginal, urinary, and bowel bleeding can be mistaken for uterine
2. Age of the patient	Consider
	<20 y: perimenarcheal: mostly anovulatory, bleeding diathesis needs to be ruled out
	20–40 y: predominantly anovulatory rule out systemic conditions
	<40 y: perimenopausal distinctions between menopausal transition vs. benign or malignant lesions
3. Pregnancy and associated complications (e.g., spontaneous abortion, ectopic, missed abortion, and trophoblastic disease)	Must be ruled out in any patient
4. Systemic illness	Weight changes: thyroid, liver, kidney
5. Personal/family history	Bleeding disorder
6. Iatrogenic	Anticoagulant therapy may exacerbate, copper-containing intrauterine devices, hormonal contraception, etc.

III. EVALUATION

A. History

1. **A menstrual and reproductive history is necessary.** Ask about previous patterns of the menstrual cycle: the regularity, duration, and frequency of all bleeding, including any intermenstrual flow. Determine if dysmenorrhea is present and attempt to quantify the number of pads or tampons per period.

2. **Pregnancy should always be considered and excluded.** All contraceptive methods, even permanent ones such as tubal sterilization, are subject to failure; women may not reveal sexual activity.

3. **Weight change, excessive patterns, anxiety or stress disorders, as well as symptoms of systemic disease** (e.g., coagulopathy, and thyroid, renal, and hepatic diseases) should be evaluated.

4. **Medication history** should include the use of contraceptives (3), anticoagulants, selective serotonin reuptake inhibitors, corticosteroids, antipsychotics, tamoxifen, and herbal modalities such as ginseng, gingko, and soy.

5. **Presence of easy bruising or any abnormal bleeding** such as with toothbrushing or minimal trauma may indicate a bleeding disorder.

6. **The presence of moliminal symptoms** (e.g., edema, abdominal bloating, pelvic cramping, and breast fullness) is more likely with ovulatory cycles; however, these symptoms are not reliable enough to be truly diagnostic.

7. **Psychosocial factors should be considered.** One third of women with menorrhagia have menstrual blood loss within a normal range. Anxiety, unemployment, and abdominal pain are more common in these women, and these factors may have influenced their decision to seek health care.

8. **Probable etiologies can be classified by age (4).**
   a. **Neonatal period.** Although not "menorrhagia" in this age group, vaginal bleeding may occur during the first few days of life as the infant experiences a rapid decrease in maternal-derived estrogen levels. This is generally treated with reassurance if no other signs or symptoms are present.

b. Neonatal period to menarche. Similarly, prepubertal bleeding is not "menorrhagia" but should be carefully evaluated to exclude sexual abuse and assault, malignancy, sexually transmitted infections, and trauma.

c. Early menarche. With no moliminal symptoms and irregular menses, anovulatory cycles are likely. Almost all normal adolescents experience some degree of menstrual irregularity; "heavy periods" should be evaluated. Pregnancy should be excluded if there is any question of sexual activity. Abnormal bleeding may also occur as a side effect for contraceptive hormonal methods taken correctly or incorrectly. Fever and pelvic pain can indicate PID. Easy bruising or bleeding may indicate a bleeding disorder. With neurologic symptoms such as blurred vision, visual field defects, headache, and the presence of galactorrhea, a pituitary lesion should be considered.

d. Late menarche to late thirties. Exclude pregnancy and contraceptive-related causes. Anovulation is less common. Polycystic ovarian syndrome (the most common endocrine disorder affecting 6% of reproductive age women) (5), the female athlete triad, and stress-induced conditions, such as eating disorders, may be present. Other gynecologic conditions include endometriosis, endometrial hyperplasia, endometrial polyps, PID, and endocrinopathies (both hypo- and hyperthyroidism, as well as pituitary and hypothalamic conditions).

e. Late thirties and older. Exclude pregnancy. If the patient is not pregnant, abnormal bleeding in this age group should arouse suspicion of cancer until proved otherwise. Women are increasingly anovulatory as they approach the perimenopause. Inquire about menopausal symptoms, exogenous use of estrogens, and personal or family history of gynecologic malignancy or genetically linked cancers, such as colon and breast. Other causes include adenomyosis.

f. Postmenopausal period. See Chapter 11.8.

9. **In >50% of women with menorrhagia, no etiology is found (4);** the diagnosis is then dysfunctional uterine bleeding.

B. Physical Examination

1. **Assess vital signs and the patient's general appearance, blood pressure, and pulse.** If orthostatic changes are present, evaluate for symptoms of shock. If present, these are usually related to pregnancy and may indicate a ruptured ectopic pregnancy; alternatively, trauma, sepsis, or cancer may be present.

2. **Pallor** with normal vital signs may be present if chronic blood loss has resulted in anemia. Anemia, if present, may be due to the blood loss itself, blood dyscrasia, systemic conditions, or malignancy.

3. **Fever and pelvic tenderness** are suggestive of acute PID.

4. **Physical examination includes the vulva, cervix uterus, and adnexa.** A pelvic mass may indicate abscess, fibroid, ectopic pregnancy, or malignancy. Exclude genital trauma.

5. **Signs of thyroid disease** (e.g., rapid or slow pulse, reflex changes, hair changes, and thyromegaly) can be associated with menstrual abnormalities.

6. **Excessive bruising** can indicate nutritional deficiency, eating disorder, trauma, abuse, medication overuse, or a bleeding disorder.

7. **Jaundice and hepatomegaly** may signify an underlying bleeding disorder.

8. **Obesity, hirsutism, acne, and acanthosis nigricans** suggest polycystic ovary disease.

9. **Galactorrhea** may indicate pituitary pathology.

10. **Edema** may signify renal and hepatic diseases and anemia.

C. Testing

1. **Laboratory tests**

   a. A baseline complete blood count and serum pregnancy test should be obtained.

   b. A platelet count, bleeding time, and other tests for bleeding disorders should be performed as indicated to exclude a bleeding disorder if no other etiology is readily apparent. Inherited bleeding disorders occur in as many as 11% of patients with menorrhagia compared with 3% of control women; most of these have von Willebrand's disease. Establishing this diagnosis is important, because many of the diagnostic and therapeutic options are surgical and may present added risk if an underlying bleeding disorder is present. The available data do not support routinely screening all women with menorrhagia (6).

   c. Screening for sexually transmitted diseases and thyroid dysfunction should be considered.

   d. A Papanicolaou smear should be performed if indicated, although cervical dysplasia rarely causes significant vaginal bleeding.

   e. Renal and liver function tests are useful if these etiologies are suspected.

2. Diagnostic imaging

   a. Any nonpregnant woman with irregular bleeding and a pelvic mass requires complete evaluation with ultrasound, computed tomography (CT) scan, or laparoscopy.

   b. Transvaginal ultrasound detects leiomyoma, endometrial thickening, and focal masses but may miss endometrial polyps and submucous fibroids. Although highly sensitive for endometrial carcinoma, it may miss 4% more cancers than a dilation and curettage (D&C) (7). An endometrial stripe of <5 mm is reassuring but does not conclusively exclude cancer.

   c. Saline-infused sonography (sonohysterography) (5 to 10 mL sterile saline infused into the endometrial cavity) with ultrasound imaging can be done. The utility of this procedure is comparable to diagnostic hysteroscopy and is more accurate than transvaginal ultrasound alone. The sensitivity is 95% to 97% and the specificity is 70% to 98% when combined with endometrial biopsy (8). A decision analysis recommends it as the procedure of first choice (8).

   d. Magnetic resonance imaging (MRI) may be useful for adenomyosis.

3. Endometrial sampling is recommended in women ≥35 years of age or those at increased risk for endometrial carcinoma. This procedure is best performed on the first day of menses to avoid unexpected pregnancy.

4. Hysteroscopy Diagnostic and/or Therapeutic.

5. D&C can be diagnostic and therapeutic.

IV. DIAGNOSIS (7). [TABLE 11.6.2]. Menorrhagia presents most frequently at the extremes of the reproductive years, during menarche and in perimenopause. Pregnancy must be excluded. Any pelvic mass must be evaluated with ultrasound, CT scan, or MRI. If no diagnosis can be made, laparoscopy or hysteroscopy may be indicated.

TABLE 11.6.2	Synopsis of Diagnostic Testing
Physical exam	• Vital signs, pallor, fever
	• Pelvic exam to confirm the source of bleeding to rule out pelvic mass
	• Signs of systemic disease affecting liver, kidney, bleeding disorders, or endocrinopathies like PCOS and thyroid disorders
Laboratory	• Pregnancy test
	• CBC (including platelet count)
	• Complete metabolic panel
	• Thyroid panel
	• Bleeding time
	• STD testing
	• Papanicolaou if indicated
Imaging	• Pelvic ultrasonography for pelvic mass
	• MRI and CT scan if indicated
Histopathology	• Endometrial sampling, hysteroscopy, D&C

PCOS, polycystic ovarian syndrome; CBC, complete blood count; CT, computed tomography; MRI, magnetic resonance imaging; STD, sexually transmitted disease; D&C, dilation and curettage.

REFERENCES

1. Zacur HA. *Chronic menorrhagia or anovulatory bleeding.* UpTodate. Accessed February 16, 2012.
2. Albers JR, Hull SK, Wesley RM. Abnormal uterine bleeding. *Am Fam Physician* 2004;69:1915–1926.
3. Schrager S. Abnormal uterine bleeding Associated with hormonal contraception. *Am Fam Physician* 2002;65(1):2073–2080.
4. Finley B, Harnisch DR, Comer B, et al. *Women's genitourinary conditions: FP essentials,* Monograph No, 314 AAFP Home Study, Leawood, Kan: American Academy of Family Physicians, 2005:28–41.
5. Goodman A. Initial approach to the premenopausal woman with abnormal uterine bleeding. UpToDate. Accessed September 24, 2010.
6. James A, Matchar DB, Myers ER. Testing for von Willebrand disease in women with menorrhagia: a systematic review. *Obstet Gynecol* 2004;104(2):381–388.
7. Roy SN, Bhattacharya S. Benefits and risks of pharmacological agents used for the treatment of menorrhagia. *Drug Saf* 2004;27(2):75–90.
8. Dijkhuizen FPHLJ, Mol BWJ, Bongers MY, et al. Cost effectiveness of transvaginal sonography and saline infused sonography in the evaluation of menorrhagia. *Int J Gynecol Obstet* 2003;83(1):45–52.

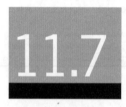

Nipple Discharge in Nonpregnant Females

Hamid Mukhtar

I. BACKGROUND. Nipple discharge is the third most commonly encountered breast complaint after pain and mass (1). Nipple discharge that is bilateral, that is multiductal, and that tends to occur after manipulation is more likely to be of benign origin. Spontaneous discharge, particularly if it is unilateral or bloody, is a source of greater concern.

II. PATHOPHYSIOLOGY

    A. Etiology. Galactorrhea results from the stimulation of breast tissue by prolactin. Prolactin is released from the anterior pituitary gland. Under normal conditions, prolactin release is inhibited by dopamine. Elevated prolactin levels, and factors that suppress dopamine, lead to the secretion of milk from the lobular and ductal epithelium of the breast.

        1. Common causes of physiologic nipple discharge include stress, nipple stimulation (including that occurring from rubbing due to jogging and straps from a backpack), as well as chest trauma or lesions such as herpes zoster, which may elevate circulating prolactin levels.

        2. Medications and other substances that affect dopamine levels, thereby resulting in increased prolactin production include phenothiazines and other antipsychotics, tricyclic antidepressants, metoclopramide, verapamil, digitalis, isoniazid, opiates, and marijuana.

        3. Other causes of nipple discharge include infections, systemic diseases, benign tumors, and malignancy. Intraductal papilloma is the most common cause of benign pathologic unilateral discharge. The discharge is typically straw colored or clear. Ductal ectasia is another cause of pathologic discharge. This condition is commoner in smokers and women in the 40- to 60-year age group.

        4. Pituitary adenoma: Classically presents with bilateral nipple discharge, amenorrhea, and/or neurologic symptoms.

        5. Thyroid disorders: Increased production of thyrotropin-releasing hormone may stimulate prolactin release.

        6. Chronic renal failure: Approximately 30% of the patients with chronic renal failure have elevated prolactin levels (2).

B. Epidemiology. Fifty percent to 80% of women will present with a nipple discharge at some point in their reproductive years. Only 5% of these women have breast cancer (3). The risk of malignant nipple discharge increases with age, unilateral and uniductal bloody discharge (3).

III. EVALUATION

A. History. Initial history should begin with queries regarding the nature of the discharge and characteristics of the patient. How old is the patient? What is the circumstance of discovery of the discharge, including spontaneity, and the presence of a palpable mass? How does the patient describe the characteristics of the discharge? A thorough history should include past breast history, chest trauma, infection, and medication and substance use. Family history of breast cancer is also critical to risk assessment. Is there a history of friction of the nipple? Does the patient smoke?

  1. Reproductive history. What is the patient's menstrual status? Has there been a recent pregnancy or abortion? This information helps identify normal lactation. Is the patient using hormonal contraception?

  2. Review of systems. Review of systems should include queries about thyroid function, renal and hepatic disease, as well as adrenal or pituitary symptoms. Does the patient have a history of headaches, visual disturbances, and associated amenorrhea or menstrual disturbance?

B. Physical Examination

  1. Breast Exam

  a. Inspection. Observe the skin of the breast for erythema, crusting, or rash on the nipple or areolar region. Document the color of the discharge if present. Look for nipple retraction. Look for any chest wall scars, rash, eczematous changes, or inflammation.

  b. Palpation. Feel the skin for warmth. Palpate both breasts for a mass or tenderness. Palpate the regional lymph nodes for lymphadenopathy. Document the size, shape, location, consistency, and mobility of any mass.

  c. Compression. Compress the base or the areolar region of the breast with thumb and index finger to try to express any discharge. A warm compress prior to examination may assist in identification of the discharge. Note the location and color of discharge and the number of ducts involved.

  2. Other Exam: A complete neurologic exam should accompany any history of headache or visual disturbance. Thyroid and abdominal exam should also be performed if the history is suggestive of pathology in these areas.

C. Laboratory Evaluation

  1. Discharge. Guaiac testing of the discharge should be performed if the discharge is not obviously bloody or serosanguineous in a unilateral, uniductal presentation. Although the role of cytology is controversial, the presence of blood increases the positive predictive value of cytology. A positive cytology is highly predictive of cancer (3).

  2. Other Tests. Laboratory tests are based on clinical assessment. A pregnancy test should be considered in all women of reproductive age. Further tests that should be considered include prolactin level, thyroid, renal, and liver function tests.

  3. Imaging. Ultrasound is a good diagnostic tool, which often provides good visualization of dilated ducts and any nodules inside of them. Mammogram is indicated in all women older than 30 years of age with a spontaneous discharge (3). The role of mammogram is to identify occult disease and help in the characterization of any palpable mass. The roles of ductography, ductoscopy, ductal lavage, and magnetic resonance imaging are under investigation.

  4. Surgery. Surgical referral for ductal exploration or further evaluation is indicated for a patient with a unilateral and uniductal nipple discharge or a nipple discharge in the presence of a mass or positive cytology.

  5. Genetic Testing. A positive family history of a parent or sibling with breast cancer or abnormal BRCA1/BRCA2 genes increases the chance that a discharge may be malignant. Otherwise, genetic testing is not indicated in the evaluation of a nipple discharge (4).

IV. DIFFERENTIAL DIAGNOSIS

The main consideration in the differential diagnosis is to distinguish between physiologic and pathologic nipple discharge. The differential diagnosis includes pregnancy, pseudodischarge, friction or manipulation, systemic disease, pituitary disease, cancer, ductal ectasia, intraductal papilloma, Paget's disease, eczema, and local inflammation secondary to trauma or infection.

REFERENCES

1. Hussain A, Policarpio C, Vincent M. Evaluating nipple discharge. *Obstet Gynecol Surv* 2006;61(4): 278–283.
2. Leung A, Pacaud A. Diagnosis and management of galactorrhea. *Am Fam Physician* 2004;70(3): 543–550.
3. Golshan M, Iglehart D. Nipple discharge. UpToDate, A. Chagpar MD, UpTodate, Waltham, MA. Accessed June 16, 2012.
4. Andolsek K, Copeland J. Conditions of the breast. In: David A, Fields S, Phillips D, Scherger J, Taylor R, eds. *Family Medicine: Principles and Practice.* 5th ed. New York, NY: Springer-Verlag; 1998:326–342.

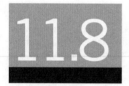

11.8 Pap Smear Abnormality

Mindy J. Lacey

I. BACKGROUND. In 2012, the American Cancer Society estimated that approximately 12,000 cases of invasive cervical cancer and 4,000 (1.5%) of cancer-related deaths annually in the United States were due to cervical neoplasia (1). While once the leading cause of cancer death in women, the incidence of squamous cell carcinoma of the uterine cervix has steadily decreased in the United States after the widespread introduction of cervical cytology screening. Approximately 60 million Pap smears are performed in the United States each year, with fewer than 4% of these revealing abnormalities that necessitate additional testing, such as colposcopy (2). Although most cytologic alterations found in Pap smears will likely regress without intervention, the risk of progression to an invasive lesion underlies the rationale for the follow-up of even low-grade lesions (3). In recent years, the introduction of a variety of molecular assays that screen for high-risk human papilloma virus (HPV) have vastly altered diagnostic and therapeutic algorithms.

II. PATHOPHYSIOLOGY

A. Etiology

1. Within the uterine cervis is the squamocolumnar junction, or transformation zone, where the columnar epithelium of the endocervical mucosa abuts the squamous epithelium of the ectocervix. This area is prone to numerous physiologic, inflammatory, and mechanical stresses that commonly result in metaplastic change. In addition, the rapid cellular turnover makes the transformation zone particularly susceptible viral oncogenesis and genetic damage by environmental agents.

2. HPV replicates within epithelial cells at various mucosal sites, that include the basal and parabasal epithelial cells. In most immunocompetent individuals, the infection is transient and clears within 8 to 24 months, particularly among women younger than 30 (4). The clinical manifestations of HPV infection are somewhat dependent on the viral subtype. Approximately 30 to 40 subtypes are known to infect the lower genital tract, usually via sexual contact, and are broadly divided into those with low and high oncogenic potential ("low risk" and "high risk," respectively as shown in Table 11.8.1).

TABLE 11.8.1	Human Papilloma Virus Types According to the Oncogenic Potential	
Oncogenic potential	**Virus type**	
Low risk	6, 11, 40, 42–44, 53, 54, 61, 72, 73, 81	
High risk	16, 18, 31, 33, 35, 39, 45, 51, 52, 56, 58, 59, 68, 82	

Low-risk viral subtypes are associated with condyloma acuminatum and other low-grade cervical abnormalities with a small potential for the development of invasive lesions. The high-risk subtypes may cause high-grade dysplasia and carry greater risk for the subsequent development of malignancy (5).

B. Epidemiology

1. HPV has an estimated prevalence of 5% to 20% in the US population and up to half of young women will develop a transient infection following the initiation of sexual activity (6). Infections with HPV in older women are much less prevalent but carry a higher risk of progression to cervical neoplasia. In most cases, progression of cytologic and histologic abnormalities is sequential (from low grade to high grade, Table 11.8.2) and takes place over a span of months to years, making it ideal for screening (7).

2. Risk factors for cervical neoplasia include HPV infection, early onset of intercourse, multiple and high-risk sexual partners, young age, low socioeconomic status, race, history of other sexually transmitted diseases, compromised immunity, cigarette smoking, and oral contraceptive use.

III. EVALUATION

A. History. Most patients with cervical dysplasia are asymptomatic. They may also present with evidence of external condyloma, vaginal discharge, or even vaginal bleeding. For most, the initial discovery of cervical neoplasia is usually as an abnormality in the Pap smear. The gynecologic and prior Pap smear history, which is essential in estimating a patient's risk, should be shared with the cytopathologist whenever possible.

B. Physical Examination. On physical examination, the cervix usually appears normal to the naked eye. Grossly visible cervical lesions should be biopsied (not Pap smeared) to obtain an accurate diagnosis.

C. Testing. The contemporary method for obtaining Pap smear specimen is a liquid-based system, which has virtually supplanted the older "conventional" method. The cervix and endocervix are sampled with a plastic "broom" or a similar apparatus and the specimen is suspended in a bottle containing the fixative and transported as a suspension. Advantages of

TABLE 11.8.2	Natural History of Cervical Dysplasia			
	Regression (%)	Persistence (%)	Progression to severe dysplasia (%)	Progression to cancer (%)
Mild dysplasia	57	32	11	1
Moderate dysplasia	43	35	22	5
Severe dysplasia	32	-56	–	12

liquid-based Pap smears include less artifact, a lower number of unsatisfactory specimens, and the ability to perform HPV DNA testing on a single sample.

1. The American Cancer Society, American Society for Colposcopy and Cervical Pathology, and American Society for Clinical Pathology released updated consensus guidelines for cervical cancer screening in 2012 (8). They state that:

   a. women should begin screening at 21 years of age with only Pap smears every 3 years.

   b. At age 30, women should receive either a Pap smear alone every 3 years, or a Pap smear combined with molecular screening for high-risk HPV every 5 years.

   c. Those older than 65 with either three negative Pap smears or two negative high-risk HPV assays in the preceeding 10 years may discontinue screening.

   d. Women who are status-post hysterectomy for benign reasons are exempt from testing.

   e. Current recommendations for women who have received the HPV vaccine are not different from that listed above.

IV. PAP SMEAR DIAGNOSES AND MANAGEMENT. It is important to remember that the Pap test is for screening only; the definitive diagnosis of preinvasive and invasive neoplastic lesions can only be made histologically. The purpose of the Pap smear is to identify abnormalities in exfoliated ecto- and endocervical cells that suggest underlying neoplastic lesions and signify the need for additional testing. The 2001 Bethesda System delineates uniform terminology for cervical cytopathology reporting. This allows for standardization of follow-up and treatment. The common cytopathologic diagnoses with typical follow-up for each are as follows (9):

A. **Atypical Squamous Cells of Undetermined Significance.** This represents abnormal squamous cells that do not meet morphologic criteria for higher grade lesions. According to 2006 ASCCP guidelines, women <30 years of age can be followed with a repeat Pap smear in 4 to 6 months or proceed to diagnostic colposcopy, depending on the clinical situation. Those older than 30 years of age are typically managed according to the high-risk HPV DNA status: if positive, colposcopy should be performed. If negative, the patient can be followed with a repeat Pap smear in 1 year.

B. **Atypical Squamous Cells (Cannot Exclude High-Grade Squamous Intraepithelial Lesion [ASC-H]).** Because 30% to 40% of patients with ASC-H demonstrate high-grade dysplasia and a very high prevalence of high-risk HPV DNA (approaching 85%), these patients should all have colposcopic evaluation and biopsies.

C. **Atypical Glandular Cells (AGCs).** This diagnosis should include a comment by the pathologist regarding the probable source of the AGCs. Patients with AGC favored to be endometrial in origin should undergo endometrial and endocervical sampling with colposcopy afterward if no endometrial pathology is noted. All other ACG diagnoses warrant immediate colposcopy with HPV testing and the addition of endometrial sampling if the patient is >35 years of age.

D. **Low-Grade Squamous Intraepithelial Lesion (LGSIL).** All patients with LGSIL results on a Pap smear should undergo colposcopy with a recommendation for endocervical curettage in non-pregnant, premenopausal patients or those with an unsatisfactory colposcopic examination. HPV DNA testing is only performed if moderate- or high-grade squamous dysplasia (CIN 2-3) is discovered on colposcopic biopsies. Pregnant women with LGSIL may defer colposcopy until at least 6 weeks following delivery.

E. **High-Grade Squamous Epithelial Lesion (HGSIL).** Most guidelines recommend that patients of any age with HSIL should undergo immediate colposcopy. If high-grade squamous dysplasia is noted on biopsy, definitive excisional therapy (such as loop electrosurgic excision) is warranted. HPV testing is not appropriate in this setting.

V. COLPOSCOPY. Colposcopy uses magnification to identify the abnormal areas of the uterine cervix. After a Pap smear is performed, the cervix is painted with a solution of 3% to 5% acetic acid, allowing for the visualization of abnormally staining areas to direct subsequent biopsy. The examination is considered satisfactory only if the entire transformation zone can be visualized and the most abnormal areas can be biopsied. A simultaneous endocervical curettage is usually performed to ensure adequate sampling of the transformation zone and to evaluate the glandular cells in the endocervical canal. If colposcopy is inadequate, there is an abnormality in the endocervical canal, or there is a suspicion of invasive cancer; further diagnostic testing should include either a conization of the cervix or a loop electrosurgical excision procedure (LEEP) to complete the workup.

REFERENCES

1. Siegel R, Naishadham D, Jemal A. Cancer statistics 2012. *CA Cancer J Clin* 2011;61:69.
2. Mahdavi A, Monk BJ. Vaccines against human papillomavirus and cervical cancer: promises and challenges. *Oncologist* 2005;10:528.
3. Holoway P, Miller AB, Rohan T, et al. Natural history of dysplasia of the uterine cervix. *J Natl Cancer Inst* 1999;91:252.
4. Ho GY, Bierman R, Beardsley L, et al. Natural history of cervicovaginal papillomavirus infection in young women. *N Engl J Med* 1998;338:423–428.
5. Kahn JA. HPV vaccination for the prevention of cervical intraepitheial neoplasia. *N Engl J Med* 2009;361:271.
6. Winer RL, Lee SK, Hughes JP, et al. Genital human papillomavirus infection: incidence and risk factors in a cohort of female university students. *Am J Epidemiol* 2003;157:218.
7. Östor AG. Natural history of cervical intraepithelial neoplasia: a critical review. *Int J Gynecol Pathol* 1993;12:186–192.
8. U.S. Preventive Services Task Force. *Screening for cervical cancer: recommendations and rationale,* http://www.ahrq.gov/clinic/uspstf/uspscerv.htm, accessed January 20, 2003.
9. Wright TC, Massad LS, Dunton CJ, et al. 2006 consensus guidelines for the management of women with abnormal cervical cancer screening tests. *Am J Obstet Gynecol* 2007;197:346–355.

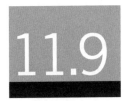

11.9

Postmenopausal Bleeding

Naureen Rafiq

I. BACKGROUND. Postmenopausal bleeding or PMB is defined as vaginal bleeding that occurs in a woman who has had amenorrhea for a year or more.

II. PATHOPHYSIOLOGY

A. Etiology. Any vaginal bleeding in a postmenopausal woman requires the clinician to strongly consider the possibility of endometrial malignancy. Women on cyclic hormone replacement therapy (HRT) are expected to have uterine bleeding; however, irregular or excessive bleeding in these patients requires investigation (Table 11.9.1).

B. Epidemiology. Abnormal vaginal bleeding is a common outpatient problem, occurring in 10% of women older than 55 years of age (1) and accounting for 70% of gynecologic visits during the perimenopausal and postmenopausal years (2).

III. EVALUATION

A. History

1. **Pattern of bleeding.** The amount of bleeding should be estimated to help assess whether and what type of intervention may be required in order to avoid anemia or hypovolemia. Vaginal and endometrial atrophy and endometrial polyps are common causes of PMB. Association of bleeding with bowel movements or urination suggests a nongenital source.

2. **Current medications.** Any use of hormonal therapy, including estrogen, progesterone, tamoxifen, thyroid replacement, or corticosteroids should be quantified and recorded.

TABLE 11.9.1	Etiology of Postmenopausal Bleeding
Gynecologic Causes	**Non-gynecologic causes**
Atrophic uterus	Hormone replacement therapy
Cervical and endometrial polyp	Thyroid replacement therapy
Endometrial hyperplasia	Corticosteroids
Uterine fibroids	Anticoagulants
Endometrial, cervical, ovarian, or Fallopian tube cancers	Obesity
Hydrometra	Dramatic weight loss
Pyometra	Infections in adjacent organs like diverticulitis leading to endometritis
Hematometra	Stress
	Diabetes, hypertension, and liver disease

a. Acyclic bleeding is common in the first 3–4 months on continuous estrogen–progestin therapy and usually does not indicate pathology. Bleeding that is excessive, persists after months of therapy, or occurs after amenorrhea has been established on these regimens should be evaluated.

b. The rate of endometrial cancer in women taking tamoxifen or unopposed estrogen is six to seven times the rate for untreated women. The frequency of endometrial polyps is also increased (3, 4).

c. Exogenous corticosteroids or thyroid abnormalities can lead to menstrual irregularities and PMB.

d. Anticoagulant therapy may cause uterine bleeding in postmenopausal women.

e. Endometritis is an uncommon cause of bleeding in postmenopausal women, but endometrial tuberculosis in developing countries may present with PMB (5–7).

3. **Past medical history.** Nulliparity, early menarche, late menopause, and history of chronic anovulation are risk factors for endometrial hyperplasia and carcinoma. Obesity, hypertension, diabetes, and liver disease are commonly associated with estrogen excess and can also increase risk. Past use of oral contraceptives is associated with a decreased risk of endometrial carcinoma.

4. **Family history.** A strong family history of endometrial, breast, or colon cancer is a risk factor for endometrial cancer.

B. **Physical examination**

1. **Vital signs.** Blood pressure and pulse can indicate the degree and acuity of blood loss; orthostatic changes can be evidence of significant volume depletion. Fever suggests infection as a potential cause (Chapter 2.6).

2. **Abdomen.** Tenderness or guarding suggests an infectious or inflammatory cause. Malignancy may also present with an abdominal mass.

3. **Pelvis.** It is necessary to examine the external genitalia, vagina, and cervix for lesions that could be the source of bleeding. The uterus and ovaries are palpated to assess for enlargement, masses, and tenderness.

4. **Rectum.** Rectal examination and anoscopy may be warranted to rule out hemorrhoids or other intestinal sources of bleeding (Chapter 9.11).

C. **Testing**

1. **Office laboratory testing.** Urinalysis, stool guaiac testing, or both can be useful to assess for nongenital sources of blood. A complete blood count may be helpful in assessing the

degree of blood loss or elevated white count due to infection. Testing for gonorrhea and chlamydia may be warranted.

2. **Papanicolaou (Pap) smear.** Many sources recommend a Pap smear as part of the evaluation, although the diagnostic yield is generally low. Cervical lesions or friability raise the possibility of a source of cervical bleeding. Endometrial cells or abnormal glandular cells of unknown significance found on the Pap smear of a postmenopausal woman not on HRT warrants further evaluation of the endometrium.

3. **Biopsy**
   a. Visible lesions of the vulva, vagina, or cervix should be sent for biopsy.
   b. In the absence of a clear nonuterine source of bleeding, endometrial biopsy is recommended. Office-based endometrial biopsy is less invasive and more cost-effective than dilation and curettage (D & C), with comparable sensitivity and specificity (8). There is excellent correlation between the histopathology of specimens taken by office biopsy and D & C (9). Blind sampling of either type is most effective when pathology is global, rather than focal.
   c. If there is persistent bleeding after a normal biopsy result, further assessment is necessary. This may include a repeat biopsy, D & C, and/or imaging.

4. **Diagnostic imaging.** Several methods are available; there is little evidence-based consensus on when each method should be used (1, 10).
   a. Transvaginal ultrasound (TVUS) is gaining popularity as an alternative or adjunct to endometrial biopsy. A clearly identifiable, homogeneous endometrial stripe ≤4 mm in thickness is highly unlikely to contain hyperplasia or carcinoma, and biopsy may not be necessary (8). TVUS is better tolerated than endometrial biopsy, with similar detection rates for endometrial abnormalities (1, 9). However, women with persistent bleeding warrant further investigation. TVUS should not be used in place of biopsy among women taking tamoxifen or women on HRT (Table 11.9.2).
   b. Saline infusion sonohysterography (SIS; ultrasound evaluation after the instillation of fluid into the endometrial cavity) allows the architectural evaluation of the uterine cavity to detect small lesions that may be missed by endometrial biopsy or TVUS. The disadvantage of this method is the absence of tissue diagnosis, so if a lesion is found, hysteroscopy is then necessary for directed biopsy.
   c. Hysteroscopy is becoming the "gold standard" against which other methods of endometrial assessment are compared. This provides direct visualization of the endometrial cavity, allowing targeted biopsy or excision of lesions. However, it is more costly and requires more special expertise than most other modalities. Because lesions are occasionally missed even with this method, some recommend performing D & C along with hysteroscopy (9).
   d. Magnetic resonance imaging is occasionally helpful in determining the presence of fibroids when sonography is not definitive.
   e. Palpable adnexal abnormalities should be evaluated by ultrasound or other imaging as appropriate.

D. **Genetics.** Genetic testing is not helpful in the evaluation of PMB. Women with a family history of gynecologic malignancy are at high risk and should be evaluated thoroughly.

IV. DIAGNOSIS

A. **Differential diagnosis.** Causes of PMB have been reported as atrophy (59%), polyp (12%), endometrial cancer (10%), endometrial hyperplasia (9.8%), hormonal effect (7%), cervical cancer (<1%), and other (2%) (8).

TABLE 11.9.2	Endometrial Thickness	
<3 mm with or without endometrial fluid	3–5 mm with endometrial fluid	5 mm with bleeding or 11 mm without bleeding
No further studies	Further studies	Further studies

B. Clinical manifestations. Initial clinical evaluation may identify a nonuterine source. Postcoital spotting in conjunction with vaginal atrophy or cervical friability suggests cervical or vaginal mucosal bleeding. If no other source is identified, the key to diagnosis is imaging and tissue sampling of the endometrium. A thin endometrial stripe in a woman in a low-risk category suggests endometrial atrophy. If neither biopsy nor TVUS provides sufficient information, SIS and/or hysteroscopy with directed biopsy may be used. D & C should be reserved for cases in which other methods are unsuccessful or unavailable.

REFERENCES

1. Goldstein RB, Bree RL, Benson CB, et al. Evaluation of the woman with postmenopausal bleeding: society of radiologists in ultrasound-sponsored consensus conference statement. *J Ultrasound Med* 2001;20:1025–1036.
2. Clark TJ, Mann CH, Shah N, et al. Accuracy of outpatient endometrial biopsy in the diagnosis of endometrial cancer: a systematic quantitative review. *BJOG* 2002;109:313–321.
3. Fisher B, Costantino JP, Redmond CK, et al. Endometrial cancer in tamoxifen-treated breast cancer patients: findings from the National Surgical Adjuvant Breast and Bowel Project (NSABP) B-14. *J Natl Cancer Inst* 1994;86:527.
4. Chalas E, Costantino JP, Wickerham DL, et al. Benign gynecologic conditions among participants in the Breast Cancer Prevention Trial. *Am J Obstet Gynecol* 2005;192:1230.
5. Sabadell J, Castellví J, Baró F. Tuberculous endometritis presenting as postmenopausal bleeding. *Int J Gynaecol Obstet* 2007;96:203.
6. Mengistu Z, Engh V, Melby KK, et al. Postmenopausal vaginal bleeding caused by endometrial tuberculosis. *Acta Obstet Gynecol Scand* 2007;86:631.
7. Güngördük K, Ulker V, Sahbaz A, et al. Postmenopausal tuberculosis endometritis. *Infect Dis Obstet Gynecol* 2007;2007:27028.
8. Goodman A. *Evaluation and management of uterine bleeding in postmenopausal women.* Accessed at UpToDate online (www.uptodate.com) on July 2005, last update October 2004.
9. Feldman S. *Diagnostic evaluation of the endometrium in women with abnormal uterine bleeding.* Accessed at UpToDate (www.uptodate.com) on July 2005, last update January 2005.
10. Clark TJ, Voit D, Gupta JK, et al. Accuracy of hysteroscopy in the diagnosis of endometrial cancer and hyperplasia: a systematic quantitative review. *JAMA* 2002;288(13):1610–1621.

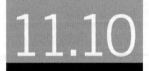

11.10 Vaginal Discharge

Sanjeev Sharma

I. BACKGROUND. Vaginal discharge can be physiologic or pathologic. When pathologic, it is reported that 90% of affected women have bacterial vaginosis (BV), vulvovaginal candidiasis (VVC), or trichomoniasis (1–3). Other pathologic causes include vaginal infections such as chlamydia and gonorrhea, malignancies, and allergic conditions.

II. PATHOPHYSIOLOGY. BV is not a sexually transmitted disease. It is characterized by a reduction in the number of vaginal *Lactobacillus* species with subsequent overgrowth of *Gardnerella vaginalis*, *Mobiluncus* species, *Mycoplasma hominis*, or anaerobic Gram-negative rods. This disruption of the normal vaginal microflora has been associated with multiple or new sex partners, antimicrobial use, douching, smoking, or pregnancy. These predisposing factors have been reported in up to 33% of women suffering from BV (4).

Candida species are a part of the normal vaginal flora among many healthy asymptomatic females. Vulvovaginitis is most commonly due to *Candida albicans*. Less commonly, it may be due to *C. glabrata* or *C. parapsilosis*. The exact mechanism by which it causes symptomatic disease is complex and involves host inflammatory responses and virulence factors in the organism. Risk factors for vaginal candidiasis include diabetes mellitus, antibiotic use, and immunosuppression.

Trichomoniasis vaginalis is a flagellated protozoan parasite contracted almost exclusively through sexual contact. *Trichomoniasis* is responsible for 10–25% of vaginal infections (4).

In the United States, infection with *Chlamydia trachomatis* is prevalent. Between 5 and 15% of pregnant women may be infected with this organism (5). *Neisseria gonorrhoeae* is the second most commonly reported bacterial sexually transmitted infection (STI) (6). *N. gonorrhoeae* and *C. trachomatis* infections both present with cervicitis, although *N. gonorrhoeae* typically presents more acutely. Other common causes of vaginal discharge include noninfectious causes such as atrophy and allergies, chemical irritation (2), neoplasia, and foreign bodies such as retained tampons (5) or intrauterine devices.

III. EVALUATION

A. History. A good clinical history is helpful in clarifying the cause of vaginal discharge. Many women take over-the-counter medications before presenting to the physician, and this may affect patient presentation or subsequent evaluation. The history should focus on the age of the patient, relationship status, sexual history, number and gender of sexual partners, menstrual history, vaginal hygiene practices including douching, recent medication, instrumentation or surgery, current health and smoking, contraceptive history, and the characteristics of the discharge.

Young women, especially those younger than 30 years, may be at increased risk for STIs (7, 8). In elderly patients, a persistent vaginal discharge may indicate atrophy or neoplasia.

The patient's general health status is important; frequent problems with discharge, particularly recurrent candidiasis, may suggest the presence of a systemic illness such as diabetes or human immunodeficiency virus.

B. Discharge Characteristics. Physiologic discharge is most commonly described as being clear and thin. Typically, the amount of discharge varies with the menstrual cycle. Pathologic discharge is more frequently described as copious, having a particular color and may have an odor.

The discharge of BV is classically a homogenous white, noninflammatory discharge that smoothly coats the vaginal walls. The discharge can be fishy or musty before or after the addition of potassium hydroxide (KOH; a positive "whiff" test); see Section III.C (3).

The discharge of VVC is often thick, clumpy, white, and odorless, and it can be associated with vaginal pruritus, erythema, and edema. The discharge of trichomoniasis may be diffuse, malodorous, and yellow-green, with vulvar irritation (3).

C. Associated Symptoms. These can include itching, soreness, dysuria, or postcoital bleeding, lower abdominal pain, pelvic pain, and dyspareunia.

D. Physical Examination. A complete physical examination should be considered if the patient appears to be acutely ill, has signs of systemic illness, including abdominal pain, rash, fever, or other complaints. When preparing to examine the genitalia, care must be given to patient comfort, privacy, and the sensitive nature of the lithotomy position. Attention should be given to the presence of cervical or vulvar inflammation and the presence of cervical motion tenderness.

E. Testing. (Refer Table 11.10.1.) Office laboratory testing is easy and usually available in the outpatient clinical setting. KOH test, pH, and microscopic examination of the vaginal discharge can determine the cause of vaginal discharge in most cases.

IV. DIAGNOSIS.

BV is commonly diagnosed by using Amsel's criteria. These include the presence of a characteristic discharge, the presence of clue cells on microscopic examination, discharge pH > 4.5, and a positive "whiff" test. Diagnosis of vaginal trichomoniasis is usually made by microscopic examination of a wet mount of the discharge. However, the sensitivity of microscopic exam has been reported to be only 60–70% , and a fresh specimen yields better results (8). Culture is a sensitive method of diagnosing trichomoniasis. A polymerase chain reaction assay for the detection of gonorrhea and chlamydia is widely available.

If all laboratory tests are negative and signs of local inflammation are present, noninfectious causes of vaginitis should be considered. These include mechanical friction, as well as chemical irritation (often seen with the use of douching) or allergic causes, often seen among those using certain soaps, scented menstrual pads, or fabric softeners.

TABLE 11.10.1	Differential Diagnosis and Clinical Manifestations in Vaginal Discharge		
	Bacterial vaginosis	**Vulvovaginal candidiasis**	**Trichomoniasis**
Discharge characteristics	Homogenous, white, noninflammatory	Thick, white, cottage cheese-like	Yellow-green copious, watery, pooling, frothy (4)
Odor	Fishy before and after KOH + "whiff" test	Not typical	Malodorous (10%)
Physical examination	Discharge coats vaginal wall	Excoriation edema, erythema	Strawberry cervix (2% of patients) (4)
Precipitating factors	Changes to vaginal flora, pregnancy, condoms, douching, new or multiple partners (1)	Antibiotics, systemic illness, medication, immunocompromise	Sexually transmitted infection
pH	>4.5	Normally <4.5	>4.5 in 90%
Microscopy/ Gram stain	Amsel's diagnostic criteria[a]	Budding yeast or hyphae after 10% KOH	60–70% sensitive
			Culture most sensitive (3)
	Presence of clue cells highly suggestive (1)		
			Moving flagellae (2)
Associated symptoms	May be asymptomatic	Pruritus, vaginal irritation, dysuria (1)	Vulvar irritation and dysuria, lower abdominal pain; may be asymptomatic (4)

[a]Thin homogenous discharge, positive "whiff test," clue cells, vaginal pH >4.5—three out of four is highly suggestive of BV (1).

REFERENCES

1. Egan ME, Lipsky MS. Diagnosis of vaginitis. *Am Fam Physician* 2000;62(5):1095–1104.
2. Miller KE, Ruiz DE, Graves JC. Update on the prevention and treatment of sexually transmitted diseases. *Am Fam Physician* 2003;67(9):1915–1922.
3. Accessed at http://www.cdc.gov/mmwr/preview/mmwrhtml/rr5106a1.htm on August 11, 2012.
4. Accessed at www.infopoems.com on May 11, 2012.
5. Mitchell H. Vaginal discharge—causes, diagnosis and treatment. *BMJ* 2004;328:1306–1308.
6. Mejeroni U. Screening and treatment for sexually transmitted infections in pregnancy. *Am Fam Physician* 2007;76:265–270.
7. *Diseases characterized by vaginal discharge.* Treatment guideline. Accessed at www.cdc.gov/std/trichomonas/treatment.htm on August 12, 2012.
8. Department of Health and Human Services. Centers for Disease Control and Prevention. *Morbidity and mortality weekly report: recommendations and reports. Sexually transmitted diseases treatment guidelines, 2006.* August 4, 2006, Volume 55, Number RR-1.

CHAPTER 12

Musculoskeletal Problems
Allison M. Cullan

12.1 Arthralgia
Richard H. Rutkowski

I. **BACKGROUND.** Arthralgia means joint pain. It is a symptom, not a diagnosis. Arthralgia may affect a single joint or several joints. The symptom may arise from bones or periarticular structures (such as muscle, ligament, or tendon). Arthralgia is sometimes equated with "arthritis," although the terms are not synonymous. Arthritis typically causes arthralgia, but not all arthralgia is caused by arthritis (1).

II. **PATHOPHYSIOLOGY.** Arthralgia can be a manifestation of a variety of causes, including mechanical trauma to a joint, degenerative joint disease (DJD)/osteoarthritis, infection, and local or systemic inflammation. Twenty percent of all primary care visits worldwide are related to joint and muscle pains. In the elderly, the most common cause of arthralgia is DJD, affecting about one-third of those over age 65 years; in middle-aged patients, inflammatory conditions (various arthritides) predominate; in the young, systemic conditions, such as viral infections, are more likely (2–4).

III. **EVALUATION.** The differential diagnosis is broad; thus, it is useful to target the history and examination upon several key elements: duration of arthralgia, the presence or absence of signs of joint inflammation, distribution of affected joints, systemic symptoms, patient gender/age/ medical history (5). The consideration of these factors can substantially narrow the range of possible diagnoses and help establish the cause. Laboratory testing and imaging may be necessary in some instances to clarify or confirm a final diagnosis.

A. **Duration of Arthralgia (5, 6)**
   1. Abrupt onset of significant pain in a single joint immediately following trauma highlights the probable cause.
   2. Acute onset of pain, with signs of inflammation and fever, points to an infectious or perhaps crystal-induced arthropathy.
   3. Indolent onset of arthralgia in several joints over weeks or months would make infection or crystal-induced disease improbable.
   4. Acute onset may reflect an acute, self-limited process or simply the first recognition of what will become a chronic condition.

B. **Presence or Absence of Inflammation (5, 6)**
   1. Warm, swollen, erythematous, tender joints point to "arthritis" as a result of bacterial or viral infection, crystal arthropathy, or connective tissue disease and would be less likely to represent osteoarthritis.
   2. Morning stiffness, especially that lasting for over 30 minutes, would support a diagnosis of rheumatoid arthritis.

C. Distribution of Joints (5, 6)

1. Symmetric involvement of the metacarpophalangeal (MCP) joints would suggest consideration of rheumatoid arthritis.
2. Symptoms in weight-bearing joints such as the knees and hips raise suspicion of DJD.
3. Symptoms in the first metatarsophalangeal (MTP) joint with signs of local inflammation support a diagnosis of gout.

D. Systemic Symptoms (5, 6)

1. Current symptoms of upper respiratory infection or recent history of measles mumps rubella vaccine and polyarthralgia point to reactive arthralgia.
2. Urethritis, conjunctivitis, and large lower extremity joint involvement in a young male raises the likelihood of Reiter's syndrome or perhaps gonococcal infection.
3. Associations with fatigue, myalgias, and sleep disturbance may indicate a diagnosis of fibromyalgia, depression, hypothyroidism, or hypercalcemia.

E. Age/Gender/Family History (5)

1. Most connective tissue diseases are more prevalent in females.
2. Gout is more common in males and uncommon in premenopausal females.
3. Osteoarthritis (DJD) is the most common cause of arthralgia in the elderly population. Polymyalgia rheumatica may present with arthralgias, particularly in the axial skeleton in individuals over the age of 50 years.
4. Multiple joint inflammation in a female with a malar rash and a family history of systemic lupus erythematosus (SLE) would suggest a likely diagnosis of SLE.

F. Physical Examination—Some Helpful Findings (5, 6)

1. Vital signs/general: weight loss, fever, lymphadenopathy.
2. Head, eyes, ears, nose, throat: conjunctivitis, decreased tears/saliva, thyroid enlargement.
3. Skin: psoriatic plaques, malar rash, "viral" exanthem, erythema chronicum migrans, thickening of the skin, erythema infectiosum.
4. Cardiovascular: new heart murmur.
5. Joint examination: warmth, tenderness, joint effusion, deformity, range of motion, crepitus.
6. Tenderness in periarticular structures or trigger points in soft tissue.

G. Testing. Careful history and examination may be sufficient to confidently establish a diagnosis. However, some cases of arthralgia may require laboratory testing and/or imaging to evaluate for or confirm the presence of inflammation, infection, crystal-induced disease, or systemic conditions. Several examples include

1. **Laboratory Tests** (5–8)
   a. Complete blood count, erythrocyte sedimentation rate, and C-reactive protein are nonspecific tests but may support or refute inflammatory conditions.
   b. Analysis of synovial fluid can confirm bacterial infection, inflammation, trauma, or crystal-induced disease.
   c. Antinuclear antibody is positive in 90% of SLE cases.
   d. Rheumatoid factor or anti-citrullinated protein antibody could support a diagnosis of rheumatoid arthritis or some other autoimmune diseases.
   e. Human leukocyte antigen-B27 (HLA-B27) is often present in ankylosing spondylitis, Reiter's disease, and enteropathic arthritis.
   f. Positive rapid test for influenza supports reactive arthralgia.
   g. Positive Lyme serology in the proper context favors Lyme arthritis.
2. **Imaging** (5, 8)
   a. Plain radiographs, especially in cases of trauma or suspected DJD.
   b. Computed tomography and magnetic resonance imaging may be useful for suspected traumatic injury, possible metastatic disease, or intraarticular derangements.

IV. DIAGNOSIS. The differential diagnosis of arthralgia, highlighting the types more commonly encountered in a primary care setting, and classified by usual presentation as monoarticular or polyarticular (or both), is presented in Table 12.1.1.

TABLE 12.1.1	Differential Diagnosis of Arthralgia, by Usual Presentation (5, 6, 8)
Monoarticular	**Polyarticular**
Trauma	DJD/osteoarthritis
Overuse injury	Fibromyalgia
DJD/osteoarthritis	Rheumatoid arthritis
Septic arthritis/osteomyelitis	Psoriatic arthritis
Crystal-induced arthropathy (e.g., gout)	Reiter's syndrome
Lyme disease	Viral reactive arthritis (e.g., parvovirus)
Hemoglobinopathy (e.g., sickle cell)	Lyme disease
Metastatic tumor	Systemic lupus erythematosus and other
Stress fracture	connective tissue diseases
	Adverse drug reaction

DJD, degenerative joint disease.

REFERENCES

1. Hardin JG. Arthralgia. In: Walker HK, Hall WD, Hurst JW, eds. *Clinical methods: the history, physical, and laboratory examinations*, 3rd ed. Boston, MA: Butterworths, 1990:Chapter 160.
2. Morris D. Osteoarthritis. *Prim care Update* 2005;3(1):20–26.
3. Lawrence RC, Felson DT, Helmick CG, et al. Estimates of the prevalence of arthritis and other rheumatic conditions in the United States. Part II. *Arthritis Rheum* 2008;58(1):26–35.
4. Dillon CF, Rasch EK, Gu Q, Hirsch R. Prevalence of knee osteoarthritis in the United States: arthritis data from the Third National Health and Nutrition Examination Survey 1991-1994. *J Rheumatol* 2006;33(11):2271–2279.
5. Richie AM, Francis ML. Diagnostic approach to polyarticular joint pain. *Am Fam Physician* 2003;68(6):1151–1160.
6. Sergent JS, Fuchs HA. Polyarticular arthritis. In: Firestein GS, et al., eds. *Kelley's textbook of rheumatology*, 8th ed. Philadelphia, PA: Saunders Elsevier, 2008:273–289.
7. Britten N, Culpepper L, Gass D, et al., eds. *Volume 2: clinical management from Oxford textbook of primary medical care*, 3rd ed. New York, NY: Oxford University Press, 2005.
8. Golbus J. Monoarticular arthritis. In: Firestein GS, et al., eds. *Kelley's textbook of rheumatology*, 8th ed. Philadelphia, PA: Saunders Elsevier, 2008;230–272.

12.2

Calf Pain
Michael J. Bryan

I. **BACKGROUND.** Calf pain is a common problem that can result from an array of causes that range from benign to life threatening.

II. **PATHOPHYSIOLOGY.** A number of conditions can result in calf pain (see Table 12.2.1). Musculoskeletal causes account for 40% of calf pain (1). Pain can be referred from the back, such as an S1–S2 radiculopathy. Deep vein thrombosis (DVT) is one of the most serious causes

TABLE 12.2.1	Differential Diagnosis of Calf Pain

Vascular
  Venous
    Deep venous thrombosis
    Superficial thrombophlebitis
    Varicose vein
  Arterial
    Claudication
    Ischemia/embolus
Neurologic
  Referred pain
    Hip
    Back
  Peripheral neuropathy or nerve entrapment
  Restless leg syndrome
Musculoskeletal
  Calf muscle strain
  Calf tendon rupture
  Baker's cyst
  Delayed-onset muscle soreness
  Compartment syndrome
  Muscle cramps/myalgia
    Electrolyte imbalance
    Rhabdomyolysis
  Trauma
    Fracture
    Bruise/hematoma
Infectious

of calf pain. Risk factors for DVT include elements of Virchow's triad (venous wall damage, stasis, and hypercoagulability); therefore, immobilization, pregnancy, and recent surgery are classic antecedents. Compartment syndrome usually results from swelling, typically from trauma, and can affect any of the four fascial compartments of the lower leg. This results in increased intracompartmental pressure, ischemia, and irreversible loss of neuromuscular function if not promptly recognized and treated. Rhabdomyolysis can be triggered by trauma, ischemia, drugs, or infection. Restless leg syndrome may be described as pain (2). Peripheral neuropathy can be caused by nerve entrapment or medical causes such as diabetes, vitamin B12 and folate deficiencies, thyroid disease, alcoholism, human immunodeficiency virus, or syphilis and may be painful.

III. EVALUATION

A. History. The history is critical in narrowing the differential diagnosis. Pertinent information includes the exact location of the pain, as well as quality, severity, duration, and aggravating or alleviating factors. Other symptoms include swelling, color changes, warmth, numbness, weakness, and fever or chills. Related trauma or exercise must be noted, as well as a recent history of immobilization. Current medications, including hormones, statins, or drugs that affect electrolytes such as diuretics, bisphosphonates, and alcohol should be recorded.

Peripheral arterial disease (PAD) typically presents with intermittent claudication that resolves rapidly upon rest. Restless leg syndrome presents with an uncomfortable sensation, associated with an uncontrollable urge to move the legs, usually at night. Sudden calf pain in an active patient often represents a muscle strain or tendon rupture. The gastrocnemius is the most commonly injured muscle.

B. Physical Examination. The examination begins by assessing vital signs, specifically blood pressure, temperature, heart rate, and pain level. The lower extremities should be examined for swelling (DVT and trauma), color changes (uremia, anemia, cellulitis, DVT, and ischemia), wounds, trophic changes in nails or hair (chronic ischemia), and symmetry. The calf circumferences may be measured. Palpation evaluates warmth, tenderness, edema, and bone or muscle defects. Range of motion of the knees, ankles, and toes is noted. Suspicion that the pain is referred should result in evaluation of the back (e.g., straight leg raise) and hips. Vascular examination includes evaluation for venous insufficiency, tender varicosities, venous cords, arterial pulses, and capillary refill. Neurologic examination includes lower extremity evaluation of motor and sensory function, as well as reflexes. The ability to bear weight, patient stance, and gait are observed. Special tests for DVT exist, including Homan's sign (pain on passive dorsiflexion of the foot). However, the positive predictive value of physical examination findings is only 55%. Thompson's test (squeezing of the proximal gastrocnemius and soleus tendons, observing for ankle plantar flexion) evaluates possible rupture of the Achilles tendon.

C. Testing. Duplex ultrasound is used to diagnose superficial thrombosis and DVT (sensitivity 89% and specificity 94%) (3). Contrast venography is the gold standard (sensitivity 95% and specificity 97%), but is more invasive (3). The ankle-brachial index (sensitivity 95% and specificity 99%) (4) with duplex ultrasound is used to diagnose PAD. Angiography is considered the gold standard. Plain radiographs are unnecessary unless there is suspicion of fracture, foreign body, or malignancy. Magnetic resonance imaging (MRI) can be used for the diagnosis of muscle and soft tissue injuries, as well as suspected radicular symptoms. Ultrasound or MRI can evaluate muscle tears and tendinopathy. Compartment pressure testing is performed to confirm the diagnosis of compartment syndrome. Electromyogram can be performed for suspected radiculopathy or neuropathy. Restless leg syndrome may be further investigated with iron studies and evaluation of renal function.

IV. DIAGNOSIS. Pertinent examination findings for DVT include swelling, warmth, tenderness, and discoloration. Rupture of the Achilles tendon leads to inability to actively plantar flex the ankle and a positive Thompson's test. A ruptured Baker's cyst may cause swelling and discoloration that advances distally into the calf. Exertional, or chronic, compartment syndrome usually occurs with exercise. The patient has pain or numbness that resolves after cessation of exercise. The anterior compartment is involved 70% of the time (5). In acute compartment syndrome, increased pain on passive stretching of the long muscles passing through a compartment is an important sign. Severe pain, pallor, and paralysis are signs of advanced ischemic compartment syndrome. Muscle cramps and soreness may also result from dehydration, overexertion, or rhabdomyolysis. Cellulitis causing redness, pain, warmth, and swelling is usually due to an obvious local area of skin disruption on the calf or foot, but occasionally the infection originates in an area such as the interdigital web space and may be missed unless specifically sought for.

REFERENCES

1. Kahn SR. The clinical diagnosis of deep vein thrombosis: integrating incidence, risk factors, and symptoms and signs. *Arch Intern Med* 1998;158(21):2315–2323.
2. O'Keefe ST. Restless leg syndrome. A review. *Arch Intern Med* 1996;156:243.
3. Line BR. Pathophysiology and diagnosis of deep vein thrombosis. *Semin Nucl Med* 2001;31(2):90–101.
4. Comerota AJ. The case for early detection and integrated intervention in patients with peripheral artery disease and intermittent claudication. *J Endovasc Ther* 2003;10:601–613.
5. Korkola M, Avandola A. Exercise induced leg pain. *Phys Sportsmed* 2001;29(6):35–50.

12.3 Hip Pain
Destin Hill

I. BACKGROUND. The hip joint is one of the largest joints in the entire body. It is surrounded by 17 muscles and 3 extremely strong ligaments that provide the hip with a great deal of power and range of motion. It also has more bony support than any other joint in the body. Hip pain is a common chief complaint in the clinical setting.

II. PATHOPHYSIOLOGY. The differential diagnosis for the patient with hip pathology (Table 12.3.1) is significantly influenced by age. Young children are more likely to suffer from septic arthritis, transient synovitis, and referred pain from the knee. Preadolescent and adolescent patients are more likely to have hip pain secondary to slipped capital femoral epiphysis (SCFE) and Legg-Calve-Perthes disease (avascular necrosis of femur). Young athletes and active patients typically present with etiologies such as traumatic fracture, stress fracture, muscular strain, and intra-articular etiologies including labral tear and femoroacetabular impingement (FAI) (1). Elderly patients more commonly have hip pain related to degenerative arthritis, greater trochanteric bursitis, iliopsoas bursitis, fracture, and referred pain from the low back.

III. EVALUATION

A. History. The history should include specifics about pain onset, location, duration, severity, quality, and exacerbating and ameliorating factors. Questioning a young child's parents or guardian for any recent trauma or illness is necessary (1). An active patient should be probed about contributing activities, trauma, and any previous injury or surgeries. The most common ailment causing hip pain in the mature patient is osteoarthritis. However, fracture, bursitis, and referred lumbar pain are important to consider as the treatments for these diagnoses are quite different (2). It is also important for clinicians to question the patient about associated gastrointestinal symptoms (change in stool frequency, rectal bleeding, and abdominal pain), genitourinary symptoms (dysuria, hematuria, and menstrual irregularity), or systemic symptoms (night sweats, weight loss, and fever) that may alert them to alternative diagnoses.

B. Physical Exam. Although the hip joint is obscured by bone and soft tissue, it is not difficult to examine. As with any musculoskeletal exam, a systematic approach to the physical exam of the hip can assist the examiner in obtaining an accurate diagnosis.

1. Ask the patient to locate where they feel the hip pain. Intra-articular hip pain is commonly described as groin pain. Lateral hip pain can direct the clinician to suspect muscle, ligaments, or bursa as the cause for pain.

2. Inspect for any ecchymosis, swelling, erythema, or rashes.

3. Palpate the hip for tenderness over the soft tissue and bony landmarks including the hip flexors, adductors, gluteal musculature, iliotibial band, greater trochanter and overlying bursa, and pelvis.

4. Test range of motion of the hip with the patient supine including hip flexion, internal rotation, and external rotation. Extension can be tested by having the patient lie on the contralateral side.

5. Test strength with resisted hip flexion, extension, adduction, and abduction with the patient supine.

6. There are many specialized tests for the hip. A few of these include:

   a. **Log Roll.** The patient is supine with the leg resting on the examination table. The femur is internally and externally rotated by the examiner by rolling the leg, similar to a rolling pin motion. Decreased or painful internal rotation or external rotation can indicate intra-articular pathology.

TABLE 12.3.1	Differential Diagnosis of Hip Pain	
Diagnosis	**Patient age**	**Suggestive findings**
Septic arthritis	Infants and toddlers	Pseudoparalysis, irritability, limp, fever
Transient synovitis	Children, preadolescent	Pain, limp, decreased ROM, fever
Legg-Calve-Perthes disease	Preadolescent	Limp, decreased ROM, males
SCFE	Adolescent	Limp, decreased internal rotation, males, obesity, bilateral 50% of the time
Avulsion fracture	Young adult, athlete	Sudden onset, "pop" heard or felt, pain at origin/insertion of tendon
Femoral neck stress fracture	Young adult, athlete	Insidious onset; associated with increased activity, eating disorders, menstrual irregularities, and distance runners
Osteoid osteoma	Young adult	Vague pain, nocturnal pain, decreased ROM
Iliotibial band syndrome	Young adult, athlete	Lateral thigh/leg pain, snapping sensation, positive Obers, radiation to lateral knee
Sports hernia	Young adult, athlete	Groin pain, worse with full exertion activities, painful resisted abdominal crunch
FAI	Adult	Groin pain, restricted ROM and crossing legs, positive FAI test
Greater trochanteric bursitis	Adult	Lateral thigh pain over greater trochanter
Avascular necrosis of femoral head	Adult	Dull pain with weight bearing, decreased ROM
Iliopsoas tendinitis	Adult	Medial thigh/groin pain or snapping, pain with standing
Hip labral tear	Adult, athlete	Sudden onset, painful clicking in medial hip/groin, decreased ROM
Adhesive capsulitis of the hip	Adult, especially middle-aged women	Restricted and painful ROM in the absence of osteoarthritis or other cause for pain, associated with diabetes
Meralgia paresthetica	Adult	Anterior/lateral thigh numbness, obesity, compressive clothing, no weakness
Degenerative joint disease	Adult	Progressive pain, decreased internal rotation, worse with weight-bearing activity

FAI, femoroacetabular impingement; ROM, range of motion; SCFE, slipped capital femoral epiphysis.

    b. FABER Test. The hip is placed in the *F*lexed, *AB*ducted, and *E*xternally *R*otated position. This is compared with the contralateral side. Decreased or painful hip motion can point to an intra-articular process or iliopsoas muscular strain.

    c. FAI Test. The patient is supine and the hip is flexed to 90°. The hip is then internally rotated. Reproduction of the patient's hip pain is suggestive of possible FAI.

   7. Watch the patient walk, if possible.

   8. One of the most important portions of the hip exam is the patient's neurologic exam including reflexes, sensation, and muscular strength. This portion of the exam can reveal a neurologic disorder.

9. Palpate lower extremity pulses.
10. Also consider examination of the knees (especially in pediatric patients), lumbar spine, and sacroiliac joints.

C. Testing

1. Plain X-rays of the hip (anteroposterior pelvis, anteroposterior and frog-leg, or lateral views of hip) are the first radiographic test completed in most presentations of hip pain.
2. Magnetic resonance imaging (MRI) or computed tomography (CT) scan can be helpful if the diagnosis remains unclear after a thorough history, physical exam, and plain radiographs. These can be used to reveal radiographically occult fractures, stress fractures, labral injuries, chondral degeneration, intra-articular loose bodies, and evaluation of cystic or lytic lesions seen on X-rays. An MRI with intra-articular contrast should be considered if labral pathology, Legg-Calve-Perthes disease, or avascular necrosis is high on the examiner's differential (3).
3. Ultrasound can be helpful in detecting small joint effusions when the suspicion of transient synovitis or septic arthritis is high.
4. Bone scanning can be useful in diagnosing stress fracture, Legg-Calve-Perthes disease, and avascular necrosis.
5. Complete blood count, erythrocyte sedimentation rate, and C-reactive protein can be helpful in patients with suspected inflammatory disorders.
6. Occasionally, hip joint aspiration is necessary to make a diagnosis. Fluid should be sent for cell count, Gram stain, culture, crystals, and other studies as appropriate.

IV. DIAGNOSIS. Accurate diagnosis of hip pain can be quite challenging for clinicians. A focused physical exam can be extremely helpful in narrowing the differential diagnosis. Tenderness over the greater trochanter directs the clinician to bursitis, while a positive FAI test points toward femoroacetabular impingement. Plain radiographs are an important tool in evaluating patients with hip pain. These can be used to assess for some of the most common causes of hip pain including osteoarthritis and fracture. MRI, CT scans, and ultrasound can also be used to further evaluate for intra-articular pathology or when the diagnosis is unclear after initial testing. Table 12.3.1 lists the differential diagnosis for common hip conditions.

REFERENCES

1. Hill DE, Whiteside JW. Evaluation of the limping child. *J Fam Pract* 2011;60:193–197.
2. Hoppenfield S. *Physical examination of the spine and extremities.* New York, NY: Appleton-Century-Crofts, 1976:133–169.
3. Madden CC, Putukian M, Young CC, McCarty EC. *Netter's sports medicine.* Philadelphia, PA: Saunders, 2010:404–416.

12.4 Knee Pain

Michael L. Grover

I. BACKGROUND. Knee symptoms are the tenth most common reason for outpatient office visits in the United States. Primary care physicians evaluate about four million patients per year for knee pain (1). Knee pain will be experienced by nearly one-half of all US adults in their lifetime (2). Most nontraumatic anterior knee pain in adults seen in primary care clinics is due to patellofemoral syndrome.

II. PATHOPHYSIOLOGY

A. Etiology. Knee pain has many causes: acute injury, overuse, inflammatory or degenerative arthritis, infection, and other miscellaneous problems. Referred pain from the hip or low back may also result in knee pain.

B. Epidemiology. The age of the patient, location of pain, and temporal onset are all essential elements of the history taking to focus the physical examination and differential diagnosis. In children, knee pain is most often caused by minor trauma. However, other likely causes include patellar subluxation, patellar tendonitis (Jumper's knee), and tibial apophysitis (Osgood-Schlatter disease) (3). In pediatric patients, the clinician should also have a low index of suspicion for conditions such as osteomyelitis, osteosarcoma, and referred pain from pathology in the hip. In adolescents and adults, traumatic and overuse injuries become more common. Knee pain in adults and seniors is more commonly due to osteoarthritis, degenerative meniscal tears, and inflammatory arthritis from gout or pseudogout.

III. EVALUATION

A. History

1. **Pain Onset, Character, Location, and Mechanism of Injury.** Overuse injuries and arthritic conditions tend to have an insidious onset, with gradually progressive pain that is characterized as dull or aching. With acute-onset pain caused by injury, pain may be sharp in quality. In injured patients, determining the location of pain (anterior, medial, lateral, or posterior) can guide physical examination. Knowledge of the mechanism of injury is very important. Lateral blows may be associated with medial collateral ligament and medial meniscus tears. Hyperextension or quick deceleration (particularly with direct trauma) may injure the cruciate ligaments. Twisting and pivoting may injure the menisci due to shear forces (4).

2. **Associated Symptoms.** One should inquire about mechanical symptoms such as locking (menisci), popping (ligament), and giving way of the knee (ligament) (4). Self-noted swelling is important as well. Ligamentous injuries and fractures tend to have rapid-onset effusion due to acute hemarthrosis. Effusions tend to develop more slowly with arthritic conditions and meniscal injuries. The presence of an effusion is a predictor of derangement of ligaments or menisci. Up to 90% of patients with traumatic injury and effusion have internal derangement of the knee (5).

B. Physical Examination.
Developing the ability to perform a good knee examination is important as up to a third of patients with internal derangement of the knee will seek care from their primary care physician (2).

1. **Inspection and Palpation.** Comparing the painful knee to the contralateral side may allow for recognition of swelling, erythema, bruising, or asymmetry (4). Palpation for bony point tenderness may increase suspicion for fracture. Joint line tenderness is often related to meniscal injury. Injured collateral ligaments are often tender with palpation and have associated soft tissue swelling.

2. **Range of Motion.** Active and passive range of motion should be assessed. Inability to actively extend the knee raises concerns for quadriceps tendon rupture, while restricted passive or active flexion or extension may be related to injury of menisci (6). Observation of abnormal patellofemoral tracking and presence of crepitation with range of motion may be seen in patients with patellofemoral syndrome and chondromalacia.

3. **Collateral Ligaments.** Valgus and varus stress testing applied to the knee while it is in slight flexion can reproduce pain from medial and lateral collateral ligament injury. A firm end point of motion should be appreciated if the ligament is intact (4).

4. **Cruciate Ligaments.** The pivot shift, Lachman, and anterior drawer tests are helpful to assess for anterior cruciate ligament injury. The posterior drawer test is used to assess for posterior cruciate ligament injury. The pivot shift test has better positive predictive value (i.e., a positive test is helpful for ruling in injury), and a Lachman test has a greater negative predictive value (i.e., a negative test is helpful for ruling out injury) (Table 12.4.1).

5. **Menisci.** Multiple systematic reviews have looked at the diagnostic accuracy of examination maneuvers in evaluating for meniscal tears (6). The Thessaly test has been proven to be more accurate in predicting injury than a positive McMurray test or joint line tenderness (6).

6. **Presence of Effusion.** If patients report noticing swelling and the examiner finds a positive ballottement test, the probability of internal derangement of the knee is greatly increased (6).

TABLE 12.4.1	Knee Physical Examination Tests

Test	Description
Meniscal tear	
Joint line tenderness	Palpate medially or laterally along the knee to the joint line between the femur and tibial condyles. Pain on palpation is a positive finding.
McMurray test	Flex the hip and knee maximally. Apply a valgus (abduction) force to the knee while externally rotating the foot and passively extending the knee. An audible or palpable snap during extension suggests a tear of the medial meniscus. For the lateral meniscus, apply a varus (adduction) stress during internal rotation of the foot and passive extension of the knee.
Thessaly test	Hold patient's outstretched hands while he or she stands flat-footed on the floor, internally and externally rotating three times with the knee flexed 20°.
Anterior cruciate ligament tear	
Anterior drawer test	With the patient supine on the examining table, flex the hip to 45° and the knee to 90°. Sit on the dorsum of the foot, wrap hands around the hamstrings (ensuring that these muscles are relaxed), then pull and push the proximal part of the leg, testing the movement of the tibia on the femur. Do these maneuvers in three positions of tibial rotation: neutral, 30° externally rotated, and 30° internally rotated. A normal test result is no more than 6 to 8 mm of laxity.
Lachman test	With the patient supine on the examining table and the leg at the examiner's side, slightly externally rotated and flexed (20–30°), stabilize the femur with one hand and apply pressure to the back of the knee with the other hand, with the thumb on the joint line. A positive test result is movement of the knee with a soft or mushy end point.
Pivot shift test	Fully extend the knee and rotate the foot internally. Apply a valgus (abduction) force while progressively flexing the knee, watching and feeling for translation of the tibia on the femur.

Based on Grover M. Evaluating acutely injured patients for internal derangement of the knee. *Am Fam Physician* 2012;85(3):247–252. Test descriptions from Jackson JL, O'Malley PG, Kroenke K. Evaluation of acute knee pain in primary care. *Ann Intern Med* 2003;139(7):575–588 and Harrison BK, Abell BE, Gibson TW. The Thessaly test for detection of meniscal tears: validation of a new physical examination technique for primary care medicine. *Clin J Sport Med* 2009;19(1):9–12.

C. Testing

1. **Laboratory Testing.** A hot, red, and very tender knee raises concerns for acute inflammatory arthritis (gout, pseudogout, and rheumatic fever) and, particularly if these findings are associated with a history of skin trauma or fever, septic arthritis (4). A complete blood count and sedimentation rate may be helpful. Arthrocentesis to obtain joint aspirate for Gram stain, culture, cell count, and crystals is of paramount importance. In patients with acute effusion after traumatic injury, a finding of hemarthrosis is associated with a high probability of internal derangement (6).

TABLE 12.4.2	Differential Diagnosis of Knee Pain
Overuse	Patellofemoral pain, patellar tendinopathy, quadriceps tendinopathy, iliotibial band syndrome, apophysitis (Osgood-Schlatter most common), pes anserine bursitis, synovial plica, bipartite patella
Traumatic	Anterior cruciate ligament rupture, collateral ligament sprain (medial and lateral collateral, fracture (bony and/or chondral), meniscal tear, patellar subluxation or dislocation, prepatellar bursitis, posterior cruciate ligament rupture, quadriceps tendon rupture, patellar tendon rupture
Arthritic	Osteoarthritis, inflammatory (rheumatoid, gout, pseudogout, other)
Infectious	Septic joint
Referred	Back or hip
Miscellaneous	Osteonecrosis, osteochondritis dessicans, Baker (popliteal) cyst, tumor, deep vein thrombosis (presenting as popliteal pain), benign or malignant tumor, pigmented villonodular synovitis

Other systemic causes (complex regional pain syndrome, fibromyalgia)

2. **Imaging.** Determining whether a patient may have a fracture is critical during the initial evaluation after trauma.
   a. **X-Ray.** By use of clinical information, application of the Ottawa Knee Rule can guide X-ray utilization. X-rays are indicated in the following situations: the patient is aged 55 or older, inability to bear weight for four steps, unable to flex the knee to 90°, or presence of tenderness over the head of the fibula or patella (without other bony point tenderness) (7).
   b. **MRI.** While magnetic resonance imaging (MRI) can diagnose internal derangement very effectively, normal findings with clinical examination maneuvers can effectively rule out cruciate or meniscal injury for many patients (8). MRI may be best utilized in those with equivocal findings acutely (in an effort to rule out derangement) or in those who have reassuring initial findings but who fail conservative treatment measures (to rule them in).

IV. DIAGNOSIS. See Table 12.4.2.

REFERENCES

1. Cherry DK, Woodwell DA, Rechtsteiner EA; Centers for Disease Control and Prevention. *National Ambulatory Medical Care Survey: 2005 summary.* http://www.cdc.gov/nchs/data/ad/ad387.pdf
2. Baker P, Reading I, Cooper C, Coggon D. Knee disorders in the general population and their relation to occupation. *Occup Environ Med* 2003;60(10):794–797.
3. Calmbach M, Hutchens M. Evaluation of patients presenting with knee pain: part II. differential diagnosis. *Am Fam Physician* 2003;68:917–922.
4. Calmbach W, Hutchens M. Evaluation of patients presenting with knee pain: part I. History, physical examination, radiographs, and laboratory tests. *Am Fam Physician* 2003;68:907–912.
5. Kastelein M, Luijsterburg PA, Wagemakers HP, et al. Diagnostic value of history taking and physical examination to assess effusion of the knee in traumatic knee patients in general practice. *Arch Phys Med Rehabil* 2009;90(1):82–86.
6. Grover, M. Evaluating acutely injured patients for internal derangement of the knee. *Am Fam Physician* 2012;85(3):247–252.
7. Stiell IG, Greenberg GH, Wells GA, et al. Derivation of a decision rule for the use of radiography in acute knee injuries. *Ann Emerg Med* 1995;26(4):405–413.
8. Jackson JL, O'Malley PG, Kroenke K. Evaluation of acute knee pain in primary care. *Ann Intern Med* 2003;139(7):575–588.
9. Harrison BK, Abell BE, Gibson TW. The Thessaly test for detection of meniscal tears: validation of a new physical examination technique for primary care medicine. *Clin J Sport Med* 2009;19(1):9–12.

12.5 Low Back Pain

Carolyn Carpenter Moats

I. BACKGROUND. Low back pain is common in developed countries, affecting approximately 70% of the adult population (1) at some stage during their life. In the primary care setting, however, fewer than 15% of patients with back pain have an identifiable underlying disease or spinal abnormality (2).

II. PATHOPHYSIOLOGY. The cause of pain is nonspecific in the majority of people present-ing with acute low back pain; serious conditions are rare. Low back pain is generally self-limited (3), but diagnosis must exclude rarer but potentially serious, life-threatening causes (see Table 12.5.1).

III. EVALUATION
   A. History. The clinician needs to be alert to the presence of indications of potentially serious low back conditions, often called "red flags" (see Table 12.5.2).
      1. Pain Characteristics. Assess the nature of the pain, along with the position, onset, and duration of the symptom. Is there any radiating pain, leg weakness, or paresthesia? Does

---

TABLE 12.5.1   Causes of Low Back Pain

Common causes

Muscle and soft tissue strain

Degenerative disease, including osteoarthritis and spondylosis

Vertebral dysfunction, including facet joint and lumbar disc involvement

Lumbar or sacral nerve root compression: disc herniation, cauda equina syndrome, sciatica, spinal stenosis

Vertebral fracture or subluxation

Inflammatory conditions

Rheumatologic conditions (e.g., rheumatoid arthritis, ankylosing spondylitis)

Sacroiliac joint sprain or degenerative disease

Other less common causes that may also be life threatening

Infection: osteomyelitis, discitis, epidural abscess

Hematologic

Multiple myeloma, myelodysplasia

Cancer (primary or metastatic)

Benign tumors

Aortic aneurysm

Retroperitoneal pathology

Pyelonephritis, renal calculus, cancer

Abdominal pathology

Perforated viscus, pancreatitis

TABLE 12.5.2	**"Red Flags" That Indicate Potentially Serious Lower Back Conditions**

Age >50 y

History of malignancy

Temperature >37.8°C

Constant pain

Weight loss

History of trauma (may be minor in patients with osteoporosis)

Features of spondyloarthropathy

Neurologic signs

Alcohol or drug disorder

Recent invasive urologic procedures

Sudden onset of sharp back pain with uneven pulses (abdominal aneurysm)

History of anticoagulant use

History of corticosteroid use

Pain not improved after 1 mo

Signs of cauda equina syndrome

- saddle anesthesia
- recent onset of bladder dysfunction
- severe or progressive neurologic deficit

Adapted from Murtagh J. *General practice.* Australia: McGraw-Hill, 2003.

the pain limit the patient physically or socially? Is there a history of previous back problems or back surgery?

2. **Review of Systems.** Look for any red flag indicators of serious disease (Table 12.5.2). Gastrointestinal and genitourinary symptoms are particularly important, especially incontinence.

3. **Psychosocial Information.** Look for any "red flag" indicators of serious disease (Table 12.5.2). Have there been any recent events or activities that may be associated with the pain? If work related, assess workplace activities. Assess urinary and sexual function, which can be affected by neurologic compromise. Perform a psychiatric and psychosocial assessment; depression may also occur as a consequence of chronic back pain. Disrupted sleep patterns are common in both depression and back pain. Patients seeking drugs of dependence may present with back pain, and addiction or pseudoaddiction may be present.

B. **Physical Examination.** Examination aims to identify the location, level, and cause of discomfort, in part by reproducing the pain. For this reason, the most painful parts of the examination are left to the end of the assessment.

1. **General.** Initial impressions of how the patient moves may give important diagnostic clues. Patients with disc lesions may prefer to stand. Gait can be observed as the patient moves about the exam room, and level of function or disability can be observed when the patient sits in a chair or climbs onto the examination table. Sufficient exposure of the back and lower limbs should be achieved to allow close examination of the back and inspection of the gait. Abdominal examination should focus on possible causes of back pain (Table 12.5.1). Systemic examination, especially neurologic examination, is also important to exclude other serious causes of back pain.

2. **Musculoskeletal**

a. **Inspection.** Inspect the contour and shape of the back, looking for scoliosis, lordosis, spasm, and muscle wasting. Assess the range of motion of the spine and lower extremities through flexion, extension, and lateral flexion. Perform the straight leg raising (SLR) test passively with the patient supine. Note the angle of leg elevation precipitating pain. A positive test for sciatica is buttock pain radiating to the posterior thigh and perhaps to the lower leg and foot. The SLR test is usually negative in spinal stenosis (4).

b. **Palpation.** Palpation and percussion of the spine and upper pelvis help identify areas of localized tenderness, as seen in myofascial conditions, fracture, metastatic disease, and some inflammatory conditions. Include an examination of the hip and sacroiliac joint.

3. **Neurologic.** Neurologic examination is especially important in the presence of paresthesia, weakness, and radiating pain. Assess strength by having the patient walk on their heels (L5), walk on their toes (S1), and testing for specific nerve root motor, sensory, and reflex function for each lumbar level. The lower extremity examination includes motor strength, deep tendon reflexes, sensation, proprioception, and certain functional maneuvers (see Table 12.5.3). Romberg and Babinski reflexes may also be assessed. Rectal examination may be done to assess sphincter tone, which can be compromised in sacral root dysfunction. In the primary care setting, most clinically significant disc herniations are detected by the following limited examination: dorsiflexion of the great toe and ankle, Achilles reflex, light touch sensation of the medial (L4), dorsal (L5), and lateral (S1) aspect of the foot, and the SLR test (1, 3).

C. **Testing**

1. **Clinical Laboratory Tests**

a. Testing is influenced by the differential diagnosis after the history and physical examination. The majority of low back pain evaluations do not require laboratory or imaging evaluation. In the presence of "red flag" indicators, tests may include urinary examination, complete blood count, erythrocyte sedimentation rate, electrolytes, including serum calcium, serum alkaline phosphatase, or prostate-specific antigen. Pain suspected to be caused by a "red flag" condition may also require other urgent tests (3).

b. Specific tests for inflammatory conditions (such as rheumatoid arthritis or ankylosing spondylitis) or infections may also be needed if indicated from history and examination.

2. **Diagnostic Imaging.** In low-risk patients, diagnostic imaging is unlikely to be helpful. A posteroanterior and lateral radiograph of the lumbosacral spine may be used to delineate bony structure and alignment but does not provide diagnostic information regarding many serious causes of back pain. Patients with a potential "red flag" condition, such

TABLE 12.5.3	**Neurologic Findings Seen with Disc Herniation**		
Disc pain/numbness	**Motor weakness**	**Functional maneuver**	**Reflex**
L3–4/anteromedial thigh and knee	Quadriceps	Deep knee bends	↓ Patellar
L4–5/lateral leg, first three toes	Dorsiflexion of foot or great toe	Heel walking	↓ Achilles
L5–S1/posterior leg, lateral heel	Plantar flexion of foot or great toe	Toe walking	

From Davis S. Low back pain. In: Taylor RB, ed. *Musculoskeletal problems. The 10 minute diagnosis manual.* Philadelphia, PA: Lippincott Williams & Wilkins, 2006.

as spinal trauma, or suspected cauda equina syndrome may require computed tomography scanning and/or magnetic resonance imaging (MRI). MRI is usually the preferred modality if available and the patient is stable. A bone scan may be used when tumor or infection is suspected. Electromyography may rarely be useful to assess for nerve root dysfunction when symptoms are questionable. Persistent, chronic pain may require further diagnostic imaging.

IV. DIAGNOSIS

A. The most common cause of low back pain in primary care is myofascial dysfunction with subsequent muscle spasm. The physical examination reveals limitation of motion of the affected area, with tenderness and increased tone in the affected muscle groups. Spondylolisthesis (displacement of a vertebra in relation to the vertebra below) typically presents in adolescence, particularly in athletes. Low back pain, loss of lumbar lordosis, and a palpable "step off" are classic findings. Lumbar degenerative disc disease may present in older age groups, with localized or radicular pain due to nerve root compression. Pain radiating below the knee is more likely to be a true radiculopathy.

B. Aching, throbbing pain of insidious onset that is worse in the morning and is unrelieved by rest and worse at night suggests an inflammatory origin of the pain. A deep, dull pain, with intermittent stiffness relieved by rest and worse after activity or the end of the day associated with a precipitating event or a previous history of back pain suggests mechanical origin. Increased pain from standing or walking suggests spinal stenosis, whereas pain on sitting is often due to disc disease. Pain and stiffness in the morning suggest inflammatory disease, whereas continuous pain is more suggestive of neoplasm or infection. Mechanical disease often coexists with inflammatory disease, resulting in a more complicated mixed pattern.

REFERENCES

1. Deyo RA, Rainville J, Kent DL. What can the history and physical examination tell us about low back pain? *JAMA* 1992;268:760–765.
2. Van Tudler MW, Assendelft WJ, Koes BW, et al. Spinal radiographic findings and nonspecific low back pain. A systematic review of observational studies. *Spine* 1997;22:427–434.
3. Casazza BA. Diagnosis and treatment of acute low back pain. *Am Fam Physician* 2012;85(4):343–350.
4. McCoy, R. (2007). Low Back Pain. In P. M. Paulman, A. A. Paulman, & J. D. Harrison, Taylor's 10-Minute Diagnosis Manual: Symptoms and Signs in the Time-Limited Encounter (2nd ed., pp. 279–282). Philadelphia: Lippincott Williams & Wilkins.

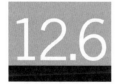

Monoarticular Joint Pain
David Patchett

I. BACKGROUND. Pain in a single joint is a common presenting complaint.

II. PATHOPHYSIOLOGY

A. Etiology. Monoarticular joint pain has many etiologies. Acute monoarticular joint pain is most commonly due to trauma, infection, osteoarthritis, or crystal-induced conditions. Other causes of monarticular joint pain are rheumatic diseases and neoplasm. Further, pain may arise from bursae, ligaments, and tendons or be referred from myofascial trigger points.

B. Epidemiology. Musculoskeletal complaints account for greater than 315 million outpatient clinic visits per year and 20% of outpatient visits in the United States (1); 49.9 million (22%) Americans older than age 18 years report having arthritis (2). This is expected to rise to 67 million (25%) Americans by 2030 (3).

III. EVALUATION

A. History. It is important to first determine whether the joint pain is acute or chronic. Acute monoarthritis is defined as an inflammatory process that develops over the course of a few days or has been present for less than 2 weeks (4). If the joint pain is acute, then determine if the pain stems from trauma. A history of trauma or an inability to bear weight indicates the possibility of fracture, dislocation, or soft tissue injury. Of note, there may be a history of minimal or no trauma in patients with fractures secondary to osteoporosis (5). Excessive use of a joint or a rapid increase in physical activity may indicate a stress fracture (6).

Atraumatic acute monoarthritis is most commonly associated with crystals or infection. In young adults, disseminated gonococcal infection is the most common cause (5). Gout occurs most commonly in males, affects the first metatarsophalangeal joint, ankle, mid foot, or knee (5). Pseudogout is most common in the elderly and is indistinguishable in presentation to gout in the acute setting (7). Both present with joint pain, erythema, and decreased joint range of motion (ROM).

Risk factors for septic arthritis include intravenous drug use, immunosuppression, and sexual activity (8). Constitutional symptoms such as fevers, chills, and rigors present in 57%, 27%, and 19% of patients, respectively (9). These symptoms may also be present in acute crystal joint disease.

Other atraumatic causes of monoarticular joint pain include degenerative joint disease, rheumatic disease, and malignancy (see Table 12.6.2).

B. Physical Examination

1. A general physical examination is important. Vital sign abnormalities can point to infection or systemic disease as the cause of joint pain. Elements of the musculoskeletal physical examination should always include inspection, palpation, ROM, and special tests. When evaluating an individual for joint pain, you must first determine if the source is articular or arising from the periarticular soft tissue. Joint pain commonly results from

TABLE 12.6.1	Diagnoses Consistent with Findings from Synovial Fluid Analysis				
Condition	Appearance	White blood cells/mm	Polymorphonuclear neutrophils (%)	Glucose (% serum level)	Crystals under polarized light
Normal	Clear	<200	<25	95–100	None
Noninflammatory (e.g., Degenerative joint disease (DJD))	Clear	<400	<25	95–100	None
Acute gout	Turbid	2,000–5,000	>75	80–100	Negative birefringence; needle-like crystals
Pseudogout	Turbid	5,000–50,000	>75	80–1,000	Positive birefringence; rhomboid crystals
Septic arthritis	Purulent/turbid	>50,000	>75	<50	None
Inflammatory (e.g., rheumatoid arthritis)	Turbid	5,000–50,000	50–75	~75	None

Adapted from Roberts JR, Hedges JR, eds. *Clinical procedures in emergency medicine,* 3rd ed. Philadelphia, PA: WB Saunders, 1998.

tendonitis or bursitis. Pain may also be referred from myofascial trigger points (10). Asking the patient to point with one finger to the exact site of pain can be helpful. Intra-articular problems cause restriction in both active and passive ROM, whereas periarticular problems favor restrictions in active ROM. In tendonitis or bursitis, pain is elicited with joint motion against resistance (5).

   2. Erythema, edema, and warmth signal inflammation of a joint. This can be due to infection, crystal-induced disease, trauma, or rheumatic conditions (11). Crepitus of a joint indicates a derangement of bone, cartilage, or menisci (12).

C. Testing. Laboratory testing with a complete blood count, sedimentation rate, or C-reactive protein can help to distinguish inflammatory from noninflammatory disorders. Uric acid levels may be helpful in diagnosing and monitoring gout (1). Other lab tests such as antinuclear antibody and rheumatoid factor are useful if there is a high degree of suspicion of a specific diagnosis.

   1. Arthrocentesis is indicated when there is a warm, red joint with effusion, especially when there is no history of trauma (13). Absence of fever does not exclude the presence of a septic joint and should not influence this decision (14). Synovial fluid should be sent for the "3 Cs": cell count, culture (Gram's stain), and crystals. Table 12.6.1 reviews the diagnoses consistent with findings on synovial fluid analysis.

   2. Plain radiographs remain the initial imaging of choice in most bone and joint disorders. X-rays should be ordered for patients with chronic pain, suspected arthritits, chondrocalcinosis, fractures, or dislocations. Computed tomography is helpful at detecting occult fractures and other bony abnormalities (15). Magnetic resonance imaging (MRI) is superior at detecting septic arthritis and meniscal, tendinous, and ligamentous injuries.

   3. MRI with gadolinium injection (MRI arthrography) can visualize intra-articular structures. This modality is used commonly to detect labral tears of the hip and shoulder.

IV. DIAGNOSIS

A. Differential Diagnosis. Table 12.6.2 illustrates the differential diagnosis for monoarticular joint pain (16).

TABLE 12.6.2 — Differential Diagnosis of Joint Pain

Trauma	Infection	Other
Sprain	Gonococcal	Reflex sympathetic dystrophy
Strain	Nongonococcal: viral, mycobacterial, or fungal	Sjögren's syndrome
Fracture	Lyme disease	Polymyositis
Dislocation	Subacute bacterial endocarditis	Scleroderma
Tear of ligament, tendon, or meniscus	Secondary to enteric and urogenital infections	Sarcoidosis
Tendinitis		Fibromyalgia
		Erythema nodosum
		Sickle cell disease
		Aseptic necrosis
		Charcot's disease
		Drug reaction
		Hypothyroidism
		Irritable bowel syndrome
		Osteochondritis dissecans

(Continued)

TABLE 12.6.2	Differential Diagnosis of Joint Pain *(Continued)*	
Crystal-induced arthropathy	**Degenerative joint disease**	**Malignant**
Gout	Osteoarthritis	Tumor
Pseudogout		Metastases
Leukemia		
	Rheumatic	
	Rheumatoid arthritis	
	Reiter's syndrome	
	Psoriatic arthritis	
	Lupus erythematosus	
	Ankylosing spondylitis	

B. Clinical Manifestations

1. Osteoarthritis is a common cause of monoarticular joint pain in older patients. It occurs most commonly in large weight-bearing joints or joints used repetitively. It may manifest initially or during flares as monoarticular joint pain and is usually worse at the end of the day or after prolonged weight-bearing. There may be some swelling, usually without erythema or warmth in the affected joint.

3. Gout occurs rapidly over hours to days and often during the night. An affected great toe may be tender, swollen, and erythematous. Affected joints are often exquisitely tender.

4. Septic arthritis typically presents with fever, joint pain, swelling, and erythema. Absence of fever should not preclude joint aspiration. Infants may present atypically with non-specific symptoms such as irritability, fever, crying with movement of the hip (as with diaper changes), or refusal to bear weight.

REFERENCES

1. Longo DL, Fauci AS, Kasper DL, et al., eds. *Harrison's principles of internal medicine*, 18th ed. New York, NY: McGraw-Hill, 2012.
2. Bolen J, Schieb L, Hootman JM, et al. Differences in the prevalence and impact of arthritis among racial/ethnic groups in the United States, National Health Interview Survey, 2002, 2003, and 2006. *Prev Chronic Dis* 2010;7(3):A64.
3. Hootman JM, Helmick CG. Projections of U.S. prevalence of arthritis and associated activity limitations. *Arthritis Rheum* 2006;54(1):226–229.
4. Sack K. Monarthritis: differential diagnosis. *Am J Med* 1997;102:30S.
5. Civa C, Valazquez C, Mody A, Brasington R. Diagnosing acute monoarthritis in adults: a practical approach for the family physician. *Am Fam Physician* 2003;68:83–90.
6. Reeder M, Dick B, Atkins J, et al. Stress fractures. Current concepts of diagnosis and treatment. *Sports Med* 1996;22(3):198–212.
7. Rosenthal, AK. Pseudogout: presentation, natural history, and associated conditions. In: Wortmann RL, Schumacher HR Jr, Becker MA, Ryan LM, eds. *Crystal-induced arthropathies. Gout, pseudogout and apatite-associated syndromes*. New York, NY: Taylor & Francis Group, 2006:99.
8. Horowitz D, Katzap E, Horowitz S, Barilla-Labarca M. Approach to septic arthritis. *Am Fam Physician* 2011;84(6):653–660.
9. Margaretten ME, Kohlwes J, Moore D, Bent S. Does this adult patient have septic arthritis? *JAMA* 2007;297(13):1478–1488.
10. Simons DG, Travell JG, Simons LS, Cummings BD. *Travell and Simons' myofascial pain and dysfunction: the trigger point manual*, 2nd ed. Baltimore, MD: Lippincott Williams and Wilkins, 1998.

11. Sarwark JF. *Essentials of musculoskeletal care,* 4th ed. Rosemont, IL: American Academy of Orthopaedic Surgeons, 2010.
12. Richie A, Francis M. Diagnostic approach to polyarticular joint pain. *Am Fam Physician* 2003;68(6):1151–1160.
13. Till SH, Snaith ML. Assessment, investigation, and management of acute monoarthritis. *J Accid Emerg Med* 1999;16(5):355–361.
14. Learch TJ. Imaging of infectious arthritis. *Semin Musculoskelet Radiol* 2003;7(2):137–142.
15. Conway WF, Totty WG, McEnery KW. CT and MR imaging of the hip. *Radiology* 1996;198:297.
16. Paulman PM, Paulman AA, Harrison JD, et al., eds. *Taylor's 10-minute diagnosis manual,* 2nd ed. Baltimore, MD: Lippincott Williams and Wilkins, 2006.

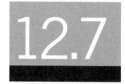

Neck Pain
Richard L. Engle

I. **BACKGROUND.** Neck pain is defined as pain occurring anywhere between the base of the skull and thorax. This pain can occur anteriorly, posteriorly, or laterally. The cervical spine is one of the most mobile and complex joints in the body. Considering that, on average, the neck moves over 600 times an hour (1), it is no wonder that it is a common source of pain. Most episodes of neck pain are short lived and resolve spontaneously. The examiner must be cautious about ascribing the etiology of pain as intrinsic to the neck without evaluating the patient for risk factors and conditions that cause pain referred to the neck region such as angina, aortic dissection, or other mediastinal pathology.

II. PATHOPHYSIOLOGY
A. Etiology
1. Trauma, job-related causes (e.g., manual labor, driving for long periods, head forward positioning while typing), smoking, and a previous history of low back pain are considered risk factors for neck pain. Often, no specific cause can be elicited.
2. Symptoms due to cervical pathology can be referred to other areas of the body, most commonly the upper back, chest, and arms. Likewise, pain from shoulder or chest pathology can be referred to the neck.

B. Epidemiology.
Neck pain is extremely common in the general population, with a 40–70% lifetime prevalence. Cervical arthritis is seen in 80% of individuals over 50 years of age and cervical radiculopathy in 83.2/100,000 of the general population, with most of them in the C6–7 distribution (2).

III. EVALUATION
A. History.
Characterizing the location, quality, intensity, radiation, duration, and associated symptoms helps determine the likely cause of neck pain.
1. Key associated neck complaints are radicular symptoms, such as paresthesias, sensory loss, muscle weakness, which can indicate nerve root compression; lower extremity symptoms, such as lower extremity paresthesias, bowel/bladder dysfunction, which can indicate cauda equina syndrome; and fever, weight loss, and other joint involvement that can indicate inflammatory arthritis, infection, or neoplasm.
2. Unusual symptoms can be related to neck pathology and should not be discounted. Sympathetic nervous system activation can cause eye pain, increased tearing, and blurry vision. Irritation of the C3–5 nerve root (due to phrenic nerve involvement) can cause respiratory symptoms such as shortness of breath (3).

TABLE 12.7.1	Special Physical Examination Tests of Cervical Spine		
Test	**Evaluation for**	**How performed**	**Positive test**
Spurling's test	Nerve root compression (disc herniation)	Head in mild extension and flexion toward side of radicular symptoms	Pain in dermatomal pattern on affected side
Distraction test	Nerve root compression (disc herniation)	Head lifted axially with one hand under chin and other hand around occiput	Pain relief with lifting head
Adson's maneuvers	Thoracic outlet syndrome	Extend patient's symptomatic shoulder while patient rotates neck toward affected side. Pulse is checked during deep inspiration	Loss of pulse in affected extremity
Lhermitte's sign	Spinal canal narrowing (spinal stenosis), multiple sclerosis	Patient sitting with legs extended; ask patient to flex neck forward	Shock-like sensation into lower back and/ or extremities

B. **Physical Examination.** Examination should include inspection, palpation for tenderness in both midline and paraspinous areas, range of motion, neurovascular examination, and special tests. Inspection of the neck should evaluate for loss of normal lordosis, rash, or other abnormalities. Active range of motion is observed. Reduction of active range of motion may be associated with underlying bony pathology such as arthritis or may be due to muscle spasm. Loss of passive range of motion is usually due to underlying bony pathology. Neurovascular examination includes the evaluation of motor strength, sensation, and deep tendon reflexes. Special tests for cervical pathology are reviewed in Table 12.7.1.

C. **Testing.** Laboratory tests are rarely needed in patients with neck pain. Suspicion of a malignancy or inflammatory arthritis, such as rheumatoid arthritis or ankylosing spondylitis, may prompt tests such as rheumatoid factor, sedimentation rate, complete blood count, and/or HLA B27.

1. Radiographs are frequently helpful in cases of trauma, radicular symptoms, or prolonged (3–6 weeks) symptoms. Typical views include anteroposterior, odontoid (open-mouth view), and lateral radiographs of the cervical spine. All seven cervical vertebrae should be visualized in the lateral radiograph. Oblique views assist in the evaluation of the neural foramina and posterior elements. Flexion and extension views are obtained when instability of the cervical spine is suspected. It is important to remember that radiographic abnormalities are common in the general population and may not be the cause of the symptoms.

2. Computerized tomography is best used for identifying bony pathology such as subtle fractures, whereas magnetic resonance imaging is ideal for soft tissue pathology, such as disc disease and spinal stenosis. The use of discography to localize the exact disc causing pain is controversial (1). Nerve conduction velocity and electromyogram may be helpful in differentiating the nerve root from peripheral nerve pathology.

D. **Genetics.** Cervical degenerative disc disease may have a genetic component (4). Genetic predisposition to inflammatory disorders such as rheumatoid arthritis, ankylosing spondylitis, and osteoarthritis is well established (1).

TABLE 12.7.2	Differential Diagnosis of Neck Pain			
Musculoskeletal	**Neurologic**	**Infectious**	**Neoplastic**	**Referred**
Cervical strain or sprain	Thoracic outlet syndrome	Discitis	Spinal cord tumor	Rotator cuff tendinopathy
Disc herniation	Peripheral neuropathy	Osteomyelitis	Primary neck neoplasm	Myocardial ischemia
Degenerative disc disease	Myelopathy	Meningitis	Malignant neoplasm	Pneumonia
Inflammatory arthritis (rheumatoid, ankylosing spondylitis)	Radiculopathy	Cervical lymphadenitis		
Cervical fracture				
Cervical instability				
Cervical stenosis				
Fibromyalgia				
Whiplash				
Diffuse idiopathic skeletal hyperostosis				
Torticollis				

IV. DIAGNOSIS

    A. Differential Diagnosis. See Table 12.7.2.

    B. Clinical Manifestations. See Table 12.7.3.

TABLE 12.7.3	Most Common Causes of Neck Pain		
Etiology	**Typical history**	**Key physical examination findings**	**Key lab findings**
Spondylosis	Dull neck ache	Tender to palpation midline	Radiograph (X-ray) shows degenerative changes that can include narrowing of disc space, sclerosis of posterior elements, and osteophytes
	Older age group	Decreased active and passive ROMs	
	Occipital headache and/ or radicular symptoms		

(Continued)

TABLE 12.7.3   **Most Common Causes of Neck Pain *(Continued)***

Etiology	Typical history	Key physical examination findings	Key lab findings
Cervical disc herniation	Sharp neck pain	Decreased active ROM	MRI shows disc protrusion or extrusion into spinal canal
	Burning or tingling in upper extremities	Reduced deep tendon reflexes	
	Pain with neck motion	Decreased strength in upper extremities	
	Upper extremity weakness	Positive Spurling's test	
Cervical strain/sprain	Intermittent dull neck pain	Normal ROM	X-ray is normal or shows loss of lordosis
	And/or occupational related (postural)	Loss of lordosis	Consider computed tomography to rule out bony injury in trauma
	And/or trauma history (motor vehicle accident, fall)	Palpable tightness	
	Muscle spasm	Occasional acute edema	
		Muscle spasms	
Fibromyalgia	Diffuse axial skeletal pain	Normal passive ROM	No laboratory test to confirm
	Sleep disturbance	Trigger points	
	Fatigue		
Inflammatory arthritis such as RA or AS	Dull ache	Decreased active and passive ROMs	RA: increased rheumatoid factor and erythrocyte sedimentation rate
	Morning stiffness >1 h	Other joint inflammation	AS: positive HLA B27
	Other joint involvement		
Referred pain	Symptoms from other sites (e.g., chest pain, shoulder pain)	Normal ROM of neck	X-ray of other sites, electrocardiogram, MRI potentially helpful
		Physical examination findings at other sites (e.g., shoulder strength loss, chest rales)	

AS, ankylosing spondylitis; MRI, magnetic resonance imaging; RA, rheumatoid arthritis; ROM, range of motion.

REFERENCES

1. Nankano KK. Neck pain. In: Harris E, Budd R, Firestein G, et al., eds. *Kelley's textbook of rheumatology,* 7th ed. Philadelphia, PA: Elsevier Saunders, 2005:537–554.
2. Devereaux MW. Neck pain. *Prim Care Clin Office Pract* 2004;31:19–31.
3. Bland JH. Disorders of the cervical spine. In: Noble J, ed. *Textbook of primary care medicine,* 3rd ed. St Louis, MO: Mosby, 2001:1125–1137.
4. MacGregor AJ, Andrew T, Sambrook PN, et al. Structural, psychological, and genetic influences on low back and neck pain: a study of adult female twins. *Arthritis Rheum* 2004;51:160–167.

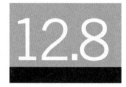

12.8 Polymyalgia

Shannon C. Scott

I. BACKGROUND. Multiple (*poly*) muscle aches (*myalgia*) are a common presentation in primary care with a broad differential diagnosis. The challenge for the physician lies in distinguishing benign and self-limiting causes, such as a benign viral infection, from more serious illnesses. In most cases, diagnosis remains primarily a clinical one.

II. PATHOPHYSIOLOGY. A number of conditions can result in polymyalgia (see Table 12.8.1). The most common causes are polymyalgia rheumatica and inflammatory conditions (e.g., polymyositis/dermatomyositis and fibromyalgia). Table 12.8.2 summarizes how these may be distinguished. The etiology and epidemiology are dependent upon the cause. In many cases, the precise etiology is unknown.

III. EVALUATION. The key to the evaluation of this condition lies in a careful history and physical examination (1). Frequently, laboratory investigations are inconclusive, and there is a danger that patients may be overinvestigated.

A. History

1. Ask about onset (acute or insidious) and the muscles affected (diffuse, proximal muscles of shoulder/hip girdle). To assess proximal muscle weakness, ask about difficulty going up stairs, getting up from chairs, and raising hands above the head.
2. Inquire about the presence of systemic symptoms; such as fever, weight loss, and fatigue. Is there joint involvement? If so, which ones?

TABLE 12.8.1 Differential Diagnosis of Polymyalgia

Systemic rheumatic disease	Infection	Endocrine
Polymyalgia rheumatica	Viral or bacterial	Hypothyroid
Polymyositis/dermatomyositis	Spirochetal	Adrenal insufficiency
Rheumatoid arthritis		
Systemic lupus erythematosus	**Noninflammatory**	**Medications**
Spondyloarthropathy	Fibromyalgia	Statins
Vasculitis	Chronic fatigue syndrome	
		Metabolic
		Osteomalacia (7)

TABLE 12.8.2 Most Common Causes of Polymyalgia

	Polymyalgia rheumatica (1–4)	Fibromyalgia (5)	Inflammatory conditions (e.g., polymyositis/ DM) (6)
Epidemiology	Most common >50 y	Middle age, usually <50 y	Most common 40–60 y
	2:1 women:men 58/100,000 (1)	Affects women more than men 2–8% (where studied)	2:1 women:men 1/100,000
Pathophysiology	Cause unknown	Unclear	Inflammation of striated muscle
	Systemic inflammation commonly found in proximal joints surrounding tendons, bursa, and soft tissues	Sensitization of central nervous system	DM, also involves skin
	Large vessel vasculitis		
History	Sudden onset	Chronic widespread	Slowly progressive
	>2 wk duration	Nonarticular pain and muscle tenderness	Systemic: fever, malaise, weight loss
	Systemic: fever, malaise, anorexia, weight loss, depression	Systemic: fatigue, sleep disturbance, headaches, frequently multiple symptoms	Specific: proximal symmetric muscle and truncal weakness over weeks to months (worse after use)
	Specific: proximal symmetric shoulder and/or hip girdle pain with AM **stiffness** (lasting >45 min)		Dysphagia (50%)
Physical	**Proximal tenderness (bilateral)** upper arms and thighs, limited range of motion in neck, shoulders, and hips secondary to pain	**Tender "trigger" points (11 of 18 points)**	Proximal tenderness AND weakness (bilateral)
		No weakness	Muscle atrophy
			Rash (DM), Gottron's papules, heliotrophe rash on eyelids
	NO weakness		
Laboratory tests	Elevated ESR >50 mm/h (often ESR 100 mm/h)	No specific test	ESR
		Normal ESR	Creatine kinase
	Normochromic normocytic anemia		Aldolase
			Autoantibodies: anti-Jo-1
			Electromyography
			Muscle biopsy

(Continued)

TABLE 12.8.2	**Most Common Causes of Polymyalgia** *(Continued)*		
	Polymyalgia rheumatica (1–4)	**Fibromyalgia (5)**	**Inflammatory conditions (e.g., polymyositis/ DM) (6)**
Treatment	Rapid response to oral prednisone (10–20 mg/d)	No response to steroids	Admission, steroids, cytotoxics
		Multifaceted individualized program	Splinting of joints and gradual rehabilitation
		Medications: muscle relaxants, antidepressants	
		Exercise	
Associations	Temporal arteritis (giant cell arteritis)	Irritable bowel syndrome	Systemic lupus erythematosus, rheumatoid arthritis, systemic sclerosis
	25/100,000 (1)	Sleep disorders	
	Symptoms: headache, scalp pain, temporal artery tenderness (beading or diminished pulse), visual disturbance, jaw or tongue claudication	Restless leg syndrome	Malignancy (lung, ovary, breast, stomach)
		Depression/anxiety	
		Myofascial pain syndrome	Extramuscular manifestations: cutaneous (DM), cardiac, pulmonary, gastrointestinal
		Chronic fatigue syndrome	

DM, dermatomyositis; ESR, erythrocyte sedimentation rate.

3. Is there a significant past medical history? Ask about medications and family history. In the social history, it is important to inquire about occupation and sources of stress.

B. **Physical Examination.** Pay particular attention to the musculoskeletal system. Inspect for muscle atrophy and palpate for muscle tenderness (including the scalp and temporal artery). The presence or absence of muscle weakness is the *key* clinical finding. Even patients with significant pain can perform a brief maneuver at maximum effort to assess strength. Distinguish between soft tissue pain (myalgia) and joint pain (arthralgia). Are the tender points located in a significant pattern (fibromyalgia)? Is a rash present?

C. **Testing.** Frequently, laboratory tests fail to elucidate the cause. Baseline investigations may include a complete blood count, erythrocyte sedimentation rate, C-reactive protein, glucose, liver function tests, creatine kinase, thyroid function tests, electrolytes, rheumatoid factor, urinalysis, and a chest radiograph. If muscle weakness is present, consider obtaining serum aldolase, anti-Jo-1 antibodies, electromyelogram, and/or muscle biopsy. Consideration may be given to obtaining serologies for infectious diseases, depending on risk factors (1).

IV. **DIAGNOSIS.** The differential diagnosis is wide ranging (Table 12.8.1). It is important to review the patient's history and perform a complete physical examination to most accurately delineate the cause of polymyalgia.

REFERENCES

1. Donnelly JA, Torregiani ST. Polymyalgia rheumatica and giant cell arteritis. *Clin Fam Pract* 2005;7(2):225–246.
2. Dasgupta B, Borg FA, Hassan-N, et al. BSR and BHPR guidelines for the management of polymyalgia rheumatica *Rheumatology* 2010;49:186–190.
3. Spiera RF, Paget SA. Polymyalgia rheumatica and temporal arteritis. In: Goldman L, Schafer A, eds. *Goldman's Cecil textbook of medicine*, 24th ed. Pennsylvania, PA: Elsevier Saunders, 2011:1728–1731.
4. Unwin B, Willimas C, Gilliland W. Polymyalgia rheumatica and giant cell arteritis. *Am Fam Physician* 2006;74(9):1547–1554.
5. Chakrabary S, Zoorob R. Fibromyalgia. *Am Fam Physician* 2007;76(2):248–254.
6. Khan S, Christopher-Stine L. Polymyositis, dermatomyositis, and autoimmune necrotizing myopathy clinical manifestations. *Rheum Dis Clin North Am* 2011;37:143–158.
7. Lyman D. Undiagnosed vitamin D deficiency in the hospitalized patient. *Am Fam Physician* 2005;71(2):299–304.

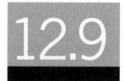

Shoulder Pain

Kevin J. Benson

I. BACKGROUND. Shoulder pain is a common musculoskeletal complaint. Eighty-five percent of patients with pain have a problem that is intrinsic to the shoulder. Understanding the functional anatomy and biomechanic properties will help determine the etiology and appropriate treatment (1).

II. PATHOPHYSIOLOGY

   A. Pathologic processes cannot be evaluated in isolation because of the complex relationship of the shoulder girdle with other structures. The shoulder is composed of three bones (clavicle, scapula, and proximal humerus) and four articular surfaces (sternoclavicular (SC), acromioclavicular (AC), glenohumeral (GH), and scapulothoracic (ST)). The GH joint is loosely constrained by muscles and ligaments within a thin capsule. The rotator cuff (RC) is composed of four muscles (supraspinatus, infraspinatus, subscapularis, and teres minor), which serve as a dynamic stabilizer. The function of the subacromial bursa is to lubricate and protect the RC tendons from the pressure and friction of the underside of the acromion. Shoulder motion is dependent on the AC and SC joints and the ST articulation. Repetitive overhead activities, trauma, or instability can result in impingement, which is associated with pain and inflammation.

   B. Younger patients, especially those who participate in sports requiring overhead motion, have pain and instability secondary to repetitive microtrauma of the labrocapsular structures. Psychosocial factors may play a role in chronic pain. Focal degeneration and ischemia of the RC occurs with advancing age. Other sites of significant pain due to trauma include the biceps tendon, AC joint, and brachial plexus. Pain can be referred from the cervical spine, chest, and abdomen to the shoulder.

III. EVALUATION

   A. History. Pain should be described accurately (onset, duration, palliation, provocation, quality, location, and radiation). Inquire about previous injuries, past surgery, and other comorbidities. A fall on an outstretched hand (FOOSH) can give rise to instability in a younger patient and RC tear in the elderly. A fall on the point of the shoulder may result in an RC tear or AC joint injury. Throwing injuries stress the labrocapsular complex and ligamentous attachments and give rise to RC tendonitis and bicipital tendonitis. Referred pain may arise from other sources like myocardial ischemia, hepatobiliary disease, and nerve entrapments.

B. Physical Exam. It should be guided by history and approached in a step-wise fashion. Is it traumatic versus nontraumatic, extrinsic versus intrinsic, GH versus extra-GH? Inspection should include all aspects of the shoulder. Palpation should reveal tenderness, swelling, or instability. Range of motion should be both active and passive. Check abduction, adduction, flexion, extension, and internal and external rotation. See special tests to confirm shoulder pathology as noted in Table 12.9.1 (2). The sensitivity and specificity of these tests is questionable (1).

1. GH pathology is unlikely in the presence of normal range of passive motion. There are tests for impingement (Neer and Hawkin's sign), RC pathology (empty can test, lift-off test, and drop arm test), AC joint pathology (cross-body adduction test), biceps tendon injury (Yergason and Speed's tests), and instability (apprehension test).
2. The painful arc (pain with abduction between 60° and 120°) suggests impingement (3).
3. Limited active abduction associated with weakness against resistance suggests an RC tear.

TABLE 12.9.1   Special Tests to Confirm Shoulder Pathology

Test	Maneuver	Pathology
Neer test (impingement sign)	Examiner stabilizes patients acromion with one hand, performs maximum passive shoulder abduction and internal rotation with the other.	Subacromial inflammation, impingement
Hawkin's impingement sign	Forced internal rotation with the shoulder flexed forward to 90°	Impingement
Jobe's test (empty can test)	Deltoid assessed with arm at 90° abduction and neutral rotation. Shoulder then internally rotated and angled forward 30°; thumbs pointing toward the floor. Downward pressure of examiner's hand resisted.	Supraspinatus weakness due to injury, pain due to rotator cuff pathology
Cross-body adduction test	Shoulder flexed to 90° and adducted across the patient's body	Rotator cuff/acromioclavicular pathology
Lift-off test	Patient's arm behind back, with volar surface of the hand resting on the sacrum. Weakness in lifting the hand away from the spine	Subscapularis muscle weakness/injury
Yergason test	Supination of the pronated forearm against resistance with the elbow flexed at 90°	Biceps tendonitis/tear
Speed's test	Extension and supination of the elbow as the examiner resists flexion of the humerus	Biceps tendonitis/tear
Apprehension test	Abduction to 90° and external rotation of the shoulder with the examiner's hand applying forward pressure to the scapula. The patient resists further shoulder extension	Positive anterior instability
Drop arm test	The arm is passively abducted to 90° and the support is suddenly discontinued. A positive test is reported if the arm drops abruptly	Rotator cuff tear or axillary nerve injury

4. AC joint pathology is accompanied by pain on top of the shoulder, localized tenderness, and possible pain referral to the neck.
5. Crepitus is associated with GH osteoarthritis.

C. Testing

1. **Lab Tests**. A CBC and synovial fluid analysis for cell count, Gram stain, and culture are obtained if infection is suspected. Consider checking erythrocyte sedimentation rate, C-reactive protein (CRP), antinuclear antibody (ANA), and joint aspirate for crystals in an inflammatory process.
2. **Imaging Studies**. There are no specific guidelines. Plain radiography including anterior–posterior, lateral, and scapular views may be beneficial if there is loss of range of motion, severe pain, or known trauma. The following may be identified: fracture of the proximal humerus, clavicle, and scapula, GH dislocation, AC joint pathology, and SC joint pathology (requires apical lordotic view of chest). Magnetic resonance imaging (MRI) is preferred with suspected impingement and RC injury. If it is normal, there is less than a 10% chance of a tear. MRI is useful in the evaluation of avascular necrosis, biceps tendinopathy or rupture, and inflammatory processes. Ultrasound is helpful in identifying RC tear, labral tear, and biceps tendon tears and dislocation. MR arthrography can be useful in evaluating and treating frozen shoulder (4). Computerized tomography (CT) scan may be an option if there is a contraindication to using MRI (5). CT is preferred for imaging tumors and occult fractures. CT arthrography may play a role in suspected RC tears in patients with claustrophobia (4).

IV. DIAGNOSIS

A. Specific Conditions

1. **Subacromial bursitis** is a term used when describing the pathology of impingement. It is usually associated with RC tendonitis.
2. **RC tendonitis** has three stages (edema and hemorrhage of tendon, fibrosis of subacromial bursa, eventual rupture of tendon if not responsive to treatment). Fifty percent of patients over age 70 years have RC tears. RC tears may eventually lead to cuff arthropathy (5).
3. **Bicipital tendonitis** is associated with overuse and commonly occurs in weight lifters. Rupture of the long head of the biceps (Popeye sign) is often present. Weakness is seldom significant, since 85% of the power associated with elbow flexion comes from the short head of the biceps and brachioradialis (3).
4. **Adhesive capsulitis** is a painful restriction of shoulder movement of soft tissue origin. It is associated with diabetes, thyroid disease, pulmonary disorders, stroke, and Dupuytren's disease. The diagnosis is clinical (6).
5. **AC syndromes** can be acute or chronic and are usually posttraumatic in the young. AC osteoarthritis usually follows AC separation or excessive repetitive training. It is common after age 40 years.
6. **Calcific tendonitis**. Calcification occurs as part of a degenerative process of the RC tendons. It usually occurs in the fourth decade. Twenty-one percent have complete RC tears associated with it. The condition is associated with HLA-A1 (1).
7. **ST bursitis**. This condition is often seen among patients with habitually poor posture. Crepitus is usually present at the superior medial angle of the scapula.
8. **GH instability** represents a spectrum of disorders from unidirectional dislocation to multidirectional instability. It could be from repetitive overhead activity, FOOSH, or anterior dislocation of the shoulder. It usually occurs in athletes.
9. **Polymyalgia rheumatica** is seen in older patients who have pain and stiffness in both shoulders. The sedimentation rate (and more commonly CRP level) is elevated in these patients.
10. **Temporal arteritis** may present with shoulder pain associated with headache and visual changes or jaw claudication.
11. **Fibromyalgia, cervical radiculopathy**, and **thoracic outlet syndrome** are also common sources of shoulder pain (4). If the pain radiates below the elbow and possibly into the hand, consider a source of pain extrinsic to the shoulder.

REFERENCES

1. Dalton SE. The shoulder. In: Hochberg MC, Silman AJ, Smolen JS, Weinblatt ME, Weisman MH, eds. *Rheumatology*, 5th ed. Philadelphia, PA: Mosby Elsevier, 2011:683–699.
2. Ramakrishnan K, Jones AD. Shoulder pain. In: Paulman, ed. *Taylor's 10-minute diagnosis manual*, 3rd ed. Philadelphia, PA: Lippincott Williams and Wilkins, 2077:292–295.
3. Waldman SD. *Physical diagnosis of pain: an atlas of signs and symptoms*. Philadelphia, PA: Elsevier Saunders, 2006.
4. Burbank KM, Stevenson JH, Czarnecki GR, Dorfman J. Chronic shoulder pain. *Am Fam Physician* 2008;77(4):453–460.
5. Anderson BC, Anderson RJ. *Evaluation of the patient with shoulder complaints*, 2012. Retrieved from http://www.uptodate.com
6. Ewald A. Adhesive capsulitis: a review. *Am Fam Physician* 2011;83(4):417–422.

CHAPTER **13**

Dermatologic Problems

Hassan Galadari

<table>
<tr><td>

13.1

</td><td>

Alopecia

Khawla Rashid Alnuaimi and Hassan Galadari

</td></tr>
</table>

I. BACKGROUND. Hair-related problems are common medical complaints encountered by physicians. Among the most common problems presenting to the primary care provider are telogen effluvium and androgenic alopecia (1).

The human scalp has an average of 100,000 hairs (2). The hair follicle goes through three stages of growth. The initial growth phase, a process that lasts an average of 2–6 years, is termed the anagen phase (2). At any one time, 90–95% of scalp hair is in the anagen phase. This is followed by the catagen phase, which is a transitional stage, in which the hair follicle enters a process of involution (2). This stage lasts for 2–3 weeks. Less than 1% of scalp hair is in the catagen phase (2). Approximately 5% of hair follicles enter a resting stage, at the end of which they are shed. This process may last 2–3 months and is known as the telogen phase (2).

II. PATHOPHYSIOLOGY

A. Etiology. Alopecia can be classified by its clinical presentation, that is, according to whether the alopecia is localized or generalized. Alternatively, the classification can be based on the pathology of the condition causing the alopecia. This classification divides alopecia into scarring (cicatricial) and nonscarring (noncicatricial) alopecia (3). In scarring alopecia, hair loss occurs due to inflammation, leading to permanent follicular damage (2). Scarring alopecia generally causes localized hair loss. Examples of scarring alopecia include infections such as severe folliculitis, dissecting cellulitis, and kerion; inflammatory disorders affecting the hair follicle and scalp such as discoid lupus erythematosus, lichen planopilaris, and bullous diseases; other disorders such as tumors, acne keloidalis, frontal fibrosing alopecia, and pseudopelade of Brocq (2). In nonscarring alopecia, the hair loss is not permanent and regrowth is generally possible after treatment. Examples of nonscarring alopecia include telogen effluvium, androgenetic alopecia, anagen effluvium, alopecia areata, and traumatic or chemical alopecia (3). Telogen effluvium is the most common cause of diffuse hair loss (3). It occurs after a stressful event such as surgery, childbirth, crash dieting, or psychological illness (4). It often occurs 3 months following the inciting event and resolves spontaneously after 3–4 months (4). Anagen effluvium involves loss of anagen hair and usually occurs 10–24 days after starting chemotherapeutic agents (3). Androgenetic alopecia or male pattern baldness occurs in genetically susceptible individuals in a process known as hair miniaturization, resulting in shortened anagen phase and subsequently shorter, thinner hair shaft (1). While both sexes may be affected by androgenetic alopecia, the condition is much more commonly seen in men. Fifty percent of males over the age of 50 years will have some degree of androgenetic alopecia. Alopecia areata is an autoimmune disorder affecting hair follicles, resulting in nonscarring hair loss (3). The clinical picture varies from localized patches of hair loss to total body involvement termed alopecia universalis (3). Chemical and physical trauma to hair follicles secondary to the use of hot combs, hair straighteners, and traction may occur (2). Prolonged or repeated trauma to the hair follicle may permanently damage the hair follicles, resulting in scarring alopecia (2).

B. **Epidemiology.** Alopecia is a common problem affecting all genders, all races, and all ages. A variety of illnesses result in alopecia, each with its own distinct age, sex, and race characteristics and patterns of morbidity. The most common causes of alopecia are androgenetic alopecia and telogen effluvium (1).

III. EVALUATION

A. **History.** To assess patients with hair loss, a careful medical history and examination can help avoid expensive, unnecessary evaluation, and laboratory tests. In the history, physicians should inquire about onset and duration of hair loss, any preceding stressful event, medications, and diet. In the review of systems, physicians should ask specifically for thyroid symptoms. Family history of hair loss, androgenetic alopecia, and autoimmune disorders should be determined (2).

B. **Physical Examination.** Examine the scalp and hair shaft carefully. Determine whether the hair loss is diffuse or localized, look for signs of inflammation, and determine hair density. The texture, length, and thickness of individual hairs may suggest the cause of hair loss. Shorter, fine hairs may be found in areas affected by androgenic alopecia. "Exclamation point hairs," which have a distal broken shaft and a proximal club-shaped hair root, are seen at the periphery of hair loss in alopecia areata (5). Short, broken hairs in the area of hair loss are seen with trichotillomania and tinea capitis. All areas of the body must be carefully examined for hair growth patterns and changes. Trichotillomania can be seen in the scalp, eyebrow areas, and even the eyelashes. Patterns of hair loss in male pattern androgenic alopecia typically range from bitemporal recession, to frontal and vertex thinning, and to loss of all hair except for the occipital and temporal fringes. Female pattern alopecia classically presents as diffuse thinning that is more prominent in the frontal or parietal areas, with sparing of the frontal fringe (5). In women, signs of virilization associated with androgenic alopecia may be seen. Virilization can also cause acne, hypertrichosis in other areas, deepening of the voice, and clitoromegaly. Rashes or other changes in the skin either in the area of hair loss or elsewhere may suggest various causes. Scaling and flaking suggest tinea, psoriasis, or drying of the skin as a result of heat or chemicals. Scarring of the areas of hair loss suggest trauma, infection, or discoid lupus. A "moth-eaten" pattern of hair loss on either the scalp or face should suggest syphilis and sarcoid or discoid lupus. Telogen effluvium can be detected by the "pull test," which is performed by grasping approximately 60 hairs between thumb and fingers and exerting traction to determine degree of shedding and anagen to telogen hair ratio (2). Normal shedding should yield six or fewer hairs. The patients' hair should not have been shampooed in the 24 hours prior to this test (6).

C. **Testing**

1. Any laboratory testing should be ordered on the basis of clinical findings. A typical androgenic alopecia pattern of hair loss with normal skin in men and women without evidence of virilization requires no further testing. Women who show evidence of virilization should have serum free testosterone, total testosterone, prolactin, and dehydroepiandrosterone sulfate levels drawn first. If these are abnormal, then workup should continue, focused on the specific findings. Patients with nonandrogenic patterns of alopecia should have thyroid function tests, a complete blood count, a ferritin level, and an antinuclear antibody done. The need for syphilis serology should also be considered on the basis of the history and examination. If these tests are all normal, other nutritional deficiencies, such as zinc, may be considered (7). Bacterial and fungal cultures of any drainage should be obtained. Potassium hydroxide microscopic evaluation of skin scrapings for fungal elements and/or fungal cultures of scaling areas can confirm the diagnosis of fungal infection.

2. Scalp biopsy for histopathology may be useful in suspected cases of scarring alopecia for definitive diagnosis (5).

D. Genetics. Inherited or congenital hair disorders affecting the scalp and hair can result in structural defects with or without hair fragility (4). There are more than 300 genetic disorders that affect the hair (8).

IV. DIAGNOSIS

A. Differential Diagnosis. The key consideration in diagnosis is whether the hair loss is localized or generalized or scarring versus nonscarring. Subsequent examinations as noted earlier allow a definitive diagnosis.

B. Clinical Manifestations. Most cases of alopecia are caused by either androgenic alopecia or telogen effluvium. Early diagnosis and intervention can be critical in the remaining cases if caused by thyroid disorder, carcinoma, metastatic adenocarcinoma, melanoma, syphilis, or human immunodeficiency virus. Permanent hair loss may be prevented or limited by early institution of therapy. If alopecia is caused by a drug, hair loss can be reversible if the drug is stopped early in the process. Treatment, if desired, for androgenic alopecia works best if started early on in hair loss.

REFERENCES

1. Beth G, Adam O. Androgenetic alopecia. www.Uptodate.com. Accessed July 21, 2012.
2. Habif T. *Clinical dermatology*, 5th ed. Philadelphia, PA: Elsevier, 2010:916–938.
3. Bth G, Adam O. *Nonscarring alopecia*. www.Uptodate.com. Accessed July 21, 2012.,
4. Anthony D. *Atlas of clinical dermatology*. Philadelphia, PA: Elsevier, 2002:631–634.
5. James WD, Berger TG, Elston D. *Andrew's diseases of clinical dermatology*. Philadelphia, PA: Elsevier, 2006:749.
6. Bertolino A. Alopecia areata. *Postgrad Med* 2000;107(7):81–90.
7. Irvine A, Christiano A. Hair on a gene string: recent advances in understanding the molecular genetics of hair loss. *Clin Exp Dermatol* 2001;26:59–71.
8. Thiedke C. Alopecia in women. *Am Fam Physician* 2003;67(5):1017–1018.

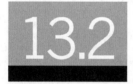

13.2 Erythema Multiforme

Amr Salam and Ophelia E. Dadzie

I. BACKGROUND. Erythema multiforme (EM) and related diseases are a group of mucocutaneous disorders believed to be a hypersensitivity reaction triggered by various stimuli, including infectious agents and drugs (1–4). The clinical classification of this group of diseases is complicated partly due to controversies regarding the precise etiologies of some of the conditions and the clinical manifestation of the disease along a spectrum. However, EM broadly consists of the syndromes EM minor, EM major (EMM), Stevens-Johnson syndrome (SJS), and toxic epidermal necrolysis (TEN) (Table 13.2.1). EM minor represents the mild end of the spectrum, presenting as an acute self-limiting eruption. It is primarily confined to acral sites, with minimal to no mucosal involvement. In contrast, EMM, SJS, and TEN are more serious diseases, with associated morbidity and/or mortality. EMM is characterized by more extensive mucosal involvement as compared with EM minor. SJS and TEN are considered to represent a single disease entity distinguished only by the severity of the illness. Both are also considered to be related to EMM.

II. PATHOPHYSIOLOGY

A. Etiology. EM minor, EMM, SJS, and TEN are believed to be hypersensitivity reactions triggered by various stimuli. These include infectious agents and drugs (1–4). Recent herpetic infections (herpes simplex virus, HSV 1 and 2) are the most common triggers of EM minor and EMM; recent work implicates transport of viral particles to the skin by CD34 cells (5). Other infectious agents may also trigger EM. These include Epstein-Barr virus,

Table 13.2.1	Overview of EM and Related Diseases
Condition	**Defining Features**
EM minor	Typical target lesions (≥3 zones), mainly cutaneous (acral sites), rarely involves mucous membrane but if so usually mouth only
	infective triggers > drug triggers
	BSA <10%
EMM	skin lesions as with EM + ≥2 mucosal sites, may have associated
	infective triggers > drug triggers
	BSA <10% (but more severe than EM)
SJS	Atypical target lesions (2 zones), purpuric macules on face and trunk, severe mucosal erosions, systemic symptoms
	drug triggers > infective triggers
	BSA <10% (but more severe than EMM)
SJS/TEN overlap	As with SJS
	drug triggers > infective triggers
	BSA = 10–30%
TEN	Poorly defined erythematous macules and atypical target lesions
	Early mucosal erosion, detachment of epidermis, systemic symptoms
	drug triggers > infective triggers
	BSA >30%

BSA, body surface area; EM, erythema multiforme; EMM, erythema multiforme major; SJS, Stevens Johnson syndrome; TEN, toxic epidermal necrolysis.

cytomegalovirus, Mycoplasma pneumonia (especially in children), mycobacterium tuberculosis (TB), β-hemolytic streptococcus, *Histoplasma capsulatum*, and *Coccidioides immitis* (3). Drugs may also trigger EM minor and EMM; however, this accounts for a minority of cases.

In contrast, medications are a major trigger for the development of SJS/TEN. These include allopurinol, carbamazepine, cotrimoxazole (and other anti-infective sulfonamides and sulfasalazine), lamotrigine, nevirapine, nonsteroidal anti-inflammatory drugs (especially oxicams), phenobarbital, and phenytoin (4). Drug-related illness appears to invoke a pathway that involves tumor necrosis factor, whereas HSV-related illness does not (6).

B. Epidemiology. EM minor, EMM, SJS, and TEN occur worldwide, in individuals of all ages, although most are under 40 years old (2–4). Significant ethnic variation in the incidence of SJS/TEN has been observed (7).

III. EVALUATION

A. History. Pertinent aspects of the clinical history which must be obtained include the presence of prodromal symptoms, any concurrent or preceding illness, and recent drug exposure (2, 4). EM minor is often asymptomatic, although some patients may experience itching or tenderness. The condition is of sudden onset and generally does not cause systemic symptoms. Herpetic infection is an important etiologic factor in the setting of EM minor and EMM; thus, the history should specifically explore the presence or absence of recent infection. In SJS/TEN, prodromal symptoms may occur. These include fever, malaise, and myalgias. Recent exposure to medications (especially in the preceding 1–3 weeks) is of relevance in the setting of SJS/TEN.

B. Physical Examination. The morphology of the cutaneous eruption, distribution and estimated percentage body surface involvement, presence of mucosal disease, and/or systemic signs are important determinants of disease subtype and severity (2–4). EM minor manifests as target or iris lesions that are symmetrically distributed and are found primarily on the extremities (e.g., palms, soles) and sometimes on the face or trunk. The lesions develop over 10 days or more and resolve on their own, usually in 1–6 weeks. Recurrences are common and may continue for years. EMM spans a wide range of presentations ranging from a severe variant of EM minor to mild SJS. There is, however, more extensive mucosal involvement. Lesions that are irregular or occur in large erythematous patches, blister, or bullae with sloughing in large sheets are highly suggestive of SJS and the more severe TEN.

Systemic signs, such as a high fever, are seen primarily in SJS and/or TEN. In richly pigmented skin, erythema may be underappreciated.

C. Testing. The diagnosis of EM and the closely related conditions discussed above are based primarily on clinical findings. Nevertheless, histologic assessment (3) of lesional skin may be of help, especially when the morphology of the cutaneous lesions are atypical and/or to exclude other diagnoses. Other ancillary tests that may be helpful, especially if an underlying infectious etiology is suspected, include a complete blood count, throat culture, antistreptolysin-O titer, testing for infectious mononucleosis, HSV serology (immunoglobulin (Ig) M and IgG), and a hepatitis screen. A chest radiograph may be obtained if *Mycoplasma pneumoniae*, histoplasmosis, coccidiomycosis, or TB is suspected.

D. Genetics. There is no well-defined genetic basis to EM and its related group of diseases. The exception is SJS/TEN secondary to carbamazepine and allopurinol in persons of Chinese and South Asian origin, where specific HLA haplotypes (HLA-B*1502 and HLA-B*5801, respectively) have been found to be of relevance (4, 7).

IV. DIAGNOSIS

A. Differential Diagnosis. A fixed, discrete, annular, erythematous eruption, which lasts for 1–6 weeks from onset to healing and is self-limited, acute, or episodic, satisfies the clinical criteria for EM minor. A systemic, erythematous eruption, with irregular and target lesions, blisters, sloughing, and a systemically unwell patient, is much more indicative of SJS/TEN. Other differential diagnoses to consider in the setting of EM and its related group of diseases include autoimmune bullous disease, other drug eruptions (e.g., morbilliform drug eruptions), figurate erythema, connective tissue disease (e.g., lupus erythematosus), pityriasis rosea, polymorphic light eruption, urticaria, urticarial vasculitis, and even viral exanthems. Clinical features and histologic findings may be of help in excluding these conditions, as may collegial help from a dermatologist in difficult cases.

B. Clinical Manifestations. Determining which subtype of EM is present helps dictate treatment and anticipate prognosis. EM minor is a limited illness with little morbidity and mortality, although recurrences are common. SJS/TEN are often life-threatening illnesses with considerable morbidity and even mortality.

V. TREATMENT.
The management of EM and related diseases lacks significant evidence-based data and is based primarily on anecdotal evidence (3, 4). Identification of the underlying triggering factor and prompt withdrawal or treatment is key to management of these patients. EM minor does not always require therapeutic intervention, but supportive therapy is important, including the use of antihistamines and topical corticosteroids to alleviate cutaneous symptoms and local anesthetic/antiseptic mouthwash for oral mucosal involvement. In the setting of HSV-associated EM minor, antiviral therapy (e.g., oral aciclovir) has been shown to be effective. In particular, long-term low-dose prophylactic antiviral therapy, such as oral aciclovir, in the setting of recurrent EM minor, is efficacious. The principles of managing SJS and TEN include prompt withdrawal of the implicated drug(s), as well as supportive care. Management is best undertaken in a hospital setting rather than in the community. Other ancillary measures include use of systemic antibiotics, corticosteroids, and/or other immune modulating drugs. Where there is extensive cutaneous and/or mucosal ulceration, patients are best managed in an intensive care/burns unit, ideally by a multidisciplinary medical team. The management of EMM is determined by the severity, being similar to EM minor or SJS.

REFERENCES

1. Auquier-Dunant A, Mockenhaupt M, Nalda L, et al. Correlations between clinical patterns and causes of erythema multiforme majus, Stevens-Johnson syndrome, and toxic epidermal necrolysis: results of an international prospective study. *Arch Dermatol* 2002;138:1019–1024.
2. Lamoreux MR, Sternbach MR, Hsu WT. Erythema multiforme. *Am Fam Physician* 2006;74(11): 1883–1888.
3. Al-Johani KA, Fedele S, Porter SR. Erythema multiforme and related disorders. *Oral Surg Oral Med Oral Pathol Oral Radiol Endod* 2007;103(5):642–654.
4. Mockenhaupt M. The current understanding of Stevens-Johnson syndrome and toxic epidermal necrolysis. *Expert Rev Clin Immunol* 2011;7(6):803–813; quiz 14–15.
5. Ono F, Sharma B, Smith C, et al. CD34+ cells in the peripheral blood transport Herpes simplex virus DNA fragments to the skin of patients with erythema multiforme (HAEM). *J Invest Dermatol* 2005;124(6):1215–1224.
6. Kokuba H, Aurelian L, Burnett J. Herpes simplex virus associated erythema multiforme (HAEM) is mechanistically distinct from drug-induced erythema multiforme: interferonis expressed in HAEM lesions and tumor necrosis factor in drug-induced erythema multiforme lesions. *J Invest Dermatol* 1999;113(5):808–815.
7. Roujeau, J.-C. (2013). Drug eruptions and ethnicity. In O. Dadzie, A. Petit, & A. Alexis, *Ethnic Dermatology: Principles and Practice*. Oxford: John Wiley & Sons.

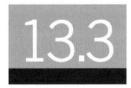

13.3 Maculopapular Rash
Naama Salem Al Kaabi

I. BACKGROUND. Maculopapular rash is a term used to describe any skin rash that contains both macules and papules. The affected skin appears red and has multiple confluent bumps.

II. PATHOPHYSIOLOGY

   A. Etiology. When a maculopapular rash is associated with fever, an infectious cause should be suspected. If no fever is present, allergic reaction is usually the cause. Serious infections, such as meningococcemia, disseminated gonorrhea, and Rocky Mountain spotted fever (RMSF), may present with an acute onset of fever and a maculopapular rash (1, 2). Occasionally, anaphylaxis starts as maculopapular rash with palmar or pharyngeal itching (3). Maculopapular rash is rarely a presenting sign of internal malignancy (1).

   B. Epidemiology. Maculopapular rash is associated with many different diseases. The prevalence, morbidity, and mortality in various ages, sexes, and race populations reflect the underlying disease.

III. EVALUATION

   A. History. A detailed history of present illness should be obtained. The location that was first affected, the course of spread, associated symptoms such as fever, itch, burn, or pain, and any similar previous attacks are determined. If the patient had similar rash before, the previous treatment and response to the treatment should be determined. A history of contact with individuals affected by a similar rash should be considered. The history should also include any chronic medical illnesses and treatments the patient is already using or has just started. Treatments should include any prescribed medication, over-the-counter medicine, and herbal preparations. A history of allergy to foods or drugs should be included. The social history is also important; this includes occupation, hobbies, smoking, drug abuse, new sexual partners, and travel (1).

   B. Physical Examination. A thorough physical examination should be performed. The distribution of the rash should be noted when conducting the skin exam (1, 4). Viral exanthems such as rubeola and rubella usually start centrally on face and trunk, then spread centrifugally. The rash of meningococcemia tends to start peripherally. It usually begins as a macule with central petechiae which then progress to a nodule followed by a widespread rash. Lesions of gonorrhea start acrally on limbs and digits. If a maculopapular rash manifests on the palms and soles, conditions such as syphilis, rocky mountain spotted fever (RMSF), and disseminated gonorrhea should be considered (1–3).

1. **Head, Eyes, Ears, Nose, and Throat Examination.** Examination of the scalp to detect ticks is important if RMSF is suspected. Swelling of mucous membranes may be indicative of early anaphylaxis. Koplik's spots of measles may appear on oral mucosa (3).

2. **Lung Examination.** Wheezing may be associated with anaphylaxis (1).

3. **Genitourinary Examination.** Primary syphilis presents with chancre on genitals. After chancre heals, the palmar lesions of secondary syphilis appears (1, 4). Purulent discharge or evidence of pelvic inflammation may indicate gonorrhea (3).

4. **Extremities Examination.** Joint swelling is often present in meningococcemia, gonococcemia, and rheumatologic conditions (3).

5. **Neurologic Examination.** Signs of meningitis may indicate meningococcemia or RMSF (3).

C. **Testing.** The complete blood count (CBC) is valuable. An elevated white blood cell count with a left shift may indicate a bacterial infection; lymphocytosis may indicate a viral infection; eosinophil counts are sometimes increased with allergic reactions; and rarely, myelogenous leukemias can present with rash and abnormalities on CBC. Other testing should be performed on the basis of the most likely causes of the rash. Consider the rapid plasma reagin test and testing for gonococcemia in sexually active patients. Consider a smear and culture of any pustules, especially if meningococcemia or gonococcemia is suspected. Cerebrospinal fluid examination is useful if meningococcemia is suspected; it is usually negative in RMSF. Consider an erythrocyte sedimentation rate in the presence of joint involvement.

D. **Genetics.** Maculopapular rash is mostly caused by infectious or allergic causes; therefore, genetic factors are not likely to play a strong role in this condition.

IV. DIAGNOSIS

A. **Differential Diagnosis.** Maculopapular eruptions are seen in infections including viral, bacterial, spirochetes, and rickettsial infections. They are also seen in immune-mediated syndromes and rheumatologic diseases.

1. **Viral Exanthems.** Viral infections that usually present with maculopapular rash include rubeola (measles), rubella (German measles), Fifth disease, and roseola (5). Rubeola starts with cough, conjunctivitis, and coryza, with a maculopapular rash appearing around the fourth day of fever. Rash starts on the hairline and then it spreads downward, sparing the palms and soles. It lasts 4–6 days before it fades, leaving yellow-tan pigmentation and some desquamation. Koplik's spots are often seen on the oral mucosa, particularly during the prodrome (1, 5). Rubella is similar to measles but is less severe, lasts for shorter period of time, and is associated with prominent occipital adenopathy. Severe birth defect can result from rubella infection of pregnant women (1, 3). Roseola is caused by human herpes virus 6, starting with a febrile prodrome of 3–4 days. Within 2 days of defervescence, the rash starts. It is a diffuse rash that spares the face and hands and resolves spontaneously (5).

2. **Allergic Eruptions.** They usually appear as dull rash that contains vesicles or bullae. It is intensely pruritic and tends to appear on hands, arms, knees, and genitals symmetrically. It starts within 1 week of starting the offending medication and resolves gradually after stopping it (1, 4).

3. **Bacterial Infection.** Meningococcal and gonococcal bacteremia should be suspected in acutely ill patients presenting with fever, tachycardia, tachypnea, hypotension, leukocytosis, and meningeal signs (2). Secondary syphilis presents with a diffuse rash or localized rash mainly on head, neck, palms, and soles. It is often preceded by a chancre, and it usually takes 2–10 weeks after appearance of the chancre for the rash to appear (3, 4). Lesions appear as brown-red or pink macules and papules. Scaly papules, pustules, and

acneiform lesions can also be found. Fever, lymphadenopathy, and splenomegaly may accompany the eruption. Secondary syphilis may have recurrent symptomatic attacks interspersed by symptom-free periods (1, 4).

4. **Rocky Mountain Spotted Fever.** It is caused by *Rickettsia rickettsii*. It has an abrupt onset with fever, headache, myalgia, bradycardia, and leukopenia. The rash usually starts at the fourth day of illness as pinkish-red maculopapules on the wrists and ankles. It spreads toward the trunk and progresses to petechiae. Late on the disease, palms and soles become involved (1–3).

5. **Kawasaki's Disease.** A disease of unknown cause, occurring almost exclusively among young children. It is characterized by high-grade fever, lasting 5 days or longer, conjunctivitis, lymphadenopathy, and desquamation of the hands. Strawberry tongue is a common finding. Skin findings include a maculopapular to scarlatiniform rash with mucous membrane involvement (1, 3).

REFERENCES

1. James W, Berger T, Elston D. *Andrews' diseases of the skin: clinical dermatology*, 10th ed. Canada: Saunders Elsevier, 2006.
2. Richard P, Natasha S, Dermatologic emergencies. *Am Fam Physician* 2010;82(7):773–780.
3. Ali A. *Specialty board review: dermatology, a pictorial review*, 2nd ed. New York, NY: McGraw Hill, 2010.
4. Bolognia J, Jorizzo J, Rapini R. *Dermatology*, 2nd ed. Philadelphia, PA: Mosby Elsevier, 2008: vol 1.
5. Wolff K, Lowella A, Katz SI, et al. *Fitzpatrick's dermatology in general medicine*, 7th ed. New York, NY: McGraw Hill, 2008: vol 2.

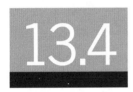

13.4 Pigmentation Disorders

Fatima Al Faresi

I. **BACKGROUND.** Disorders of pigmentation present as skin that is darker or lighter than normal. The major determinant of skin color is the activity of the melanocytes, i.e., the quantity and quality of melanin production. These disorders can be localized or generalized. Disorders of hyperpigmentation include melasma, freckles, lentigines, ashy dermatosis, *café au lait* macules, pityriasis versicolor, phytophotodermatitis, acanthosis nigricans, drug eruptions, and postinflammatory hyperpigmentation. Disorders of hypopigmentation include vitiligo, pityriasis alba, pityriasis versicolor, ash leaf macules, halo nevus, idiopathic guttate hypomelanosis, postinflammatory hypopigmentation, and hypomelanosis from physical agents.

II. **PATHOPHYSIOLOGY**

A. **Etiology.** With some pigmentary disorders, the cause may be readily identified as hereditary, sun induced, due to a medication, infectious, or inflammatory. In some cases, the cause is less clear.

B. **Epidemiology.** The prevalence of these conditions varies widely with the specific disease. However, these disorders affect all races, ages, and both genders.

III. **EVALUATION**

A. **History.** The first step in the diagnosis of these disorders is to classify the problem as one of hyperpigmentation or hypopigmentation (1). Table 13.4.1 contains historic data, including onset, exacerbating and relieving factors, as well as associated symptoms.

B. **Physical Examination**

1. **Disorders of Hyperpigmentation.** Melasma is a common, acquired disorder, characterized by symmetric, hyperpigmented patches with an irregular outline that occur most commonly on the face. Exacerbating factors include pregnancy, oral contraceptives,

TABLE 13.4.1	Factors Used to Differentiate Between Hyperpigmentation and Hypopigmentation			
	Onset	Exacerbating factors	Relieving factors	Associated symptoms
		Hyperpigmented disorders		
Café au lait spots	Birth or early childhood	None	Regress over time	None
Melasma	Onset of liver dysfunction, pregnancy, phenytoin use, oral contraceptive use	Worsening liver disease or ongoing exposure	May improve with removal of offending agents, but rarely disappears entirely	Usually none
Acanthosis nigricans	Increased weight, insulin use	Weight gain or the use of insulin, nicotinic acid, glucocorticoids, or estrogens	Improves with weight loss and removal of offending agents	Diabetes-related symptoms
Halo nevus	Severe sun exposure in a youth, especially in Turner's syndrome	Ongoing sun exposure	Tends to disappear with time	Usually none
Solar lentigines	Older age with earlier age sun exposure	Ongoing sun exposure	None	Usually none
Pityriasis versicolor	Exposure to humidity and heat	Ongoing exposure to humidity and heat	Lower humidity, treatment	Occasionally mild pruritus
Drug-induced hyperpigmentation	Drug exposure, especially to minocycline or zidovudine	Reexposure to causative agent	Occasionally fades with removal of offending agents. Minocycline-induced changes are often permanent	Usually none
Fixed-drug eruption	Drug exposure, (phenolphthalein, salicylates, tetracyclines, and sulfonamides)	Reexposure to causative agent	May fade with removal of offending agents, but often remains	Sometimes painful

(Continued)

TABLE 13.4.1   Factors Used to Differentiate Between Hyperpigmentation and Hypopigmentation *(Continued)*

	Onset	Exacerbating factors	Relieving factors	Associated symptoms
Phytophotodermatitis	Exposure to topical agents containing furocoumarins (oil of bergamot, psoralens, limes)	Ongoing exposure to topical agents containing furocoumarins (oil of bergamot, psoralens, limes)	Topical or oral steroids, antihistamines	Sometimes painful
Inflammation	With inflammation	Ongoing inflammation	Relief of inflammation	Pain from inflammation
Pityriasis alba	Young children (especially those with eczema)	Drying agents, sunlight	May fade with moisturizers, tends to disappear at puberty	Occasionally itchy or burning
Ash leaf macule	Childhood	None	None	If underlying tuberous sclerosis: mental retardation, seizures, and adenoma sebaceum
Vitiligo	10–30 y of age	Stress, illness, personal crises, skin trauma	Progressive illness	
Guttate hypomelanosis	Middle age and older	None (idiopathic lesions)	None (idiopathic lesions)	None

and sun exposure. Freckles are small, red or light brown macules that are promoted by sun exposure. They are most commonly found on the face, arms, and back. They occur as an autosomal dominant trait and are most often found in individuals with fair complexions. Lentigines are similar to freckles; however, these are persistent in the absence of sun exposure (2). Café au lait spots are uniformly pale-brown macules that vary in size from 0.5 to 20 cm and can be found on any cutaneous surface. Five or more spots greater than 5 mm in diameter in prepubertal person or 15 mm in a postpubertal person suggest the diagnosis of neurofibromatosis. Acanthosis nigricans, though not primarily a disorder of pigmentation, appears as grayish brown velvety plaques in a symmetric pattern in the axillae, neck, and folds of the breast and groin. It may be a cutaneous marker of insulin resistance, malignancy, or obesity. Pityriasis versicolor is a common fungal infection of the skin. Lesions begin as multiple small, circular macules of various colors (white, pink, or brown) that enlarge radially located on the upper back, shoulders, upper arms, neck, and chest. Drug-induced hyperpigmentation occurs with minocycline, bleomycin, amiodarone, clofazamine, 5-fluorouracil, cyclophosphamide, hydroxyurea, and others. Phytophotodermatitis initially resembles sunburn, subsequently becoming hyperpigmented. Postinflammatory hyperpigmentation represents an acquired and localized increase in melanin following cutaneous inflammation or injury.

2. **Hypopigmented Disorders.** Vitiligo is an acquired loss of pigmentation characterized histologically by the absence of epidermal melanocytes. There is a fairly symmetric pattern of white macules with well-defined borders affecting any part of the skin. Over time, the macules often coalesce into larger depigmented areas. Vitiligo often occurs at sites of trauma (Koebner phenomenon), such as around the elbows and in sunburned skin. Pityriasis alba presents as nonspecific erythema and gradually becomes scaly and hypopigmented. The face, neck, and arms are the most common sites. Ash leaf macules are hypopigmented macules (oval, ash leaf shaped, or stippled) that are concentrated on the arms, legs, and trunk and are associated with tuberous sclerosis. A halo nevus is an area of depigmentation surrounding a typical pigmented nevus. Guttate hypomelanosis is seen as small, 2–5 mm porcelain-white macules with sharply demarcated borders. They are located on the exposed areas of hands, forearms, and lower legs of middle-aged and older people. Various types of physical injuries induce cutaneous hypomelanosis or amelanosis, including thermal burns, freezing, UV radiation, lasers, ionizing radiation, and physical trauma from surgical procedures.

C. Testing

1. Obtaining skin scrapings from pityriasis versicolor may reveal the characteristic "spaghetti and meatball" appearance of *Malassezia furfur* on a KOH prep. Wood's light often reveals pale yellow fluorescence.

2. Neurologic examination should be considered in individuals with café au lait or ash leaf macules.

3. A complete physical examination and evaluations should be considered for patients with acanthosis nigricans to assess for the presence of a systemic process, such as diabetes or a malignancy.

4. Examination of vitiligo with Wood's light in a dark room accentuates the hypopigmented areas. Vitiligo can be associated with other autoimmune disorders, such as thyroid dysfunction (e.g., Graves' disease, Hashimoto's thyroiditis). Others include insulin-dependent diabetes, pernicious anemia, Addison's disease, and alopecia areata.

D. Genetics.
Examples of the many known genetic defects causing hypomelanosis include oculocutaneous albinism, piebaldism, Waardenburg syndrome, hypomelanosis of Ito, and tuberous sclerosis. Some defects resulting in hypermelanosis include neurofibromatosis, incontinentia pigmenti, LEOPARD syndrome, and Peutz-Jeghers syndrome.

IV. DIAGNOSIS

A. **Differential Diagnosis.** Patients with pigmentary disorders are initially best classified into disorders of excessive pigmentation or hypopigmentation. The history is useful in eliciting inciting factors, especially drug- or inflammation-induced changes. Characteristic appearances of the lesions further define the disorder. Biopsy of lesions is generally not necessary, although selected lesions may require further testing to clarify the condition or a suspected underlying disorder.

B. **Clinical Manifestations.** These vary according to the disorder.

REFERENCES

1. Hori Y, Takayama O. Circumscribed dermal melanoses. Classification and histologic features. *Dermatol Clin* 1988;6:315.
2. Plensdorf S, Martinez J. Common pigmentation disorders. *Am Fam Physician* 2009;79(2):109–116.

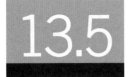

13.5 Pruritus

Nawar Al Falasi

I. BACKGROUND

Pruritus or itch is a sensation that provokes the desire to scratch. Pruritus is transmitted through slow-conducting unmyelinated C-polymodal and possibly type A delta nociceptive neurons with free nerve endings located near the dermoepidermal junction or in the epidermis (1).

II. PATHOPHYSIOLOGY

A. Etiology. Many skin diseases present with localized or generalized pruritus. These include contact dermatitis, dermatitis herpetiformis, atopic dermatitis, pediculosis, bullous pemphigoid, mycosis fungoides, and psoriasis. In addition to primary dermatologic conditions, many systemic disorders, such as renal failure, hepatitis, and hypothyroidism, can cause pruritus (Table 13.5.1).

B. Epidemiology. Systemic causes of pruritus are more common among older individuals, particularly those with other comorbidities. Otherwise, the prevalence of the particular dermatologic condition will vary by age group and setting.

III. EVALUATION

A. History. A thorough history and physical examination will usually distinguish between presentations associated with dermatologic or systemic disease and will further direct the

TABLE 13.5.1	Causes of Pruritis
	Examples
Skin diseases (4)	Contact dermatitis, dermatitis herpitiformis, eczema, bullous pemphigoid, mycosis fungoides, psoriasis, urticaria, pruitic urticarial papules and plaques of pregnancy (PUPPP), xerosis, dermatophyte infections
Endocrine disorders	Carcinoid syndrome, diabetes mellitus (DM), thyroid disease, parathyroid diseases (4)
Infectious diseases	Hepatitis, HIV, pediculosis, scabies
Renal diseases	Chronic renal failure, hemodialysis
Hematologic diseases	Iron deficiency, polycythemia rubra vera (5), hypereosinophilic syndrome, essential thrombocythemia, myelodysplastic syndrome (6)
Cholestatic pruritus (7)	Primary biliary cirrhosis, primary sclerosing cholangitis, chronic hepatitis C, choledocholithiasis, obstructive carcinoma of the pancreas/biliary system, cholestasis of pregnancy
Malignancies	Hodgkin disease, non-Hodgkin lymphoma, leukemias, paraproteinemias and myeloma, Carcinoid syndrome, Sipple syndrome (multiple endocrine neoplasia), solid tumors, including GI malignancies, CNS tumors, and lung cancer
Drugs	Chlorpropamide, tolbutamide, phenothiazines, erythromycin, anabolic steroids, oral contraceptives
Psychiatric diseases	Anxiety, depression, delusion of parasitosis

CNS, central nervous system; GI, gastrointestinal; HIV, human immunodeficiency virus.

physical examination and indicate the need for laboratory evaluation. A history of an insidious onset of generalized pruritus is more consistent with a systemic disorder. A detailed drug history will help to exclude medication-induced pruritus. A history of alcohol abuse may indicate chronic liver disease. A review of potential emotional stresses and the mental health history may suggest a psychiatric cause (1, 2).

B. Physical Examination. Physical examination assists in differentiating between systemic causes of pruritus and that of primary dermatologic conditions. In the case of systemic disease, patients may have normal-appearing skin or secondary lesions, such as excoriations, lichenification, prurigo nodules, or signs of a secondary bacterial infection (2, 3). Jaundice, thyromegaly, or a plethoric appearance may indicate a particular systemic condition. Alternatively, characteristic skin lesions in a particular distribution may be pathognomonic for a specific dermatologic condition.

C. Testing. In a suspected primary dermatologic cause of pruritus, investigations and skin biopsy may be required to make a specific diagnosis (4).

In suspected dermatophyte infections, skin scrapings or hair samples often reveal the presence of hyphae or spores on potassium hydroxide (KOH) testing with microscopic examination.

In cases of systemic causes of pruritus, investigations appropriate to the condition are indicated. Examples include the following:

1. Liver function tests in cholestatic pruritus.
2. Renal function tests in chronic renal failure.
3. Thyroid function tests in thyroid disease.
4. Iron studies in iron deficiency anemia.
5. Blood morphology in iron deficiency anemia, polycythemia vera, and paraneoplastic pruritus (4, 5).
6. Viral load, serologic testing, and CD4 count in suspected human immunodeficiency virus infection.

D. Genetics. Certain conditions that cause pruritus, such as atopic dermatitis, may be hereditary, and a positive family history is often present.

IV. DIAGNOSIS

A. Differential Diagnosis. It is important to differentiate whether the cause of pruritus is primary or systemic in nature. Further evaluation proceeds from this point. In primary dermatologic conditions, characteristic primary skin lesions or a characteristic distribution of lesions is often present.

The differential diagnosis of pruritus is extremely broad (Table 13.5.1). Common dermatologic causes of pruritus in the primary care setting include xerosis, or excessive dryness of the skin, eczematous or contact dermatitis, psoriasis and urticaria, as well as dermatophyte infections. Xerosis tends to present in older patients, during the winter, in areas of low ambient humidity and with frequent bathing. Eczematous dermatitis tends to occur on the flexural surfaces of the arms and legs and the volar surfaces of the wrists and neck, particularly in children. Among young infants, the cheeks or forehead and the lateral surfaces of the extremities are often involved. Psoriasis is often associated with a characteristic scaly rash, and urticaria is characterized by the presence of erythematous wheals and plaques. Dermatophyte infections typically present with characteristic skin lesions or reveal the causative agent on skin scrapings. A careful, stepwise approach to the patient with pruritus will reward the primary care clinician and patient with an accurate diagnosis in almost all cases.

REFERENCES

1. Bernhard JD. Endocrine and metabolic itches. In: *Itch: mechanisms and management of pruritus.* New York, NY: McGraw Hill, 1994:251–260.
2. Krajnik M. Understanding pruritus in systemic disease. *J Pain Symptom Manage* 2001;21(2):151–168.
3. Yosipovitch G. Itch associated with skin disease: advances in pathophysiology and emerging therapies. *Am J Clin Dermatol* 2003;4(9):617–622. *Ann Dermatol* 2011;23(1):1–11.

4. Bellmann R, Feistritzer C, Zoller H, et al. Treatment of intractable pruritus in drug induced cholestasis with albumin dialysis: a report of two cases. *ASAIO J* 2004;50(4):387–391.
5. Yosipovitch G. Chronic pruritus: a paraneoplastic sign. *Dermal Therapy* 2010;23(6):590–596.
6. Bernhard JD. General principles, overview, and miscellaneous treatments of itching. In: *Itch: mechanisms and management of pruritus*. New York, NY: McGraw Hill, 1994:367–381.
7. Tejesh P. Therapy of pruritus. *Expert Opin Pharmacother* 2010;11(10):1673–1682.

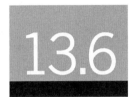

Rash Accompanied by Fever

Mohammad Balatay

I. BACKGROUND. Fever with an accompanying rash represents diagnostic challenge for even the most experienced clinician because this combination of signs may represent either a trivial or a life-threatening illness.

II. PATHOPHYSIOLOGY. A useful way of approaching the differential diagnosis is to distinguish among the various entities that cause fever and illness by the types of rash they commonly cause. Although various febrile illnesses may present with more than one type of rash, this grouping allows the clinician to look at fewer causes rather than the entire spectrum of possible causes (1).

A. Petechial rashes are commonly associated with the following:

1. Treatable infections, including endocarditis, meningococcemia, gonococcemia, septicemia from any bacteria, Rickettsiosis (especially Rocky mountain spotted fever) (2).
2. Infectious causes not subject to acute treatment, including enterovirus, dengue fever, hepatitis B virus, rubella, and Epstein-Barr virus.
3. Noninfectious causes including deep venous thrombosis, superficial thrombophlebitis, relapsing polychondritis, and erythema nodosum.

B. Maculopapular rashes are commonly associated with the following:

1. Treatable infections, including typhoid, secondary syphilis, meningococcemia, gonococcemia, Mycoplasma, and Lyme disease.
2. infectious causes not subject to acute treatment, including enterovirus, parvovirus B 19, human herpes virus 6, rubeola, rubella, adenovirus, and primary human immunodeficiency virus (HIV).
3. Noninfectious causes, including allergy, erythema multiforme, systemic lupus erythematosus, dermatomyositis, serum sickness, and juvenile rheumatoid arthritis.

C. Vesiculobullous rashes are commonly associated with the following:

1. Treatable infections, including staphylococcal large vesicle impetigo and toxic shock syndrome, gonococcemia, rickettsial pox, herpes zoster, herpes simplex virus, *Vibrio vulnificus* sepsis, and folliculitis.
2. Infectious causes not subject to acute treatment, including enterovirus, parvovirus B 19, and HIV (although none of these three commonly present in this manner).
3. Noninfectious causes including eczema vaccinatum, and erythema multiforme bullosum.

D. Diffuse erythematous rashes are commonly associated with the following:

1. Treatable infections, including streptococcal scarlet fever, toxic shock syndrome, ehrlichosis (3), and Kawasaki disease.
2. Infectious causes not subject to acute treatment, including enterovirus infections.
3. Noninfectious causes of erythema are only rarely associated with fever.

III. EVALUATION

A. History. History is quite important and should include standard items, such as onset, duration, aggravating factors, relieving factors, and associated symptoms. Additionally, other factors should be considered, such as the following:

1. **Exposure History.** Are any other family members or close contacts ill? Is there a history of exposure to standing water, mosquitoes, or foreign travel?

2. **Are there underlying illnesses** or is there a significant chance of immunologic compromise, such as undiagnosed HIV infection?

B. Physical Examination

1. **The lesions in the distribution should be carefully examined.** The rash should be classified as petechial, maculopapular, vesiculobullous, erythematous, or urticarial. The distribution of the rash should be noted. For instance, rubella and rubeola generally begin on the face and spread to the trunk, whereas the petechiae of Rocky mountain spotted fever tend to occur on the ankles and wrists first.

2. **A general physical examination should be conducted.** Areas of particular concern are as follows:

   a. **Head, eyes, ears, nose, and throat examination.** Koplik spots are pathognomonic for rubeola. The discovery of a tick tends to support the diagnosis of Rocky mountain spotted fever. Sinusitis may present as a source for meningococcemia. Pharyngitis in the young adult with diffuse erythema may be due to *C. haemolyticum*. The presence of mucous membrane swelling may indicate early anaphylaxis.

   b. **Lung examination.** Wheezing on examination, especially in a patient who has recently received medications or contrast dye, can indicate anaphylaxis. Evidence of pneumonia is consistent with psittacosis and Mycoplasma.

   c. **Cardiac examination.** Cardiovascular collapse is associated with meningococcemia another sepsis. A new murmur may indicate subacute bacterial endocarditis in the patient with subungual or scleral petechiae.

   d. **Genital examination.** Purulent urethral drainage or evidence of pelvic inflammatory disease supports the consideration of gonorrhea. A chancre supports a diagnosis of syphilis, although palmar lesions often occur well after the healing of the initial chancre.

   e. **Joint examination and extremities.** A petechial rash near the ankles and wrists is suggestive of Rocky Mountain spotted fever. Evidence of joint swelling supports diagnosis of meningococcemia or gonococcemia. A maculopapular rash may be seen in juvenile rheumatoid arthritis and other rheumatologic conditions as well.

   f. **Neurologic examination.** Evidence of meningitis supports a diagnosis of meningococcemia. Patients with Rocky Mountain spotted fever may also have meningeal signs.

C. Testing. Testing should be directed by the suspected illnesses, with life-threatening illnesses being tested for upon reasonable suspicion. A complete blood count is generally useful, although life-threatening sepsis often presents without significant elevation of the white blood cell count. In general, a blood culture should be obtained in all patients with petechial rashes and in those with signs of cardiovascular collapse.

IV. DIAGNOSIS.
On the basis of the history and physical examination, the likelihood of various illnesses can be assessed. Patients who appear toxic should be treated as septic until initial laboratory tests and culture results can be evaluated (4).

REFERENCES

1. Schlossberg D. Fever and rash. *Infect Dis Clin North Am* 1996;10(1):101–110.
2. Drolet BA, Baselga E, Esterly NB. Painful, purpuric plaques in a child with fever. *Arch Dermatol* 1997;133(12):1500–1501.
3. American Journal of Medicine. Fever, nausea, and rash in a 37-year-old man [clinical conference]. *Am J Med* 1998;104(6):596–601.
4. Dellinger RP. Current therapy for sepsis. *Infect Dis Clin North Am* 1999;13(2):495–509.

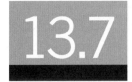

Urticaria

Omar Shamsaldeen

I. BACKGROUND. Urticaria is composed of wheals, which are transient erythematous, edematous, pruritic papules and plaques. They are usually surrounded by a red or white halo caused by the release of histamine and other vasoactive substances from mast cells. Lesions usually are itchy and last less than 24 hours.

II. PATHOPHYSIOLOGY

A. Etiology. Urticaria is classified as immunologic, nonimmunologic, or idiopathic. Immunologic Type I or Type III immunoglobulin (Ig)E-mediated reactions are the main causes of acute urticaria. Circulating antigens such as foods (milk, eggs, wheat, shellfish, nuts) and drugs (penicillins, cephalosporins) interact with membrane-bound IgE to release histamine which cause localized vasodilation. Nonimmunologic causes such as aspirin or nonsteroidal anti-inflammatory drugs can cause direct release of histamine (1).

B. Epidemiology. Urticaria is a common condition; 1–5% of the population may suffer from this condition during their lifetime. It is more common in women (2).

Urticaria is defined as "acute" (new onset or recurrent episodes, of less than 6 weeks duration) or "chronic" (recurring episodes of more than 6 weeks duration).

III. EVALUATION

A. History. History is an important part of diagnosis, because the lesions are often not present at the clinic visit. When assessing a patient presenting with possible urticaria, a helpful approach to the problem is as follows:

1. Ask the patient if he or she knows what triggers the hives. Often the patient has already determined the cause or has narrowed down the list of possibilities.
2. Take a detailed history for specific foods, any known food additives, medications, recent respiratory infections, bites, contact, inhalants, or a history of systemic disease, particularly autoimmune diseases or neoplasms.
3. Ask about the timeline of the disease. When does it occur? How long does it last? Is it related to cold, exertion, heat, or physical trauma or sun exposure?
4. Ask if there is any related swelling of soft tissue, such as the eyelids and lips.
5. Ask about history of personal/family history of atopy or a family history of autoimmune disease.

B. Physical Examination. Look for well-defined, erythematous, edematous papules or plaques, often with a pale center. Individual lesions last less than 24 hours. In contrast, in urticarial vasculitis, individual lesions are fixed and persist beyond 24 hours. Lesions may differ in size from 2–5 mm to over 30 cm and may be annular, serpiginous, or irregularly shaped. Edema of the mucous membranes may be present.

Angioedema, which manifests with swelling of the face, bowel, or part of an extremity, is seen in approximately 50% of urticaria cases and can last for several days.

C. Testing

1. Laboratory testing is not routinely indicated for acute urticaria.
2. In chronic urticaria, perform a complete blood count with differential, sedimentation rate, liver function testing, a urinalysis, and consider thyroid function tests.
3. If individual lesions persist for more than 24 hours, it may be helpful to biopsy a lesion to rule out urticarial vasculitis. If a vasculitis is present, additional testing should include C3, C4, CH50 levels, hepatitis B and C serologies, antinuclear antibody (ANA), cryoglobulins, immunoglobulin levels, serum protein electrophoresis and urine protein electrophoresis.
4. Provocative tests (such as the ice cube test or strenuous exercise) may help establish a diagnosis of cold or physical urticaria. However, the provider should be cognizant of the risk of precipitating anaphylaxis.

5. Imaging studies such as sinus, dental films and chest X-ray may help to rule out infection or neoplasms.

6. Skin testing or radioallergosorbent assays are ordered if hypersensitivity to a particular allergen is suspected.

IV. DIAGNOSIS

A. Differential Diagnosis. The diagnosis of urticaria is made clinically. Other skin problems that present with urticarial lesions include urticarial vasculitis (painful, purpuric, and last >24 hours), drug eruptions, viral exanthema, bullous pemphigoid in elderly patients, erythema multiforme (acral, and lasting >24 hours) and angioedema.

B. Clinical Manifestations. Although the lesions of urticaria are distinctive, the various underlying conditions that trigger the skin's response are numerous and varied in their clinical manifestations. Virtually all patients with urticaria complain of pruritus in addition to the rash.

REFERENCES

1. Habif TP, Urticaria and angioedema. In: *Clinical dermatology*, 5th ed. Mosby, Elsevier, 2009:181–193.
2. Grattan, C., & Kobza-Black, A. (2007). Urticaria and angioedema. In J. Bolognia, J. Jorizzo, & R. Rappini, *Dermatology* (2nd ed., pp. 261–276). St. Louis: Elsevier-Mosby.

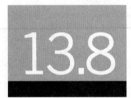

Vesicular and Bullous Eruptions

13.8

Ahmed Salem Al Dhaheri and Hassan Galadari

I. BACKGROUND. A vesicle is a liquid-filled cavity that is less than 1 cm in diameter. A bulla is a similar lesion larger than 1 cm in diameter. Vesiculobullous eruptions (VBE) are commonly termed blistering diseases.

II. PATHOPHYSIOLOGY

A. Etiology. There are many causes of VBE. These include infectious conditions such as herpes simplex (HS) infection, inflammatory causes like dyshidrotic eczema (DE) and contact dermatitis, autoimmune causes such as bullous pemphigoid (BP), and hereditary causes like epidermolysis bullosa (EB). Systemic conditions, such as allergic vasculitis, and porphyria cutanea tarda (PCT) often present with VBE. Drug-induced conditions, such as Stevens-Johnson syndrome/toxic epidermolysis necrolysis (SJS/TEN) are also seen. Environmental factors can contribute to the development of VBE. For example, sun exposure, alcohol ingestion, as well as certain medications and infections are thought to contribute to the induction of PCT (1). Sun exposure, stress, menses, smoking, and alcohol ingestion can induce recurrent HS infection.

B. Epidemiology

1. The patient age group can provide the physician with clues to the diagnosis:

   a. Newborns. Most commonly present with hereditary or infectious conditions. Examples include EB, pemphigus neonatorum, and syphilitic pemphigus.

   b. Children. The most common causes in this age group are infections. These include varicella, primary HS, hand, foot, and mouth (HFM) disease, and bullous impetigo (BI).

   c. Adults. Infectious causes continue to predominate, but inflammatory and autoimmune causes become increasingly common. These include PCT, pemphigus vulgaris (PV), DE, and dermatitis herpetiformis (DH). A variant of BP, pemphigoid gestationis may occur during pregnancy or the puerperium.

In addition, rarer causes, such as linear immunoglobulin A disease (linear IgA bullous dermatosis) may be seen.

d. Elderly. Autoimmune diseases become commoner in this age group. For example, the median age of presentation of BP is 80 years.

2. Examples of conditions that occur commonly in all age groups include allergic contact dermatitis, allergic vasculitis, SJS/TEN, insect bites, and partial thickness (second-degree) burns.

III. EVALUATION

A. History

1. **Pain or Pruritus.** Most of the VBE are asymptomatic; however, some are associated with discomfort. For example, contact dermatitis and DH are commonly associated with pruritus (1). Herpes zoster (HZ) can cause pain and/or a burning sensation preceding the skin eruption.

2. **Family History.** A positive family history of a blistering disease in a newborn may suggest a particular diagnosis. A history of similar eruptions among other siblings or classmates implicates an infectious etiology of VBE.

3. **Onset and Duration.** VBE can be acute or chronic. Causes of VBE that are more likely to present acutely include SJS/TEN, varicella, BI, HZ, allergic vasculitis, HFM disease, and PV. Conditions that are more likely to present indolently include DH, DE, BP, EB, and PCT. Some causes can be episodic and recurrent, such as acute contact dermatitis and HS infection.

B. Physical Examination

1. **Appearance.** In patients who appear systemically ill, or toxic, consider SJS/TEN, PV, or primary HS infection as possible etiologies.

2. **Presence of Fever.** Patients with infectious etiologies, particularly those with varicella, HFM, primary HS or BI may have a fever, as may patients with SJS/TEN.

3. **Presence of Oral Lesions.** The presence of oral lesions should be sought in every patient, since some serious VBEs can involve the oral cavity, such as STS/TEN. It also can guide the provider to the diagnosis of PV, varicella, or HFM. The skin lesions of PV may appear months after the onset of oral lesions (2).

4. **Vesicles versus Bullae.** Vesicles and bullae are the primary lesions in VBEs. Clinically, the size of the lesions may overlap, and it may be difficult to distinguish whether the lesions are vesicular or bullous. This is particularly true when, as frequently happens, the lesions rupture, and the patient will present with secondary lesions such as erosions, ulcers, and/or crusts.

   Conditions such as HS infection, varicella, HZ, contact dermatitis, DE, hemorrhagic vasculitis, HFM disease, Kaposi's varicelliform eruption (KVE or eczema herpeticum), and DH tend to present with vesicles. PV, BP, BI, PCT, SJS/TEN, TEN, and EB tend to present with bullae. The presence of larger bullae or erosions tends to occur more commonly in bullous diseases.

5. **Lesion Characteristics and Distribution.** Blisters of BI rupture easily and often form a honey-colored crust. BI most frequently affects the face, particularly around the mouth and nose, or at sites of trauma. In PV, intact flaccid blisters are occasionally found. Involvement of the scalp, face, upper torso, and oral mucosa is common. In BP, blisters are tense and large, urticarial patches and plaques often precede the blister formation. The trunk, extremities, and flexures are commonly involved. Linear IgA disease presents with small vesicles and/or large bullae in the groin, buttocks, trunk, and extremities, with occasional oral involvement. In PCT, the patient usually presents with erosions and blisters on sun-exposed areas, such as the dorsum of the hands. Often these form painful sores that heal slowly, resulting in depigmentation and scarring (1). Contact dermatitis occurs at sites of contact with allergenic materials, and DE tends to involve the lateral sides of the fingers and the palms. HFM syndrome presents with lesions on the hands, feet, in the mouth, and on the buttocks. HZ is generally confined to one or two adjacent dermatomes and is unilateral. KVE will occur in areas of existing dermatitis.

   C. Testing
   1. **Tzanck Smear**. This test is done by unroofing an intact blister and scraping its base. The material is smeared on a slide, stained, and examined under microscopy for the presence of multinucleated giant cells (3).
   2. **Biopsy**. When the clinical diagnosis is uncertain, a skin biopsy is helpful. When biopsying vesicles, a biopsy of the entire vesicle with adjacent normal skin when possible is ideal. With bullae, the edge of the lesion should be biopsied, with the roof of the bulla included, as well as some adjacent normal skin (1). Direct immunofluorescence microscopy, and other techniques are helpful in distinguishing between various VBEs in the clinical setting.

IV. DIAGNOSIS
   A. Differential Diagnosis. An accurate differential diagnosis and subsequent diagnosis is greatly facilitated by obtaining a thorough history and physical examination. If the diagnosis remains unclear, particularly if a potentially serious condition may exist, biopsy or referral may be helpful to confirm a diagnosis.

REFERENCES
1. Welsh B. Blistering skin conditions. *Aust Fam Physician* 2009;38(7):484–490.
2. Bickle KM, Roark TR, Hsu SH. Autoimmune bullous dermatoses: a review. *Am Fam Physician* 2002;65(9):1861–1870.
3. Brodell RT, Helms SE, Devine M. Office dermatologic testing: the Tzanck preparation. *Am Fam Physician* 1991;44(3):857–860.

CHAPTER 14

Endocrine and Metabolic Problems

Arwa Abdulhaq Nasir

14.1 Diabetes Mellitus

Michael J. Hovan and Curtiss B. Cook

I. BACKGROUND. Diabetes mellitus (DM) refers to a group of metabolic disorders characterized by hyperglycemia resulting from deficient insulin secretion and/or insulin action. The clinical classes of DM are type 1, type 2, gestational, and other specific types secondary to a variety of causes. The classification of DM is based on the etiology of the disorders as currently understood (1). Inadequate glucose control leads to both micro- and macrovascular complications (2). The Centers for Disease Control and Prevention lists diabetes as the seventh leading cause of death in the United States (3).

II. PATHOPHYSIOLOGY

A. Etiology

    1. Type 1. Type 1 diabetes is further categorized as type 1A or type 1B diabetes. Both result from autoimmune or idiopathic destruction of pancreatic beta cells and result in absolute insulin deficiency. Type 1A is associated with human leukocyte antigen (HLA)-related genes DQA and DQB and is suggested by the presence of numerous autoantibodies. These include anti-glutamic acid decarboxylase (GAD), anti-islet cell autoantigen 512, and anti-insulin antibodies. Type 1B is idiopathic, lacking any identifiable autoimmune markers or HLA association.

    2. Type 2. Type 2 becomes manifest after several years of progressive insulin resistance within muscle, fat, and liver cells. To maintain fasting euglycemia, endogenous insulin secretion is often increased early in the prediabetic phase. Over time, insulin production can subsequently decline, postprandial glucagon becomes increasingly nonsuppressible, and patients may require a transition to insulin therapy. Glucagon-like peptide 1 (GLP-1) is secreted by intestinal L cells during digestion, and it influences gastric emptying, promotes insulin secretion, and decreases glucagon secretion. It, too, behaves aberrantly in type 2 DM.

B. Epidemiology

Currently, 25.8 million adults and children in the United States are estimated to have diabetes, with the number of cases increasing at a rate of 1.5 million per year (3). One-third of the people born in the United States in 2000 are projected to develop diabetes during their lifetime. As measured by fasting glucose values or hemoglobin A1C levels studied between 2005 and 2008, 35% of US adults aged 20 years or older were prediabetics. Among those 65 years or older, up to 50% are prediabetic. Collectively, this means that roughly 79,000,000 American adults aged 20 or older are at significant risk for diabetes (3).

A. Type 1. Type 1 diabetes accounts for approximately 5% of all diagnosed cases in adults. About 215,000 US residents under 20 years of age have diabetes and the vast majority are classified as having type 1 diabetes (3). Despite the increasing rate of type 2 diabetes among children, type 1 diabetes still accounts for approximately two-thirds of new cases of diabetes in patients under 20 years of age (4). In the United States, Caucasians face the highest risk for type 1 diabetes among ethnic and racial groups, with an incidence of 23.6 per 100,000 (5). In contrast, type 1B diabetes occurs more often in individuals of Asian or African descent.

B. Type 2. Type 2 DM accounts for 95% of diabetes overall and remains rare in individuals under age 20 years, although the rising rates of obesity among US youths have led to a corresponding increase in the rates of type 2 DM among younger patients in the last decade. Among Caucasians aged 10–19 years, the rate of new cases remains higher for type 1 than for type 2 diabetes. For blacks and Hispanics aged 10–19 years, the rates of new cases are equally split between types 1 and 2. In Asian, Pacific Islander, and Native Americans aged 10–19 years, the rates of new cases of type 2 exceed those of type 1. Type 2 remains rare under age 10 years in all groups.

C. Gestational DM. Approximately 2–10% of pregnancies are complicated by gestational diabetes. In the 20 years subsequent to the pregnancy, 35–60% will develop diabetes (3).

III. EVALUATION

Although type 1 and type 2 diabetes can present with similar symptoms of polyuria and polydipsia, the onset of type 1 typically occurs more precipitously. Accurate screening and diagnosis is important in order to identify those at risk and to reduce diabetic complications.

A. Physical Examination

The physical findings and diabetes are influenced by the duration and severity of the disease. With acute hyperglycemia, tachycardia, poor skin turgor, dry mucous membranes, and orthostasis result from glucose-induced osmotic diuresis. Ketonemia may be identified by a fruity odor of respiratory expiration and an altered mental status if severe. With longer, more established disease, diminished lower extremity sensory function measured by monofilament testing and altered vibratory sensation detected with a 128 Hz tuning fork suggests neuropathy. Hypertension and edema suggest possible nephropathy. Visual impairment is a late finding in individuals with diabetic retinopathy, and the physical exam may show nerve fiber infarcts, cotton wool spots, intraretinal hemorrhages, hard exudates, and dilated or tortuous vessels.

B. Testing

The 2011 American Diabetes Association (ADA) guidelines define diabetes with any one of the following parameters, as long as confirmed with repeat testing (unless unequivocal hyperglycemia): hemoglobin A1C > 6.5%, fasting glucose >126 mg/dL, a 2-hour plasma glucose ≥200 mg/dL following a 75 g anhydrous glucose challenge, or classic symptoms and a random glucose ≥200 mg/dL (6). Prediabetes is defined as fasting glucose values between 100 and 125 mg/dL, a 2-hour oral glucose tolerance test value of 140–199 mg/dL, or a hemoglobin A1C of 5.7–6.4%. The hemoglobin A1C is the least sensitive diagnostic test, while the oral glucose tolerance test remains the most sensitive. In the setting of discordant values, the most abnormal test takes precedent over other values. Hemoglobin A1C is excluded from diagnostic criteria in pregnancy.

For gestational diabetes, the ADA and the American College of Obstetrics and Gynecology (ACOG) differ in their diagnostic approaches. The ADA suggests that a universal 75 g oral glucose tolerance test be performed between weeks 24 and 28 of gestation. A fasting value ≥92 mg/dL, a 1-hour value ≥180 mg/dL, or a 2-hour value ≥153 mg/dL confirms gestational DM. ACOG proposes a two-step process and states that very low-risk individuals do not require testing. A 1-hour 50 mm oral glucose tolerance test is first given, and if the plasma glucose is >140 mg/dL, then a confirmatory test is performed. This consists of a 3-hour 100 g oral glucose tolerance test. Diagnostic cutoffs include a fasting value >95 mg/dL, a 1-hour value ≥180 mg/dL, a 2-hour value ≥155mg/dL, or a 3-hour value ≥140 mg/dL. All women with gestational DM should be retested in 6–12 weeks postpartum and every 3 years thereafter because of their lifelong increased risk of diabetes.

C. Genetics

Type 1A DM has HLA associations with linkages to the DQA and DQB genes, while type 1B is idiopathic. Type 2 diabetes is influenced by both modifiable and non-modifiable risk.

Non-modifiable risks include family history, ethnicity, and advanced age. Modifiable and nongenetic factors include sedentary lifestyle, high body mass index, and central adiposity (7).

IV. DIAGNOSIS

    A. Clinical manifestations. Determination of the specific type of diabetes is essential to providing appropriate treatment. Prior to the development of acute hyperglycemia (manifested as polyuria, polyphagia, and usually ketosis), most type 1 patients appear healthy prior to the diagnosis.

        1. Type 1. Nonobese children, adolescents, and young adults account for most cases of type 1 diabetes. Since beta-cell destruction most often occurs rapidly over the course of days or weeks, diabetic ketoacidosis (DKA), abrupt weight loss, polyuria, polydipsia, and lethargy usually herald the diagnosis. The most serious presentation, DKA, is more likely to occur in children (8). DKA is defined as a glucose exceeding 200 mg/dL and metabolic acidosis is designated by a pH <7.3 or bicarbonate <15 mEq/L. Additional common features include fatigue, dehydration, nausea, anorexia, hyperventilation (Kussmaul respiration), and acute visual and mental status changes. Asymptomatic hyperglycemia as a silent presentation is rare in type 1 diabetes, due to the rapid destruction of beta cells and because polyuria usually ensues once the serum glucose exceeds 180 mg/dL.

        2. Type 2. Individuals with acanthosis nigricans, obstructive sleep apnea, hypertension, vascular disease, positive family history, hyperuricemia, polycystic ovarian disease, and nonalcoholic steatohepatitis face a greater risk of type 2 diabetes. At the time of diagnosis, many individuals already have evidence of neuropathy, nephropathy, or retinopathy. The typical type 2 diabetic patient is overweight or obese and older than 40 years. Patients usually present with characteristic features of hyperglycemia, including polyuria, polydipsia, and nocturia. Less specific and subtle clues to the diagnosis might include poor wound healing, recurrent infections, and/or candidal vulvovaginitis. An urgent presentation of type 2 diabetes involves a hyperosmolar hyperglycemic state with marked glucose elevation, profound dehydration, but little or no ketonemia. On rare occasions, DKA can occur in type 2 DM and is more likely to occur in African American children (9).

        3. Gestational DM. Pregnancy can precipitate an acute state of insulin resistance. Since its pathogenesis is similar to type 2 DM, the clinical features are similar, though polyuria is sometimes mistakenly attributed to the gravid uterus's effects on the bladder rather than hyperglycemia. Delivery of an infant weighing >4.1 kg (9 lb) poses a future risk of diabetes.

    B. Differential diagnosis. Autoimmune antibody markers and a C-peptide assay help distinguish type 1 from type 2 diabetes. C-peptide confirms whether endogenous insulin production exists. Since proinsulin consists of insulin peptide and C-peptide, C-peptide is removed from the proinsulin peptide when active insulin is generated. The absence of C-peptide suggests total beta-cell failure. Its presence supports the production of endogenous insulin. Caution in the interpretation of C-peptide results is necessary since some patients with type 1 diabetes, at least early in the course of autoimmune beta-cell destruction, may still produce some insulin secretion and therefore have measurable levels of C-peptide. The presence of hyperglycemia and autoantibodies suggests type 1 disease, but is not necessary for the diagnosis. These markers include islet cell autoantibodies, insulin autoantibodies, autoantibodies targeting the 65 kDA isoform of GAD, and autoantibodies targeting the phosphate-related 1A-2 molecule (10).

        Clinical entities other than DM that present with polyuria include central and nephrogenic diabetes insipidus, various hypothalamic disorders, psychiatric polydipsia, postobstructive diuresis, and the effects of certain medications such as lithium. Transient hyperglycemia can occur with acute severe illness, especially with the use of corticosteroids and vasopressor/catecholamine agents, such as in the ICU setting. A new diagnosis of diabetes in this setting is cautioned, and new hyperglycemia detected in a hospitalized patient, particularly if mild, should be reevaluated in an outpatient setting.

REFERENCES

1. American Diabetes Association. Diagnosis and classification of diabetes mellitus. *Diabetes Care* 2008 Jan;31(Suppl 1):S58.
2. Wingard DL, Barrett-Conner, E. Heart disease and diabetes. In: *Diabetes in America*, Washington, DC: US Government Printing Office (NIH Publ no 95-1468). 1995:429–448.
3. U.S. Department of Health and Human Services CfDCaP. *National diabetes fact sheet: National estimates and general information on diabetes and prediabetes in the United States,* 2011, Atlanta, GA: U.S. Department of Health and Human Services, Centers for Disease Control and Prevention. 2011.
4. Liese AD, D'Agostino RB, Jr., Hamman RF, et al. The burden of diabetes mellitus among US youth: prevalence estimates from the SEARCH for Diabetes in Youth Study. *Pediatrics* 2006 Oct;118(4):1510–1518.
5. Bell RA, Mayer-Davis EJ, Beyer JW, et al. Diabetes in non-Hispanic white youth: prevalence, incidence, and clinical characteristics: the SEARCH for Diabetes in Youth Study. *Diabetes Care* 2009 Mar;32(Suppl 2):S102–S111.
6. American Diabetes Association. Standards of medical care in diabetes-2011. *Diabetes Care* 2011 Jan;34(Suppl 1):S11–S61.
7. Nyenwe EA, Jerkins TW, Umpierrez GE, Kitabchi AE. Management of type 2 diabetes: evolving strategies for the treatment of patients with type 2 diabetes. *Metabolism* 2011 Jan;60(1):1–23.
8. Mallare JT, Cordice CC, Ryan BA, Carey DE, Kreitzer PM, Frank GR. Identifying risk factors for the development of diabetic ketoacidosis in new onset type 1 diabetes mellitus. *Clin Pediatr (Phila)* 2003 Sep;42(7):591–597.
9. Sapru A, Gitelman SE, Bhatia S, Dubin RF, Newman TB, Flori H. Prevalence and characteristics of type 2 diabetes mellitus in 9-18 year-old children with diabetic ketoacidosis. *J Pediatr Endocrinol Metab* 2005 Sep;18(9):865–872.
10. Handelsman Y, Mechanick JI, Blonde L, et al. American Association of Clinical Endocrinologists Medical Guidelines for Clinical Practice for developing a diabetes mellitus comprehensive care plan. *Endocr Pract* 2011 Mar-Apr;17(Suppl 2):1–53.

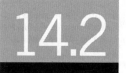

14.2 Gynecomastia

Michelle L. Benes

I. BACKGROUND. The male breast consists of minimal amounts of adipose and glandular tissues. An altered estrogen-to-testosterone ratio in a male may lead to gynecomastia, or proliferation of the glandular breast tissue (1).

II. PATHOPHYSIOLOGY. Gynecomastia is caused by a relative increase of estrogen in relationship to androgens.

A. Physiologic gynecomastia has three peaks of age distribution: the newborn period, adolescence, and men older than 50 years.

1. Newborn gynecomastia, which occurs in up to 90% of newborn boys, is due to the transplacental transfer of maternal estrogens. This type of gynecomastia typically resolves spontaneously within the first four weeks of life (2).

2. Pubertal gynecomastia occurs in about 50% of boys, presenting in the early teens and corresponding to Tanner stage 3 or 4. This is due to an increase in estradiol concentration, delayed testosterone production, and increased sensitivity to estrogen at the tissue level (2).

3. One-third to two-thirds of older adult males develop physiologic gynecomastia as a result of age-related decreasing levels of circulating free testosterone (1).

B. Nonphysiologic gynecomastia can occur at any age due to medication use, substance abuse, and several medical conditions.

1. Persistent pubertal gynecomastia is diagnosed when present in an adolescent male for more than 2 years or past the age of 17 years and is not associated with other causes.

2. Medication and substance use are the most common causes of nonphysiologic gynecomastia. Long-term use of cimetidine, antipsychotics, antiretrovirals, prostate cancer therapies, and spironolactone are commonly identified as transient causes, typically resolving within 3 months of drug discontinuation. Anabolic steroid use, marijuana, heroin, and amphetamines may lead to persistent gynecomastia (3).

3. Medical conditions such as cirrhosis, primary hypogonadism, malignant tumors, hyperthyroidism, and malnutrition may cause about 25% of nonphysiologic cases of gynecomastia (4, 5). Over 50% of patients on hemodialysis for chronic renal failure will develop gynecomastia.

4. Obesity is commonly associated with pseudogynecomastia, or proliferation of the adipose component of the breast. Obesity may also lead to increased circulating estrogens leading to true gynecomastia (2).

5. Approximately 25% of cases of gynecomastia are idiopathic (2).

III. EVALUATION

A. History. A thorough history should be obtained. Other specific identifiable causes such as medications, supplements, or illicit drug use should be sought. Systemic symptoms such as weight loss should direct concern to the possibility of a malignancy, endocrinopathy, or other underlying disease processes (1, 2).

B. Physical examination. A palpable, firm, glandular tissue mass under the nipple areolar complex is consistent with gynecomastia. Increased deposition of adipose tissue is consistent with pseudogynecomastia. Hard, irregular, or immobile masses, masses with associated skin changes, nipple retraction, nipple discharge or adenopathy should alert the clinician to the possibility of malignancy. Physical exam should also include a search for testicular changes, liver disease, and thyroid abnormalities, indicating the presence of underlying disease process as the cause of the gynecomastia (1, 2).

C. Laboratory testing. If findings from the history and physical exam suggest nonphysiologic causes, targeted testing of liver, kidney, and thyroid function should be performed. Serum β-hCG, dehydroepiandrosterone sulfate, and urinary 17-ketosteroid may be obtained to help identify testicular or adrenal tumors. Elevated prolactin levels are associated with pituitary adenoma. Low luteinizing hormone and testosterone levels characterize secondary hypogonadism. High luteinizing hormone levels in conjunction with low levels of testosterone indicate primary hypogonadism (1).

D. Imaging and cytologic studies. Breast imaging, including mammography and ultrasound, is indicated when breast cancer is suspected. Fine needle aspiration for cytologic sampling should be included in the evaluation if the concern for malignancy is not resolved.

IV. CLINICAL MANIFESTATIONS.
Gynecomastia is bilateral in more than 50% of affected men, but it may be unilateral or symmetric. It presents as a firm, mobile, or rubbery mass that may be slightly tender and forms a symmetrical mount around the nipple. Most patients with normal physiologic gynecomastia can be readily identified, and no further evaluation is required. If the condition does not resolve with observation, if it is progressive or rapid onset, or if history and examination suggest a general medical disorder, then an underlying pathologic process should be sought.

REFERENCES

1. Braunstein GD. Gynecomastia. *N Engl J Med* 2007;357(12):1229–1237.
2. Dickson A. Gynecomastia. *Am Fam Physician* 2012;85(7):716–722.
3. Eckman A, Dobs A. Drug-induced gynecomastia. *Expert Opin Drug Saf* 2008;7(6):691–702.
4. Lawrence SE, Faught KA, Vethamuthu J, Lawson ML. Beneficial effects of raloxifene and tamoxifen in the treatment of pubertal gynecomastia. *J Pediatr* 2004;145(1):71–76.
5. Derkacz M, Chmiel-Perzynska I, Nowakowski A. Gynecomastia—a difficult diagnostic problem. *Endokrynol Pol* 2011;62(2):190–202.

14.3

Hirsutism

Razan Taha and Reshma Gandhi

I. BACKGROUND. The presence of abundant terminal hair in women in a male pattern is known as hirsutism. The degree of hirsutism is based upon the level of androgen in the body. It is important to differentiate hirsutism from hypertrichosis, which can be defined as the presence of nonterminal hair in a generalized pattern and unrelated to the effect of androgens (1, 2). Hirsutism can signal a pathologic disorder and also have a negative impact on a patient's self-esteem, so recognizing the etiology and assessing this condition are important.

II. PATHOPHYSIOLOGY

    A. Etiology. Hirsutism can be caused by either excessive androgen production or excessive sensitivity of hair follicles to normal levels of androgen (2).

        The majority of cases of hirsutism are caused by functional hyperandrogenism, which includes conditions such as polycystic ovarian syndrome (PCOS), idiopathic hyperandrogenism, idiopathic hirsutism, and congenital adrenal hyperplasia (3).

        Less commonly, other adrenal pathology, ovarian issues, medications, and pituitary and gestational hyperandrogenism are the cause of hirsutism (3). Adrenal causes include congenital adrenal hyperplasia, Cushing's syndrome, and adrenal virilizing tumors. Ovarian causes include hilus cell tumors, granulosa cell tumors, and Sertoli-Leydig cell tumors. Drugs that induce hirsutism include high-dose glucocorticoids, anabolic steroids, valproic acid, phenytoin, danazol, and minocycline. Pituitary causes include hyperprolactinemia and Cushing's disease (4).

        Table 14.3.1 lists the causes of hirsutism.

    B. Epidemiology. The prevalence of hirsutism in the United States is estimated to involve about 7% of women (1). Between 70 and 80% of the cases of hirsutism are caused by PCOS (1).

III. EVALUATION

    A. History. The first step in evaluating hirsutism includes a detailed history. Details of the history should include the onset and progression of hair growth, sites of hair growth, pubertal, menstrual, and reproductive history, a family history of hirsutism, and any potentially virilizing alterations in voice, abdomen, breasts, weight, and acne (1). History should also include the use of anabolic steroids and the psychosocial effects of hirsutism on the patient (4).

    B. Physical examination. The evaluation should include height, weight, and body mass index. The severity of hirsutism can be assessed using the Ferriman-Gallwey scale. This scoring system assesses nine areas of the body (upper lip, chin, chest, abdomen, superior pubic triangle, upper arms, thighs, upper back, and buttocks) using a score of 1–4. Hirsutism is diagnosed as mild with a score of 8–15 and moderate to severe if the score is more than 15. A score less than 8 is considered normal (1).

        To assess signs of virilization, a clinician should look for clitoromegaly, acne, male pattern hair loss, deepened voice, breast atrophy, and increase in muscle mass. A detailed skin exam may reveal acne, acanthosis nigricans, seborrhea, and androgenic alopecia (1,4). A thorough abdominal and pelvic bimanual exam should always be performed to exclude ovarian and adrenal tumors (1). A breast exam can help detect galactorrhea (1). Signs of conditions like Cushing's syndrome, acromegaly, thyroid dysfunction, and hyperprolactinemia can sometimes be detected by detailed physical examination.

    C. Testing. If the patient's history and physical examination are unremarkable, serum levels of total testosterone and dehydroepiandrosterone sulfate can be obtained to exclude an androgen-producing tumor. Elevated levels of androgens over twice the normal values should prompt an evaluation for an ovarian or adrenal tumor. High-resolution pelvic

TABLE 14.3.1 **Diagnostic Features and Clinical Manifestations**

Common causes of hirsutism	Percentage	Clinical manifestations	Laboratory tests
Polycystic ovarian syndrome "PCOS"	72–82%	Menstrual irregularity or amenorrhea Insulin resistance Infertility Sonographic evidence of ovarian cysts Truncal obesity	Variations in androgen levels (normal or elevated)
Idiopathic hyperandrogenemia	6–15%	Normal menstrual period No evidence of cysts on ultrasonography Etiology not explained by other causes	High levels of androgen
Idiopathic hirsutism	4–7%	No menstrual abnormalities No evidence of cysts on ultrasonography Etiology not explained by other causes	Normal androgen levels
Adrenal hyperplasia	2–4%	Two forms: 1) Classic: early onset, characterized by ambiguous genitalia in newborns 2) Non classic: late onset, menstrual irregularities, infertility Hispanics and Ashkenazi Jews are at higher risk Positive history of congenital adrenal hyperplasia (CAH) in the family	Confirm by high levels of 17-hydroxyprogesterone before and after corticotrophin stimulation test
Androgen secreting tumors	0.2%	Abdominal or pelvic mass on physical exam Virilization Dramatic onset of hirsutism Worsening of hirsutism in spite of treatment	Elevated early morning total testosterone more than 200 ng/dL
Iatrogenic hirsutism	Relatively rare	Medications like systemic and topical corticosteroids, clonazepam, isotretinoin, paxil, etc.	

(Continued)

TABLE 14.3.1	Diagnostic Features and Clinical Manifestations *(Continued)*		
Common causes of hirusutism	**Percentage**	**Clinical manifestations**	**Laboratory tests**
Acromegaly	Rare incidence with isolated hirsutism	Coarse facial features, enlargement of hands and feet	
Cushing syndrome	Rare incidence with isolated hirsutism	Moon faces, central obesity, hypertension	High 24-h urine free cortisol level
Hyperprolactinemia	Rare incidence with isolated hirsutism	Menstrual irregularities, infertility	High prolactin levels
Thyroid dysfunction	Rare incidence with isolated hirsutism	Hypothyroidism or hyperthyroidism	Abnormal thyroid function tests

Above table has been modified from AAFP (1)

ultrasonography with a transvaginal probe can identify ovarian follicles and cysts as small as 3–5 mm in diameter. Basal body temperature charts and serum progesterone levels in the luteal phase (20–24 days) of the menstrual cycle can be used to document the normal ovarian function of women who are thought to have idiopathic hirsutism. A clinical suspicion of hypothyroidism, hyperprolactinemia, or Cushing's disease requires confirmatory testing. Referral and further diagnostic testing may be warranted for patients with early-onset, severe, or rapidly progressive hirsutism.

IV. DIAGNOSIS

A. Differential diagnosis. PCOS and idiopathic hyperandrogenemia cause the majority of cases of hirsutism (1). See Table 14.3.1 for diagnostic features and clinical manifestations.

REFERENCES

1. Bode D, Seehusen DA, Baird D. Hirsutism in women. *Am Acad Family Pract* 2012;3:374–377.
2. Sathyapalan T, Atkin SL. Investigating hirsutism. *BMJ* 2009;338:912.
3. Escobar-Morreale HF. Diagnosis and management of hirsutism. *Ann N Y Acad Sci* 2010;4:166–174.
4. Somani N, Harrison S, Bergfeld WF. The clinical evaluation of hirsutism. *Dermatol Therapy* 2008;7:376–391.

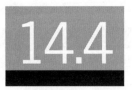

14.4 Hypothyroidism
Riad Z. Abdelkarim

I. BACKGROUND. Hypothyroidism is a common clinical syndrome resulting from thyroid hormone deficiency.

II. PATHOPHYSIOLOGY. Thyrotropin-releasing hormone (TRH), secreted by the hypothalamus, stimulates the anterior pituitary to produce thyroid-stimulating hormone (TSH), which mediates the production of thyroxine (T4) and triiodothyronine (T3) by the thyroid gland. T4 is converted into T3 (the active form of thyroid hormone) in the peripheral tissues. Hypothyroidism can be classified into primary, secondary, or tertiary conditions. *Primary hypothyroidism*—the most common type—results when inadequate amounts of thyroid hormone are produced by the thyroid gland due to a localized gland disorder. Thus, primary hypothyroidism is the result of thyroid gland failure (1). In a primary hypothyroid state, the decreased production of T4 results in increased pituitary secretion of TSH, which in turn stimulates thyroid gland hypertrophy and hyperplasia. *Secondary hypothyroidism* occurs when inadequate amounts of thyroid-stimulating hormone (TSH, or thyrotropin) are secreted from the pituitary gland, leading to diminished thyroid hormone release from the thyroid gland. *Tertiary hypothyroidism* results when the hypothalamus secretes insufficient amounts of TRH, leading to inadequate pituitary secretion of TSH, which in turn results in reduced thyroid gland production of thyroid hormone. *Subclinical hypothyroidism*, diagnosed on the basis of laboratory test results, is defined as a normal serum T4 level in the presence of an elevated serum TSH concentration.

Thyroid hormones stimulate diverse metabolic activities in most tissues and have profound effects on many major physiologic processes, such as development, growth, and metabolism. Thus, regardless of the cause, deficiency of thyroid hormone has numerous systemic effects.

III. EPIDEMIOLOGY. Overt primary hypothyroidism is prevalent in 0.3% of the US population, while subclinical hypothyroidism has a prevalence of 4.3%. The combined prevalence of overt and subclinical hypothyroidism is 5.1% in Caucasians, 4.2% in Hispanics, and 1.7% in blacks (1). The prevalence is higher in women than in men, and it increases with age. In women aged 18–24 years, the prevalence is 4%, while prevalence in women older than 74 years is 21%, according to one US study of over 25,000 people (2). Additionally, hypothyroidism is more common in women with small body size at birth and during childhood (3).

IV. ETIOLOGY. The most common cause of primary hypothyroidism is autoimmune thyroiditis, or Hashimoto disease, which results from the gradual destruction of the thyroid by T cells. Up to 95% of individuals with Hashimoto disease will have circulating antibodies to thyroid tissue. Another common cause is subacute granulomatous thyroiditis, in which viral syndromes or other inflammatory conditions can be associated with a transient hyperthyroid state followed by transient hypothyroidism (de Quervain thyroiditis). The patient with subacute thyroiditis may have fever and a painful thyroid gland. Various drugs have been associated with primary hypothyroidism, including amiodarone, interferon alpha, lithium, and stavudine. Iatrogenic hypothyroidism from either radioactive iodine or surgery can also occur. Radioactive iodine used for the treatment of Graves' disease usually causes permanent hypothyroidism within 1 year. Radiation of the external neck for neoplastic disease may also result in hypothyroidism. While still common in the developing world, goitrous hypothyroidism from iodine deficiency is rare in the United States and other developed countries since the introduction of iodized salt. Secondary or tertiary hypothyroidism is caused by pituitary or hypothalamic disease, respectively. The most common cause of secondary hypothyroidism is a pituitary adenoma. Other causes include tumors impinging on the hypothalamus; pituitary surgery; cranial radiation therapy; postpartum hemorrhage (Sheehan's syndrome); head trauma; granulomatous diseases; metastatic disease (breast, lung, colon, and prostate); infectious diseases (tuberculosis and others); and genetic disorders (4). Multiple endocrine end-organ failure caused by the autoimmune destruction of endocrine glands (Schmidt's syndrome) is a rare cause of primary hypothyroidism that mimics secondary disease.

V. EVALUATION

    A. History. Hypothyroidism can be asymptomatic, but often manifests as diminished physical and mental activity. Symptoms generally correspond directly to the duration and severity of disease, and the probability of thyroid disease is directly related to the number of typical symptoms manifested by the patient. Signs and symptoms include weakness, lethargy or fatigue, constipation, hair loss, muscle or joint pain, depression or slowed mentation, and menstrual disturbances. Neonates may present with prolonged jaundice, macroglossia, enlarged fontanelles, growth failure, failure to attain developmental milestones, or altered school performance.

Symptoms more specific to Hashimoto's thyroiditis include painless enlargement of the thyroid; a feeling of fullness in the throat; low-grade fever; neck pain and/or sore throat; and exhaustion. Symptoms suggestive of secondary or tertiary hypothyroidism include loss of axillary or pubic hair; headaches; visual field defects; amenorrhea, galactorrhea, or postural hypotension. Clinicians should determine whether patients they are evaluating for possible hypothyroidism fall into any of the following higher risk groups: women 4–8 weeks postpartum; women older than 50 years of age; patients with immunologically mediated diseases (including type 1 diabetes mellitus, pernicious anemia, vitiligo, Addison's disease, and rheumatoid arthritis); and persons with a family history of thyroid disease.

B. Physical examination. Physical examination findings can be quite subtle. Thus, clinicians must conduct a careful and detailed physical examination if hypothyroidism is suspected. A systematic head-to-toe examination is helpful, because all major organ systems are affected by thyroid hormone deficiency.

1. **Observation.** A welcoming handshake may reveal cold, dry skin, and further observations might uncover altered affect; a hoarse voice while relating the history; facial or eyelid edema; hair loss (scalp and eyebrows); and apparent physical or mental slowing.

2. **General examination.** Specific findings may include
   - Vital sign abnormalities
     o Hypothermia
     o Elevated diastolic blood pressure
     o Decreased systolic blood pressure
     o Bradycardia
     o Orthostatic hypotension (in secondary or tertiary hypothyroidism)
     o Increased weight
   - Head, ears, eyes, nose, throat, and neck
     o Coarse, brittle hair; loss of scalp hair
     o Dull facial expression/affect
     o Coarse facial features
     o Periorbital puffiness
     o Macroglossia
     o Hoarseness
     o Goiter (diffuse or nodular)
   - Cardiac
     o Cardiac rub or distant heart sounds (due to pericardial effusion)
   - Breasts
     o Galactorrhea (in secondary or tertiary hypothyroidism)
   - Abdomen
     o Abdominal distension or ileus
     o Ascites (uncommon)
   - Extremities/skin
     o Dry skin
     o Jaundice
     o Pallor
     o Loss of axillary and/or pubic hair
     o Nonpitting edema (myxedema); pitting edema of lower extremities
   - Neurologic
     o Slowed speech and movements
     o Hyporeflexia, prolonged relaxation phase of deep tendon reflexes
     o Carpal tunnel syndrome
     o Visual field defects (in secondary or tertiary hypothyroidism)

3. **Thyroid examination.** The thyroid gland itself should always be examined if hypothyroidism is suspected. The location, size, consistency, mobility, and tenderness of any nodules should be noted.

C. **Testing**

1. **Laboratory Studies.** The widely available third-generation TSH assays serve as the most useful and sensitive screening test for primary hypothyroidism (5). If a screening TSH is found to be above the reference range, a free T4 level can be checked. Primary hypothyroidism is characterized by an elevated TSH level with decreased free T4 levels. An elevated TSH level in the presence of normal free T4 levels is indicative of subclinical hypothyroidism. As TSH levels increase in early disease, T3 levels are maintained by an increased conversion of T4 to T3. Thus, early hypothyroidism may be characterized by elevated TSH, normal or low T4, and normal T3.

Although the TSH is characteristically elevated in primary hypothyroidism, pitfalls can occur. Starvation, corticosteroid administration, and use of dopamine can lower TSH, even in patients with hypothyroidism. In some hospitalized patients with severe nonthyroidal illness, low peripheral thyroid hormone levels may suggest hypothyroidism, although the TSH may be normal or decreased in this setting. In such patients, with the so-called euthyroid sick syndrome, the primary abnormality is the decreased peripheral conversion of T4 to T3, as well as an increased reverse T3 level (which can be measured). Additionally, during recovery from acute illness, some patients may exhibit transient elevations in TSH levels. Thus, thyroid function should not be tested in critically ill individuals unless there is a high index of suspicion for thyroid disease (5).

2. **Imaging Studies.** Ultrasound scans of the neck and thyroid are useful to detect nodules, but such studies are not indicated for routine evaluation of hypothyroidism. Radioactive iodine uptake and thyroid scanning are not generally helpful in evaluating hypothyroidism, because these tests require some level of endogenous functioning (6).

D. **Genetics.** Molecular defects have been identified in only a few causes of human hypothyroidism (7). Hypothyroidism remains primarily an acquired disease associated with aging.

IV. **DIAGNOSIS**

A. **Differential diagnosis.** Because the symptoms of hypothyroidism are nonspecific, its differential diagnosis is large and includes such variable entities as depression, sleep apnea, fibromyalgia, chronic infections, autoimmune disorders, anemia, menopause, cardiovascular disease, occult malignancies, adverse reactions to medication, and other endocrine disorders such as Addison disease, panhypopituitarism, and diabetes.

B. **Making the diagnosis.** Most patients have only mild or moderate disease at the time of diagnosis. *Subclinical hypothyroidism* occurs when the TSH is mildly elevated and there are no associated signs or symptoms. *Primary hypothyroidism* can be diagnosed by the typical findings on history and physical examination, coupled with an elevated TSH and a low free T4. *Secondary hypothyroidism* should be suspected when both the TSH and the free T4 are low. *Myxedema coma* is a life-threatening complication of long-standing hypothyroidism. These patients may present with stupor, areflexia, respiratory depression, hypercapnia, and profound hypothermia. Prompt diagnosis, hospitalization, and rapid treatment are required to prevent death.

REFERENCES

1. Hollowell JG, Staehling NW, Flanders WD, et al. Serum TSH, T4, and thyroid antibodies in the United States population (1988 to 1994): National Health and Nutrition Examination Survey (HHANES III). *J Clin Endocrinol Metab* 2002;87:489–499.
2. Canaris GJ, Manowitz NR, Mayor G, et al. The Colorado thyroid disease prevalence study. *Arch Intern Med* 2000;160:526–534.
3. Kajantie E, Phillips DI, Osmond C, Barker DJ, Forsen T, Eriksson JG. Spontaneous hypothyroidism in adult women is predicted by small body size at birth and during childhood. *J Clin Endocrinol Metab* Dec 2006;9(12):4953–4956.

4. Yamada M, Mori M. Mechanisms related to the pathophysiology and management of central hypothyroidism. *Nat Clin Pract Endocrinol Metab* Dec 2008;4(12):683–94.
5. U.S. Preventive Services Task Force. *Recommendation statement: screening for thyroid disease (January 2004).* Available at: http://www.uspreventiveservicestaskforce.org/uspstf/uspsthyr.htm, accessed on July 29, 2012.
6. Moreno JC, de Vijlder JJ, Vulsma T, et al. Genetic basis of hypothyroidism: recent advances, gaps and strategies for future research. *Trends Endocrinol Metab* 2003;14(7):318–326.
7. American Association of Clinical Endocrinologists. American Association of Clinical Endocrinologists medical guidelines for clinical practice for the evaluation and treatment of hyperthyroidism and hypothyroidism. *Endocr Pract* Nov–Dec 2002;8(6);457–469.

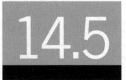

Polydipsia

Mohammed Zalabani

I. BACKGROUND. Polydipsia is a symptom in which the patient displays excessive thirst. The word derives from the Greek word polys, meaning "much, many" and dipsa, "thirst" and is attributed to medical or psychogenic causes.

II. PATHOPHYSIOLOGY

A. Epidemiology. Polydipsia is a common symptom among patients with diabetes mellitus (DM) and is prominent in patients with diabetes insipidus (DI). Polydipsia has a prevalence of 3–39% among chronic psychiatric inpatients (1).

B. Etiology. Polyuria is the most common symptom associated with polydipsia. There are several causes of polydipsia associated with polyuria:

1. **Poorly resorbed solutes**—Glucose, mannitol, or sorbitol can cause an osmotic diuresis. DM should be suspected in any patient with polydipsia and polyuria of recent onset.
2. **Primary Polydipsia**—Psychiatric patients infrequently suffer from polydipsia, because of dry mouth from medications with anticholinergic properties and/or delusions. Another term that has been used for primary polydipsia is psychogenic water drinking (2).
3. **Diabetes Insipidus (DI)**—This may be due to either a central (neurogenic DI) or a renal (nephrogenic DI) cause. Central DI is associated with deficient secretion of antidiuretic hormone (ADH). This condition can be idiopathic, genetic, or secondary to intracranial pathology such as a brain tumor, head trauma, toxic brain injury, metastatic cancer, and granulomatous disease (tuberculosis, sarcoidosis) or from a complication of a neurosurgic procedure. Vasopressinase-induced DI occurs in the last trimester of pregnancy and is often associated with preeclampsia. Nephrogenic DI is characterized by normal ADH secretion but varying degrees of renal resistance to its water-retaining effect. Nephrogenic DI presenting in childhood is almost always due to inherited defects, e.g., mutations in the AVPR2 gene and mutations in the aquaporin-2 (water channel) gene. It can also be secondary to medications (lithium, methoxyflurane, demeclocycline) or secondary to systemic disease (hypokalemia, hypercalcemia) (3).

III. EVALUATION

A. History. In eliciting the history, the clinician should take note of the onset of symptoms. Symptoms presenting at an early age may indicate a hereditary nature of the disease, while symptoms occurring after neurosurgery or a history of cancer may suggest the cause of the symptoms. Presence of neurologic symptoms (problems with visual fields, headaches) must be assessed and a detailed history of cancer, particularly metastatic brain cancer, or encephalitis must be obtained. The patient's psychiatric history may also be relevant (4).

B. Physical examination. A good general physical examination, including vital signs, is helpful in making the diagnosis, but the emphasis is on the neurologic examination (i.e., visual fields, cranial nerve deficits, oculomotor palsies, and reflexes). Signs of recent weight loss or the presence of peripheral neuropathy suggests the diagnosis of DM.

C. Testing

1. **Laboratory tests**—A urinalysis needs to be performed to check for glucosuria or low specific gravity associated with DI. A chemistry panel is helpful in checking for elevated serum glucose levels or elevated creatinine seen with renal disease and nephrogenic DI. A calcium level could be useful if hypercalcemia is suspected. Serum and urine osmolality are useful in differentiating between DI and primary polydipsia. DI presents with increased serum osmolality and a low urine osmolality (specific gravity <1.005), while primary polydipsia presents with low or normal serum osmolality and an appropriately low urine osmolality. Normal serum values are between 285 and 295 mOsm/L.

2. **Imaging**—Magnetic resonance imaging (MRI) of the head may be indicated to exclude pituitary or hypothalamic tumors. In DI associated with pituitary disease, MRI is quite specific, because the normal bright spot of a functioning pituitary gland is absent (5).

3. **Water deprivation test**—This test may be useful in the diagnosis of DI and to differentiate between neurogenic and nephrogenic DI by determining the effects of water deprivation (mild dehydration) on ADH secretion by measuring serum, urine osmolarity, urine specific gravity, and serum sodium in a controlled environment. This test needs to be carefully supervised by someone able to treat severe hypertonic dehydration, if necessary. Patients with mild polydipsia are placed on a fluid restriction starting at midnight prior to testing, but in those with severe polydipsia, fluids are restricted only during the day. Baseline body weight, plasma osmolality, serum sodium, and urine osmolarity are determined. Urine osmolarity and weight are assessed on an hourly basis. Adequate dehydration is noted by a decrease in body weight by 5% and serum osmolarity greater than 275 mOsm/L. A normal response would show normal plasma osmolarity and sodium concentration with decreased urine output and increasing urine osmolarity to greater than 800 mOsm/L (i.e., two to four times greater than the plasma). In contrast, healthy patients with DI cannot concentrate their urine in response to dehydration. Patients with central DI respond to desmopressin (a synthetic analog of vasopressin) administered intranasally, whereas patients with nephrogenic DI do not. Patients may not fall into a definite category sometimes (e.g., partial central DI). The direct form of testing where ADH levels are measured after infusing hypertonic saline is rarely performed (6).

D. Genetics. An inherited autosomally dominant form of neurogenic DI is caused by mutations in the *AVP neurophysin II* gene (*AVP-NPII* gene), and hereditary nephrogenic DI can be caused by V2 receptor problems (X-linked mode of inheritance or a defect in the ADH-sensitive aquaporin-2 water channels) (5).

IV. DIAGNOSIS

A. Differential diagnosis. Often, important clues about the cause of polydipsia can be obtained with a directed clinical history with particular attention to the onset of symptoms, the presence of nocturia, and the medication history. The value of the physical examination is limited unless there are signs of defects due to a pituitary tumor (e.g., progressive headaches, visual field defects) or endocrinologic symptoms (e.g., amenorrhea, galactorrhea, acromegaly, Cushing's syndrome). The diagnosis is often made with routine laboratory tests. Sometimes, a water deprivation test needs to be performed to make the diagnosis, but this test should be performed in a hospital setting with the patient monitored closely for signs of dehydration.

B. Clinical manifestations. Thirst associated with polyuria is the chief complaint in patients with DM, DI, and psychogenic polydipsia. Nocturia occurs more frequently with DM and DI than with psychogenic polydipsia. Patients with psychogenic polydipsia may have delusions leading to increased fluid intake of up to 20 L/d (1).

REFERENCES

1. Greendyke RM, Bernhardt AJ, Tasbas HE, et al. Polydipsia in chronic psychiatric patients: therapeutic trials of clonidine and enalapril. *Neuropsychopharmacology* 1998;18:272–281.
2. Schrier RW, Body water homeostasis: clinical disorders of urinary dilution and concentration *J Am Soc Nephrol* Jul 2006;17(7):1820–1832.
3. Miller, M., Dalakos, T., Moses, A., Fellerman, H., & Streeten, D. (1970). Recognition of partial defects in antidiuretic hormone secreation. *Annals of Internal Medicine*, 73(5), 721–729.
4. Olapade-Olaopa EO, Morley RN, Ahiaku EK, et al. Iatrogenic polydipsia: a rare cause of water intoxication in urology. *Br J Urol* 1997;79:488.
5. Robertson GL. Disorders of the neurohypophysis. In: Kasper DL, Fauci AS, Longo DL, eds. *Harrison's principles of internal medicine,* 16th ed. New York, NY: McGraw-Hill, 1998:2098–2103.
6. Adam P. Evaluation and management of diabetes insipidus. *Am Fam Physician* 1997;55:2146–2153.

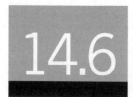

14.6

Thyroid Enlargement/ Goiter

Toby D. Free

I. BACKGROUND. Goiter, an enlarged thyroid gland, is the most common thyroid abnormality. The mean weight of the thyroid gland in iodine-sufficient populations is 10 g, with the upper limit of the normal being 20 g (1). Goiter is termed *endemic* if it occurs in more than 10% of the population. Endemic goiter most commonly results from dietary iodine deficiency and is extremely rare in the United States. Goiter is termed *sporadic* if it arises in nonendemic areas and from various causes (2). *Simple* goiter describes a diffusely enlarged thyroid gland and *multinodular* goiter is an enlarged gland with multiple areas of nodularity. Finally, functional status of a goiter is considered *nontoxic* if the patient is in a euthymic state, but is *toxic* in a patient who is hyperthyroid.

II. PATHOPHYSIOLOGY

A. Etiology. Any process that impedes thyroid hormone synthesis or release can cause goiter. By far the most important risk factor for the development of goiter is iodine deficiency. Some situations exacerbate iodine deficiency. For example, cigarette smoking has been linked to the development of goiter in iodine-deficient areas and is believed to interfere with iodine uptake of the thyroid gland. Also, pregnancy-induced goiter is related to the exacerbation of existing iodine deficiency and proliferative effect of estrogen on the thyroid gland. (However, the use of oral contraceptives has been found to be associated with reduced incidence of goiter) (3). Goitrogens, substances that interfere with thyroid hormone production and action, can cause sporadic goiter. This category includes certain drugs (thioamide derivatives, lithium, iodides, amiodarone, and others) and foods (rutabagas, cabbage, turnips, soybeans, kelp, and others) (2).

B. Epidemiology. The prevalence of goiter in the United States is estimated to be 4–7% but varies widely, depending on the regional iodine intake. One autopsy study of thyroid glands that were thought to contain no pathology demonstrated a 38% incidence of multinodular goiter, showing the prevalence of substantial, subclinical disease (1). Goiter prevalence does increase with age and is 5–10 times more common in women than in men (2).

III. EVALUATION

A. History. Although simple goiters are usually euthyroid, typical symptoms of hypothyroidism or thyrotoxicosis should be sought. Asking about pain and the quality of pain is helpful. Generalized thyroid pain suggests subacute thyroiditis, whereas sudden localized pain and swelling are consistent with hemorrhage into a nodule (4). A family history of goiter and a personal history of residing in an endemic area or ingesting goitrogens may be significant.

B. **Physical examination.** Full extension of the neck enhances the visibility of the gland. Inspection from the side with measurement of any prominence of the normally smooth and straight contour between the cricoid cartilage and the suprasternal notch is useful. Inspect the neck below the thyroid cartilage from the front, using cross-lighting to accentuate shadows and masses. Palpation is performed using the technique with which the examiner is most experienced and skilled. The thyroid is palpated by using the fingers or thumbs while standing in front of or behind the patient. If felt between the cricoid cartilage and the suprasternal notch, the thyroid isthmus can be used to help locate the gland. Palpation of the lobes can be improved by relaxation of the sternocleidomastoid; for example, the left lobe can be defined better by having the patient slightly flex and rotate the neck to the left. Other useful maneuvers include measuring the circumference of the neck or the dimensions of each lobe. The location, size, consistency, mobility, and tenderness of any nodules should be noted. Having the patient swallow during both inspection and palpation causes the thyroid to move and aids in developing a three-dimensional impression of the gland's shape and size. This maneuver can also make a low-placed gland accessible. The patient should be placed in the supine position to determine the inferior extent of the gland (1, 5). *Pemberton's sign* can be induced by having the patient raise both arms above the head for 1 minute. The patient develops facial and neck plethora if venous outflow is obstructed by the thyroid gland. Physical signs consistent with hypothyroidism or thyrotoxicosis may be present.

C. **Testing**

1. **Laboratory tests.** The highly sensitive thyroid-stimulating hormone (TSH) assay is the single best test to evaluate the thyroid status. An elevated TSH is highly suggestive of hypothyroidism. If TSH is suppressed, an elevated free thyroxine index (FTI) or free thyroxine (fT_4) measured directly confirms thyrotoxicosis. In a patient with a suppressed TSH and a normal FTI or fT_4, serum triiodothyronine (T_3) should be measured to assess for possible T_3 thyrotoxicosis. Antithyroid antibodies can help predict those patients at a higher risk for developing thyroiditis, hypothyroidism, or Graves' disease.

2. **Imaging.** Nuclear scans are not warranted in the routine evaluation of simple or multinodular goiter. Ultrasonography should be used in cases of multinodular goiter to rule out a dominant nodule and may be helpful in patients with equivocal findings on palpation (6). Symptoms suggestive of substernal mechanical pressure require evaluation, usually by computed tomography or magnetic resonance imaging (4).

3. **Other tests.** Fine needle biopsy should be performed in cases of a solitary or dominant nodule found by palpation or ultrasound. Pulmonary function tests are warranted if there is a question of inspiratory impairment. Barium swallow is indicated to evaluate goiter-associated dysphagia (4).

D. **Genetics.** Currently, no genetic markers are used in evaluating goiter. Family and twin studies have demonstrated that genetic factors play a role in the development of goiter, but at present, the results cannot be extrapolated to the general population (5).

IV. DIAGNOSIS

A. **Differential diagnosis.** A cystic hygroma or a thyroglossal duct cyst, which may transilluminate, and lymphadenopathy can be confused with goiter. Primary thyroid cancers, lymphomas, or metastatic cancers may present as a firm mass in the neck. Patients with thyroiditis (Hashimoto's, subacute, or silent) can present with an enlarged thyroid gland. An asymptomatic patient with a simple or multinodular goiter associated with a normal metabolic state does not necessarily require further diagnostic studies or treatment. Periodic assessment, at least annually, to evaluate growth, function, and symptoms is warranted. In two studies, it was shown that 10% of patients with nodular goiter developed thyrotoxicosis during a 7- to 10-year follow-up period (2).

B. **Clinical manifestations.** In simple goiter, patients are asymptomatic or, if the gland is sufficiently enlarged, present with symptoms caused by mechanical pressure. Substernal goiters are frequently responsible for tracheal pressure symptoms, including dyspnea and inspiratory stridor. They can also obstruct the large cervical veins at the thoracic inlet, causing suffusion of the face, giddiness, and syncope (Pemberton's sign). Esophageal compression can lead to dysphagia. Hoarseness caused by compression of or traction on the recurrent laryngeal nerve is rare in simple goiter and suggests a malignancy. Goiter with compressive or cosmetic symptoms usually requires surgical consultation, but referral for radioiodine therapy could be considered, especially in older patients. The natural history of simple goiter may include spontaneous resolution or no clinical change but may also involve gradual thyroid growth, nodule formation, and the development of functional autonomy. The use of thyroid hormone suppression in goiter is controversial. Nodules within a multinodular goiter may become toxic in the presence of a supplemental thyroid hormone (4,5).

REFERENCES

1. Day TA, Chu A, Hoang KG. Multinodular goiter. *Otolaryngol Clin North Am* 2003;36:35–54.
2. Hermus AR, Huymans DA. Pathogenesis of nontoxic diffuse and nodular goiter. In: Braverman LE, Utiger RD, eds. *Werner and Inbar's the thyroid,* 9th ed. Philadelphia. PA: Lippincott Williams & Wilkins, 2005:873–878.
3. Knudsen N, Laurberg P, Perrild H, et al. Risk factors for goiter and thyroid nodules. *Thyroid* 2002;12:879–888.
4. Hermus AR, Huymans DA. Clinical manifestations and treatment of nontoxic diffuse and nodular goiter. In: Braverman LE, Utiger RD, eds. *Werner and Inbar's The Thyroid,* 9th ed. Philadelphia, PA: Lippincott Williams & Wilkins, 2005:879–885.
5. Hegedus L, Bonnema SJ, Bennedbaek FN. Management of simple nodular goiter: current status and future perspectives. *Endocr Rev* 2003;24:102–132.
6. Bahn RS, Castro MR. Approach to the patient with nontoxic multinodular goiter. *J Clin Endocrinol Metabol* 2011;96(5):1202–1212.

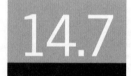

14.7 Thyroid Nodule
M. Jawad Hashim

I. **BACKGROUND.** A thyroid nodule is a palpable swelling in an otherwise normal thyroid gland. Only about 5–10% of nodules are cancerous (Figure 14.7.1). The most common nodule is the colloid nodule, which is not associated with an increased risk of cancer.

II. **PATHOPHYSIOLOGY**

A. **Etiology.** Exposure to ionizing radiation or external beam radiation therapy (especially before 20 years of age) increases the incidence of both benign and malignant thyroid nodules at a rate of 2% annually and peaks 15–20 years after exposure (2). Iodine deficiency results in increased thyroid-stimulating hormone (TSH) levels, increased thyroid cell replication, and an increased incidence of nodules.

B. **Epidemiology.** Palpable nodules are present in 4–7% of adults (3). Nodules found incidentally on ultrasound are estimated to occur as often as 19–67%. Age younger than 20 years or older than 65 years, male gender, exposure to radiation, and previous history of thyroid cancer are risk factors for thyroid cancer. Benign thyroid nodules are present four to five times more often in women, but are more likely to be cancerous in men.

III. **EVALUATION.** The evaluation of nodular thyroid disease focuses on the functional status of the gland and detection of thyroid cancer. Hypothyroidism or hyperthyroidism may be suggested by the history and physical examination.

A. **History.** Rapid growth of a nodule or symptoms of local invasion (hoarseness, neck pain, dysphagia, stridor, or dyspnea) increase the suspicion of cancer. Sudden onset of localized swelling, pain, or tenderness suggests hemorrhage into a preexisting nodule or cyst.

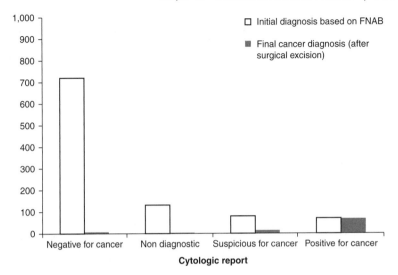

Figure 14.7.1. Risk of cancer in thyroid nodules

FNAB, fine needle aspiration biopsy. Modeled data based on experience at one center.
Source: reference (1)

B. Physical examination. The neck is inspected below the thyroid cartilage from the front and side, using cross-lighting to accentuate shadows and masses. Full extension of the neck enhances the visibility of the gland. The patient is approached from either the front or behind during palpation, which is accomplished using the fingers or thumbs. Having the patient swallow during both inspection and palpation causes the thyroid to move and aids in developing a three-dimensional impression of the gland. The location, size, consistency, mobility, and tenderness of all nodules should be documented. A nodule that is hard, irregular, nontender, >4 cm, fixed to surrounding structures, associated with local lymphadenopathy or vocal cord immobility suggests malignancy (3).

C. Testing

1. Laboratory tests. Serum TSH should be assessed in every patient. It is the best screening test for both hypothyroidism (elevated TSH; Chapter 14.4) and thyrotoxicosis (suppressed TSH; Chapter 14.8). A family history of medullary thyroid cancer or multiple endocrine neoplasia type II warrants a basal serum calcitonin.

2. Fine needle aspiration biopsy. In euthyroid patients with a nodule, a fine needle aspiration biopsy (FNAB) should be performed. FNAB has demonstrated a sensitivity of 68–98% and a specificity of 72–100% (2). After applying local anesthetic, a 25-G needle, guided by palpation (or ultrasound if the nodule is smaller than 1 cm) is used to obtain two to five specimens (4). Even in experienced hands, biopsies are often unsatisfactory and need to be repeated. A thyroid lobectomy with frozen section analysis may be required if FNAB is repeatedly nondiagnostic and the clinical pretest probability of cancer is high.

3. Imaging studies. Ultrasound cannot reliably differentiate benign from malignant nodules, although features such as microcalcifications and irregular margins are suggestive of cancer (3). Although less frequently used, radioisotope scanning with radioiodine can differentiate between active ("hot nodules") and non-functional ("cold") nodules (3). About 5% of nodules are active and are less likely to be malignant. Similarly, computed tomography and magnetic resonance imaging have limited value in the initial diagnostic workup except in cases of local compression.

D. Genetic biomarkers. The presence of certain genetic mutations has been correlated with thyroid cancers, proving to be clinically useful when FNAB is indeterminate (3). These mutations occur in the genes for tyrosine kinase receptors (RET/PTC, NTRK), nuclear proteins (PAX-8-PPARγ), and signaling proteins (RAS, BRAF). The latter alterations along with RET/PTC mutations are frequent in papillary carcinomas while follicular cancers bear RAS proto-oncogenes and PAX-8-PPARγ defects. These genetic markers are expected to be incorporated into diagnostic algorithms as more data are accumulated and the assays become more widespread in availability (3). Approximately 4–8% of cases of papillary cancer are familial, and a high incidence has been reported in patients with adenomatous polyposis coli (Gardner's syndrome) and multiple hamartoma syndromes (Cowden disease). Medullary cancer, usually as part of multiple endocrine neoplasia type II, often occurs in a hereditary pattern.

IV. DIAGNOSIS

A. Differential diagnosis. If the results of FNAB demonstrate a malignancy or are suspicious, indeterminate, or repeatedly unsatisfactory, then an immediate surgical referral is warranted. Sometimes, radionuclide scanning is used to evaluate a suspicious biopsy result, and hyperfunctioning nodules are observed rather than removed. If the biopsy is clearly benign, a careful examination of the nodule and surrounding structures, an ultrasound, and a TSH measurement should be performed every 12 months (3). While nodules that are more than 4 cm have a 19% risk of cancer, the decision for surgery should not be based on nodule size alone.

B. Clinical manifestations. The presence of hyperthyroidism or hypothyroidism lowers the suspicion of cancer but does not exclude it. Any nodule that enlarges or becomes clinically suspicious should be rebiopsied.

REFERENCES

1. Sebo TJ. Thyroid fine needle aspiration cytology: nothing new except a re-emphasis on a back-to-basics and cost-effective approach to interpretation in the era of ultrasound examination and molecular diagnostics. *Clin Endocrinol*. Available at: http://onlinelibrary.wiley.com/doi/10.1111/j.1365-2265.2012.04404.x/abstract. Accessed May 9, 2012.
2. Welker MJ, Orlov D. Thyroid nodules. *Am Fam Physician* 2003;67(3):559–566.
3. Bomeli SR, LeBeau SO, Ferris RL. Evaluation of a thyroid nodule. *Otolaryngol Clin North Am* 2010;43(2):229–238, vii.
4. Layfield LJ, Cibas ES, Gharib H, Mandel SJ. Thyroid aspiration cytology: current status. *CA: A Cancer J Clin* 2009;59(2):99–110.

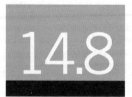

14.8 Hyperthyroidism/ Thyrotoxicosis

Rodolfo M. Sanchez

I. BACKGROUND. Hyperthyroidism is excessive thyroid hormone secretion. Thyrotoxicosis is the state of *symptomatic* thyroid hormone excess.

II. PATHOPHYSIOLOGY. Causes of thyrotoxicosis are summarized in Table 14.8.1.

A. Etiology

1. **Graves' disease,** an autoimmune disorder and the most common cause of hyperthyroidism, results when thyrotropin receptor antibodies stimulate thyroid growth, leading to the synthesis and release of the thyroid hormones T3 and T4, usually resulting in a goiter.

TABLE 14.8.1 Causes of Thyrotoxicosis and Associated Radioactive Iodine Uptake Findings

Cause	Radioactive iodine uptake
Graves' disease (most common)	Homogeneous increase
Toxic multinodular goiter	Increased heterogeneous pattern
Toxic adenoma	One area increased, rest of the gland suppressed
Exogenous	Low or absent uptake
Iatrogenic (overtreatment)	
Factitious (patient taking excess)	
Thyroiditis	
Acute suppurative (rare)	Normal
Subacute (de Quervain's)[a]	Low (transient)
Silent thyroiditis[a]	Low (transient)
Excess iodine	Low or absent
Thyroid carcinoma	Variable
Functioning bone metastases	Absent
TSH-secreting pituitary tumor	Increased
Struma ovarii	Reduced in thyroid (increased over pelvis)
Activating mutation of TSH receptor	Increased
Thyroid hormone resistance syndrome	Increased

[a]Transient, followed by hypothyroidism, then return to normal. TSH, thyroid-stimulating hormone.

2. **Toxic adenoma and toxic multinodular goiter** are characterized by the development of areas of focal or diffuse hyperplasia of thyroid follicular cells, which function without regulation by thyroid-stimulating hormone (TSH). In trophoblastic tumors, TSH receptors may be stimulated by the overproduction of the human chorionic gonadotropin or other placental proteins.
3. **Thyroiditis** results in the release of preformed thyroid hormone from the thyroid gland. It is of viral or postviral origin (subacute granulomatous thyroiditis) or from an autoimmune process (subacute lymphocytic thyroiditis). Subacute thyroiditis can also be caused by chemical toxicity from drugs such as amiodarone, by radiation, or by drugs that interfere with the immune system, such as interferon alfa.

B. **Epidemiology.** Hyperthyroidism affects up to 2% of women and 0.2% of men. The prevalence increases with age and is highest in patients older than 80 years of age (1). Graves' disease accounts for 60–80% of cases of thyrotoxicosis, occurs typically in patients between 20 and 50 years of age, and is less prevalent in areas of low iodine intake (2). Toxic nodular goiter is the next most common cause of thyrotoxicosis (10–40%) and is the most common cause of thyrotoxicosis in patients older than 40 years of age. Thyroiditis accounts for 5–20% of the cases. The other causes of thyrotoxicosis are much less common.

III. EVALUATION
A. **History.** Symptoms vary from dramatic to absent. In severe hyperthyroidism, anxiety, emotional ability, commerce, weakness, heat intolerance, weight loss, and increased perspiration are common. Milder symptoms include unexplained weight loss, myopathy, menstrual disorders, new onset of atrial fibrillation, and gynecomastia.

B. Physical examination. Vital signs may reveal weight loss, tachycardia, and systolic hypertension with a widened pulse pressure. Patients may appear nervous or restless. Sinus tachycardia is the most frequent arrhythmia. Atrial fibrillation occurs in 5–15% and may be the presenting problem. The risk of atrial fibrillation or flutter is higher in men than in women (1.8:1) and increases with age (3). Despite complaints of exertional dyspnea, the lung examination is usually normal unless there is concomitant congestive heart failure. The skin may be warm and moist with palmar erythema. Pretibial myxedema, painless raised swelling of subcutaneous tissues, most often found on the anterior lower leg or dorsal foot of patients with Graves' disease, causes a *peau d'orange* texture, which can be pruritic and hyperpigmented. A fine tremor is most evident in the fingertips when the hands are extended. Hypokalemic periodic paralysis is most commonly seen in Asian men. Auscultation of a bruit over the gland correlates with increased vascularity.

C. Testing. Measuring serum (TSH) is the most sensitive test to screen for primary hyperthyroidism. A normal TSH virtually excludes hyperthyroidism, serum TSH < 0.01 mIU/L confirms hyperthyroidism, and an elevated free T_4 would further confirm the diagnosis of hyperthyroidism. If the free T_4 is normal and suspicion is high, a serum free triiodothyronine (T_3) should also be measured to rule out T_3 toxicosis. Drugs such as glucocorticoids, levodopa, and dopamine can cause a low TSH in patients who are euthyroid. A low TSH with a normal free T_4 and T_3 may indicate subclinical hyperthyroidism. A thyroid scan with radioactive iodine uptake can help differentiate the causes of thyrotoxicosis as indicated in Table 14.8.1 (4). Ultrasonic examination of the thyroid is useful to detect the presence of nodules or cysts.

D. Genetics. A combination of genetic factors, including HLA-DR and CTLA-4 polymorphisms, and environmental factors contributes to Graves' disease. Activating mutations of Gs-α proteins have been identified in many toxic adenomas. Activating somatic mutations of the genes for TSH receptor have been identified in both toxic adenomas and toxic multinodular goiters.

IV. DIAGNOSIS

A. Differential diagnosis. Thyrotoxicosis must be differentiated from other causes of unexplained weight loss, including malignancies, psychiatric disorders, alcohol or drug abuse, diabetes, occult infections, gastrointestinal disorders, and chronic renal, hepatic, cardiac, or pulmonary disease.

B. Clinical manifestations. The signs and symptoms are extremely variable.

1. **Graves' disease** is suggested by widened palpebral fissures, lid lag, and visualization of the sclera on all sides of the iris. Typically, the thyroid is increased in size and is smooth and nontender. A bruit is present in 50% of patients.

2. **Toxic nodular goiter** presents with a gland that is typically enlarged and non-tender with multiple nodules. A single toxic nodule is more common in younger people.

3. **Thyroiditis,** which usually refers to subacute granulomatous thyroiditis (de Quervain's thyroiditis), presents with an enlarged, tender thyroid. In subacute lymphocytic thyroiditis (painless or silent thyroiditis), the gland is enlarged but nontender.

REFERENCES

1. Flynn RWV, MacDonald TM, Morris AD, et al. The thyroid epidemiology, audit, and research study: thyroid dysfunction in the general population. *J Clin Endocrinol Metab* 2004;89:3879–3884.
2. Cooper DS. Hyperthyroidism. *Lancet* 2003;362:459–468.
3. Frost L, Vestergaard P, Mosekilde L. Hyperthyroidism and the risk of atrial fibrillation or flutter: a population based study. *Arch Intern Med* 2004;164:1675–1678.
4. Intenzo CM, dePapp AE, Jabbour S, et al. Scintigraphic manifestations of thyrotoxicosis. *Radiographics* 2003;23:857–869.

14.9 Vitamin D Deficiency

Amy L. McGaha

I. BACKGROUND. Vitamin D (Vit D) is a fat-soluble vitamin, the main function of which is to regulate calcium levels in the blood. Vit D in its active form increases the absorption of calcium from the intestine. Vit D has receptors on most cells in the body, suggesting a wide range of functions some of which are not yet fully elucidated. Recent research findings suggest that Vit D plays a major role in immune regulation and thus may be of critical importance in infections, autoimmune disorders, as well as possibly playing a role in the genesis of malignant disease. Calcium is a critical mineral in the body and is important to cellular function, especially in muscle and neural cells.

Humans obtain 90% of their Vit D from sunlight and skin synthesis. It is difficult to maintain adequate levels of Vit D from dietary sources alone, as Vit D is not naturally present in a wide variety of foods. There are two kinds of Vit D: ergocalciferol (D2) from irradiation of yeast and plant sterols and cholecalciferol (D3) from skin synthesis and also present in some kinds of fish. Although only a small number of foods naturally have Vit D, many US foods are fortified, usually in the form of cholecalciferol. Naturally occurring dietary sources of Vit D (cholecalciferol) include breast milk (if the woman is not deficient), tuna, mackerel, salmon, sardines, cod liver oil, and egg yolks (ergocalciferol).

II. PATHOPHYSIOLOGY

A. Etiology. When intestinal absorption of calcium does not provide sufficient calcium to maintain normocalcemia, Vit D will then suppress osteocytes and activate osteoclasts to mobilize calcium from bones. Parathyroid hormone (PTH) is released in response to hypocalcemia and acts by stimulating the conversion of Vit D to its active form in both liver and kidneys.

B. Epidemiology. More than half of the persons older than 65 years in North America and 66% of all persons internationally failed to maintain healthy bone density and tooth attachment because of inadequate Vit D. Risk factors for Vit D deficiency include age >65 years, exclusively breast-fed infants, persons with dark skin, decreased sunlight exposure, obesity, sedentary lifestyle, and some medications (glucocorticoids, anticonvulsants). In addition, patients with a history of gastric bypass or malabsorption, liver disease, or renal failure are at higher risk for Vit D deficiency.

The incidence of rickets has declined in most industrialized countries (including the United States) due primarily to fortification of food and beverages. However, there has been a resurgence in some susceptible populations. These include exclusively breast-fed infants, especially those born to Vit D-deficient mothers, and among vegetarian and vegan populations.

III. EVALUATION

A. History. Although most commonly Vit D deficiency is asymptomatic, and only discovered after the development of a fracture or another disorder such as rickets, the clinician should maintain a high index of suspicion, particularly among patients with darker skin, on chronic anticonvulsants or steroids, with unexplained elevations in serum alkaline phosphatase, or in children presenting with irritability, or growth delay. Bone (particularly low back pain, sternum, or tibia) and muscle pain and weakness can also be manifestations of Vit D deficiency.

B. Physical exam. Clinical manifestations of Vit D deficiency can be classified as skeletal and extraskeletal. They can also be classified as manifestations of negative calcium balance or direct Vit D deficiency.

Negative calcium balance in the growing skeleton produces rickets. Manifestations of rickets include bone deformity, as well as symptomatic hypocalcemia, manifesting as seizures or hypocalcemic tetany. Widening of the wrists, bowing of legs, delayed closure of fontanels, craniotabes, and rachitic rosary (widened costochondral junctions) are classic and advanced bone manifestations of rickets. Extraskeletal symptoms of rickets include motor delay and dental maldevelopment. In addition, infants and children with rickets have increased susceptibility to infections such as pneumonia.

In the mature skeleton, Vit D deficiency results in osteopenia, osteomalacia, or osteoporosis. These manifest both as skeletal deformities such as "Dowager's hump" and increased susceptibility to fractures.

IV. DIAGNOSIS

The diagnosis of Vit D deficiency should be considered in patients presenting with complaints of widespread bone discomfort, muscle aches, or proximal muscle weakness.

A. Testing. Serum testing for 25-OH Vit D, the major circulating form of Vit D, is used to diagnose Vit D insufficiency or deficiency. Although there is little agreement on optimal Vit D levels, it has been suggested that 20 ng/mL (50 nmol/L) may be appropriate as a target to indicate sufficiency (1,2).

Parathyroid Hormone. May be measured if there is a question of insufficiency; levels of PTH tend to be inversely proportional to the levels of 25-OH Vit D in the body.

Measurement of serum levels of alkaline phosphatase, calcium, and phosphorus may be considered if osteomalacia or rickets are a possibility. Bone density testing may also be helpful (3).

After treatment, repeated measurements of 25-OH Vit D levels are carried out at intervals and then yearly to document continued sufficiency. Radiologic healing should also be documented in children who are treated for rickets.

REFERENCES

1. Pazirandeh S, Burns DL. Overview of Vitamin D, from www.uptodate.com. Accessed September 27, 2012.
2. Misra M, Pacaud D, Petryk A, Collett-Solberg PF, Kappy M. Vitamin D deficiency in children and its management: review of current knowledge and recommendations. *Pediatrics* 2008;122(2):398.
3. Holick MF, Vitamin D deficiency. *N Engl J Med* 2007;357:266–281.

CHAPTER 15

Vascular and Lymphatic System Problems

Ashley Falk

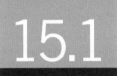

Lymphadenopathy, Generalized

Kristy D. Edwards

I. **BACKGROUND.** Lymphadenopathy, enlarged, tender, or inflamed lymph nodes, is a common presenting complaint. In primary care, patients presenting with nonspecific lymphadenopathy are mainly younger than 40 years of age, and one-fourth of the patients have generalized lymphadenopathy. Generalized lymphadenopathy is diagnosed when abnormal lymph nodes are identified in two or more noncontiguous areas (e.g., neck and groin). Generalized lymphadenopathy should prompt further investigation of systemic disease by the physician.

II. **PATHOPHYSIOLOGY.** Infectious, autoimmune, granulomatous, malignant diseases or medication reactions can cause generalized lymphadenopathy. The overall risk of cancer in patients with generalized lymphadenopathy is low; however, the risk of malignancy increases with age. There is a 4% cancer risk in those patients older than 40 years of age with generalized lymphadenopathy (1). A good complete history and physical examination can often lead to a diagnosis of the cause of lymphadenopathy.

III. **EVALUATION**

   A. **History.** The history should focus on the common causes of generalized lymphadenopathy.

   1. **History of present illness** should focus on the duration, location, quality, and context of the lymphadenopathy. Enlarged, tender lymph nodes present for <2 weeks are often due to infectious causes. Lymphadenopathy present for more than a year is usually from nonspecific causes. Associated signs and symptoms such as rash, fever, night sweats, weight loss, sore throat, and arthralgias may help identify a specific cause of the generalized lymphadenopathy (2).

   2. **Past medical history** should focus on known illness and medication usage. Common chronic illnesses (e.g., lupus erythematosus, rheumatoid arthritis, and human immuno-deficiency virus [HIV]) can also cause generalized lymphadenopathy. Drug reactions resulting in lymphadenopathy can occur with certain antibiotics and seizure and hypertension medications (1).

   3. **Social history** may identify risk factors for hepatitis B, secondary syphilis, and early HIV. All of these diseases can present with generalized lymphadenopathy.

   4. **Family history** is important to identify illness with a genetic predisposition such as lipid storage diseases and immunologic diseases (e.g., Niemann-Pick disease and rheumatoid arthritis). Any known exposures to family members with infectious diseases (e.g., tuberculosis, infectious mononucleosis, or hepatitis B) can also yield important information when trying to identify a causative etiology of lymphadenopathy.

5. **Review of systems** should focus on constitutional symptoms such as weight loss, fatigue, night sweats, malaise, arthralgias, nausea, and vomiting.

B. **Physical examination**

1. **General.** A comprehensive physical examination should be performed on all patients with generalized lymphadenopathy. It should focus on identifying systemic diseases. Vital signs are important, because fever may suggest infectious etiology and weight loss may suggest systemic disease. Skin rashes or lesions, mucous membrane ulcers, and inflammatory arthritis are important physical findings in establishing a differential diagnosis for the adenopathy. An abdominal examination for splenomegaly can yield useful information. Generalized lymphadenopathy with splenomegaly implies systemic illness (e.g., infectious mononucleosis, lymphoma, leukemia, lupus, sarcoidosis, toxoplasmosis, or cat-scratch disease) and virtually excludes nonhematologic metastatic disease (1,2).

2. **Nodal examination.** In generalized lymphadenopathy, lymph node size, location, and consistency can help in establishing a diagnosis.

   a. **Size.** Lymph nodes >1.5 cm in diameter have a 38% risk of cancer involvement and require further workup (2). Lymph nodes 1 cm in diameter and smaller can be normal and can usually be observed.

   b. **Location.** The anatomic location of lymphadenopathy is sometimes helpful in establishing a diagnosis. However, with generalized lymphadenopathy, the anatomic location is less helpful. Anterior cervical, submandibular, and inguinal nodes may normally be palpable. However, lymph nodes palpated in certain areas are always alarming. For example, supraclavicular lymphadenopathy has a 90% risk of cancer in patients older than 40 years of age.

   c. **Consistency.** Rock hard nodes particularly in older patients are worrying for metastatic disease (2). Firm rubbery nodes are found with lymphomas. Soft tender nodes tend to occur with infectious causes; however, this should not be considered diagnostic. Pain is not a reliable indicator of the cause of lymphadenopathy.

C. **Testing**

1. **Laboratory tests.** Laboratory testing in patients with generalized lymphadenopathy should be purposeful and specific. Tests should be directed by the patient's signs and symptoms of an underlying disease process (3). A complete blood count (CBC) with peripheral smear is almost always indicated (4). Elevated neutrophils suggest pyogenic etiologies, lymphocytosis suggests viral infection, and pancytopenia suggests leukemia or HIV infection. An erythrocyte sedimentation rate is nonspecific, but if it is persistently elevated, further investigation is indicated. Disease-specific serologic tests, including antibody testing for Epstein-Barr virus, cytomegalovirus, HIV, rubella virus, syphilis (FTA-ABS), and others, are useful. Antibody testing can be diagnostic and can differentiate between acute and chronic illnesses. Chest X-rays are rarely positive but should be ordered to look for mediastinal lymph node involvement in sarcoid disease, metastatic disease, lymphomas, or granulomatous disease. Purified protein derivative (PPD) testing is used to identify tuberculin disease (2).

2. **Lymph node biopsy.** If the laboratory testing is nondiagnostic, then lymph node biopsy should be considered if the enlarged lymph node persists for more than a month. The largest and most pathologic node should be removed. Axillary and inguinal nodes should be avoided, because they often reveal only reactive hyperplasia. Biopsy should be avoided in cases of suspected infectious mononucleosis and drug reaction because the histologic picture is easily confused with malignant lymphoma (2). Experienced hematologists or hematopathologists should handle all specimens. The value of fine needle aspiration is controversial, with reasonable arguments both for and against this procedure (5).

IV. **DIAGNOSIS.** The thorough history and examination should establish a differential diagnosis including infectious, autoimmune, granulomatous, and malignant etiologies. Investigation should be limited to specific diseases because generalized lymphadenopathy is often a sign of a specific systemic illness. In the event that the cause is unclear, infectious etiologies must be considered and a CBC and mononucleosis spot ordered. If these are negative, then immunologic and granulomatous etiologies are considered with serologic testing, a chest X-ray, and PPD. A lymph node biopsy must be considered in those cases where the node is rock hard or larger than 1.5 cm × 1.5 cm in size (1). Biopsy should be avoided in those cases in which viral causes are clinically suggested.

REFERENCES

1. Ferrer R. Lymphadenopathy: differential diagnosis and evaluation. *Am Fam Physician* 1998;58: 1313–1320.
2. Pangalis GA, Vassilalopoulos TP, Boussiotis VA, et al. Clinical approach to lymphadenopathy. *Semin Oncol* 1993;20:570–582.
3. Williamson HA. Lymphadenopathy in a family practice. *J Fam Pract* 1985;20:449–452.
4. Simon HB. Evaluation of lymphadenopathy. In: Goroll AH, Mulley AG, eds. *Primary care medicine: office evaluation and management of the adult patient,* 6th ed. Philadelphia, PA: JB Lippincott Williams & Wilkins, 2009:82-86.
5. Henry PH, Longo DL. Chapter 59. Enlargement of lymph nodes and spleen. In: Longo DL, Fauci AS, Kasper DL, Hauser SL, Jameson JL, Loscalzo J, eds. *Harrison's Principles of internal medicine.* 18th ed. New York, NY: McGraw-Hill; 2012. http://www.accessmedicine.com/content.aspx?aID=9113581.

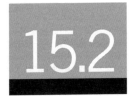

Lymphadenopathy, Localized

Kristy D. Edwards

I. BACKGROUND. Lymph nodes are normally palpated in children and may be normally felt in the neck, axilla, and inguinal regions of adults. Three-fourths of primary care patients presenting with unexplained lymph node enlargement have regional lymphadenopathy and less than 1% will have a malignancy (1). Localized or regional lymphadenopathy occurs when enlarged lymph nodes are identified in one anatomic location. The most common anatomic locations for localized lymphadenopathy are the head and neck (55%) and inguinal (14%) regions, but it may also be found in the axillary, epitrochlear, supraclavicular, and other regions. Once lymphadenopathy is identified, a complete lymph node examination should be performed to rule out generalized lymphadenopathy. A thorough history and physical examination including regions drained by the lymph nodes should be performed (2).

II. PATHOPHYSIOLOGY. The cause of localized lymphadenopathy can be separated by the age of the patient and its location. Reactive hyperplasia and benign etiologies make up 80% of the causes of lymphadenopathy in children and adults younger than 30 years of age. Older patients, especially those older than 40 years of age, are at increased risk for malignancy (3). In localized lymphadenopathy, the location can aid in determining a causative etiology. Knowledge of the patterns of lymphatic drainage and region-specific conditions is essential in the investigation of localized lymphadenopathy (4). The context in which lymphadenopathy occurs is very important in establishing a differential diagnosis. A detailed history including present illness, review of systems, past medical history, social history, and thorough physical examination of the region should be performed.

III. EVALUATION

　　A. History. It is important to elicit a detailed history. Lymphadenopathy that is present for months to years suggests underlying malignancy or systemic disease, whereas lymphadenopathy that is present for a few weeks is usually due to infectious etiologies. History of exposure to a cat scratch or sexually transmitted disease can explain lymphadenopathy in the axilla or inguinal regions. History of recent cold symptoms or local signs of redness, swelling, or discharge may suggest infection, whereas nonspecific signs of fever, chills, or night sweats may suggest systemic illness.

B. Physical examination. The examination of lymph nodes should include size, location, pain, consistency, and whether matting is present (2).

1. **Size.** As with generalized lymphadenopathy, lymph nodes >1 cm in diameter should arouse suspicion.

2. **Location.** The location of the abnormal lymph node helps focus the examination. A thorough examination of the anatomic region drained by the affected lymph node is of the highest yield for diagnosis. Cervical lymph nodes drain the oropharynx, tongue, and ears. Cervical lymphadenopathy without a known source should be treated with antibiotic coverage for *Staphylococcus aureus* and group A β hemolytic streptococci. However, bilateral cervical lymphadenopathy is often caused by viral or streptococcal pharyngitis (5). Lymphadenopathy in the neck posterior to the sternocleidomastoid muscle is a more ominous finding and warrants further evaluation (4). Palpated supraclavicular lymph nodes (SCLNs) are also worrisome. Left SCLNs drain intra-abdominal regions and right SCLNs drain the lungs, mediastinum, and the esophagus. Inguinal lymph nodes heighten the concern for venereal disease or lower extremity infection. Axillary lymph nodes suggest breast pathology or upper extremity infection. Other areas of lymphadenopathy, such as abdominal or mediastinal lymph nodes, may not be palpable but may be identified with radiologic studies.

3. **Pain.** Pain is often associated with lymphadenitis, tender, warm, soft, enlarged lymph nodes. This is usually a result of pyogenic infection (3).

4. **Consistency.** Consistency of lymph nodes is difficult to assess. Traditionally, firm and hard nodes are associated with malignancy and rubbery nodes suggest lymphoma. Matted or fixed nodes are particularly worrisome for metastatic disease (6).

C. Testing. Laboratory testing is often performed to uncover pathology involving the region of the body drained by the affected lymph nodes. For example, a monospot for Epstein-Barr virus or throat culture for streptococcal pharyngitis may be obtained in a patient with cervical lymphadenopathy. A mammogram may be ordered in older females with axillary lymphadenopathy. Screening for sexually transmitted diseases should be performed in patients with persistent inguinal lymphadenopathy. If the initial evaluation for localized lymphadenopathy does not reveal a diagnosis, it is usually acceptable to observe the patient for 2–4 weeks rather than perform unnecessary tests (7). Any testing performed should be specific to identify regional pathology. The test of choice is an excisional biopsy of the node or nodes involved when the diagnosis is unknown and a serious condition is suspected. Usually, the biopsy site is determined by location and size. Large nodes that have recently enlarged are preferred for biopsy (6).

IV. DIAGNOSIS. Localized lymphadenopathy is a common presenting complaint in clinical practice. Usually, a thorough history and physical examination lead to a diagnosis. If the diagnosis is not readily identifiable, then disease-specific tests may be helpful. Biopsy is a last resort if serious disease is suspected. Watchful waiting is acceptable and preferred as long as a serious condition is not suspected.

REFERENCES

1. Buis J. deJongh: Examining the lymph nodes. *Ned Tijdschr Geneeskd* 2001;155:A2652.
2. Ferrer R. Lymphadenopathy: differential diagnosis and evaluation. *Am Fam Physician* 1998;58: 1313–1320.
3. Simon HB. Evaluation of lymphadenopathy. In: Goroll AH, Mulley AG, eds. *Primary care medicine: office evaluation and management of the adult patient, 6th ed.* Philadelphia, PA: JB Lippincott Williams & Wilkins, 2009:82–86.
4. Sills R, Jorgensen S. Lymphadenopathy. *eMedicine* from WebMD. Available at: http://www.emedicine.com/ped/topic1333.htm. Last updated May 4, 2012.
5. Leung AK, Robson WL. Childhood cervical lymphadenopathy. *J Pediatr Health Care* 2004;18(1): 3–7.
6. Pangalis GA, Vassilalopoulos TP, Boussiotis VA, et al. Clinical approach to lymphadenopathy. *Semin Oncol* 1993;20:570–582.
7. Williamson HA. Lymphadenopathy in a family practice. *J Fam Pract* 1985;20:449–452.

15.3 Petechiae and Purpura

John L. Smith

I. BACKGROUND. Purpura are discolorations in the skin as a consequence of red blood cells extravasating into the skin or the mucous membranes. A petechia is a purpura that is <2 mm in diameter, and an ecchymosis is a purpura that is >1 cm in diameter.

II. PATHOPHYSIOLOGY. Petechiae most often result from a platelet disorder—either too few (usually <50,000/μL) or abnormally functioning platelets. Localized increases in intravascular pressure or capillaritis may also be responsible. Ecchymoses are usually due to a disorder in the coagulation cascade. Disorders of the vascular system as well as connective tissue disease can also occasionally result in purpura (1).

III. EVALUATION

A. History

1. A time sequence and past history of purpura as well as any indications of abnormal bleeding are important, because the cause of purpura can be either congenital or acquired. A recent viral or bacterial infection may affect platelets or the vessel integrity. Establish a history of easy or prolonged bleeding or bruising, or menorrhagia in women. von Willebrand's disease is the most common inherited disorder of hemostasis and occurs in up to 1% of the population. The disease is symptomatic in up to 10% of these (2). Ten to 20% of early-onset menorrhagia may be associated with an inherited bleeding disorder.

2. Although possible with many medications, drug-induced thrombocytopenia is an immune-mediated reaction. Trimethoprim-sulfamethoxazole and quinine have been most frequently reported as causative. Recovery begins within 1–2 days after withdrawal of the offending agent (3). A family history of inherited bleeding tendencies or indicators of liver disease may be clues to a coagulation disorder.

B. Physical examination. Initially, determining that the patient is stable and checking vital signs is imperative, because life-threatening causes of purpura such as disseminated intravascular coagulation (DIC), Rocky Mountain spotted fever, meningococcemia, sepsis from *Staphylococcus aureus*, and thrombotic thrombocytopenic purpura (TTP) may be present. Attention should then be directed at the purpuric lesions themselves and also at the location of the lesions. Palpable petechiae are seen with various forms of vasculitis. Purpura do not blanch like intravascular blood seen in angiomas, telangiectasias, and hyperemia. Purpura isolated to eyelids may be secondary to coughing, vomiting, or straining as in childbirth or weight lifting. Purpura limited to forearms are most likely secondary to poor stromal support as is frequently seen in senile purpura in the older population or those with much previous sun exposure. Facial or periorbital purpura may be secondary to cryoglobulinemia or amyloidosis.

C. Testing

1. Initial laboratory tests should include a complete blood count, platelet count, peripheral smear, prothrombin time (PT), and activated partial thromboplastin time (APTT). If these tests are normal, but the patient still has signs of bleeding, a bleeding time and von Willebrand's ristocetin cofactor activity may be appropriate as further evaluation of von Willebrand's disease and other platelet function abnormalities (4).

2. If the lesions are palpable, and vasculitis is a consideration, a sedimentation rate or C-reactive protein determination should be obtained.

3. In vasculitis, a skin biopsy may need to be obtained because the laboratory findings are often nonspecific.

4. Urinalysis and serum creatinine screen must be performed for any renal involvement and liver function tests for liver abnormalities.

D. Genetics. The multitude of disorders causing purpura may be acquired or congenital. Antibodies to factors in the coagulation cascade, as well as infectious diseases, and medications are examples of acquired abnormalities. Hereditary disorders are present with von Willebrand's disease and hemophilia.

IV. DIAGNOSIS

A. Differential diagnosis. The causes of purpuric lesions are numerous and have clinical implications, which may potentially be lethal. A thorough history and physical examination along with some basic laboratory studies and occasional skin biopsy are all that are frequently needed to establish a likely diagnosis.

1. In patients with isolated thrombocytopenia and prolonged bleeding time, idiopathic thrombocytopenic purpura is the probable diagnosis after ruling out drug-induced thrombocytopenia, human immunodeficiency virus infection, and pregnancy-induced thrombocytopenia.

2. An isolated increased APTT is seen in deficiencies or inhibitors of factors VIII, IX, and XI. A spontaneous factor VIII inhibitor can be seen in elderly patients with connective tissue disorders such as systemic lupus erythematosus and in postpartum women. von Willebrand's disease may have an increased bleeding time with an increased APTT (5). Heparin administration is included in the differential diagnosis.

3. An isolated PT elevation usually indicates a partial factor VII deficiency.

4. When the PT and APTT are both elevated, consider DIC, liver disease, vitamin K deficiency, and massive transfusion. Various deficiencies in the coagulation cascade are significantly less common.

5. In newborns with purpura, evaluation for sepsis, serologies for the TORCH (toxoplasmosis, other infections, rubella, cytomegalovirus infection, and herpes simplex syndrome), and coagulation factors are recommended. Purpura fulminans and leukemia are also included in the differential diagnosis (4).

B. Clinical Manifestations

1. In addition to those manifestations noted above, certain constellations of clinical and laboratory findings should be mentioned. TTP and hemolytic uremic syndrome (HUS) are seen in many clinical situations, including pregnancy, cancer, infections, and chemotherapy. The signs include the pentad of fever, thrombocytopenia, microangiopathic hemolytic anemia, hemorrhage (including purpura), and neurologic abnormalities. Because of serious consequences, diagnosis should be considered if thrombocytopenia and fragmented red blood cells are seen on the peripheral smear. TTP-HUS has a normal PT, APTT, and D-dimer as opposed to DIC.

2. With regard to coagulation factor abnormalities, hemophilia A and B can cause increased bruising and ecchymoses but not nearly as frequently as von Willebrand's disease. Patients with mild cases of von Willebrand's disease may have a normal bleeding time. Because this disease is caused by a glycoprotein that helps protect factor VIII from breakdown and interferes with platelet aggregation, the APTT is sometimes elevated. With the sudden onset of large ecchymoses and hematomas in an adult with normal platelets, an acquired factor VIII deficiency (autoantibody) should be investigated in cases of a prolonged PT and APTT.

3. Vasculitis causing palpable purpura in children is most common with Henoch-Schönlein purpura (6).

REFERENCES

1. Cox NH, Piette WW. Disorders of lymphatic vessels. In: Burns T, Breathnach S, Cox N, et al., eds. *Rook's textbook of dermatology*, 7th ed. Oxford: Blackwell Publishing, 2004.
2. Ewenstein B. von Willebrand's disease. *Annu Rev Med* 1997;48:525–542.
3. Drug Induced Thrombocytopenia: Pathogenesis, Evaluation, and Management. *Hematology* (ASH Education Program Book) Dec. 10, 2011;384–390.
4. Seligsohn U, Daushansky K. Classification, clinical Manifestations, and evaluation of disorders of hemostasis. In: Lichtman MA, Kipps TJ, et al. eds. *Williams hematology*, 8th ed. China: McGraw-Hill. 2010.
5. Schmaier A. Laboratory evaluation of hemostatic and thrombotic disorders. In: Hoffman R, ed. *Hematology: basic principles and practice*, 5th ed. Philadelphia, PA: Churchill Livingstone Elsevier, 2008.
6. Baselga E, Drolet BA, Esterly NB. Purpura in infants and children. *J Am Acad Dermatol* 1997;37:673–705.

15.4 Splenomegaly

Kimberly J. Jarzynka

I. BACKGROUND

A. Definition. Splenomegaly refers to the enlargement of the spleen to a craniocaudal measurement of 11–13 cm or more (1–3) or to a weight of >400–500 g. When the spleen reaches >20 cm in length or 1,000 g, it is termed *massive splenomegaly* (2).

B. Anatomy and physiology. The spleen is a reticuloendothelial organ located in the left upper quadrant of the abdomen at the level of the 9th to 11th ribs in the midaxillary line (3, 4). It lies adjacent to the diaphragm, stomach, splenic flexure of the colon, left kidney, and tail of the pancreas (3). The normal spleen typically weighs less than 250 g, measures less than 11–13 cm in greatest diameter (2, 4, 5), and is palpable in only 2–5% of the population (5). Essential functions of the spleen include the clearance of senescent and defective red blood cells, microorganisms, and other particulate matter from circulation (5) and iron recycling (red pulp) (6); generation of a cellular and humoral immune response (white pulp); extramedullary hematopoiesis; platelet and granulocyte sequestration; and some production of factor VIII and von Willebrand factor for hemostasis (6). As the spleen enlarges, it serves as a reservoir for blood volume and erythrocytes (6).

II. PATHOPHYSIOLOGY

A. Etiology. Enlarged spleen is not a disease state in itself, but usually indicates the underlying pathology (6). The many causes of splenomegaly can be grouped into the following categories: anatomic, hematologic, infectious, immunologic, neoplastic, infiltrative, and congestive. *Anatomic* abnormalities causing splenomegaly are typically developmental, such as hamartomas and cysts. *Hematologic* causes (due to "work hypertrophy") result from the normal sequestration of increased amounts of abnormal or lysed blood cells or from extramedullary hematopoiesis. *Infectious* causes include bacteria, mycobacteria, spirochetes, viruses, rickettsia, fungi, and parasites. *Immunologic* splenomegaly is due to reticuloendothelial cell proliferation and lymphoid hyperplasia from an increase in the antigen clearance and antibody production. This occurs in collagen vascular diseases, immunodeficiencies, and immune/inflammatory responses. *Neoplastic* causes include primary or metastatic malignancies. Macrophages can become engorged with indigestible material, which causes *infiltrative* splenomegaly. Increased venous pressure results in *congestive* splenomegaly (1, 6).

B. Epidemiology. Epidemiologic data depend on the primary etiology (1, 5–7).

III. EVALUATION

A. History. A thorough past medical, family, and social history including a history of recent travel can often reveal a possible cause of splenomegaly. Splenomegaly itself is often asymptomatic. However, symptoms of vague, colicky left upper quadrant pain and fullness, early satiety, and pain while lying on the side may be present (5, 7). Acute pleuritic left upper quadrant pain which sometimes radiates to the left shoulder can suggest perisplenitis, splenic abscess, infarction, or rupture (7). Hyperplastic splenomegaly is often associated with symptoms of cytopenia including pallor, dyspnea, easy bruising, or petechial rash (1). Other historic clues and symptoms related to the primary illness causing splenomegaly may be present.

B. Physical examination

1. Examination of the spleen is performed with the patient supine, lying at a slight incline, and/or in the right lateral decubitus position with the knees, hips, and neck flexed and the arms down at the sides. From the patient's right side, lightly palpate under the left

costal margin with the right hand while lifting the left costovertebral angle with the left hand. During deep inspiration, palpate gently inward toward the descending spleen. It is often necessary to also palpate from the left lower quadrant up toward the costal margin, as well as in the midline, to identify the lower pole and medial border of a severely enlarged spleen (4–8). The ability to palpate the spleen usually suggests splenomegaly, although 2–5% of normal spleens are palpable (5,6).

2. Dullness to percussion in the lowest intercostal space in the anterior axillary line on full inspiration and expiration suggests splenomegaly (Castell's method) (4,5).

3. Findings of splenomegaly on physical examination are recorded in centimeters below the left costal margin at a point specified by the examiner (i.e., in the midclavicular line) (6–8).

4. A venous hum or friction rub may be present (5,7).

5. With a massively enlarged spleen, left upper quadrant fullness that descends on inspiration may be present upon abdominal inspection (5).

6. Examine the skin for signs of pallor, petechiae, and bruising (secondary to hypersplenism) (1).

7. Other physical examination is directed at identifying the potential etiology of splenomegaly (4).

C. Testing

1. Complete blood count with differential and platelet count: variable results.

2. Peripheral smear: Howell-Jolly bodies (nuclear remnants); pappenheimer bodies (siderotic granules); acanthocytes and target cells; >2% pitted or pocketed erythrocytes (all are normally removed from circulation by a functioning spleen) (6).

3. Appropriate lab tests to determine primary disease: as directed by other historic and clinical findings. Consider the following for initial evaluation: liver function tests, erythrocyte sedimentation rate, C-reactive protein, clotting screen, electrolytes, renal function, monospot, hepatitis serology, antinuclear antibody (ANA), rheumatoid factor, vitamin B12, and folate (1); further testing in selected patients depending on clinical features.

D. Imaging studies

1. Ultrasound for initial evaluation: to evaluate size, shape, and other aspects of splenic anatomy, including the presence of cysts and abscesses (3,6).

2. Computed tomography (CT) for more detailed evaluation: better for detecting lesions, masses, inflammation, or accessory spleens. CT can be used to direct therapeutic intervention, i.e., CT-guided drainage of cysts, abscesses, hematomas, etc. It is the study of choice for diagnosing splenic lacerations or hematomas in the setting of trauma (3).

3. Magnetic resonance imaging: useful for identifying vascular lesions (which would otherwise require angiography) and splenic infections and to obtain quantitative measurement of iron burden (3,6).

4. Radionucleotide scans: to determine spleen size and function and to detect focal lesions, accessory spleens, and portal hypertension (3,6).

5. Positron emission tomography scan: to diagnose, stage, and monitor lymphomas and other diseases with splenic involvement (3,6).

6. Angiography for detecting circulation abnormalities (3).

E. Genetics. Splenomegaly itself has no genetic link. However, many of the primary diseases that cause splenomegaly do (e.g., hereditary spherocytosis) (1,5–7).

IV. DIAGNOSIS

A. Differential diagnosis. The differential diagnosis of diseases causing splenomegaly is presented in Table 15.4.1.

B. Clinical manifestations. Hypersplenism is an increase in normal splenic function associated with splenomegaly. It results in varying degrees of anemia, leukopenia, and/or thrombocytopenia due to the increased destruction and sequestration of cells. The bone marrow is either normal or hyperplastic, and improvement in cell counts is seen postsplenectomy (5). Other clinical manifestations depend on the primary etiology.

TABLE 15.4.1 Differential Diagnosis of Splenomegaly (1,5–7)

Anatomic	Cysts, pseudocysts, hamartomas, peliosis, hemangiomas, fibromas, lymphangiomas
Hematologic	Sickle cell anemia, thalassemia major, ovalocytosis, spherocytosis, elliptocytosis, HbSC disease, and other hemoglobinopathies; paroxysmal nocturnal hemoglobinuria; nutritional anemias; myeloproliferative diseases/myelodysplasias; myelofibrosis; polycythemia vera; essential thrombocytosis; osteopetrosis; marrow damage by toxins, radiation, or strontium
Infectious	(Bacteria) Acute and chronic systemic infection, abscess, subacute bacterial endocarditis; (mycobacterial) miliary tuberculosis; (spirochetes) congenital syphilis, Lyme disease, leptospirosis; (viruses) Epstein-Barr virus, cytomegalovirus, human immunodeficiency virus, viral hepatitis; (rickettsia) Rocky Mountain spotted fever, Q fever, typhus, ehrlichiosis, cat scratch disease; (fungi) disseminated candidiasis, histoplasmosis, blastomycosis; (parasites) toxoplasmosis, malaria, babesiosis, toxocara canis/cati, leishmaniasis, schistosomiasis, trypanosomiasis
Immunologic	Rheumatoid arthritis (Felty's syndrome), systemic lupus erythematosus, mixed connective tissue disorder, systemic vasculitis, Sjogren syndrome, systemic mastocytosis, common variable immunodeficiency, other collagen vascular diseases, autoimmune hemolytic anemias, immune thrombocytopenias, immune neutropenias, graft-versus-host disease, serum sickness, LGL lymphocytosis, Weber Christian histiocytoses, Langerhans cell histiocytosis, sarcoidosis, berylliosis, drug/toxin reactions, angioimmunoblastic
Neoplastic	Lymphomas, leukemias, metastatic tumors from skin (melanoma), breast, lung, ovary and colon; angiosarcomas
Infiltrative	Hyperlipidemias, amyloidosis, Gaucher's disease, Niemann-Pick disease, Tangier disease, histiocytosis X, Hurler's syndrome and other mucopolysaccharidoses; eosinophilic granulomas. Berylliosis, glycogen storage disease type IV, Wolman disease, hyperchylomicronemia type I and IV
Congestive	Hepatic, portal, and splenic vein obstruction; congestive heart failure, cirrhosis, splenic artery aneurysm, hepatic schistosomiasis, hepatic echinococcosis; portal hypertension of any etiology
Other	Tropical splenomegaly, hyperthyroidism

REFERENCES

1. Pozo AL, Godfrey EM, Bowles KM. Splenomegaly: investigation, diagnosis and management. *Blood Rev* 2009;23(3):105–111.
2. Motykova G, Steensma DP. Why does my patient have lymphadenopathy or splenomegaly? *Hematol Oncol Clin N Am* 2012;26(2):395–408.
3. Aslam S, Sohaib A, Reznek RH. Reticuloendothelial disorders: the spleen. In: Adam ed. *Grainger & Allison's diagnostic radiology,* 5th ed. London: Churchill Livingstone, An Imprint of Elsevier, 2008;1759–1770.
4. Brown NF, Marks DJ, Smith PJ, Bloom SL. Splenomegaly. *Br J Hosp Med (Lond)* 2011;72(11):M166–M169.
5. Henry PH, Longo DL. Enlargement of lymph nodes and spleen. In: Longo DL, Fauci AS, Kasper DL, Hauser SL, Jameson JL, Loscalzo J, eds. *Harrison's principles of internal medicine,* 18th ed. New York, NY: McGraw-Hill, 2012.
6. Shurin SB. The spleen and its disorders. In: Hoffman ed. *Hematology: basic principles and practice,* 5th ed. London: Churchill Livingstone, An Imprint of Elsevier, 2008;2419–2429.
7. Armitage JO. Approach to the patient with lymphadenopathy and splenomegaly. In: Goldman ed. *Goldman's cecil medicine,* 24th ed. Philadelphia, PA: Saunders, An Imprint of Elsevier, 2011;1107–1111.
8. LeBlond RF, DeGowin RL, Brown DD. The abdomen, perineum, anus, and rectosigmoid. In: LeBlond RF, DeGowin RL, Brown DD, eds. *DeGowin's diagnostic examination,* 9th ed. New York, NY: McGraw-Hill, 2009;445–526.

CHAPTER **16**

Laboratory Abnormalities: Hematology and Urine Determinations

Carol A. LaCroix

16.1

Anemia
Carol A. LaCroix

I. **BACKGROUND.** Anemia, simply put, is too few red blood cells (RBCs). In men, it is usually defined as hemoglobin <13.5 g/dL or a hematocrit <41.0% and in women as hemoglobin <12.0 g/dL or a hematocrit <36.0% (1). It is important to remember that anemia is only a symptom of a disease, not the disease itself. Whenever anemia is found, the cause must be sought.

II. **PATHOPHYSIOLOGY.** The causes for anemia can be broken down into three main categories:
   A. **Decreased Production.** Anemia results when the rate of RBC production is less than the rate of RBC destruction. Decreased production may be due to many causes, including lack of nutrients. Decreased intake or malabsorption of nutrients such as iron, vitamin B12, or folate may cause decreased RBC production. A bone marrow disorder such as aplastic anemia, myelodysplasia, or tumor infiltration may decrease RBC production as well. Patients who are undergoing chemotherapy or radiation may have bone marrow suppression (2–4).
   B. **Increased RBC Destruction.** The normal RBC life span is 120 days; certain situations may decrease the survival of RBCs. Hemolytic anemia is the result of increased RBC destruction. There are hereditary causes of hemolytic anemia, including hereditary spherocytosis, sickle cell anemia, and thalassemia. Acquired hemolytic anemias include autoimmune, thrombotic thrombocytopenic purpura, and hemolytic uremic syndrome (2–4).
   C. **Blood Loss.** Blood loss is by far the most common cause of anemia. Sometimes, the source of bleeding may be obvious, such as in a trauma, or it may be occult such as in a gastrointestinal bleed. In women, menstrual bleeding should always be considered (2–4).

III. **EVALUATION**
   A. **History.** A thorough history should include questions regarding symptoms such as fatigue, light-headedness, fever, weight loss, and night sweats. A gynecologic history should be taken in women. Patients should be asked whether they have ever been anemic before or have a family history of anemia or bleeding disorders. A nutritional history should also be obtained to evaluate for possible malnutrition; this is especially important in elderly and alcoholic patients. Concomitant conditions that may also contribute to the development of anemia include renal failure, cancer treatment, and immunosuppression. A thorough medication history should also be taken; any herbal supplements taken by the patient should be noted (2–4).
   B. **Physical Examination.** Pertinent findings include pallor of the skin and conjunctivae. The skin or sclera may be discolored due to jaundice. Petechiae may indicate a platelet

abnormality as well. Cardiovascular examination may reveal a systolic flow murmur or tachycardia. Abdominal examination may be significant for splenomegaly, which may suggest a lymphoproliferative disorder (2–4).

C. **Testing.** A complete blood count (CBC) is essential. This not only gives the value of hemoglobin and hematocrit but also gives the white blood cell count and platelet count. These are important in the evaluation of pancytopenia. The CBC should also include the mean corpuscular volume (MCV), which indicates the average size of the RBCs and helps with diagnosis. Additional testing may include iron studies: ferritin, total iron-binding capacity (TIBC), and percent iron saturation. Vitamin deficiencies may be evaluated by vitamin B12 and RBC folate levels. A reticulocyte count is also helpful in determining whether the bone marrow is responding appropriately to the level of anemia. If a hereditary disorder is suspected, hemoglobin electrophoresis may be required. A peripheral blood smear is also helpful in many cases (2–4).

IV. DIAGNOSIS

A. The simplest way to determine the diagnosis in anemia is to follow a three-step approach.
1. **Step One.** Categorize the anemia as microcytic, normocytic, or macrocytic on the basis of the MCV (see Table 16.1.1).
2. **Step Two.** Determine whether pancytopenia is present. If there is also a decrease in the number of white blood cells and platelets, this indicates a depression of all cell lines produced by bone marrow. If pancytopenia is found, a bone marrow examination is almost always necessary.
3. **Step Three.** Determine a cause for the anemia by evaluating the reticulocyte count. This value helps determine whether the bone marrow response to the anemia is appropriate (2–4).

B. **Differential Diagnosis**
1. **Microcytic Anemias**
   a. **Anemia of chronic disease.** Decreased iron and decreased TIBC; increased ferritin.
   b. **Sideroblastic anemia.** Increased iron and normal TIBC; increased ferritin. Peripheral smear shows basophilic stippling and ringed sideroblasts.
   c. **Iron deficiency anemia.** Decreased iron and increased TIBC. Ferritin <12 μg/L is very suggestive of iron deficiency.
   d. **Thalassemia.** Very low MCV (usually <70 fL); normal iron studies. The peripheral smear may reveal basophilic stippling. Hemoglobin electrophoresis is needed for diagnosis (2–4).

TABLE 16.1.1	Etiology of Anemia Based on Mean Corpuscular Volume (4)		
Mean Corpuscular Volume (fL)	**<80**	**80–100**	**>100**
Possible etiology	Iron deficiency	Acute hemorrhage	Vitamin B12 deficiency
	Thalassemia	Chronic renal insufficiency	Folate deficiency
	Myelodysplastic syndrome		Sickle cell disease
		Chronic disease	Reticulocytosis
	Sideroblastic anemia	Iron deficiency (early)	Liver disease
	Chronic disease		Endocrine dysfunction
			Alcohol abuse

2. **Normocytic Anemias**
   a. **Hemorrhage.** Look for source of blood loss. Perform a hemoccult of the stool
   b. **Glucose-6-phosphate deficiency.**
   c. **Autoimmune hemolytic anemia.** Positive Coombs
   d. **Membranopathies.** Hereditary spherocytosis with splenomegaly may be present on physical examination (2–4)
3. **Macrocytic Anemias**
   a. **Vitamin B12 or folate deficiency.** Low serum vitamin B12 and folate levels. The peripheral smear reveals hypersegmented neutrophils. Vitamin B12 deficiency may also have neurologic findings.
   b. **Liver disease.** Elevated liver function tests, aspartate aminotransferase, and alanine aminotransferase. The peripheral smear may reveal target and spur cells (2–5).

REFERENCES

1. Beutler E, Waalen J. The definition of anemia: what is the lower limit of normal of the blood hemoglobin concentration? *Blood* 2006;107:1747.
2. Tefferi A. Anemia in adults: a contemporary approach to diagnosis. *Mayo Clin Proc* 2003:78;1274–1280.
3. Hillman RS, Ault KA, eds. Clinical approach to anemia. In: *Hematology in clinical practice*. New York, NY: McGraw Hill, 2001:29.
4. Schrier, SL. Approach to the adult patient with anemia. *UpToDate* May 21, 2012, Topic 7133, Version 13.0.
5. Davenport J. Macrocytic anemia. *Am Fam Physician* 1996;53:155.

16.2 Eosinophilia

Carol A. LaCroix

I. BACKGROUND. Eosinophilia refers to an elevated eosinophil count. It occurs in a wide variety of diseases, ranging from allergic to infectious to neoplastic to idiopathic causes. These range in severity from self-limited to life threatening. Eosinophilia in the blood can be classified as mild (350–1,500 eosinophils/μL), moderate (1,500–5,000 cells/μL), or severe (greater than 5,000 cells/μL). Hypereosinophilia refers to counts of 1500 or higher (1). Hypereosinophilic syndrome (HES) currently is defined as eosinophil count over 1500/μL without discernible evidence of a secondary cause. Previously the definition required the presence of eosinophilia for more than 6 months and evidence of end-organ damage (2).

II. PATHOPHYSIOLOGY
   A. Etiology
   1. Eosinophils develop from myeloid precursors in the bone marrow through the action of at least three hematopoietic cytokines. Interleukin-5 (IL-5) is specific for eosinophil differentiation. Recent research has focused on why the dysregulated overproduction of eosinophils occurs. Eosinophilic infiltration and release of mediators often cause organ damage. Generally, the concentration of eosinophils is much higher in the tissues of the host than it is in the peripheral blood, so end-organ effects must be monitored (2).
   2. The causes have been divided into primary, secondary, and idiopathic.
      The most common secondary causes are allergic, infectious, and neoplastic (1). The idiopathic group is a heterogeneous group called HESs. It is subdivided into six variants: myeloproliferative forms, lymphocytic forms, familial, overlap, associated, and undefined (2).
   B. Epidemiology. In the United States, the most common cause of eosinophilia is allergic diseases. In developing countries, parasites are the most common etiology (3).

III. EVALUATION

A. History. Travel history, medications, family history, and review of systems are especially important (3).

B. Physical. Patients with HES may have physical findings involving the skin, lungs, heart, gastrointestinal tract, and the nervous system. Skin problems include eczema, erythroderma, recurrent urticaria, and angioedema. The main pulmonary complaints are cough and breathlessness. Gastrointestinal problems may cause abdominal pain, weight loss, vomiting, or diarrhea. Cardiac involvement results in necrosis followed by fibrosis and can be a major cause of morbidity. Neurologic manifestations may include cerebral emboli, encephalopathy, or peripheral neuropathy (2).

C. Testing. Because eosinophilia in the peripheral blood can be sporadic, more than one CBC may be needed to verify the degree of severity.

1. If allergic conditions are suspected, obtain nasal smear and sputum for eosinophils.

2. If parasites are suspected, workup begins with three stool specimens for ova and parasites. If these are not diagnostic, consider serology as indicated, urinalysis for schistosome eggs, and biopsy of the small bowel or muscle for trichinosis.

3. To assess end-organ involvement, obtain blood chemistries, especially liver enzymes, creatine kinase, renal function, and troponin. Electrocardiogram, echocardiogram, and chest X-ray help screen for cardiac and pulmonary involvement. CT scan of the chest or abdomen may identify tumors.

4. Bone marrow biopsy should be done to evaluate for clonal disorders.

D. Referral. Identifying the diagnosis for the eosinophilia is important because the treatment and prognosis vary greatly, depending on the cause. If the diagnosis remains elusive after workup, consider referral to a specialist in hematology or infectious disease (3).

IV. DIAGNOSIS

A. Differential Diagnosis

1. **Primary**. Included are acute leukemias and chronic myeloid disorders which have evidence of clonal expansion. Acute eosinophilic leukemia has a chromosomal 16 abnormality involving FAB M4. Other cancers involve abnormalities of interleukin 3 and 5 (3).

2. **Secondary**

   a. Infection

      i. Tissue-invasive parasites: Eosinophilia is most likely when the helminthic larvae or adults are migrating within the tissues of the host. Screen for *Strongyloides stercoralis*, hookworm, filariae, and *Toxocara canis*. Single-cell protozoans, such as *Giardia lamblia* and *Entamoeba histolytica*, do not cause eosinophilia. However, two significant exceptions are *Dientamoeba fragilis* and *Isospora belli*. Serologic tests are available for Trichinella, Wuchereria, Toxocara, Schistosoma, and Echinococcus.

      ii. Fungal: Aspergillosis and coccidiomycosis.

      iii. Viral: Viral infections cause eosinopenia except for the retroviruses. Screen for HIV-1, Human T lymphotropic virus (HTLV-1), and especially HTLV-2.

   b. Allergic disorders: atopic dermatitis, asthma, and rhinitis. Eosinophilia of both blood and sputum occurs with asthma. Differential includes COPD and eosinophilic bronchitis. Nasal eosinophilia is seen with allergic rhinitis but is not diagnostic.

   c. Drug reactions

   d. Vasculitis. Churg-Strauss syndrome (allergic granulomatosis)

   e. Cancers such as lymphomas where there is eosinophilia but no clonal disorder. Systemic mastocytosis

   f. Adrenal insufficiency: Addison's disease *or* a relative deficiency of cortisol

   g. Autoimmune diseases (3)

3. **Idiopathic.** Hypereosinophilic syndromes

   a. T-cell lymphocytic variants (L-HES): Skin problems, polyclonal hypergammaglobulinemia due to aberrant IL-5 producing T cells

   b. Myeloproliferative variants (M-LES): Elevated serum B12, elevated serum tryptase, and hepato- or splenomegaly. Chromosomal abnormality called F1P1L1-PDGRFalpha fusion. Occurs almost exclusively in males

  c. Familial: Autosomal dominant (5q 31–33)

  d. Undefined: Ranges from benign to complex to episodic involvement May have episodic angioedema

  e. Overlap: Eosinophilia affects only one organ, such as chronic eosinophilic pneumonia and eosinophilic gastrointestinal disease

  f. Associated: Eosinophilia is due to a second disease such as ulcerative colitis, sarcoid, or collagen vascular disease (2–5).

REFERENCES

1. Tefferi A. Blood eosinophilia: a new paradigm in disease classification, diagnosis, and treatment. *Mayo Clin Pro* 2005;80:75–83.
2. Roufosse F, Klion AD, Weller PF. Clinical manifestations, pathophysiology, and diagnosis of the hypereosinophilic syndromes. *Up To Date* Topic 2211, version 8.0. January 25, 2012. 23 pages.
3. Weller, PF. Approach to the patient with eosinophilia. *Up To Date* Topic 7133, Version 13.0. April 27, 2011.
4. Simon HU, Rothenberg ME, Bochner BS, et al. Refining the definition of hypereosinophilic syndrome. *J Allergy Clin Immunol* 2010;126:45.
5. Swerdlow SH, Campo E, Harris NL, et al. *World Health Organization classification of tumours of haematopoietic and lymphoid tissues*. Lyon: IARC Press, 2008.

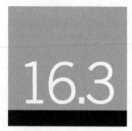

Erythrocyte Sedimentation Rate and C-Reactive Protein

16.3

Elisabeth L. Backer

I. BACKGROUND. The erythrocyte sedimentation rate (ESR) and C-reactive protein (CRP) are currently the most widely used indicators of the acute-phase protein response used to detect illnesses associated with acute and chronic infection, inflammation, trauma, tissue destruction, infarction, and advanced neoplasm. The CRP test is a more sensitive and rapidly responding indicator than the ESR, often showing an earlier and more intense increase than the ESR in an acute inflammatory process. With recovery, the disappearance of the CRP precedes the normalization of the ESR (1).

II. PATHOPHYSIOLOGY. The acute-phase response is a major pathophysiologic phenomenon that accompanies inflammation and other disorders (2). Focus on this phenomenon first occurred with the discovery of elevated serum concentrations of CRP during the acute phase of pneumococcal pneumonia (3). The initial concept of an ESR dates back to 1918. The Westergren method is still considered the gold standard for measuring the ESR (4).

III. EVALUATION

  A. History and Physical Examination. Acute-phase reactant measurements are useful in conjunction with a thorough history and physical examination. Since the ESR and CRP levels are influenced by multiple factors, the results should be interpreted in the light of the clinical findings.

  B. Testing

    1. The ESR, which measures the distance in millimeters that erythrocytes fall during 1 hour, is a simple but nonspecific lab test ordered frequently in clinical practice. The CRP is a nonspecific (3) acute-phase reactant protein used to diagnose infectious and inflammatory disorders; it also serves as a cardiovascular disease (CVD) marker (5). The ESR has the advantages of familiarity, simplicity, and extensive literature compiled over many decades (3). The CRP test is standardized, inexpensive, and widely available. High-sensitivity CRP does not differ from CRP, but refers to the assay used, which is capable of measuring very low levels of CRP.

2. Although elevations in multiple components of the acute-phase response commonly occur together, not all happen uniformly in all patients, and discrepancies between ESR and CRP are found fairly frequently (2) (e.g., an elevated ESR together with a normal CRP may reflect a false-positive value for the ESR; in lupus, the CRP response, but not the ESR, may be muted). Currently, the optimal use of acute-phase reactants may be to obtain several measurements and interpret the results in light of the clinical context (3,5).

IV. DIAGNOSIS

A. Differential Diagnosis

1. CRP levels can be affected by lifestyle choices, concurrent disease, pharmacotherapy, age, gender (female), and possibly ethnicity (e.g., African Americans).

   a. Factors known to increase CRP values include smoking, elevated body mass index, elevated blood pressure, dyslipidemia, metabolic syndrome, type 2 diabetes, hormone use, chronic infections (bronchitis), and chronic inflammations (rheumatoid arthritis) (5).

   b. Factors known to decrease CRP values include moderate alcohol consumption, physical exercise, weight loss, and medications (statins, fibrates, thiazolidinediones, anti-inflammatory agents, salicylates, and steroids) (5).

2. ESR levels can be affected by menstruation and pregnancy, hematologic disorders, medications, gender, age, ethnicity, and obesity (1,3). Conditions with an ESR > 100 mm/h include abscess formation, subacute bacterial endocarditis, osteomyelitis, temporal arteritis, collagen vascular disease, multiple myeloma, leukemia/lymphoma, neoplasms, and drug hypersensitivity reactions.

   a. Factors known to increase ESR values include chronic renal failure (nephritis, nephrosis), macroglobulinemia, hyperfibrinogenemia, iron/B12 deficiency anemias, medications (dextran, heparin, methyldopa, oral contraceptives, penicillamine, procainamide, theophylline, vitamin A), female gender, advanced age, African American ethnicity, and hyperlipidemia (1).

   b. Factors known to decrease ESR levels include sickle cell anemia, spherocytosis, hypofibrinogenemia, polycythemia vera, medications (aspirin, cortisone, quinine), and chronic heart failure (1).

B. Clinical Manifestations

1. Despite the lack of diagnostic specificity, measuring acute-phase protein levels is useful in differentiating between inflammatory and non-inflammatory conditions and in evaluating the response to and need for therapeutic interventions. In general, the ESR increases as the disease worsens and decreases as it improves. Whereas the ESR changes relatively slowly, the CRP concentration does so more rapidly. The CRP may be useful when the ESR is equivocal or inconsistent with the clinical impressions (1). Results should be expressed as the average of two tests performed 2 weeks apart. Patients with levels above 10 mg/L should be examined for sources of inflammation before repeating the test (5). Acute-phase reactants should not be ordered for screening purposes in asymptomatic patients (1).

   a. Normal ESR rates for men between the ages of 20 and 65 years can be empirically calculated as age/2; for women, it would be (age plus 10)/2 (1). Most normal subjects have a CRP level of <3 mg/L. Levels of 3-10 mg/L may indicate minor degrees of inflammation or other influences, such as metabolic dysfunction, obesity, and insulin resistance. Levels >10 mg/L suggest significant inflammation (3) or infections, especially of bacterial origin.

   b. CRP testing is also recommended as an adjunct to traditional risk factor assessment in CVD. It has been found to be the strongest marker for future CVD, de novo atherosclerosis, and plaque rupture. Additionally, it has independent prognostic value for future strokes and peripheral vascular disease (5). The relative risk category based on CRP levels is shown in Table 16.3.1.

TABLE 16.3.1	Risk of Cardiovascular Disease Based on C-Reactive Protein (CRP) Level
Risk	**CRP level (mg/L)**
Low	<1
Average	1.0–3.0
High	>3.0

2. Specific applications of acute-phase reactant measurements include monitoring of disease processes such as Crohn's disease, rheumatoid arthritis (CRP superior to ESR), polymyalgia rheumatica and giant cell arteritis (ESR often above 100 mm/h, but CRP may be more sensitive for disease detection), and the noninvasive prognostic assessment in patients with malignancy (3). Systemic lupus erythematosus represents an exception in that CRP levels are often not elevated, except during bacterial infections (3).

REFERENCES

1. Pagana KD, Pagana TJ. *Mosby's manual of diagnostic and laboratory tests.* St. Louis, MO: Mosby, 1998.
2. Kushner I. The phenomenon of the acute phase response. *Ann N Y Acad Sci* 1982;389:39–48.
3. www.UpToDate.com. Accessed April 27, 2012.
4. Bedell SE, Bush BT. Erythrocyte sedimentation rate. From folklore to facts. *Am J Med* 1985;78(6 Pt 1): 1001–1009.
5. Brunton S. The value of C-reactive protein in the clinical assessment of cardiovascular disease risk. *Female Patient* 2005;30:11–16.

16.4 Neutropenia
Anna Maruska

I. BACKGROUND. Neutropenia is defined as an absolute neutrophil count (ANC) of <1,500 cells/μL. Severe neutropenia is defined as an ANC of <500 cells/μL. The risk of infection increases with levels <1,000 cells/μL and is dependent on the cause and length of the neutropenia. As the ANC only represents 3% of the body's neutrophils, neutropenia in the presence of preserved marrow function poses a decreased risk of infection. Infection in severe neutropenia is most commonly caused by normal flora (1–3).

II. PATHOPHYSIOLOGY
  A. Etiology. Neutropenia may be congenital or acquired. Three basic processes leading to acquired neutropenia include (a) decreased production, (b) enhanced peripheral destruction, and (c) pooling of neutrophils in the vascular endothelium or tissue. Infection most commonly causes acquired neutropenia (2).
  B. Epidemiology. ANC may vary by race and ethnicity. Blacks and some Jewish populations may normally have ANCs as low as 1,500/μL and have no clinical manifestations (1,3).

III. EVALUATION
  A. History. A history of frequent or recurrent infections should be elicited, as well as symptoms of fevers, chills, night sweats, easy bleeding or bruising, and unintended weight loss.

Race, ethnicity, prior and current medications, alcohol abuse, toxin exposure, and family history should be sought (1).

B. Physical Examination. The oral cavity should be explored, as gingivitis and stomatitis may be the first presenting symptoms of neutropenia. Splenomegaly and lymphadenopathy may be present. In children, evidence of failure to thrive may indicate a congenital disorder. Examine sinuses, ears, and the perirectal area for active infection (1,2).

C. Testing. A manual differential and peripheral blood smear confirm the diagnosis of neutropenia. If pancytopenia exists, a bone marrow biopsy is required. If the patient has mild neutropenia and an absence of infection, ANC measurements up to three times per week may be performed to monitor for resolution or to diagnose cyclic neutropenia (2). If counts normalize, surveillance for the next year should include a complete blood count at the first sign of infection to look for recurrence. If neutropenia fails to resolve after 8 weeks, recurrent infections develop, or lower ANC ($<1,000/\mu L$) counts are noted, further workup is needed. Additional laboratory tests may include bone marrow biopsy (even if not pancytopenic), antinuclear antibodies, complement levels, rheumatoid factor, antineutrophil antibodies, reticulocyte count, lactate dehydrogenase, erythrocyte sedimentation rate, thyroid-stimulating hormone, immunoglobulins, human immunodeficiency virus serology, vitamin B12 and folate levels, and bone marrow culture (1,2).

D. Genetics. Hereditary neutropenia is rare. Two main forms include cyclic neutropenia and severe congenital neutropenia (Kostmann's syndrome). *ELA2* and *HAX1* gene mutations have been linked to these disorders (4).

IV. DIAGNOSIS

A. Differential Diagnosis. See Table 16.4.1.

TABLE 16.4.1	Differential Diagnosis of Neutropenia	
Acquired Neutropenia		**Congenital Neutropenia**
Infectious		
EBV, HBV, CMV, parvo virus, varicella, measles, HIV, any infection causing sepsis, TB, tularemia, ehrlichiosis, rickettsia		Ethnic neutropenia
Medication induced		
Clozapine, sulfasalazine, thioamides		Severe congenital neutropenia
Chronic idiopathic neutropenia		Cyclic neutropenia
Primary immune		
Antineutrophilic antibodies, seen in children		Shwachman-Diamond syndrome
Secondary Immune		
RA, SLE, hyperthyroid, Felty syndrome, Wegener's granulomatosis		Fanconi anemia
Malignant		
MDS, leukemia		Chédiak-Higashi syndrome
Nutritional deficiency		
B12, folate, copper		Barth's syndrome
Hypersplenism (sequestration)		X-linked neutropenia

CMV, cytomegalovirus; EBV, Epstein-Barr virus; HBV, hepatitis B virus; HIV, human immunodeficiency virus; MDS, myelodysplastic syndrome; RA, rheumatoid arthritis; SLE, systemic lupus erythematosus; TB, tuberculosis.

Information pooled from references 1–4.

B. Clinical Manifestations. Signs and symptoms are generally based on the underlying etiology of neutropenia; however, moderate to severe neutropenia may present with recurrent infection. The inflammatory response is blunted, decreasing radiographic signs, peritoneal signs, pyuria, or pyrexia. As a result, the patient's infection may go undetected until late in the course (3).

V. TREATMENT

A. Initial Treatment. Fever and neutropenia warrant immediate treatment with empiric antibiotics (2,5).

B. Risk Assessment. Determination of patient risk will determine inpatient versus outpatient and oral versus parenteral treatment. Patients with brief durations of neutropenia (<7 days) and no comorbidities are generally considered low risk. Patients with longer durations of neutropenia, comorbidities, ANCs <100 cells/µL, or neutropenia due to chemotherapy are considered high risk (5).

C. Prophylaxis. Prophylactic fluoroquinolone administration is indicated in high-risk patients (2,5).

D. Long-Term Therapy. Treatment with granulocyte colony-stimulating factor (G-CSF) is indicated in severe congenital neutropenias and chemotherapy-induced neutropenia. Stem cell transplants may offer curative treatment for those who respond poorly to G-CSF (2,4).

REFERENCES

1. Reagan JL, Castillo JJ. Why is my patient neutropenic? *Hematol Oncol Clin North Am* 2012;26(2): 253–266.
2. Bonilla MA. Neutropenia. In: *Bope and Kellerman: Conn's current therapy 2012.* St. Louis, MO: W.B. Saunders, 2012:825–827.
3. Berliner N. Leukocytosis and leukopenia. In: *Goldman: Goldman's Cecil medicine.* St. Louis, MO: W.B. Saunders, 2011:1101–1106.
4. Boztug K, Welte K, Zeidler C, Klein C. Congenital neutropenia syndromes. *Immunol Allergy Clin North Am* 2008;28:259–275.
5. Freifeld AG, Bow EJ, Sepkowitz KA, et al. Clinical practice guideline for the use of antimicrobials in neutropenic patients with cancer: 2010 Update by the Infectious Diseases Society of America. *Clin Infect Dis* 2011;52:56–93.

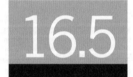

Polycythemia

Carol A. LaCroix

I. BACKGROUND. Polycythemia is defined as an increased number of red blood cells (RBCs) in the blood. This condition is diagnosed when a man has a hemoglobin over 18.5 and a hematocrit over 52% or a woman has a hemoglobin over 16.5 and a hematocrit over 48%. This elevation in hemoglobin or hematocrit may be relative or absolute. Absolute polycythemia occurs when there is a true increase in the RBC mass due to either primary or secondary causes. Relative polycythemia occurs when a contraction in plasma volume causes an apparent increase in RBC mass (1).

II. PATHOPHYSIOLOGY

A. Etiology

1. Primary polycythemia is due to genetic mutations. Polycythemia vera (PV) is related to a genetic mutation in the *JAK2* gene on the short arm of chromosome 9. Primary familial and congenital polycythemia is due to a mutation in the *EPOR* gene. In both diseases, there is an increased sensitivity in the bone marrow to epopoietin (EPO), resulting in

increased RBC production. In PV, there may also be increased production of white blood cells or platelets (2–4).

2. Secondary polycythemia occurs in response to increased levels of circulating erythropoietin. This may occur with chronic hypoxia which causes low blood oxygen levels), abnormal RBCs (which results in poor delivery of oxygen), or EPO-secreting tumors.

   EPO is produced in the kidneys in response to hypoxia. The increase in cell mass results in hyperviscosity of the blood. This causes most of the symptoms experienced by the patient such as headaches, dizziness, pruritus especially after a shower, and stroke (2–4).

III. EVALUATION

A. History. Since the most common cause of polycythemia is related to hypoxia, a thorough evaluation of the respiratory status should be done. Patients should be asked if they have a history of asthma or chronic obstructive pulmonary disease (COPD), shortness of breath, dyspnea on exertion, or cyanosis. A thorough smoking history should be obtained, including how much tobacco is smoked daily and how many years the patient has smoked. If the person is no longer smoking, document how many years ago he/she stopped. Occupational history is important because many jobs predispose patients to environmental exposures, especially carbon monoxide (2,3,5).

B. Physical Examination. The physical examination in patients with polycythemia may be notable for cyanosis of lips, earlobes, and extremities. Clubbing may also be evident. A thorough abdominal examination for hepatosplenomegaly and a heart examination evaluating for murmurs or bruits should be performed (2,3,5).

C. Testing. The most important laboratory tests are hemoglobin, hematocrit, and RBC count. These values should be adjusted for the sex and age of the patient. One should also obtain a white blood cell count and platelet count. A urinalysis should be obtained, looking for hematuria. Liver function tests should also be obtained. If the patient has significant history of carbon monoxide exposure, a serum carboxyhemoglobin should be obtained. Once elevation of the RBC mass has been confirmed, the next two tests should be carboxyhemoglobin and erythropoietin (2,3,5).

D. Imaging Studies. If cardiopulmonary disease is suspected, a chest X-ray may be helpful to assess the patient for COPD or congestive heart failure. Ultrasound or CT scan of the abdomen can be utilized to evaluate for EPO-secreting tumor (4,5).

IV. DIAGNOSIS

A. Differential Diagnosis

1. Elevated carboxyhemoglobin. If the occupational exposure can be stopped, the carboxyhemoglobin level should return to normal within 3 months.

2. Decreased (or normal) erythropoietin level, increased RBC mass, and presence of the JAK2 mutation V617F are diagnostic of PV. There is a 10–25% chance that the person will progress from this myeloproliferative neoplasm into myelofibrosis over the next 25 years.

3. If the person has COPD, congestive heart failure, pulmonary hypertension, or obstructive sleep apnea, the serum EPO is appropriately elevated in an effort to compensate for chronic hypoxemia. No further evaluation is needed although management is important.

4. EPO-secreting tumors include renal cell carcinoma, hepatocellular carcinoma, adrenal tumors, and uterine cancer (2–5).

REFERENCES

1. Rakel RE, Rakel DP. *Textbook of family medicine,* 8th ed. Philadelphia, PA: WB Saunders, 2011:887–888.
2. Adamson JW, Longo DL. Chapter 57. Anemia and polycythemia. In: Longo DL, Fauci AS, Kasper DL, Hauser SL, Jameson JL, Loscalzo J, eds. *Harrison's principles of internal medicine,* 18th ed. New York, NY: McGraw-Hill, 2012, http://www.accessmedicine.com/content.aspx?aID=9113377.
3. Tefferi A. Diagnostic approach to the patient with polycythemia. *UpToDate.* Topic 7075, Version 8.0. Jan 18, 2012.
4. Tefferi A. Overview of the myeloproliferative neoplasms. *UpToDate.* Topic 4511, Version 27.0, June 6, 2012.
5. Nabili ST. Polycythemia. *WebMD.* Feb 26, 2010. http://www.emedicinehealth.com.

16.6 Proteinuria

Carol A. LaCroix

I. BACKGROUND. Normal adults excrete less than 150 mg of protein per day with up to 20 mg of albumin. The rate of albumin excretion is 4–7 mg/d in an young adult. It increases with age and body weight. It is also higher in non-Hispanic blacks and Mexican Americans. Persistent excretion of albumin between 30 and 300 mg/d (20–200 μg/min) is called microalbuminuria, while values above 300 mg/d are called macroalbuminuria (1,2).

II. PATHOPHYSIOLOGY. There are three types of proteinuria: glomerular, tubular, and overflow. Glomerular proteinuria involves increased permeability to plasma proteins, especially albumin, across the glomerulo-capillary membrane and may range from the minimal to the nephrotic range. Tubular proteinuria occurs when tubulointerstitial disease interferes with reabsorption of small molecular weight proteins in the proximal tubule. Overflow proteinuria results from an overproduction of immunoglobulins, particularly in multiple myeloma.

Proteinuria may be transient or persistent. Transient proteinuria can occur with exercise, cold exposure, fever, and congestive heart failure. Persistent proteinuria is diagnosed when a value of >300 mg/dL has been documented in three urine specimens (1,3).

III. EVALUATION

  A. History. Annual screening for proteinuria in healthy people below age 60 years is not cost-effective (3). However, urinalysis is warranted if the person has a history of diabetes, hypertension, polycystic kidney disease, or autoimmune disease.

  B. Physical Examination. Check vital signs, especially blood pressure. Perform a funduscopic examination, checking for diabetic retinopathy or vascular changes from hypertension. Edema of the legs or face may be due to hypoalbuminemia. Check the abdomen for renal artery bruits and masses such as polycystic kidneys.

    Rheumatoid arthritis may be accompanied by amyloid deposition in the kidneys (3,5).

  C. Testing

    1. The standard urine dipstick identifies only albumin, and it does not detect microalbuminuria. It can be falsely negative when the urine is dilute (specific gravity <1.015) and when the proteins are of low molecular weight. The dipstick can be falsely positive for 24 hours after a contrast dye study or with alkaline urine, gross hematuria, pus, semen, vaginal secretions, and the presence of penicillin and sulfonamides. Proteinuria is graded as 30 (1+), 100 (2+), 300 (3+), and 1,000 mg/dL (4+).

    2. The gold standard has been to evaluate persistent proteinuria with a 24-hour urine collection. However, two spot urine tests have been found to be generally as valid and much easier to obtain. The albumin-to-creatinine ratio is used to screen for microalbuminuria. The threshold for concern is 20 mg/24 h in women and 30 mg/24 h in men, due to the difference in muscle mass. The protein-to-creatinine ratio is useful in monitoring disease progression. A ratio less than 0.2 is normal, whereas a ratio over 3.0 is in the nephrotic range (3,4).

    3. If abnormal proteins are suspected but not detected on the standard dipstick, the sulfosalicylic acid test should be done. If a patient has acute renal failure, a benign urinalysis, and only trace protein on dipstick, the person is likely to have light chain immunoglobulins due to multiple myeloma (3).

    4. Any adult or child with proteinuria or hematuria without a clear diagnosis should have a nephrology consult. This is especially true if the proteinuria is >2 g/d, because the person most likely has some type of glomerular disease. Most of these patients will need a renal biopsy. One exception is patients with postinfectious glomerulonephritis, which is usually self-limited (4).

IV. DIAGNOSIS
A. Differential Diagnosis

1. Dehydration, fever, intense physical activity, emotional stress, and seizures can cause benign proteinuria. Transient proteinuria does not require further evaluation or monitoring.

2. Orthostatic proteinuria accounts for up to 60% of asymptomatic proteinuria in individuals 6–30 years of age. This is seen when the first-morning spot urine is negative but a specimen later in the day after the person has been upright is dipstick positive (at least 1+). This condition appears to be benign.

3. Secondary glomerulonephropathy occurs with diabetes mellitus, hypertension, lupus, amyloidosis, preeclampsia, recent streptococcal infections, endocarditis, human immunodeficiency virus, and hepatitis B and C. Patients should be closely monitored for proteinuria and hyperlipidemia.

4. If hematuria is present, further evaluation is needed. The most common causes are urinary tract infection, stones in the kidney or bladder, nephritis, and tumor. Red cell casts are seen in glomerulonephritis.

5. Tubular nephropathy may be due to hypertension, sickle cell disease, or urate stones.

6. Gold, penicillamine, lithium, and heroin can cause glomerulonephropathy. Nonsteroidal anti-inflammatory drugs and heavy metals can damage both the glomeruli and the tubules.

7. Multiple myeloma causes proteinuria with light-chain immunoglobulins, which can be detected with the sulfasalicylic acid test. Monocytic or myelocytic leukemia causes increased production and excretion of lysozyme, which can be detected on the standard dipstick (3,5).

REFERENCES

1. Rose BD, Post TW. Measurement of urinary protein excretion. *UpToDate*. Topic 3102, Version 10.0, Oct 21, 2011.
2. Molitch MR, DeFrazo RA, Franz MJ, et al. Nephropathy in diabetes. *Diabetes Care* 2004;27(suppl 1):S79–S83.
3. Rose BD, Fletcher SW. Evaluation of isolated proteinuria in adults. *UpToDate*. Topic 3101, Version 6.0, Apr 15, 2011.
4. Hassan A. Proteinuria. *Postgrad Med* 1997;101(4):173–180.
5. Carroll MF, Temte JL. Proteinuria in adults. *Am Fam Physician* 2000;62(2):1333–1342.

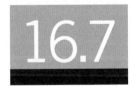

16.7 Thrombocytopenia
Mandeep Bajwa

I. BACKGROUND

A. Definition. Thrombocytopenia is defined as a pathologic decrease in platelet count. It is identified typically as a laboratory finding of a platelet count below 150,000 cells/µL (1), but it is generally not detected clinically until platelets fall below 100,000/µL. Bleeding tendencies may occur, but spontaneous bleeding generally does not occur until the platelet count is below 20,000 cells/µL unless other preexisting conditions occur that would encourage bleeding risk (1–5).

II. PATHOPHYSIOLOGY

A. Etiology. Thrombocytopenia occurs through one or more of the following mechanisms: decreased platelet production by the bone marrow, increased platelet destruction, splenic entrapment, dilutional effect, and laboratory error (2,3).

III. EVALUATION
A. History. A meticulous history must be obtained, with particular focus on the following:
1. Recent infection
2. A thorough review of all medications currently being taken and the date prescribed
3. Menstrual and pregnancy history
4. The presence of the following: epistaxis and bleeding gums, reddish or purplish discoloration of the skin, excessive bruising, hematuria, and melena or hematochezia
5. Dietary intake, alcohol use
6. Past personal medical history
7. Family history

B. Physical Examination. A thorough physical examination is warranted with special emphasis on the following:
1. Skin examination looking for petechiae, purpura, and ecchymoses
2. Abdominal examination to assess for splenomegaly and hepatomegaly
3. Neurologic examination to ascertain if hemorrhage has occurred, although rare

C. Testing
1. Complete blood count with differential and peripheral smear
2. Bone marrow biopsy is beneficial in patients with splenomegaly and in those who follow an uncharacteristic course

D. Imaging studies are rarely indicated (1,3–5).

IV. DIAGNOSIS
A. Differential Diagnosis
1. Decreased platelet production by the bone marrow
   a. Viral infections
   b. Chemotherapy/radiation
   c. Congenital bone marrow abnormalities
   d. Alcohol toxicity
   e. Vitamin B12/folate deficiency
2. Increased platelet destruction
   a. Idiopathic thrombocytopenic purpura (ITP)

   ITP is a relatively common autoimmune thrombocytopenic disease that occurs in the acute and chronic setting with a prevalence of 1 in 10,000 persons. Acute ITP is seen solely in children 2–9 years of age, with a peak incidence at 3–5 years of age. It affects boys and girls equally. Acute ITP typically follows an acute viral syndrome and has a self-limiting course. In contrast, chronic ITP affects adults 20–50 years of age, has a female predominance of 3:1, and rarely results in spontaneous remission.
   b. Drug induced

   Drug-induced thrombocytopenia may be caused by a plethora of medications. The most frequent culprit, especially in hospitalized patients, is heparin. Although drug-induced thrombocytopenia is also an antibody-mediated syndrome, it is transient, typically resolving when the offending agent is discontinued.
   c. Alloimmune destruction
   d. Disseminated intravascular coagulation
   e. Thrombocytopenic purpura/hemolytic uremic syndrome
   f. Antiphospholipid syndrome
   g. Hemolysis, Elevated Liver enzymes, Low Platelets (HELLP) syndrome
   h. Viral infections
   i. Mechanical platelet destruction
3. Splenic entrapment: may occur in cirrhosis, myelofibrosis, Gaucher's disease.
4. Dilutional effect: large blood replacement with too few platelets.
5. Laboratory error: clotted specimen, wrong patient, or technical/equipment errors (1–6).

REFERENCES

1. Rakel RE, Rakel DP *Textbook of family medicine,* 8th ed. Philadelphia, PA: WB Saunders, 2011: 892–895.
2. George JN. Evaluation and management of thrombocytopenia by primary care physicians. *UpToDate.* Topic 6864, Version 6.0, July 10, 2012.
3. Landaw SA, George JN. Approach to the adult patient with thrombocytopenia. *UpToDate.* Topic 6680, Version 14.0, May 30, 2012.
4. Thiagarajan P. *Platelet disorders.* Last updated March 29, 2011. http://emedicine.medscape.com/article/201722-overview#aw2aab6b3
5. Kaplan JL, Porter RS, eds. 2011. *Merck manual Of diagnosis and therapy,* 19th ed. Whitehouse Station, NJ: Merck Sharp & Dohme Corp., a subsidiary of Merck & Co., Inc. ISBN-10: 0-911910-19-0, ISBN-13: 978-0-911910-19-3. ISSN: 0076-6526. STAT!Ref Online Electronic Medical Library. http://online.statref.com/document.aspx?fxid=21&docid=470.
6. Kravitz MS, Shoenfeld Y. Thrombocytopenic conditions-autoimmunity and hypercoagulability: commonalities and differences in ITP, TTP, HIT, and APS. *Am J Hematol* 2005;80:232–242.

CHAPTER 17

Laboratory Abnormalities: Blood Chemistry and Immunology

Nathan Falk

17.1 Alkaline Phosphatase, Elevated

Peter F. Cronholm, Joseph Teel, and Nasreen Ghazi

I. **BACKGROUND.** Serum alkaline phosphatase (ALP) is an enzyme that arises primarily from the liver and bone, although small amounts are derived from the intestines and the vascular endothelium. The placenta is also a source of ALP in pregnant women. In the liver, ALP is bound to the cell membranes on the canalicular side of the hepatocytes. Osteoblasts and intestinal epithelial cells also produce their own ALP (1). The normal range of serum ALP varies by age and clinical history. The normal ranges for adolescents, adults older than 60 years, and pregnant women are higher than for nonpregnant women and men younger than 60 years (see Table 17.1.1) (1).

Serum ALP should be ordered only if bone or liver disease is suspected. ALP results should be compared with appropriate normal ranges on the basis of the age and clinical history. Abnormal results should be repeated, because spurious elevations can be caused by a recent albumin infusion, by the use of an anticoagulant tube for blood collection, or by serum samples left standing at room temperature for prolonged periods (2, 3).

II. **PATHOPHYSIOLOGY**

A. **Etiology**

1. Identifying the source of ALP elevation is based upon measuring γ-glutamyltransferase (GGT) or $5'$-nucleotidase levels. Elevated ALP from liver sources results in elevated GGT or $5'$-nucleotidase, while ALP elevation in the setting of normal GGT or $5'$-nucleotidase suggests a bone source (2, 3).

TABLE 17.1.1	Normal ranges for serum ALP (1)
Age Group	**Normal Range (U/L)**
Infant	50–165
Child	20–150
Adult	20–70
>60	30–75

2. Uncommon causes of ALP elevation include hyperthyroidism and intestinal conditions such as bowel obstruction, inflammatory bowel disease, and infarction. Additionally, infarction of any solid organ may cause ALP elevation owing to the presence of ALP in the vascular endothelium (2).

III. EVALUATION. Further testing should be carried out on the basis of the results of a careful history and physical examination and should be targeted at specific clinical suspicions (Table 17.1.2) (1–3).

IV. DIAGNOSIS. See Table 17.1.2 (1–3).

TABLE 17.1.2	Evaluation of the Patient with Elevated ALP (1–3)		
History	**Physical examination**	**Testing**	**Diagnosis**
A. Bone disorders (1)			
Primary bone			
• Asymptomatic or bone pain • Male • Hearing/vision problems • Headaches • Pain increased with walking (tibia involved)	• Frontal bossing • Dilated superficial vessels • Saber tibia • Deafness • Congestive heart failure	• 24-h urine hydroxyproline • Serum phosphate • Serum calcium (normal) • X-ray involved bone(s) • Bone scan	Paget's disease
• Female • >60 y • Diffuse aches and pains • Vague abdominal pain • Depressive symptoms	• Neck mass (rare) • Muscle weakness • No clinical evidence of malignancy	• Parathyroid hormone • Serum calcium • Urinary calcium/ blood • Serum phosphate • Serum chloride	Hyperparathyroidism
• 10–30 y • Male • Pain near joint • Very high ALP	• Mass near joint • Tender over mass	• X-ray area (mixed sclerotic/lytic lesion of bone) • Magnetic resonance imaging of affected region • Bone scan • Biopsy	Osteosarcoma
• Recent trauma	• Bone pain in area	• X-ray (callous formation)	Healing fracture
• Smoker • Cough	• Dull to percussion	• Serum calcium	Homer's syndrome

(Continued)

TABLE 17.1.2	Evaluation of the Patient with Elevated ALP (1–3) *(Continued)*		
History	**Physical examination**	**Testing**	**Diagnosis**
• Hemoptysis			
• Shortness of breath			
• Limited sunlight exposure	• Bowed legs (rickets)	• 25-OH vitamin D	Vitamin D deficiency
• Fatigue		• Gliadin antibody	
• Diarrhea		• Basic metabolic panel	
• Recent bariatric surgery			
• History of malabsorptive processes			
Metastatic bone			
• Female	• Breast mass	• Mammogram	Breast cancer
• >50 y	• Axillary and supraclavicular nodes	• Bone scan	
• Family history		• Serum calcium	
• Breast mass	• Liver enlargement		
• Female	• Ovarian mass	• Pelvic ultrasound	Ovarian cancer
• >45 y	• Ascites	• Pelvic CT scan	
• Family history		• CA-125	
• Abdominal bloating		• CT scan	
• Unexplained weight loss		• Serum calcium	
• Male	• Unilateral flank mass	• Urinalysis	Renal cell carcinoma
• >50 y	• Conjunctival pallor	• Abdominal CT scan	
• Hematuria		• Serum calcium	
• Flank/abdominal pain			
• Female	• Cervical mass on exam	• Pap smear or colposcopy	Cervical cancer
• Vaginal bleeding			
• Family history			
• Male	• Prostate mass on rectal examination or diffusely enlarged hard prostate	• Serum calcium	Prostate cancer
• >50 y		• Prostate-specific antigen	
• Urinary complaints		• Ultrasound-guided prostate biopsy	
• Family history		• Bone scan	

(Continued)

TABLE 17.1.2	**Evaluation of the Patient with Elevated ALP (1–3)** *(Continued)*		
History	**Physical examination**	**Testing**	**Diagnosis**
B. Biliary/liver disease (2)			
1. Obstructive processes			
• Female • >40 y • Obese • Family history of gallstones • Pain after meals/episodic • Bloating	• RUQ abdominal tenderness + Murphy's sign (only in acute cholecystitis) • Jaundice	• AST/ALT may be elevated • Bilirubin elevated • Ultrasound of gallbladder	Gallstones Biliary colic Acute cholecystitis
• Weight loss • Anorexia • Back or RUQ pain • Jaundice	• Palpable gallbladder • Cachectic • Epigastric mass • Jaundice	• Abdominal CT scan • Elevated bilirubin • CT scan or ultrasound-guided biopsy	Pancreatic carcinoma Gallbladder carcinoma
2. Intrinsic hepatic processes			
• Alcohol use/abuse (chronic) • Family history of liver disease • Risky sexual practices • Blood transfusions • Intravenous drug use • Obesity • Fatigue • Weight loss	• Spider nevi • Leukonychia • Dupuytren's contracture • Tender RUQ • Liver may be enlarged • Jaundice	• Serum AST/ALT levels: ↑ in early disease ↓↔ late disease • Bilirubin (elevated) • Hepatitis screen (A, B, C) • Coagulation screen • Liver biopsy	Cirrhosis Hepatitis Fatty liver
3. Infectious causes			
• Fatigue • Pharyngitis • 10–25 y old • Fever • Sore throat/fatigue • History of contact with infected friend/relative	• Fever • Tender RUQ • Splenomegaly • Lymphadenopathy (mainly cervical)	• Monospot test • AST/ALT • CBC • Toxoplasma titers	Infectious mononucleosis Toxoplasmosis Cytomegalovirus infection

(Continued)

TABLE 17.1.2 Evaluation of the Patient with Elevated ALP (1–3) *(Continued)*

History	Physical examination	Testing	Diagnosis
4. Drug induced (3)			
• Chlorpropamide	• Frequently normal	• AST/ALT	Drug-induced elevation of ALP
• ACE inhibitors	• RUQ tenderness	• Liver biopsy if problem persists	
• Estrogen			
• Antineoplastic agents			
• Immune modulators			
5. Immune mediated			
• 35–60 y of age (90%)	• Excoriations	• Antimitochondrial antibodies	Primary biliary cirrhosis
• Jaundice	• Jaundice	• Liver biopsy	
• Frequently asymptomatic	• Skin pigmentation	• Elevated bilirubin (late)	
	• RUQ tenderness		
	• Xanthelasma		
• Itching (palms/soles first)	• Liver/spleen enlarged	• Elevated liver enzymes (late)	
• Fatigue		• Cholesterol elevated	
• Bone pain			
• Steatorrhea			
• Male	• RUQ tenderness	• Endoscopic retrograde cholangiopan-creatography (ERCP)/ Magnetic resonance cholangiopancreatography (MRCP)	Sclerosing cholangitis (primary or secondary)
• 30–60 y of age	• Jaundice		
• RUQ pain			
• Jaundice			
• Pruritus			
• Inflammatory bowel disease			
• Fatigue			
• 10–40 y of age	• Crackles	• Chest X-ray (CXR) with bilateral hilar adenopathy	Sarcoidosis
• Cough	• Rales		
• Dyspnea	• Maculopapular rash on face		
• Chest pain			
6. Oncologic			
• Fatigue/lethargy	• Lymphadenopathy	• CBC	Lymphoma
• Fever		• Elevated uric acid	
• Anorexia/weight loss		• Elevated Lactate dehydrogenase (LDH)	
• Enlarged lymph nodes			

ALP, alkaline phosphatase; ALT, alanine aminotransferase; AST, aspartate aminotransferase; CBC, complete blood count; RUQ, right upper quadrant.

REFERENCES

1. McPherson R, Pincus M. *Henry's clinical diagnosis and management by laboratory methods,* 22nd ed. Philadelphia, PA: Elsevier, 2011.
2. Aragon G, Younossi, Z. When and how to evaluate mildly elevated liver enzymes in apparently healthy patients. *Cleve Clin J Med* 2010;7(3):195–204.
3. Giannini EG, Testa R, Savarino V, et al. Liver enzyme alteration: a guide for clinicians. *CMAJ (OTTAWA)* 2005;172-3:367–373.

Aminotransferase Levels, Elevated

Peter F. Cronholm, Giang T. Nguyen, and N. Corry Clinton

I. BACKGROUND. Liver function tests (LFTs) are common, useful tools for evaluating the differential diagnosis of hepatic pathology. The standard panel includes tests to evaluate for the presence of hepatocellular injury, disorders of bile formation and excretion, and synthetic dysfunction (1). Tests for hepatocellular injury include aspartate aminotransferase (AST) (or serum glutamic oxaloacetic transaminase) and alanine aminotransferase (ALT) (or serum glutamic pyrunic transaminase). Bile formation and excretion tests include alkaline phosphatase, total and direct serum bilirubin, and sometimes γ-glutamyl transpeptidase (GGT) or 5′-nucleotidase. Synthetic function tests include albumin, total protein, and sometimes prothrombin time. The focus of this chapter will primarily be elevation of the aminotransferases AST and ALT.

II. PATHOPHYSIOLOGY. The aminotransferases are cytosolic enzymes found in the hepatocytes; they are released into the serum as a result of hepatocellular damage, thereby elevating the serum levels from their low, but present, baseline (2). ALT is very specific to the hepatocytes, whereas AST is not specific to hepatocytes and is found in numerous other body tissues (3). The presence of elevated AST and ALT is not in and of itself specific to any condition—etiologies include viruses, toxins, alcohol, cirrhosis, neoplasm, cholestasis, and vascular/circulatory compromise (4, 5). As such, the pattern of elevation must be evaluated and considered in light of a thorough history and physical examination, as well as review of the remaining LFTs, other appropriate lab tests, and imaging.

III. EVALUATION. Evaluation of abnormalities should include an assessment of medication use (including over-the-counter and herbal medications), travel, country of origin, alcohol consumption, recreational drug use (particularly a history of intravenous drug use), sexual history, signs and symptoms of hepatic injury, and a thorough physical examination. ALT and AST may also be elevated in association with myocardial infarctions, hemolytic anemia, trauma, and intramuscular injections. A thorough clinical history and examination are essential in guiding the testing and interpretation of the results, because patterns of abnormalities in liver testing are better predictors of clinical disease than any single component.

IV. DIAGNOSIS. See Table 17.2.1.

TABLE 17.2.1 Evaluation of the Patient with Elevated Aminotransferase

History	Physical examination	Testing	Diagnosis
• Patient often asymptomatic or transient flu-like illness • Antecedent illness of several days to weeks with nausea, vomiting, anorexia, malaise, diarrhea, arthralgias, or low-grade fever • Recent shellfish ingestion • Incarceration • Multiple sexual partners • Past or present intravenous drug use • History of blood transfusions before 1992 or tattoos • From country with endemic hepatitis virus • Sexual or household contacts with hepatitis virus • HIV infection • Hemodialysis	• Jaundice • Clay-colored stools • Dark urine • Left upper quadrant tenderness • Hepatomegaly • Urticaria • Maculopapular skin eruptions • Isolated joint swelling, redness, or tenderness	• AST and ALT can be markedly elevated with ratio usually <1 • Alkaline phosphatase and serum bilirubin may be elevated or normal • Begin serial testing of AST and ALT • CBC • Hepatitis A IgM • Hepatitis B surface antigen, IgM anti-hepatitis B surface antigen antibody, and IgM anti-hepatitis B core antibody • IgG anti-hepatitis C antibody • Epstein-Barr virus or cytomegalovirus titers • Liver biopsy if diagnosis cannot be determined or to guide treatment for hepatitis C	• **Acute viral hepatitis**
• Excessive somnolence • Obtundation • History of rectal or upper GI bleeding • Rapidly progressive course in 65–95% of patients • Symptoms of sepsis with or without multi-organ failure • Prior hepatitis • History of aspirin ingestion in children younger than 17 y with influenza or chickenpox • Toxic doses of acetaminophen (paracetamol in many countries)	• Liver may be reduced in size • Ascites • Refractory hypotension • Petechiae • Bleeding from mucous membranes • Edema	• AST and ALT can be markedly elevated with ratio usually <1 • Prothrombin time (profoundly prolonged) • Low blood glucose • Low total serum protein and serum albumin • CBC • Serum ammonia (may be severely elevated)	• **Fulminant hepatitis** • **Acute hepatic failure associated with Reye's syndrome** • 1% of the elderly or immunocompromised patients with hepatitis

(Continued)

TABLE 17.2.1	Evaluation of the Patient with Elevated Aminotransferase (Continued)		
History	**Physical examination**	**Testing**	**Diagnosis**
• Chronic or acute alcohol ingestion • Younger age drinker • History of pancreatitis or erosive gastritis • Cirrhotic liver disease • Hepatitis C history • Anorexia • Nausea • Vomiting • Abdominal pain	• Jaundice • ± Fever • Weight loss • Hepatomegaly with mild tenderness • Advanced disease can be characterized by spider angiomas, ascites, palmar erythema, caput medusae, gynecomastia, parotid enlargement, and testicular atrophy	• AST:ALT > 2:1 • γ-glutamyl transferase elevation • CBC (possible anemia)	• **Alcoholic hepatitis** (5)
• Often asymptomatic • Previous episode of acute hepatitis • Coagulopathy • History of risk factors for acute hepatitis as above	• May be no findings • Thin • Jaundiced • Small, nodular liver	• AST and ALT are variably elevated • Hepatitis B surface antigen, IgM anti-hepatitis B surface antigen antibody, and IgM/G anti-hepatitis B core and envelope antibody • IgG anti-hepatitis C antibody • Albumin (often low) • Prothrombin time (may be elevated) • Liver biopsy	• **Chronic hepatitis**
• RUQ pain, often after eating fatty foods • History of gallstones • Middle aged • Overweight • Female	• Jaundice • Intermittent fever • Rigors • RUQ tenderness ± rebound	• Alkaline phosphatase elevated more than AST or ALT • Elevated serum bilirubin • CBC • RUQ ultrasound • Endoscopic retrograde cholangio-pancreatography or imaging equivalent • HIDA scan	• **Biliary tract obstruction** with or without an infection (cholestasis vs. cholangitis)

(Continued)

| TABLE 17.2.1 | Evaluation of the Patient with Elevated Aminotransferase *(Continued)* | | |

History	Physical examination	Testing	Diagnosis
• Known or unknown malignancy • Abdominal pain • Weakness • Anorexia • History of hepatitis B or C infection	• Weight loss • Ascites • GI malignancies may have left supraclavicular (Virchow's) or periumbilical (Sister Mary Joseph) lymph node enlargement • Other findings specific to the primary site malignancy	• Can present as hepatocellular injury, obstructive or a combination profile • MRI • Serum a-fetoprotein • Workup for source of primary malignancy	• **Malignancy** (primary or metastatic)
Use of • HMG-CoA reductase inhibitor • Isoniazid • Phenothiazine • Erythromycin • Progesterone • Halothane • Opiates • Indomethacin • Corticosteroids • Some herbal drugs • Polypharmacy	• Often none	• Increased AST and ALT • Repeat AST and ALT after discontinuation of the medication • Other testing specific to medication effects (e.g., creatinine kinase levels with toxicity of HMG-CoA reductase inhibitors)	• **Medication effect**
• Fatigue, malaise, and vague right upper abdominal discomfort • Hepatitis with no clear etiology	• Obesity • Hepatomegaly • Splenomegaly	• AST:ALT ratio <1 • Fasting lipids • Fasting glucose • Ultrasound, CT scan, or MRI • Liver biopsy is necessary to determine inflammation	• **Hepatic steatosis and nonalcoholic steatohepatitis**
• Family history of hemochromatosis • Polyuria, polyphagia, and polydipsia • Weakness and lethargy • Arthralgia • Impotence or decreased libido in men • Amenorrhea in women	• Weakness • Skin hyperpigmentation • Diabetes mellitus • Hepatomegaly • Electrocardiographic abnormalities	• Serum iron • TIBC • Iron saturation (ratio of serum iron to TIBC) >45% • Ferritin • Liver biopsy for determination of hepatic iron index • Family screening • HbA1c	• **Hemochromatosis**

(Continued)

TABLE 17.2.1   **Evaluation of the Patient with Elevated Aminotransferase** *(Continued)*

History	Physical examination	Testing	Diagnosis
• Muscle pain or weakness	• Muscle tenderness or weakness on examination	• Creatine kinase • Aldolase • Muscle biopsy	• **Muscle disorders**
• Unintentional weight loss or gain • Skin and hair changes • Heat or cold intolerance	• Goiter and/or thyroid nodule(s) in certain conditions • Hair loss • Abnormal reflexes	• TSH • Thyroid function testing if TSH is abnormal	• **Thyroid disorders**
• Hepatitis or liver failure • Emphysema when young or out of proportion with smoking history • Family history of pulmonary pathology	• Physical examination ranging from acute hepatitis to end-stage liver disease • Pulmonary examination suggestive of end-stage pulmonary disease	• α-1-antitrypsin level • α-1-antitrypsin phenotype • Serum protein electrophoresis	• **α-1-antitrypsin deficiency**
• Child or young adult (5–25 y) • Hepatitis • Dysarthria • Dysphagia	• Kayser-Fleischer rings in cornea • Tremor or other movement disorders • Behavioral and psychiatric symptoms	• Liver function tests often nonspecific • Ceruloplasmin (reduced in 85% of patients) • 24-h urine for quantitative copper excretion (>10 μg/d is suggestive) • Serum protein electrophoresis	• **Wilson's disease**
• Female • History of autoimmune disorder		• Antibody to liver/kidney • Microsomal antibody type 1 • ANA • Smooth muscle antibody	• **Autoimmune hepatitis**
• Diarrhea, abdominal pain, malabsorption		• Tissue transglutaminase	• **Celiac disease**
• G6PD deficiency • Sickle cell anemia • Infection		• Lactate dehydrogenase • Haptoglobin • Reticulocyte count	• **Hemolysis**

(Continued)

TABLE 17.2.1	Evaluation of the Patient with Elevated Aminotransferase *(Continued)*		
History	Physical examination	Testing	Diagnosis

• Strenuous exercise
• Muscle weakness
  or pain
		• Creatine kinase
		• Aldolase
			• Muscular
			  disorders

ALT, alanine aminotransferase; AST, aspartate aminotransferase; CBC, complete blood count; Ig, immunoglobulin; GI, gastrointestinal; RUQ, right upper quadrant; MRI, magnetic resonance imaging; HMG-CoA, 3-hydroxy-3-methylglutaryl coenzyme A; TIBC, total iron binding capacity; TSH, thyroid-stimulating hormone.

REFERENCES

1. Oh RC, Hustead TR. Liver transaminase levels. *Am Fam Physician* 2011;84(9):1003–1008.
2. Pratt DS, Marshall MK. Evaluation of liver function. In: Longo DL, Fauci AS, Kasper DL, eds. *Harrison's principles of internal medicine,* 18th ed. New York, NY: McGraw-Hill, 2011;2527–2530.
3. Pratt DS, Kaplan MM. Evaluation of abnormal liver-enzyme results in asymptomatic patients. *N Engl J Med* 2000;342:1266.
4. Crawford JM. Liver and biliary tract. In: Kumar V, Abbas AK, Fausto N, eds. *Robbins and Cotran pathologic basis of disease,* 7th ed. Philadelphia, PA: Elsevier Saunders, 2005;877–937.
5. Cohen JA, Kaplan MM. The SGOT/SGPT ratio an indicator of alcoholic liver disease. *Dig Dis Sci* 1979;24:835.

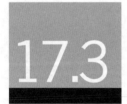

Antinuclear Antibody Titer, Elevated

Peter F. Cronholm, Rahul Kapur, and Kristina E. McElhinney

I. BACKGROUND. Antinuclear antibodies (ANAs) include antibodies to double-stranded DNA, histones, chromatin, along with other nuclear proteins and RNA–protein complexes. ANAs are associated with both systemic and organ-specific autoimmune diseases, use of certain medications, chronic systemic infections, and rarely malignancy. Due to the low specificity of a positive ANA titer (50% for all rheumatic diseases), ANA should only be checked when there is clinical suspicion of a disease process in which the ANA value plays a significant role (1). Five percent of young adults and 18% of individuals older than 65 years have a mildly elevated ANA and no disease process (2).

II. PATHOPHYSIOLOGY. ANAs produced in patients with autoimmune connective tissue disease belong predominantly to the immunoglobulin G class and are generally present at higher levels. Some ANAs contribute to inflammatory processes by forming immune complexes or cross-reacting to other antigens. Disease-specific ANA may guide further diagnostic testing and monitoring; however, clinicians should regard them as a potential indicator of disease and remember that ANA can be found in many apparently healthy individuals (3,4).

III. EVALUATION. A careful history and physical examination along with an understanding of the prevalence of systemic autoimmune diseases should guide the ordering and interpretation of ANA titers. For further details, see Table 17.3.1.

IV. DIAGNOSIS. See Table 17.3.1.

TABLE 17.3.1	**Evaluation of the Patient with an Elevated ANA Titer**		
History	**Physical examination**	**Further testing**	**Diagnosis**
A. Connective tissue disorders			
• Fatigue • Fever • Weight loss • Pain, redness, or heat in two or more joints • Photosensitivity reaction • Rash • Oral ulcers • Chest pain • Shortness of breath • Seizures or psychosis without history of offending medications or drug use • Abdominal pain • More common in women and African Americans	• Malar rash (presents in one-third to one-half of patients) • Discoid rash • Joint effusion or derangement in chronic disease (present in two-thirds of patients) • Focal neurologic deficits (15% of patients) • Pleural effusions • Cardiac or pleural rubs	• Anti-ds-DNA (high specificity for SLE) • Urinalysis with 24-h collection (look for persistent proteinuria or casts) • CBC (look for evidence of anemia) • Specialized nuclear antigen tests: ribonucleoprotein, antibodies to anti-Smith, anti-SS-A/Ro, anti-SS-B/La (patients with SLE may produce different autoantibodies) • Creatinine (look for occult renal disease) • X-rays of involved joints	• SLE
• Systemic symptoms: fever, weight loss, and fatigue • Morning stiffness • Chronic, symmetric joint complaints (three or more for 6 or more wk) • Joint symptoms are often intermittent and migratory	• ± Red, hot, swollen joint(s) (most common are the wrist, metacarpophalangeal, or proximal interphalangeal joints) • Subcutaneous nodules (usually on the extensor or pressure surfaces)	• Rheumatoid factor (20% of patients with RA are negative) • CBC (look for an anemia of chronic disease) • X-rays of involved joints (typically demonstrates erosions or bone loss) • Joint aspiration (inflammatory profile to synovial fluid)	• RA

(Continued)

TABLE 17.3.1   **Evaluation of the Patient with an Elevated ANA Titer** *(Continued)*

History	Physical examination	Further testing	Diagnosis
• Excessive dryness of eyes and/or mouth • Recurrent oral ulcers • Sensation disturbance over the hands and/or feet • Vaginal dryness and dyspareunia • Dysphagia	• Enlarged salivary glands • Dry mucous membranes • Decreased salivation • Decreased tearing • Purpura • Peripheral neuropathy	• Anti-SS-A/Ro • Anti-SS-B/La • Biopsy of salivary glands or lip to assess lymphocytic infiltration • CBC (look for anemia of chronic disease) • Cryoglobulins (if positive, should screen for hepatitis C) • Immunoglobulin electrophoresis (to demonstrate a monoclonal spike) • Objective testing of tear and saliva production (Schirmer test and salivary scintigram) • Chest X-ray to differentiate from possible sarcoidosis	• Sjögren's syndrome
• Fever and malaise • Weight loss • Muscle tenderness • Muscle weakness is usually symmetric, gradual in onset, greater loss in lower limbs • Skin rash • Arthralgia • Chest pain or shortness of breath with pulmonary involvement	• Muscle strength may be diminished • Tenderness to palpation over affected areas • Skin rashes: heliotrope rash on eyelids or erythematous papules over extensor surfaces of joints (proximal interphalangeal, elbow, or knee)	• Presence of anti-U1-RNP in MCTD • ANA likely to have a high titer and a speckled pattern in MCTD in contrast to DM or PM where high titers are suggestive of a separate overlapping inflammatory condition • Muscle biopsy can be definitive for diagnosis • Specific patterns on electromyelogram in DM	• Idiopathic inflammatory myopathy (e.g., DM, PM) • MCTD

B. Drugs (More likely to be older and male)

History	Physical examination	Further testing	Diagnosis
• Procainamide (10% develop lupus, 50% have elevated ANAs)	• Symptoms consistent with SLE described above	• Anti-histone antibodies (present in 95% of cases)	• Drug-induced lupus

(Continued)

TABLE 17.3.1	Evaluation of the Patient with an Elevated ANA Titer (Continued)

History	Physical examination	Further testing	Diagnosis
• Chlorpromazine • Quinidine • Hydralazine symptoms consistent with SLE described above		• Erythrocyte sedimentation rate is often elevated • Anti-ds-DNA testing is usually negative and can be used to differentiate this condition from SLE • Antibodies to neutrophil cytoplasmic antigens may be positive	
C. Systemic illness			
• Fever (in 50–80%) • Malaise • Weight loss • Night sweats • Cough (nonproductive in early stages, may eventually be productive of sputum and/or blood tinged) • Pleuritic pain • Dyspnea • Extrapulmonary involvement (15% of cases)	• Pleural effusion • ± Adventitial lung sounds • Lymph node enlargement with or without tenderness • Organ-specific findings	• Tuberculin skin test • Chest X-ray if positive skin test • Acid-fast staining and culture of induced sputum for mycobacteria • Possibly bronchoscopy • CBC looking for anemia • Electrolytes may demonstrate hyponatremia in patients complicated by the syndrome of inappropriate adrenocortic hormone secretion	• Tuberculosis
• Fatigue • Fever • Chills • Nonspecific sore throat	• Often normal • May have lymphadenopathy • Joint swelling	• CBC (may demonstrate lymphocytosis) • Viral titers (Epstein-Barr or cytomegalovirus)	• Chronic viral infections (e.g., Epstein-Barr virus and cytomegalovirus)
• Headache • Sleep disturbances	• Right upper quadrant tenderness or liver enlargement	• Other laboratory abnormalities are unusual but may be specific to the particular viral agent suspected	

(Continued)

TAYLOR'S DIFFERENTIAL DIAGNOSIS MANUAL

372 |

TABLE 17.3.1 Evaluation of the Patient with an Elevated ANA Titer (Continued)

History	Physical examination	Further testing	Diagnosis
• Women (95% for PBC and common for AH) and young (AH) • Abdominal pain • Fever • Amenorrhea • Diarrhea • Pleuritic pain and/or polyarthritis	• Jaundice • Hepatomegaly • Splenomegaly • Advanced disease can be characterized by spider angiomas, asterixis, palmar erythema, caput medusae, gynecomastia, parotid enlargement, and testicular atrophy	• Liver function testing (AST, ALT, gamma-glutamyl transferase, alkaline phosphatase) • Serial testing of amino-transferases if elevated • CBC • Hepatitis testing (A, B, and C) • Anti-ss-DNA and anti-smooth muscle antibody testing • Anti-mitochondrial antibodies hallmark of PBC • Liver biopsy	• Liver disease (PBC, AH, and primary autoimmune cholangitis)
• Weight loss • Fatigue • Malaise • Cigarette smoking • Family history of cancer	• Physical findings are dependent on the type of malignancy suspected	• Laboratory testing is dependent on the type of malignancy suspected	• Malignancy (positive ANA is a rare finding) (3)

AH, autoimmune hepatitis; ALT, alanine aminotransferase; AST, aspartate aminotransferase; CBC, complete blood count; RNP, antiribonucleoprotein; DM, dermatomyositis; MCTD, mixed connective tissue disorder; PBC, primary biliary cirrhosis; PM, polymyositis; RA, rheumatoid arthritis; SLE, systemic lupus erythematosus; ANA, antinuclear antibodies.

REFERENCES

1. Phan TG, Wong RC, Adelstein S. Autoantibodies to extractable nuclear antigens: making detection and interpretation more meaningful. *Clin Diagn Lab Immunol* 2002;9:1.
2. Solomon DH, Kavanaugh AJ, Schur PH. Evidence-based guidelines for the use of immunologic tests: antinuclear antibody testing. *Arthritis Rheum* 2002;47:434.
3. Lane SK, Gravel JW Jr, Clinical utility of common serum rheumatologic tests. *Am Fam Physician* 2002;65(6):1073–1080.
4. Wiik AS. Anti-nuclear autoantibodies: clinical utility for diagnosis, prognosis, monitoring, and planning of treatment strategy in systemic immunoinflammatory diseases. *Scand J Rheumatol* 2005;34: 260–268.

Brain Natriuretic Peptide

17.4

Perry W. Sexton and Dana McDermott

I. **BACKGROUND.** Brain natriuretic peptide (BNP) was discovered in the brains of pigs. Human ventricular cardiomyocytes, stretched from volume or pressure overload, synthesize a peptide which is cleaved into proBNP. This is secreted and then split into active 32-BNP and inactive N-terminal proBNP (NT-proBNP) (1). Other known human natriuretic peptides are atrial, C-type, and dendroaspis.

II. **PATHOPHYSIOLOGY.** Physiologic levels of BNP cause sodium and water excretion through the kidneys, although its primary effect is lowering cardiac preload through venous dilation. It may also inhibit cardiac collagen accumulation and pathologic remodeling, which lead to progressive heart failure (2). BNP and NT-proBNP are secreted in increasing amounts as healthy individuals age and more so in women than in men. Natriuretic peptides were initially used solely in the diagnosis of congestive heart failure (CHF); however, other uses continue to be established. They are useful in diagnosing, predicting prognosis, and managing left ventricular dysfunction (LVD) and coronary ischemia. Also, some experts suggest that these could be used to monitor symptomatic and asymptomatic patients with cardiovascular risk factors and predict their overall risk of death from cardiovascular events. Recent evidence suggests that BNP may even have a role in diagnosing and treating children with CHF in renal disease (3).

III. **EVALUATION.** Current natriuretic peptide tests are rapid immunofluorescence, which cost about $29.00 per kit. Within 15 minutes, anti-peptide antibodies bind quantitatively to BNP or NT-proBNP in the serum and fluoresce proportionally to the amount present. In patients with CHF and coronary ischemia, the use of rapid bedside tests in the emergency setting has decreased the morbidity and mortality.

When the clinical diagnosis is unclear, B-type natriuretic peptides offer a way to diagnose and therapeutically manage CHF and a wide array of other diseases with secondary cardiac effects. Other factors that may contribute to elevated or decreased levels such as genetics, sex, age, obesity, exercise, and comorbid medical conditions must also be accounted for when evaluating a patient for possible CHF. Guidelines for using BNP to diagnose and treat new-onset, acute decompensated, or chronic CHF are listed in Table 17.4.1.

IV. **DIAGNOSIS.**
  A. **Congestive Heart Failure.** BNP and NT-proBNP levels are currently used for aiding diagnosis, guiding treatment, and predicting prognosis in CHF. An elevated BNP or NT-proBNP level is highly sensitive and specific, with *96%* and *98%* negative predictive values, respectively, to rule out CHF in the patient with dyspnea (see Table 17.4.1).
    1. CHF is usually diagnosed from a detailed history, physical examination, and chest X-ray. In patients who present with cough or dyspnea, a significantly elevated level can distinguish a cardiac cause from other differential diagnoses (e.g., pneumonia or asthma). Adding BNP to the clinical judgment increases the diagnostic accuracy from *74%* to *81%*. It correlates directly to the New York Heart Association (NYHA) functional class (i.e., 244–817 pg/mL for classes I–IV) (4) and inversely to cardiac output (5). BNP and NT-proBNP may be normal at <100 and <300 pg/mL, respectively, whereas most patients with dyspnea and CHF achieve values >400 and $>1,800$ pg/mL, respectively (6,7). Each 100 pg/mL BNP elevation is associated with a *35%* increase in risk of cardiac death (8).

TABLE 17.4.1   Helpful Values for BNP

BNP level (pg/mL)	NT-proBNP (pg/mL)	Interpretation	Other
<50	<50 [a]	Primary care setting	NT-proBNP targeted for patients aged <60 y
<100 [b]	<300 [c, d]	CHF improbable	BNP NPV = 96%, NT-proBNP NPV = 98%
100–400	300–1,800	Possible CHF	BNP > 100 pg/mL has 84.3% PPV. See text for discussion of confounding factors. ECHO recommended for corroboration
>400	>1,800	CHF very probable	Patients should be under intense treatment and monitoring (see Chapter 7.5)
<500	–	Goal hospital discharge	–
>700	–	Severely decompensated CHF	–

[a]Adjust cutoff for age: <60, 60-75, and >75 y = 50, 100, and 250 pg/mL, respectively.

[b]Adjust cutoff <200 pg/mL for patients with atrial fibrillation (NPV=73%, PPV=85%).

[c]Adjust cutoff for age: <50, 50 to 75, and >75 y = 450, 900, and 1,800 pg/mL, respectively (PPV=90% and NPV=84%).

[d]Adjust cutoff <1200 pg/mL for patients presenting with eGFR <60 mL/min/1.73 m^2.

Key: BNP, brain natriuretic peptide; NT-proBNP, N-terminal propeptide BNP; CHF, congestive heart failure; NPV, negative predictive value; PPV, positive predictive value; ECHO, echocardiogram; eGFR, estimated glomerular filtration rate.

2. BNP and NT-proBNP levels usually fall after effective therapeutic intervention. A half-life is only 22 minutes; therefore, serial testing can be informative and aid in titrating therapy (9,10). Morbidity, mortality, and hospital readmission rates are dependent on aggressive treatment of CHF, and a decline in these levels often correlate with clinical improvements. A suggested goal is a BNP < 500 pg/nL at hospital discharge and <50 pg/nL in outpatient primary care settings (11).

3. A persistently elevated BNP or NT-proBNP despite optimal medical intervention carries a worse prognosis. Patients with chronic CHF may have persistent elevations and be clinically stable. Though they can provide useful prognostic information at initial clinical presentation, a series of levels is often more valuable for interpreting the relative trend in a particular patient.

B. Left Ventricular Dysfunction

1. Elevated BNP and NT-proBNP levels can predict the existence and severity of LVD in both symptomatic and asymptomatic patients (12). Some authors even suggest that levels can be used as a screening test for LVD in patients with cardiovascular risk factors. Of note, NT-proBNP concentrations rise four times higher than BNP in LVD and may prove to be more sensitive for diagnosing and treating this condition (13).

2. Elevations correlate with LV mass (i.e., hypertrophy) and LV distension and right ventricular (12), intra-ventricular, and pulmonary pressures (5); thus, other conditions (e.g., primary pulmonary hypertension, pulmonary embolism, primary hyperaldosteronism, Cushing's syndrome, athletic heart, or restrictive cardiomyopathy) may precipitate and lead to relative increases. Consequently, levels also reflect the ventricular and atrial consequences of mitral regurgitation (14) and the severity of aortic stenosis (15). They even increase as LVD worsens in severe sepsis despite preservation of ejection fraction (16).

C. Acute Coronary Syndromes and Known Coronary Ischemia. In the patient presenting with chest pain and questionable coronary ischemia, BNP and NT-proBNP may be elevated, denoting ongoing or recent ischemia if measured 6 hours to 10 days after an event. NT-proBNP has shown to have a stronger correlation with cardiovascular mortality than Troponin-C and C-reactive protein markers in cardiac ischemia (17). This can be especially helpful in patients who have nonspecific ST-T wave changes, a non-q wave myocardial infarction, or atypical chest pain. It is not yet known whether BNP predicts the severity or ultimately the prognosis of cardiac ischemia in these populations (18).

D. Special Considerations

1. Genetics, obesity, and age play a significant role in the variation of BNP and NT-proBNP among patients. In fact, genetic factors may account for almost half of the total variation (19). African American and Hispanic patients have higher levels than Caucasians within the same NYHA class (20). Exercise alone can decrease their levels by about *30%* (21). Obese patients (i.e., body mass index >30) with CHF tend to have lower levels (22). Normally women and older individuals have higher levels. Optimal plasma NT-proBNP cutoffs for ruling in CHF when accounting for ages <50, 50–75, and >75 correspond to 450, 900, and 1800 pg/mL, respectively (7).

2. BNP and NT-proBNP can be elevated in cirrhosis, renal disease, anemia (23), and cardio-renal syndrome (24). Patients with cirrhosis have levels three times those of healthy subjects in some studies. Patients with dialysis-dependent renal failure have unreliable levels, likely resulting from chronic volume expansion. However, patients with nondialysis-dependent renal dysfunction have levels that reliably correlate with echocardiographic evidence of CHF. The estimated glomerular filtration rate (eGFR) is inversely related to concentrations, and thus, for patients presenting with dyspnea and an eGFR < 60 mL/min/1.73 m^2, an NT-proBNP $> 1,200$ pg/mL indicates that CHF is probable (25).

3. Any type of cardiac inflammation, including cardiac transplant rejection, Kawasaki disease, constrictive pericarditis (26), or an arrhythmogenic ventricle with decreased ejection fraction, may lead to increased levels. Specifically, atrial fibrillation is associated with higher levels in the absence of CHF (13), and 200 pg/mL has been a proposed cutoff (27).

4. Other potential uses of BNP are being studied and developed, including nesiritide (i.e., recombinant BNP) to treat CHF, but recent studies show that in acute decompensated CHF, nesiritide therapy did not significantly change dyspnea, mortality, or 30-day hospital readmission rates (28, 29).

REFERENCES

1. Levin ER, Gardner DG, Samson WK. Natriuretic peptides. *N Engl J Med* 1998;339:321–328.
2. Tamura N, Ogawa Y, Chusho H, et al. Cardiac fibrosis in mice lacking brain natriuretic peptide. *Proc Natl Acad Sci U S A* 2000;97:4239.
3. Wieczorek SJ, Wu AH, Christenson R, et al. A rapid B-type natriuretic peptide assay accurately diagnoses left ventricular dysfunction and heart failure: a multicenter evaluation. *Am Heart J* 2002;144:834.
4. Maisel AS, Krishnaswamy P, Nowak RM, et al. Rapid measurement of B-type natriuretic peptide in the emergency diagnosis of heart failure. *N Engl J Med* 2002;347:161.
5. Silver MA, Maisel A, Yancy CW, et al. BNP Consensus Panel 2004: A clinical approach for the diagnostic, prognostic, screening, treatment monitoring, and therapeutic roles of natriuretic peptides in cardiovascular diseases. *Congest Heart Fail* 2004;10(5 Suppl 3):1–30.

6. Hobbs RE. Using BNP to diagnose, manage, and treat heart failure. *Cleve Clin J Med* 2003;70(4): 333–336.

7. Mehra MR, Uber PA, Park MH, et al. Obesity and suppressed B-type natriuretic peptide levels in heart failure. *J Am Coll Cardiol* 2004;43:1590.

8. Doust JA, Pietrzak E, Dobson A, Glasziou P. How well does B-type natriuretic peptide predict death and cardiac events in patients with heart failure: systematic review. *BMJ* 2005;330:625.

9. McCullough PA, Nowak RM, McCord J, et al. B-type natriuretic peptide and clinical judgment in emergency diagnosis of heart failure: analysis from Breathing Not Properly (BNP) multinational study. *Circulation* 2002;106:416–422.

10. Jourdain P, Jondeau G, Funck F, et al. Plasma brain natriuretic peptide-guided therapy to improve outcome in heart failure: the STARS-BNP Multicenter Study. *J Am Coll Cardiol* 2007;49:1733.

11. Cowie MR, O'Collinson P, Dargie H, et al. Recommendations on the clinical use of B-type natriuretic peptide testing (BNP or NTproBNP) in the UK and Ireland. *Br J Cardiol* 2010;17:76–80.

12. Palazzuoli A, Gallotta M, Quatrini I, Nuti R. Natriuretic peptides (BNP and NT-proBNP): measurement and relevance in heart failure. *Vasc Health Risk Manage* 2010;6:411–418.

13. Hunt PJ, Richards AM, Nicholls MG, et al. Immunoreactive amino-terminal pro-brain natriuretic peptide (NT-PROBNP): a new marker of cardiac impairment. *Clin Endocrinol (Oxf)* 1997;47:287.

14. Yusoff R, Clayton N, Keevil B, et al. Utility of plasma N-terminal brain natriuretic peptide as a marker of functional capacity in patients with chronic severe mitral regurgitation. *Am J Cardiol* 2006;97:1498.

15. Gerber IL, Stewart RA, Legget ME, et al. Increased plasma natriuretic peptide levels reflect symptom onset in aortic stenosis. *Circulation* 2003;107:1884.

16. Koglin J, Pehlivani S, Schwaiblmair M, et al. Role of brain natriuretic peptide in risk stratification of patients with congestive heart failure. *J Am Coll Cardiol* 2001;38:1934.

17. James SK, Lindahl B, Siegbahn A, et al. N-terminal pro-brain natriuretic peptide and other risk markers for the separate prediction of mortality and subsequent myocardial infarction in patients with unstable coronary artery disease: a Global Utilization of Strategies To Open occluded arteries (GUSTO)-IV substudy. *Circulation* 2003;108:275.

18. De Lemos JA, Morrow DA, Bentley JH, et al. The prognostic value of B-type natriuretic peptide in patients with acute coronary syndromes. *N Engl J Med* 2001;345:1014.

19. Wang TJ, Larson MG, Levy D, et al. Heritability and genetic linkage of plasma natriuretic peptide levels. *Circulation* 2003;108:13.

20. Daniels LB, Bhalla V, Clopton P, et al. B-type natriuretic peptide (BNP) levels and ethnic disparities in perceived severity of heart failure: results from the Rapid Emergency Department Heart Failure Outpatient Trial (REDHOT) multicenter study of BNP levels and emergency department decision making in patients presenting with shortness of breath. *J Cardiac Fail* 2006;12:281–228.

21. Passino C, Severino S, Poletti R, et al. Aerobic training decreases B-type natriuretic peptide expression and adrenergic activation in patients with heart failure. *J Am Coll Cardiol* 2006;47:1835.

22. Das SR, Drazner MH, Dries DL, et al. Impact of body mass and body composition on circulating levels of natriuretic peptides: results from the Dallas Heart Study. *Circulation* 2005;112:2163.

23. Wu AH, Omland T, Wold Knudsen C. Breathing Not Properly Multinational Study Investigations Relationship of B-type natriuretic peptide and anemia in patients with and without heart failure: a substudy from the Breathing Not Properly (BNP) Multinational Study. *Am J Hematol* 2005;80: 174–180.

24. Palazzuoli A, Silverberg DS, Iovine F, et al. Effects of beta-erythropoietin treatment on left ventricular remodeling, systolic function, and B-type natriuretic peptide levels in patients with the cardiorenal anemia syndrome. *Am Heart J* 2007;154:645.e9–e15.

25. Anwaruddin S, Lloyd-Jones DM, Baggish A, et al. Renal function, congestive heart failure, and amino-terminal pro-brain natriuretic peptide measurement: results from the ProBNP Investigation of Dyspnea in the Emergency Department (PRIDE) Study. *J Am Coll Cardiol* 2006;47:91.

26. Leya FS, Arab D, Joyal D, et al. The efficacy of brain natriuretic peptide levels in differentiating constrictive pericarditis from restrictive cardiomyopathy. *J Am Coll Cardiol* 2005;45:1900.

27. Knudsen CW, Omland T, Clopton P, et al. Impact of atrial fibrillation on the diagnostic performance of B-type natriuretic peptide concentration in dyspneic patients: an analysis from the breathing not properly multinational study. *J Am Coll Cardiol* 2005;46:838.

29. O Connor CM, Starling RC, Hernandez AF, et al. Effect of nesiritide in patients with acute decompensated heart failure. *N Engl J Med* 2011;365:32–43.

17.5 Elevated Creatinine

Nathan Falk and Aaron Goodrich

I. **BACKGROUND.** Elevated creatinine is defined as a serum creatinine >1.2 mg/dL in males and >1.1 mg/dL in females (1). Creatinine is the breakdown product of creatine from muscle metabolism and is excreted in the urine. The main use of creatinine is as a measure of kidney function by calculating the glomerular filtration rate.

II. **PATHOPHYSIOLOGY.** Elevated creatinine is due to renal insufficiency and can be divided into three etiologic groups: prerenal, intrinsic renal disease, and postrenal. These can also be broken down into acute (days to weeks) and chronic (months to years) causes. Acute kidney injury is defined as an acute rise in creatinine greater than 0.5 mg/dL above baseline or greater than 1.5-fold above baseline or oliguria (urine output less than 400 mL/d). (2) Prerenal causes account for 60–70% of cases and include decreased perfusion of the kidneys from either absolute or relative dehydration or decreased intravascular volume. Intrinsic causes account for 25–40% of cases and can be further broken down into vascular diseases, glomerular diseases, and tubulointerstitial diseases. Postrenal causes account for 5–10% of cases and are caused by any obstruction between the kidney and the end of the ureter (3). Falsely elevated creatinine can occur due to medications that interfere with assay technique (cefoxitin or other cephalosporins, flucytosine, methyldopa, levodopa, vitamin C, and barbiturates), medications that block tubular excretion of creatinine (cimetidine, pyrimethamine, and trimethoprim), toxin ingestion (methanol and isopropyl alcohol), creatine supplementation, and ketoacidosis (1).

III. **EVALUATION.** See Tables 17.5.1–17.5.3. Creatinine should be monitored in patients with certain chronic medical conditions (diabetes, hypertension, etc.) and certain medications (angiotensin-converting-enzyme (ACE) inhibitors, angiotensin receptor blockers (ARBs), diuretics, etc.). Almost all admissions to the hospital should have creatinine evaluated and should be monitored daily in patients receiving treatments known to effect creatinine (IV fluids, nephrotoxic antibiotics, and diuretics).

TABLE 17.5.1	Acute vs. Chronic Renal Failure
Acute	**Chronic**
Hypovolemia	History of CKD
Sepsis	Previously elevated creatinine in records
Acute hypertension	Normochromic normocytic anemia
Fever	Hypocalcemia
Hematuria	Hyperphosphatemia
History of taking nephrotoxic agents	Atrophic kidneys
No anemia	
No hypocalcemia	
No hyperphosphatemia	

CKD, chronic kidney disease.

TABLE 17.5.2 Evaluation of the Patient with Acutely Elevated Creatinine

History	Physical examination	Testing	Diagnosis
Prerenal			
Diarrhea, vomiting, decreased oral intake, diuretic use, fever	Dry mucous membranes, decreased urine output, reduced skin turgor	CBC, CMP, urine electrolytes, urinalysis	**Hypoperfusion due to** gastrointestinal, urinary, cutaneous losses, bleeding, or pancreatitis
Dyspnea, orthopnea, tachycardia, peripheral edema	Tachypnea, tachycardia edema, new murmur on auscultation, peripheral edema, pulmonary rales	CBC, CMP, EKG, cardiac enzymes, echocardiogram, D-Dimer, urinalysis, urine electrolytes	**Decreased cardiac output due to** heart failure, pulmonary embolus, acute myocardial infarction, severe valvular disease, abdominal compartment syndrome
Fever, fatigue, swelling, edema, drug overdose	Tachycardia, hypotension, tachypnea, fever, confusion	CBC, CMP, blood cultures, urine drug screen, urinalysis, urine electrolytes	**Systemic vasodilation:** sepsis, anaphylaxis, anesthetics, drug overdose, nephrotic syndrome, cirrhosis, adrenocortic insufficiency
ACE inhibitor, ARB or NSAID use	HTN	CBC, CMP, blood cultures, urine drug screen, urinalysis, urine electrolytes	**Drug-induced impaired renal blood flow**
Intrinsic			
Headaches, weight loss, fatigue, anorexia, rash, preeclampsia	HTN, fever, rash, peripheral edema	CBC, CMP, urinalysis, urine sediment and electrolytes, erythrocyte sedimentation rate (ESR), C-reactive protein (CRP), ANA, anti-DNA, RF, C3, C4, renal ultrasound, renal biopsy	**VASCULAR** **Microvascular disease:** atheroembolic disease (cholesterol-plaque microembolism), thrombotic thrombocytopenic purpura, hemolytic uremic syndrome, HELLP syndrome, or postpartum acute renal failure **Macrovascular disease:** renal artery occlusion, severe abdominal aortic disease (aneurysm)

(Continued)

TABLE 17.5.2 Evaluation of the Patient with Acutely Elevated Creatinine *(Continued)*

History	Physical examination	Testing	Diagnosis
Recent strep infection, arthralgias, history of rheumatologic disease	Rash, joint swelling	CBC, CMP, urinalysis, urine sediment and electrolytes, 24-h urine protein, ESR, CRP, ANA, anti-DNA, ANCA, RF, C3, C4, antibodies to streptolysin O, streptokinase, or hyaluronidase, renal ultrasound, renal biopsy	**GLOMERULAR** **Inflammatory:** *anti-glomerular basement membrane disease* (Goodpasture syndrome), *anti-neutrophil cytoplasmic antibody-associated glomerulonephritis* (Wegener granulomatosis, Churg-Strauss syndrome, microscopic polyangiitis), *immune complex GN* (lupus, postinfectious, cryoglobulinemia, primary membranoproliferative glomerulonephritis, IgA nephropathy, Henoch-Schönlein purpura, polyarteritis nodosa) **Drugs:** NSAIDs, gold, penicillamine, captopril, IVIG
Cancer, drug or alcohol ingestion history, seizure, contrast use, recent antibiotics		CBC, CMP, urinalysis, urine sediment and electrolytes, CK, myoglobin, appropriate drug levels, renal ultrasound, renal biopsy, serum protein electrophoresis	**Acute tubular necrosis caused by** *heme pigment* (rhabdomyolysis, intravascular hemolysis), *crystals* (tumor lysis syndrome, multiple myeloma, seizures, ethylene glycol poisoning, megadose vitamin C, acyclovir, indinavir, methotrexate), *drugs* (aminoglycosides, lithium, amphotericin B, pentamidine, cisplatin, ifosfamide, radiocontrast agents), *prolonged ischemia* (shock, surgery)

(Continued)

| TABLE 17.5.2 | Evaluation of the Patient with Acutely Elevated Creatinine *(Continued)* |

History	Physical examination	Testing	Diagnosis
Antibiotic use, NSAID use, fever	Rash	CBC, CMP, urinalysis, urine sediment and electrolytes, WBC casts, appropriate drug levels, renal ultrasound, renal biopsy	**Interstitial:** *drugs* (penicillins, cephalosporins, NSAIDs, proton pump inhibitors, allopurinol, rifampin, indinavir, mesalamine, sulfonamides), *infection* (pyelonephritis, viral nephritides), *systemic disease* (Sjögren syndrome, sarcoid, lupus, lymphoma, leukemia, tubulonephritis)
Postrenal			
Colicky flank pain, hematuria	Flank pain, decreased urine output	CBC, CMP, urinalysis, urine electrolytes, post-void residual, abdominal/pelvis CT or renal ultrasound	Nephrolithiasis
Male, weak stream, nocturia	Enlarged prostate on digital rectal exam, distended bladder, decreased urine output	CBC, CMP, urinalysis, post void residual, urine electrolytes, abdomen/pelvis CT scan, prostate biopsy	Benign prostatic hypertrophy (BPH), prostate cancer
Female, pelvic mass	Pelvic mass, decreased urine output	CBC, CMP, urinalysis, abdomen/pelvis CT scan, biopsy	Malignancy
Painless hematuria, weight loss, fever, night sweats	Cachexia, distended bladder, decreased urine output	CBC, CMP, urinalysis, urine electrolytes, post void residual, cystoscopy	Bladder cancer, clot, fungus ball
History of diabetes, multiple sclerosis, stroke, decreased sensation	Decreased sensation, distended bladder, decreased urine output	CBC, CMP, urinalysis, urine electrolytes, post void residual	Neurogenic bladder

CBC, complete blood count; CMP, comprehensive metabolic panel; EKG, electrocardiogram; HTN, hypertension; ANA, antinuclear antibody; RF, rheumatoid factor; C3, C4, complement factors; ANCA, anti-neutrophil cytoplasmic antibody; WBC, white blood cell; NSAIDs, nonsteroidal anti-inflammatory drugs; CK, creatine kinase; IVIG, intravenous immunoglobulin

TABLE 17.5.3	Evaluation of the Patient with Chronically Elevated Creatinine		
History	**Physical examination**	**Testing**	**Diagnosis**
History of diabetes, overweight	Overweight, retinopathy, decreased sensation in extremities, HTN	CBC, CMP, Mg, Ph, Ca, urinalysis, 24-h urine protein, renal ultrasound, fasting blood sugar, HbA1C	Diabetic nephropathy
Hypertension	HTN, retinopathy, left ventricular hypertrophy	CBC, CMP, Mg, Ph, Ca, urinalysis, 24-h urine protein, renal ultrasound, EKG	Hypertension
Rheumatologic disease, recurrent infections, arthritis, patient older than 40 y	Rash, joint swelling	CBC, CMP, urinalysis, urine sediment and electrolytes, 24-h urine, renal biopsy, ESR, CRP, ANA, anti-DNA, RF, C3, C4, antibodies to streptolysin O, streptokinase, or hyaluronidase, renal ultrasound, renal biopsy	Glomerulonephritis and vasculitis
Antibiotic use, NSAID use, fever	Rash	CBC, CMP, urinalysis, urine sediment and electrolytes, WBC casts, appropriate drug levels, SS-A, SS-B, renal ultrasound, renal biopsy	Interstitial nephritis
Urinary frequency, urgency, burning with urination	Fever	CBC, CMP, urinalysis, urine culture, voiding cystourethrography, abdomen/pelvis CT	Chronic infection
Fever, weight loss, night sweats, anemia, patient older than 40 y		CBC, CMP, urinalysis, SPEP, UPEP, calcium level, ESR	Neoplasm, paraproteinemia
Family history of polycystic kidney disease, flank pain	Palpable kidneys	CBC, CMP, urinalysis, abdomen/pelvis CT	Polycystic kidney disease
Refractory HTN, sudden-onset HTN, smoker	Abdominal bruit	CBC, CMP, urinalysis, renal Doppler ultrasound or magnetic resonance angiogram (MRA)	Renal artery stenosis

CBC, complete blood count; CMP, comprehensive metabolic panel; EKG, electrocardiogram; HTN, hypertension; HbA1C, hemoglobin A1C; ANA, antinuclear antibody; NSAIDs, nonsteroidal anti-inflammatory drugs; RF, rheumatoid factor; C3, C4, complement factors; SPEP, serum protein electrophoresis; UPEP, urine protein electrophoresis; WBC, white blood cell.

IV. DIAGNOSIS. See Tables 17.5.1–17.5.3. Elevated creatinine is usually asymptomatic in the early stages. Diagnosis is made by checking serum creatinine. Evaluation of the cause of decreased renal function should be made and can include comparison with previous creatinine, creatinine clearance (calculated with the Cockcroft-Gault formula or by 24-hour collection), urinalysis, urinary sediment, measurement of diuresis over 24 hours (if anuria), 24-hour urine collection to test for clearance of creatinine and proteins, urea, electrolytes, complete blood count, glucose, bicarbonate, calcium and phosphorus, protein and albumin, renal ultrasonography, or renal biopsy (4, 5, 6). The fractional excretion of sodium (FENa) can be used to differentiate between prerenal, intrinsic, and postrenal causes. FENa is calculated by using serum and urine sodium and creatinine. Prerenal causes will have a result of less than 1% and intrinsic and postrenal causes will be greater than 2%. The FENa equation is given as

$$\text{FENa} = \frac{\text{UNa} \times \text{PCr} \times 100}{\text{PNa} \times \text{UCr}}$$

REFERENCES

1. Donald DB, Richard LD, Richard FL. Chapter 18. *Common laboratory tests. Degowin's Diagnostic Examination*, 9th ed. New York, NY: McGraw-Hill, 2009.
2. Andrew L, Suren K. Acute kidney injury. Retrieved from Renal.org. March 8, 2011.
3. Richard T. Approach to managing elevated creatinine. *Can Fam Physician* 2004;50(5):735–740.
4. Brian A. Acute renal failure—differential diagnosis. Retrieved from Dynamed.ebscohost.com. Oct 17, 2011.
5. Malay A, Richard S. Acute renal failure. *Am Fam Physician* 2000;61(7):2077–2088.
6. Susan S, Bernadette P. Detection and evaluation of chronic kidney disease. *Am Fam Physician* 2005;72(9):1723–1732.

17.6 D-Dimer

Perry W. Sexton and Nicole Otto

I. BACKGROUND. D-dimer is a degradation product of cross-linked fibrin that has undergone fibrinolysis in the final stages of the clotting cascade (1). Although the D-dimer test is useful in the diagnosis of venous thromboembolism (VTE) (deep vein thrombosis and/or pulmonary embolism), venogram, Doppler ultrasound, V/Q scan, arteriogram, and/or high-resolution chest computed tomography (CT) scan are the definitive diagnostic tests for these conditions. The challenge of some of these diagnostic tests is that the results are operator dependent and can sometimes be "indeterminate." The D-dimer test was developed to potentially eliminate the need for further diagnostic testing in those who present with an unsure diagnosis of suspected VTE (2,3).

II. EVALUATION

   A. The first step in approaching a patient with VTE is to establish the pretest probability on the basis of clinical criteria such as the Wells Criteria (4–9) (see Tables 17.6.1 and 17.6.2). Additional clinical risk factors include the use of hormonal contraception, smoking, obesity, central venous catheters, thrombophilias, and inflammatory bowel disease (10).

   1. In patients with a low clinical pretest probability of VTE, a D-dimer level can be obtained to guide the diagnosis. A result of <500 ng/mL has a negative predictive value of 95% (see Table 17.6.3) and eliminates the need for further testing. Patients with a low pretest probability and a D-dimer of ≥500 ng/mL should go on to an appropriate imaging study.

TABLE 17.6.1 Wells Criteria for Predicting Deep Vein Thrombosis (DVT)

Criteria	Number of points
Active cancer (treatment within 6 mo or palliation)	+1
Paralysis, paresis, or immobilization of lower extremity	+1
Bedridden for more than 3 d or major surgery (within 12 wk)	+1
Localized tenderness along distribution of deep veins	+1
Entire leg swollen	+1
Unilateral calf swelling of >3 cm (measured 10 cm below tibial tuberosity)	+1
Unilateral pitting edema	+1
Collateral superficial veins (non-varicose)	+1
Previously documented DVT	+1
Alternative diagnosis as likely as or more likely than DVT	−2

Risk score interpretation (probability of DVT): 3 points = high risk (75%); 1–2 points = moderate risk (17%); <1 point = low risk (3%).

DVT, deep vein thrombosis.

2. Patients with a high pretest probability of VTE should be evaluated first by an imaging study; D-dimer is used only when the imaging results are "indeterminate."

B. It is important to note that a low D-dimer test is able to rule out VTE. By contrast, an elevated D-dimer level is not able to establish a diagnosis of VTE—this test is not sufficiently specific.

TABLE 17.6.2 Wells Criteria for Predicting Pulmonary Embolism

Criteria	Number of points
Clinical signs and symptoms of DVT	+3
An alternative diagnosis that is less likely than pulmonary embolism	+3
Pulse rate >100 beats/min	+1.5
Immobilization or surgery in the previous 4 wk	+1.5
Previous DVT/pulmonary embolism	+1.5
Hemoptysis	+1
Malignancy	+1

Risk score interpretation (probability of DVT): >6 points = high risk (78.4%); 2–6 points = moderate risk (27.8%); < 2 points = low risk (3.4%).

DVT, deep vein thrombosis.

TABLE 17.6.3	Interpreting D-dimer Results		
D-dimer value	Pretest probability for VTE (DVT or PE)	Interpretation	Diagnostic decision
<500 µg/mL	Low pretest probability	Normal	Can safely exclude the diagnosis of VTE
(Any value)	High pretest probability	VTE cannot be excluded	Need further imaging
>500 µg/mL	Any clinical probability	VTE cannot be excluded	Need further imaging

DVT, deep vein thrombosis; PE, pulmonary embolism; VTE, venous thromboembolism.

    C. There are many other systemic causes of an elevated D-dimer (see Table 17.6.4). D-dimer is primarily cleared via the kidneys and partially cleared through the liver, so dysfunction in either system can lead to decreased clearance and falsely elevated levels (11).

    D. The laboratory-based quantitative enzyme-linked immunosorbent assay provides quantitative values for interpretation, whereas the bedside immunochromatographic point of care assay provides a rapid qualitative value, with similar accuracy for low-risk patients (12,13).

    E. The D-dimer test is being investigated for potential use in other clinical settings, including
        1. Determination of the duration of anticoagulation for VTE patients (14)
        2. Diagnosis of acute aortic dissection (though a potentially delayed D-dimer measurement should not preclude imaging of this life-threatening condition) (15)
        3. Utilization of an age-adjusted D-dimer cutoff (patient's age × 10 µg/L) to increase the number of patients above 50 years in whom PE can be excluded (16–18)
        4. Inclusion of D-dimer in the laboratory evaluation of disseminated intravascular coagulation (19)

III. DIAGNOSIS. The D-dimer test is a quick, noninvasive, and non-operator-dependent laboratory test that can exclude the diagnosis of VTE when negative in patients with low pretest probability but does not have sufficient specificity to rule in VTE with certainty when positive (see Table 17.6.4 for other systemic causes of an elevated D-dimer) (11).

Table 17.6.4	Factors that Affect the Predictability of the D-dimer Test
Increased false-positive results	**Increased risk of false-negative results**
Cancer (20)	Cancer (21)
Inflammatory states	Recent surgery
Infection	Pregnancy
Sepsis (18)	Hypercoagulable state
Superficial thrombophlebitis (22)	
Trauma	
Hospitalization (23)	
Advanced age (16–18)	
Renal disease (10)	

REFERENCES

1. Adam S, Key N, Greenberg C. D-dimer antigen: current concepts and future prospects. *Blood* 2009;113:2878–2887.

2. Ramzi D, Leeper K. DVT and pulmonary embolism: part I. Diagnosis. *Am Fam Physician* 2004;90:2829–2836.

3. Qaseem A, Snow V, Barry P, et al. Current diagnosis of venous thromboembolism in primary care: a clinical practice guideline form the American Academy of Family Physicians and the American College of Physicians. *Ann Intern Med* 2007;146:454–458.

4. Wells PS, Anderson DR, Bormanis J, Guy F, Mitchell M, Gray L, et al. Value of assessment of pretest probability of the deep-vein thrombosis in clinical management. *Lancet* 1997;350:1795–1798.

5. Wells PS, Anderson DR, Rodger M, et al. Evaluation of D-dimer in the diagnosis of suspected deep vein thrombosis. *N Engl J Med* 2003;349:1227–1235.

6. Fancher TL, White RH, Kravitz RL. Combined use of rapid D-dimer testing and estimation of clinical probability in the diagnosis of deep vein thrombosis: systematic review. *BMJ* 2004;329:821–824.

7. Bates SM, Jaescheke R, Stevens SM, et al. Diagnosis of DVT: antithrombotic therapy and prevention of yhrombosis, 9th ed: American College of Chest Physicians Evidence-Based Clinical Practice Guidelines. *Chest* 2012;141(2 Suppl):e35is–e418s.

8. Wells PS, Anderson DR, Rodger M, Ginsberg JS, Kearon C, Gent M, et al. Derivation of a simple clinical model to categorize patients' probability of pulmonary embolism: increasing the model's utility with the SimpliREDD-dimer. *Thromb Haemost* 2000;83:416–420.

9. Stein P, Woodward P, Weg J, et al. Diagnostic pathways in acute pulmonary embolism: recommendations of the PIOPED II investigators. *Am J Med* 2006;119:1048–1055.

10. Caprini J. Update on risk factors for venous thromboembolism. *Am J Med* 2005;118:3–10.

11. Karami-Djurabi R, Klok FA, Kooiman J, Velthuis SI, Nijkeuter M, Huisman MV. D-dimer testing in patients with suspected pulmonary embolism and impaired renal function. *Am J Med* 2009;122:1050–1053.

12. Runyon MS, Beam DM, King MC, Lipford EH, Kline JA. Comparison of the simplify D-dimer assay performed at the bedside with a laboratory-based quantitative D-dimer assay for the diagnosis of pulmonary embolism in a low prevalence emergency department population. *Emerg Med J* 2008;25:70–75.

13. Wells PS, Anderson DR, Rodger M, Stiell I, Dreyer JF, Barnes D, et al. Excluding pulmonary embolism presenting to the emergency department by using a simple clinical model and D-dimer. *Ann Intern Med* 2001;135:98–107.

14. Palareti G, Cosmi B, Legnani C, et al. D-dimer testing to determine the duration of anticoagulation therapy. *N Engl J Med* 2006;355:1780–1789.

15. Sutherland A, Escano J, Coon TP. D-dimer as the sole screening test for acute aortic dissection: a review of the literature. *Ann Emerg Med* 2008;52:339–343.

16. Van Es J, Mos I, Douma R, et al. The combination of four different clinical decision rules and an age-adjusted D-dimer cut-off increases the number of patients in whom acute pulmonary embolism can safely be excluded. *Thromb Haemost* 2012;107:167–171.

17. Douma R, le Gal G, et al. Potential of an age adjusted D-dimer cut-off value to improve the exclusion of pulmonary embolism in older patients: a retrospective analysis of three large cohorts. *BMJ* 2010;340:1475–1481.

18. Tita-Nwa F, Bos A, Adjei A, Eshle WEB, Longo DL, Ferrucci L. Correlates of D-dimer in older persons. *Aging Clin Exp Res* 2010;22:20–23.

19. Taylor FB Jr, Toh CH, Hoots WK, et al. Towards definition, clinical and laboratory criteria, and a scoring system for disseminated intravascular coagulation. *Thromb Haemost* 2001;86:1327–1330.

20. Righini M, Le Gal G, De Lucia S, et al. Clinical usefulness of D-dimer testing in cancer patients with suspected pulmonary embolism. *Thromb Haemost* 2006;95:715–719.

21. Carrier M, Lee AY, Bates SM, Anderson DR, Well PS. Accuracy and usefulness of a clinical prediction rule and D-dimer testing in excluding deep vein thrombosis in cancer patients. *Thromb Res* 2008;123:177–183.

22. Gillet JL, FFrench P, Hanss M, et al. Predictive value of d-dimer assay in superficial thrombophlebitis of the lower limbs. *J Mal Vasc* 2007;32:90–95.

23. Brotman DJ, Segal JB, Jani JT, et al. Limitations of D-dimer testing in unselected inpatients with suspected venous thromboembolism. *Am J Med* 2003;114:276.

17.7

Hypercalcemia

Peter F. Cronholm, Mario P. DeMarco, and
Alexis M. Atwater

I. BACKGROUND. The normal range of serum calcium is 8.5–10.5 mg/dL. Hypercalcemia, defined as serum calcium concentrations above 10.5 mg/dL, occurs when the calcium enters the circulatory system more rapidly than it is excreted in the urine or deposited in bones. An initial elevated calcium level should be repeated to confirm the abnormality (1).

II. PATHOPHYSIOLOGY. Nine out of ten cases of hypercalcemia in adults are caused by either hyperparathyroidism or malignancy. Hyperparathyroidism causes most of the hypercalcemia in the outpatient setting. Malignancy causes most of the hypercalcemia found in hospitalized patients. Clinical features including presence of symptoms can help differentiate between these two main causes. Less common causes of hypercalcemia are chronic renal failure, hyperthyroidism, hypervitaminosis A, hypervitaminosis D, immobilization, Paget's disease, and granulomatous diseases (2). Pseudohypercalcemia occurs when patients have increased serum calcium-binding proteins. For example, dehydration severe enough to cause hyperalbuminemia may result in high serum calcium levels. Such pseudohypercalcemia should resolve after the hemoconcentration is corrected.

III. EVALUATION

A. History. Patients are often asymptomatic until the calcium level rises above 12 mg/dL, and the symptoms are often nonspecific: generalized muscle weakness, muscle aches, decreased coordination, decreased level of consciousness, headache, loss of appetite, nausea, vomiting, constipation, increased salivation, dysphagia, and abdominal pain or distension. A review of systems may turn up a history of a renal calculus or a history of a malignancy (3).

B. Physical Examination. Depending on the severity of hypercalcemia, physical examination may reveal mental confusion, poor memory, slurred speech, acute psychotic behavior, lethargy or coma, ataxia, poor overall muscle strength, hypotonia, hyperextensible joints, increased deep tendon reflexes, positive Babinski reflexes, incoordination, decreased pain or vibration sense, calcium deposits on the conjunctiva near the palpebral fissure or on the cornea around the iris, or an acute abdomen or an ileus. A short QT interval may also be noted on the electrocardiogram.

C. Testing. See Table 17.7.1.

TABLE 17.7.1	Evaluation of the Patient with Hypercalcemia		
History	**Physical examination**	**Testing**	**Diagnosis**
A. Spurious			
• Excessive thirst • Vomiting or diarrhea with poor oral intake	• Dry mucous membranes • Decreased skin turgor • Confusion/lethargy	• Repeat calcium after rehydration	• Pseudohypercalcemia due to dehydration
B. Endocrine disorders			
• Female • >60 y old • Aches and pains	• Neck mass (unlikely) • No clinical evidence of malignancy	• Serum calcium <14.5 mg/dL • Parathyroid hormone (elevated)	• Hyperparathyroidism (4) primary or secondary (pheochromocytoma, multiple endocrine neoplasia I, IIa)

(Continued)

TABLE 17.7.1	Evaluation of the Patient with Hypercalcemia *(Continued)*

History	Physical examination	Testing	Diagnosis
• Vague abdominal pain • Depressive symptoms • Renal calculi		• Serum chloride >102 mg/dL • Alkaline phosphatase (normal) • Serum phosphate • Bicarbonate • X-ray hands and clavicles	
• Anxiety/tremor • Weight loss • Family history • Heat intolerance • Vision problems	• Exophthalmos • Eyelid tremor • Tachycardia • Perspiration • Hyperreflexia	• Thyroid-stimulating hormone, free T4	• Thyrotoxicosis
• Fatigue • Weight loss • Family history • Nausea/vomiting	• Hypotension • Lethargy • Increased mucosal or skin pigmentation	• Elevated potassium • Decreased sodium • Decreased blood glucose • Abnormal adrenal cortical hormone stimulation test	• Addison's disease
C. Malignancy (5) • >50 y old • Weight loss • Smoker • Family history • Other symptoms specific to particular tumor site	• Weight loss • Signs specific to particular tumor site	• Serum calcium >14 mg/dL • Serum chloride <100 mg/dL • Alkaline phosphatase >2 times normal • Parathyroid hormone <2 times normal • CBC (anemia frequent) • Further workup according to the suspected site of primary tumor • Bone scan	Malignancy with or without metastasis • Lung cancer • Renal cell carcinoma • Squamous cell carcinoma

(Continued)

| TABLE 17.7.1 | Evaluation of the Patient with Hypercalcemia *(Continued)* |

History	Physical examination	Testing	Diagnosis
• >50 y old • Female	• Weight loss • Signs specific to particular tumor site	• Further workup according to the suspected primary tumor site • Alkaline phosphatase • Bone scan	• Breast cancer • Ovarian cancer • Metastatic disease
• >50 y old • Male • Urinary complaints	• Prostate mass on rectal examination or a diffusely enlarged hard prostate	• Prostate-specific antigen • Alkaline phosphatase • Bone scan • Ultrasound-guided prostate biopsy	• Prostate cancer
• >60 y old • Bone pain • Weight loss • Fatigue	• Pallor • Hepatomegaly • Splenomegaly • Tenderness over bones	• CBC (anemia) • Serum and urine protein electrophoresis • Creatinine • Erythrocyte sedimentation rate	• Multiple myeloma (6)
D. Medications/vitamins			
• Lithium • Furosemide • Thiazide diuretics • Aminophylline • Teriparatide	• Physical examination normal or shows signs of hypercalcemia	• Repeat serum calcium (elevated) • Other serum electrolyte values may be abnormal	• Medication use
• Calcium-based antacids	• Normal or shows signs of hypercalcemia	• Phosphate • BUN • Creatinine • Bicarbonate	• Milk-alkali syndrome
• Vitamin pill use • Bone pain • Headaches	• Normal physical examination or tenderness over bones • Papilledema	• Repeat serum calcium • Vitamin D level • Serum phosphate and chloride levels • For vitamin A overuse, serum retinyl esters	• Vitamin D overdose • Vitamin A overdose

(Continued)

TABLE 17.7.1	Evaluation of the Patient with Hypercalcemia *(Continued)*		
History	**Physical examination**	**Testing**	**Diagnosis**
E. Other			
• Prolonged bed rest or chair rest	• Physical examination normal or shows signs of hypercalcemia	• Consider DEXA scan for osteoporosis	• Immobilization
• History of acute renal failure	• Physical examination normal or shows signs of hypercalcemia	• BUN • Creatinine • Urinalysis	• Chronic or diuretic phase of acute renal failure
• Fever • Fatigue • Malaise • Anorexia • Cough • Dyspnea • Retrosternal chest discomfort • Polyarthritis	• Findings dependent on sites involved • Erythema nodosum • Uveitis • Lymphadenopathy	• CBC (lymphocytopenia) • Chest X-ray • Pulmonary function testing • Transbronchial biopsy	• Sarcoidosis or other granulomatous disease
• Family history of hypercalcemia	• May be normal or show signs of hypercalcemia	• Low 24-h urine calcium level	• Familial hypocalciuric hypercalcemia

CBC, complete blood count; BUN, blood urea nitrogen; CT, computed tomography; DEXA, dual-energy X-ray absorptiometry.

IV. DIAGNOSIS. See Table 17.7.1. Calcium levels above 12.5 mg/dL can be life threatening. In such situations, one should perform an electrocardiogram and begin treatment immediately, because cardiac arrest, convulsions, or coma can occur. Further testing can be performed while the serum calcium is lowered.

REFERENCES

1. Bushinsky DA, Monk RD. Calcium. *Lancet* 1998;352:306–311.
2. Potts JT, Juppner, H. Disorders of the parathyroid gland and calcium homeostasis. In: Longo DL, ed. *Harrison's principles of internal medicine*, 18th ed. New York, NY: McGraw Hill, 2011:3096–3120.
3. ASBMR (2009) Chapter 67. Non-parathyroid hypercalcemia. In: Horwitz MJ, Hodak SP, Stewart AF, eds. *Primer on the metabolic bone diseases and disorders of mineral metabolism*. Hoboken, NJ: Wiley. doi: 10.1002/9780470623992.ch67
4. Al Zahrani A, Levine MA. Primary hyperparathyroidism. *Lancet* 1997;349:1233–1238.
5. Stewart AF. Hypercalcemia associated with cancer. *N Engl J Med* 2005;352:373–379.
6. Mundy GR, Guise TA. Hypercalcemia of malignancy. *Am J Med* 1997;103:134–145.

17.8 Hyperkalemia

Nathan Falk and Joshua P. Brautigam

I. BACKGROUND. Hyperkalemia is defined as a serum potassium (K^+) >5.0 mEq/L. The prevalence of hyperkalemia in hospitalized patients is between 1% and 10% (1). Hyperkalemia can be life threatening secondary to cardiac manifestations when $K^+ > 6.5$ mEq/L (2).

II. PATHOPHYSIOLOGY. Hyperkalemia can be divided into four etiologic groups: spurious, redistribution abnormalities, renal disorders (impaired excretion), and hormone deficiencies. Spurious hyperkalemia in a healthy patient, most commonly caused by hemolysis during phlebotomy, can also be seen in cases of thrombocytosis, leukocytosis, and repeated fist clenching in blood drawing. The most common redistribution abnormality is acidosis. The most frequently occurring renal disorders leading to impaired excretion are renal failure with a concomitant potassium load and/or medication involvement. The primary cause of endocrinologic hyperkalemia is uncontrolled diabetes.

III. EVALUATION. Hyperkalemia is usually not sustained unless there is a disorder of the potassium regulatory system. In an otherwise healthy individual, routine screening of potassium is not indicated. Potassium should be monitored in patients on certain medications (see Table 17.8.1), with acid–base disorders, with abnormalities in renal function and disorders of aldosterone secretion. These patients are at risk for potentially fatal hyperkalemia (6).

IV. DIAGNOSIS. The initial diagnostic approach begins with a clinical history, review of medications, and physical examination. Hyperkalemia is usually asymptomatic; however, it can present with muscle weakness, flaccid paralysis, ileus, and characteristic electrocardiographic (ECG) changes (1). Arrhythmias occur at high levels of K^+ and if K^+ rises very rapidly in its concentration. The earliest ECG changes are tall, peaked T waves, followed by the loss of the P wave, then widening of the QRS complex, and finally development of a sine wave rhythm that can precipitate into ventricular fibrillation and asystole. Hyperkalemia can be life threatening even when the ECG is normal, as nearly one-half of patients with $K^+ > 6.0$ mEq/L will have a normal ECG (1). Laboratory testing is required to determine serum potassium level. Patients with a $K^+ \geq 6.5$ mEq/L require immediate cardiac evaluation.

TABLE 17.8.1	Evaluation of the Patient with Hyperkalemia		
History	**Physical examination**	**Testing**	**Diagnosis**
A. Spurious (3)			
Laboratory reading is "hemolysis" on electrolyte panel	Healthy patient	Repeat serum K^+ testing; normalized in redrawn sample	Hemolysis in collection tube
Platelet count >1 million	Healthy patient, except for disorder causing thrombocytosis	Repeat platelet count with heparinized specimen	Thrombocytosis (platelets release K^+ during clotting)
WBC count >200,000	Healthy patient, except for underlying disorder causing leukocytosis	Repeat WBC count with rapid processing/spinning down specimen	Leukocytosis

(Continued)

TABLE 17.8.1	Evaluation of the Patient with Hyperkalemia *(Continued)*

History	Physical examination	Testing	Diagnosis
K^+ normalized in repeat draw with careful draw technique	Healthy patient	Repeat serum K^+	Tight or prolonged tourniquet or fist clenching during blood draws
B. Redistribution (4)			
Acidosis	Often no signs specific to acidosis in an otherwise ill patient	• Immediate ECG • Monitor cardiac rhythm • ABG • Sequential testing	pH < 7.35
• β-blockers • Angiotensin-converting enzyme inhibitors • Angiotensin-receptor blockers • Cardiac glycosides • Neuromuscular blocking agents • Salt substitutes • Trimethoprim • Pentamidine	No signs of hyperkalemia. Physical examination may reveal underlying illness leading to medication use	• Immediate ECG • Cardiac rhythm should be monitored	Medication/diet effect
• Crush injury • Tissue breakdown	Bruising, other signs of trauma, or a necrotic wound	• Immediate ECG • Monitor cardiac rhythm	Cell breakdown
Rhabdomyolysis	Signs of cell injury, heat stroke, crush injury	• Urinalysis for myoglobin • BUN/creatinine • Immediate ECG • Monitor cardiac rhythm	Cell breakdown and kidney dysfunction
Large bruise or hematoma	Hematoma	• Immediate ECG • Monitor cardiac rhythm	Hematoma breakdown
Muscle contraction in marathon runners	Endurance athlete		Cell breakdown and muscle release of K^+
• Cachexia • Symptoms related to the etiology of the cachexia	• Cachectic • Signs related to reason for cachexia	• Immediate ECG • Monitor cardiac rhythm	Tissue catabolism

(Continued)

TABLE 17.8.1   **Evaluation of the Patient with Hyperkalemia** *(Continued)*

History	Physical examination	Testing	Diagnosis
Hemolytic anemia	• Pallor • Petechiae • Orthostatic hypotension • Bleeding from any orifice • Other signs as related to the etiology of hemolytic anemia	• Immediate ECG • Monitor cardiac rhythm • CBC	Hemolysis
Hyperkalemic periodic paralysis (5)	Quadriplegia with sparing of the cranial nerves		Transient hyper K+
C. Renal disorders			
Use of potassium-sparing diuretics (e.g., triamterene, spironolactone)		• BUN • Creatinine • Creatinine clearance may be low • FE_{K+}	Diuretic use
History of treatment for a *Pneumocystis carinii* infection		• BUN • Creatinine • Normal creatinine clearance	Trimethoprim or pentamidine effect
Known creatinine clearance <50		• Creatinine clearance • Immediate ECG, monitor cardiac rhythm	Renal insufficiency or failure with a potassium load
Systemic lupus erythematosus	• Malar rash • Discoid rash • Recurrent oral ulcers • Focal neurologic deficits	• ABG • Creatinine clearance • FE_{K+} • Evaluation of underlying disease	Decreased GFR
Sickle cell disease or trait		• BUN • Creatinine • Creatinine clearance may be low • Low FE_{K+} • Evaluation of underlying disease	Decreased GFR

(Continued)

TABLE 17.8.1	Evaluation of the Patient with Hyperkalemia *(Continued)*		
History	**Physical examination**	**Testing**	**Diagnosis**
Amyloidosis	• Signs due to amyloidosis	• BUN • Creatinine • Creatinine clearance may be low • Low FE_{K+} • Evaluation of underlying disease	Decreased GFR
D. Hormone deficiency			
Diabetes	• Signs of DKA	• Evaluate for DKA • Check ECG/cardiac rhythm • Sequential testing	Acidosis causing redistribution with K^+/H^+ exchange
Pseudo and actual aldosterone deficiency	• Hyperpigmentation • Hypotension • Weight loss • Vomiting	• Aldosterone levels • Renin levels • Check ECG/cardiac rhythm • Cosyntropin stimulation test	Addison's disease
Heparin use		• Aldosterone levels • Check ECG/cardiac rhythm	Aldosterone excretion low second to heparin

WBC, white blood cell; ECG, electrocardiogram; CBC, complete blood count; ABG, arterial blood gases; BUN, blood urea nitrogen; FE_{K+}, low fractional excretion of potassium; GFR, glomerular filtration rate; DKA, diabetic ketoacidosis.

REFERENCES

1. Hollander-Rodriguez JC, Calvert JF Jr. Hyperkalemia. *Am Fam Physician* 2006 Jan 15;73(2): 283–290.
2. Halperin ML, Kamel KS. Potassium. *Lancet* 1998;352(9122):135–140.
3. Wallach J, ed. *Interpretation of diagnostic tests,* 6th ed. New York, NY: Little, Brown and Company, 1996.
4. Gennari F. Disorders of potassium homeostasis: hypokalemia and hyperkalemia. *Crit Care Clin* 2002;18:273–288.
5. Evers S, Engelien A, Karsch V, et al. Secondary hyperkalemic paralysis. *J Neurol Neurosurg Psychiatry* 1998;64(2):249–252.
6. Humes HD, DuPont HL, eds. *Kelley's textbook of internal medicine,* 4th ed. Philadelphia PA: Lippincott-Raven.

17.9

Hypokalemia
Nathan Falk

I. **BACKGROUND.** Hypokalemia is one of the most common electrolyte abnormalities found in basic laboratory electrolyte panels. Although the definition varies, hypokalemia is generally said to occur when serum potassium (K^+) concentration falls below 3.6 mEq/L.

II. **PATHOPHYSIOLOGY.** With the exception of factitious causes (leukemic patients with extreme leukocytosis, where K^+ is taken up by the abnormal white blood cells), true hypokalemia results from increased potassium excretion, transcellular shift, or decreased dietary intake of potassium. Most commonly, hypokalemia is caused by abnormal losses of potassium through the gastrointestinal tract or kidney (see Table 17.9.1). The most common of these causes is iatrogenic via diuretic use leading to K^+ depletion. Both the loop (blocked resorption in the loop of Henle) and thiazide diuretics (block resorption in early distal tubule) contribute to the development of hypokalemia. Sodium and chloride delivery are increased by the diuretics, resulting in the secretion of K^+. Further K^+ loss is fostered by increased magnesium excretion, which is also linked to the loop and thiazide diuretics. Other medications, metabolic alkalosis, renal tubular acidosis, and aldosteronism due to systemic diseases and genetic disorders are implicated in the development of hypokalemia (5).

III. **EVALUATION.** See Table 17.9.1.

IV. **DIAGNOSIS.** See Table 17.9.1.

TABLE 17.9.1	Evaluation of the Patient with Hypokalemia		
History	**Physical examination**	**Testing**	**Diagnosis**
A. Gastrointestinal losses (1)			
• Emesis	• Often no signs on physical examination	• Serum electrolytes	Gastrointestinal potassium losses
• Nasogastric drainage	• Generalized muscle weakness	• Spot urine electrolytes if needed	
• Pyloric/duodenal obstruction	• Constipation	• Urine and serum osmolality as needed	
• Pancreatic fistulas	• Cachexia	• Stool electrolytes as appropriate	
• Diarrhea	• Abdominal examination for signs of peritonitis or localized pain	• Electrocardiogram (look for "U" waves or, if rapidly replacing potassium by the intravenous route, look for arrhythmias)	
• Laxative abuse			
• Colonic neoplasms			

(Continued)

| TABLE 17.9.1 | Evaluation of the Patient with Hypokalemia *(Continued)* |

History	Physical examination	Testing	Diagnosis
B. Renal losses (2)			
• Diuretics (loop or thiazide)	• As above	• As above	Renal potassium losses and congenital syndromes
• Osmotic diuresis (uncontrolled diabetes)	• May also ask about history of diabetes or use of loop or thiazide diuretics	• May also check for ketones, blood sugar, serum pH	
• Metabolic alkalosis (vomiting/diarrhea)			
• Primary hyperaldosteronism			
• Cortisol-responsive aldosteronism			
• Congenital adrenal hyperplasia			
• Liddle's syndrome			
• 11β-hydroxysteroid dehydrogenase deficiency			
• Bartter syndrome			
• Gitelman's syndrome			
• Inappropriate secretion of antidiuretic hormone			
• Hypomagnesemia			
• Licorice use			
• Corticosteroids			
• Renal tubular acidosis			
• Renal artery stenosis			
C. Transcellular shift(3, 4)			
• Bronchodilators	• As above	• As above	Drug therapy and systemic diseases
• Antihistamines	• May also ask about alcohol abuse and careful medication history	• May also check for serum alcohol level, drug screen as appropriate	
• Tocolytics			
• Theophylline			
• Caffeine			
• Insulin			
• Delirium tremens			
• Hyperthyroidism			
• Familial hypokalemic periodic paralysis			
• Barium toxicity			

(Continued)

TABLE 17.9.1 Evaluation of the Patient with Hypokalemia *(Continued)*

History	Physical examination	Testing	Diagnosis
• Pancreatitis			
• Congestive heart failure			
• Toxic shock			
• Pleural effusion			
• Ascites			
• Anasarca			
• Burns (second/third degree)			
D. Inadequate intake			
• Anorexia/bulimia	• As above	• As above	Patient excesses
• Forced vomiting or diarrhea for any reason	• May also check for evidence to support the history such as weight loss, staining, or pitting of the teeth		
• Neurotic spitting			
• Poor diet			

REFERENCES

1. Gennari F. Disorders of potassium homeostasis: hypokalemia and hyperkalemia. *Crit Care Clin* 2002;18:273–288.
2. Huang C, Kuo E. Mechanism of hypokalemia in magnesium deficiency. *J Am Soc Nephrol* 2007;18:2649.
3. Rastergar A, Soleimani M. Hypokalemia and hyperkalemia. *Postgrad Med J* 2001;77:759–764.
4. Clausen T. Hormonal and pharmacological modification of plasma potassium homeostasis. *Fundam Clin Pharmacol* 2010;24:595.
5. Gennari F. Current concepts: hypokalemia. *N Engl J Med* 1998;339(7):451–458.

CHAPTER 18

Diagnostic Imaging Abnormalities

Enrique S. Fernandez

18.1   Abnormal Mammogram

Abbie Jacobs

I. **BACKGROUND.** Breast cancer is currently the most common noncutaneous malignancy and the second leading cause of cancer death among women in the United States. Widespread screening with mammography and advances in treatment have resulted in decreased mortality from breast cancer. Currently, there are differing recommendations regarding screening and concerns about the effects of false-positive results. Since most women will have a mammogram either as a screening recommendation or a found breast mass, clinicians need to be able to discuss the role of mammography and subsequent results with patients.

II. **PATHOPHYSIOLOGY**

A. **Etiology.** The exact etiology of breast cancer is unknown but is believed to be due to aberrations in cell cycle regulation. Breast cancer can have a genetic predisposition with the most common mutations, BRCA1 and BRCA2, occurring in about 5–10% of breast cancers (1, 2). No single environmental or dietary exposure has been directly linked to a specific genetic mutation. Growth-enhancing mammotropic hormones affect the number of target cells and the likelihood of spontaneous mutations. The number of mammary tissue-specific stem cells, which are determined in early life, affect the risk of breast cancer. Their differentiation occurs during pregnancy and is protective (3).

The breasts are composed of fat, connective tissue, lymphatics, lobules which are the milk-producing glands, and ducts connecting lobules to the nipple. Breast cancers often arise from the duct or lobule and can be either in situ or invasive. Ductal carcinomas are more common, with invasive ductal carcinoma occurring in about 70% of cases (1, 3). Ductal carcinoma in situ tends to be more localized, while lobular carcinoma in situ shows a diffuse distribution in the breast.

Invasive ductal carcinoma shows the highest prevalence in women who are premenopausal or in early menopause. It is composed of heterogeneous cells arranged in single rows. Invasive lobular carcinoma is composed of small homogenous cells that invade the stroma and is often multifocal and bilateral. Estrogen, progesterone, and Herceptin protein receptors (HER2) play a role in tumorigenesis and regulation of breast cancer. They are also important markers for prognosis and used for targeted treatment. Tumors with overexpression of HER2 have a poorer prognosis (3).

Other less common types of breast cancer include inflammatory breast cancer, medullary cancer (younger women), phyllodes tumor, angiosarcoma, mucinous carcinoma (older women), mixed tumors, and Paget's disease involving the nipple.

B. Epidemiology. Breast cancer is mainly a disease affecting women, with only 1% of cancer detected in men (2). The chance of a woman having invasive breast cancer at some time during her life is approximately 1 in 8, while the chance of dying from breast cancer is approximately 1 in 35 (3). It was estimated that in 2011, there were 57,650 cases of carcinoma in situ, 230,480 cases of invasive cancer, and 39,520 deaths from breast cancer, with the majority of cases affecting women over the age of 50 years (2).

Numerous risk factors have been identified for breast cancer. The highest risk incurs for women older than 65 years, biopsy-confirmed atypical hyperplasia, presence of BRCA1/BRCA2 genetic mutations, mammographically dense breasts, and personal history of breast cancer. Women at modest risk are postmenopausal women with high bone density, history of high-dose radiation to the chest, high endogenous estrogen or testosterone levels, or two first-degree relatives with breast cancer. Other risk factors include alcohol consumption, prolonged estrogen exposure (early menarche and late menopause), recent and long-term use of estrogen and progestin, personal history of endometrial, ovarian, or colon cancer, obesity or overweight after menopause, and pregnancy-related factors including nulliparity, first pregnancy over age 30 years, and no breast-feeding. Tall height, high socioeconomic status, and Ashkenazi Jewish heritage also increase a woman's relative risk for breast cancer (2, 4).

Although the majority of breast masses are due to benign causes, breast cancer prevalence in women with a breast mass also increases with age: 1% in women younger than 40 years, 9% in women between the ages of 41 and 55 years, and 37% in women older than 55 years (5).

III. EVALUATION

A. History. Most patients who have breast cancer do not have risk factors. Nonetheless, it is important to take an appropriate history because screening recommendations and testing will be determined based on a patient's risk factors and symptoms. Ask about a family history of breast or ovarian cancer, menstrual and pregnancy history, use of oral contraceptives, prior mammogram results, previous cancer history and treatment, and lifestyle issues such as obesity and alcohol.

If the patient presents with a breast mass, in addition to evaluating breast cancer risk factors, inquire about duration, pain, skin changes and redness, relation to the menstrual cycle, history of breast cysts, masses and biopsies, and whether the breast or mass has been rapidly enlarging,

B. Physical Examination. Breast exams are relatively easy and inexpensive and are particularly important when there is a mass or the unavailability of mammography. As a screening method for breast cancer, there is controversy about the use of breast self-exams (BSE) and clinical breast exams (CBE). Studies using mammography alone compared with studies using mammography and CBE show no differences, and there are no studies that have evaluated either CBE or BSE alone. The sensitivity of CBE ranges from 40–69% and BSE from 12–41% (1).

The physical exam is essential for the evaluation of a patient presenting with a breast mass and is part of the triple approach which includes imaging with mammography/sonography and tissue sampling by aspiration/biopsy (5,6). The optimal time to do a breast exam is about 7–10 days after menstruation, when hormonal changes are low, but the exam should not be delayed. The exam includes the chest wall, breast, and lymph nodes both supraclavicular and in the axilla. Inspect the breasts visually while the patient is sitting, with arms at side and then up behind the head, looking for any asymmetry. Note the skin for dimpling, retractions, induration, or thickening. Next, palpate the breast while the patient is lying down with one arm stretched to the side or over the head. If the patient has large breasts, a towel or pillow may be used under the side to more equally distribute the breast tissue during the exam. Examine the entire breast area, preferably always following the same sequence. The clinician should palpate superficially, intermediate, and deep. Pay particular attention to any areas of possible thickening or masses, noting whether it is painful, soft or hard, and whether it is mobile or fixed. If the patient reported discharge from the breast, squeeze each nipple to establish whether the discharge is unilateral or bilateral. Palpate the axilla carefully, feeling against the chest wall and if nodes are palpated, note whether they are freely mobile or fixed, soft or hard.

C. Testing. There are several tests available to image the breast but only mammography has been shown in studies to decrease breast cancer mortality at an estimated 15% reduction (7). Screening mammography is for asymptomatic women, whereas diagnostic mammography is intended to provide specific information in patients with abnormalities on screening mammography or clinical presentation. Mammography sensitivity is 77–95% and specificity is 94–97%, with the positive predictive value increasing with age and with a family history of breast cancer (1).

The screening examination is ordinarily limited to craniocaudal and mediolateral oblique views of each breast. Supplemental views are occasionally required to visualize breast tissue completely or for women with implants. During diagnostic mammography, additional views might include spot compression with or without magnification or tangential views (8).

Screening recommendations vary among national organizations. The American Cancer Society, American College of Radiology, and American College of Obstetrics and Gynecology all recommend routine screening at age 40 years. The U. S. Preventive Services Task Force recommends biennial screening mammography in women aged 50–74 years and that physicians discuss the risks and benefits for patients 40–49 years and over 75 years. Women who have a family history of BRCA mutation should begin annual screening mammography between 25 and 35 years of age (1).

Magnetic resonance imaging (MRI) screening is more sensitive for detecting breast cancers than mammography and is being used to screen women with BRCA mutations. MRI detects smaller tumors. The sensitivity of MRI is higher than that of mammography, but has a lower specificity (9).

The Breast Imaging Reporting and Data Systems (BI-RADS) was implemented to standardize the readings of mammograms. The reporting helps guide the follow-up plan. BI-RADS 0 means the assessment is incomplete and the radiologist needs to review prior studies and/or complete additional imaging. BI-RADS 1 and 2 are considered a negative result—with 1 being normal and 2 a benign finding. With BI-RADS 1 and 2, the patient continues routine screening. BI-RADS 3 means a finding is probably benign but a shortened period of follow-up is recommended with a mammogram at 6 months, then every 6–12 months for 1–2 years. BI-RADS 4 and 5 show a suspicious abnormality, with 5 being highly suspicious. Biopsy is necessary for determination. BI-RADS 6 is a known biopsy-proven malignancy with treatment pending—to assure that treatment is completed (8).

For women with a palpable breast mass, additional imaging is required. There are differing approaches for the initial evaluation depending on the likelihood that the mass could be breast cancer. Initial steps may include fine needle aspiration, sonography, or diagnostic mammography. The American College of Radiology recommends diagnostic mammography followed by ultrasonography for a palpable mass noted in a woman over the age of 30 years. For women under 30 years, ultrasonography is the first test (10). In each situation, a determination is made to define whether the mass is benign (normal breast tissue, lipoma), cystic, or solid. A solid suspicious lesion always needs a biopsy. Most often a palpable breast mass will demonstrate benign findings on biopsy consistent with fibrocystic disease, a simple cyst, or a fibroadenoma.

IV. DIAGNOSIS. An abnormal mammogram requires follow-up. Further imaging may include additional mammographic views, ultrasound evaluation, or breast MRI. . For a non-palpable abnormality, image-guided biopsy is utilized, most commonly a stereotactic biopsy for suspicious microcalcifications. If sonography demonstrates a simple cyst, then fine needle aspiration may be appropriate, whereas a solid mass requires a biopsy. Tissue diagnosis of breast cancer will determine whether the cancer is ductal or lobular and whether receptors are present enabling a treatment plan to be established.

REFERENCES

1. Nelson HD, Tyne K, Naik A, et al. *Screening for breast cancer: systematic evidence review update for the US Preventive Services Task Force (Internet)*. Rockville, MD: Agency for Healthcare Research and Quality (US); 2009 Nov. (Evidence Syntheses, No. 74.)
2. American Cancer Society. Breast Cancer Facts & Figures 2011-2012. Atlanta: American Cancer Society, Inc.
3. Amin, S, Smith, MA. Breast cancer. *Essential Evidence Topics* Feb 14, 2012. Retrieved from http://www.essentialevidenceplus.com
4. Hauk, L. American College of Obstetricians and Gynecologists Updates Breast Cancer Screening Guidelines. *Am Fam Physician* 2012 Mar 15;85(6):654–655.
5. Kerlikowske, K, Smith-Bindman, R, Liung, BM, Grady D. Evaluation of abnormal mammography results and palpable breast abnormalities. *Ann Intern Med* 2003 Aug 19;139(4):274–284.
6. Klein S. Evaluation of palpable breast masses. *Am Fam Physician* 2005 May 1;71(9):1731–1738.
7. Wilkinson J, Effect of mammography on breast cancer mortality. *Am Fam Physician* 2011 Dec 1; 84(11):1225–1227.
8. ACR practice guidelines for the performance of screening and diagnostic mammography. Retrieved from http://www.acr.org/~/media/ACR/Documents/PGTS/guidelines/Screening_Mammography.pdf
9. Armstrong C, ACS recommendations on MRI and mammography for breast cancer screening. *Am Fam Physician* 2007 Jun 1;75(11):1715–1716.
10. Parikh JR, Bassett LW, Mahoney et al. Expert Panel on Breast Imaging. ACR Appropriateness Criteria® palpable breast masses. [online publication]. Reston (VA): American College of Radiology (ACR); 2009. 10 p. [42 references]

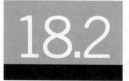

18.2 Bone Cyst

Lauri Costello

I. BACKGROUND. Simple or unicameral bone cysts are common and benign. They present either incidentally on X-rays obtained for other reasons or as the underlying cause of a pathologic fracture, usually in the proximal humerus or femur in a child. Aneurysmal bone cysts (ABCs) are uncommon and benign, although they can cause local bony destruction and may be associated with an underlying bone tumor.

II. PATHOPHYSIOLOGY

A. Etiology. The cause of bone cysts is still unknown despite the original description in 1942 (1). A simple bone cyst expands the cortex of the bone and the periosteum covers the thin cortical shell of the cyst. A membrane lines the cyst and septations may develop that give a more complex appearance on X-ray. Growth plate involvement may cause arrested or slowed long bone growth. When it involves the growth plate, the cyst is termed "active" and becomes "inactive" when the physis is no longer involved due to bone growth away from the cyst (2).

B. Epidemiology. Most simple cysts occur between the ages of 5 and 15 years and are twice as common in males as in females (3). The most common location is the humerus, followed by the femur; at least 75% of all simple bone cysts occur in these two sites (3). Simple cysts usually involve the central proximal metaphysis, but involvement of the epiphysis can occur. They can occur in virtually any bone, with the ileum and calcaneus being possible alternate sites.

ABCs typically occur in teenagers and are more common in females than in males (4). They can form in virtually any bone in the arms, legs, trunk, or skull and tend to be eccentric as opposed to the central location of simple cysts (5). ABCs are blood filled, with hemorrhage being a possible cause of rapid expansion; they are more likely to need treatment due to their increased likelihood for rapid growth and bony destruction. Some ABCs will resolve spontaneously, although they can recur after treatment (5).

III. EVALUATION

A. History. Simple bone cysts are usually asymptomatic unless a spontaneous fracture has occurred through the cyst. These fractures are typically in the proximal humerus or proximal femur and may be associated with trivial activity or more significant trauma (6). Rapid growth of a benign lesion, including an ABC but not typically a simple cyst, can produce pain by disrupting the periosteum where sensory nerve fibers are present. ABCs with rapid growth can also produce swelling and even a palpable mass.

B. Physical Examination. There are usually no associated findings on physical exam with a simple bone cyst unless there is a fracture causing some deformity and/or swelling. In this case, the physical exam should be directed at assessing for neurovascular damage as in any fracture. A limb-length discrepancy may be present, with lesions adjacent to or involving the growth plate. Tenderness and swelling associated with a rapidly expanding ABC may be noted on physical exam and possibly a palpable mass.

C. Testing. Plain X-ray is usually the only diagnostic test required to establish the diagnosis of simple bone cyst. The X-ray shows a well-defined, well-circumscribed lesion with a thin sclerotic margin without reaction or disruption of the periosteum. It is usually centrally located in the metaphysis, has a septated appearance, and is fluid filled. A large bone cyst that has expanded and thinned the overlying cortex puts the patient at risk for pathologic fracture. Suspected cysts in the spine or pelvis or cysts that appear atypical on plain X-ray may require computed tomography or magnetic resonance imaging (MRI) to elicit the anatomic detail necessary for the diagnosis. If an associated soft-tissue lesion is suspected in a long bone, an MRI can be helpful in determining the presence or absence of an associated mass.

ABCs appear more aggressive on plain films as they tend to erode the surrounding bone and are usually septated and blood filled. They also tend to be eccentric instead of central in the involved bone. ABCs are commonly associated with an underlying lesion, and in fact some investigators believe ABCs arise from underlying lesions. For these reasons, an MRI is often indicated in further evaluation of an ABC (4).

IV. DIAGNOSIS.
The diagnosis of simple bone cyst is made by plain X-ray (see above). An MRI of the affected extremity should be ordered if the bone cyst detected on X-ray is painful, is tender to palpation, or has an associated soft-tissue mass. Since ABCs can be associated with an underlying lesion including a malignant bone tumor, a biopsy should be performed when such a cyst is suspected (7).

REFERENCES

1. Jaffe HL, Lichtenstein L. Solitary unicameral bone cyst with emphasis on the Roentgen picture, the pathologic appearance and the pathogenesis. *Arch Surg* 1942;44:1004–1025.
2. Simple bone cyst. Boston Children's Hospital. Available at http://www.childrenshospital.org/az/Site642/mainpageS642P0.html
3. Randall RL, Hoang BH. Chapter 6. Musculoskeletal oncology. In: Skinner HB, ed. *Current diagnosis & treatment in orthopedics*, 4th ed. New York, NY: McGraw-Hill Medical, 2006. Available at http://www.accessmedicine.com/content.aspx?aID=2320059
4. Eastwood B, Gellman H. Aneurysmal bone cyst. eMedicine from Web MD 2011. Available at http://emedicine.medscape.com/article/1254784-overview
5. Anderson M. Aneurysmal bone cyst. Boston Children's Hospital; 2011. Available at http://childrenshospital.org/az/Site643/mainpageS643P0.html.
6. Melhman CT. Unicameral bone cyst. eMedicine from WebMD; 2011. Available at http://emedicine.medscape.com/article/1257331-overview#a01022.
7. Docquier PL, Delloye C, Galant C. Histology can be predictive of the clinical course of a primary aneurysmal bone cyst. *Arch Orthop Trauma Surg* 2012;130(4):481–487.

18.3 Mediastinal Mass

Ronnie Coutinho and Enrique S. Fernandez

I. **BACKGROUND.** Most mediastinal masses are discovered incidentally during routine radiographic studies. Because these may frequently be malignant, it is important to initiate a timely investigation of any symptoms that may be associated with a mediastinal process. When a mediastinal mass is suspected or detected, knowledge of the boundaries of individual mediastinal compartments and their contents facilitates the formulation of a differential diagnosis. Causes of a mediastinal mass are numerous, ranging from infectious etiologies to benign cystic lesions to malignancies.

The *mediastinum* is the space in the thorax between the pleural cavities. It extends from the sternum anteriorly to the vertebral column posteriorly and contains all the thoracic viscera except the lungs. Traditionally, the mediastinum has been divided into the *anterior (or anterosuperior) mediastinum* (the space in front of the pericardium), the *middle mediastinum* (the portion that contains the pericardium and its contents), and the *posterior mediastinum* (the portion behind the pericardium). It is vital to establish the location of the mass in a particular compartment, as masses in the anterior compartment are more likely to be malignant than those found in the other compartments (1).

II. **PATHOPHYSIOLOGY.** The pathophysiology of mediastinal masses is determined by both the age of the patient and the location of the mass itself. On chest X-ray, a line drawn through the anterior aspect of the trachea and the posterior aspect of the heart may be considered to be in the middle mediastinum. A line drawn through the anterior margins of the vertebral bodies is in the posterior mediastinum. It may often be difficult to tell if an abnormality is in the middle or posterior mediastinum. Therefore, these two compartments may at times be considered together when formulating a differential diagnosis.

A. **Anterior Mediastinum.** The anterior mediastinum contents include the thymus gland, a quantity of loose areolar tissue, lymphatic vessels, a few anterior mediastinal lymph glands, branches of the internal mammary artery, and the sternopericardial ligaments. Lesions seen in this region are thymic lesions (including thymic cysts), lymphoid proliferations, thyroid lesions, parathyroid lesions, and germ cell tumors. Additional tumors that may be seen in the anterior mediastinum include lymphangiomas, hemangiomas, and lipomas. One should consider infectious etiologies, such as tuberculous lymphadenitis, as well as noninfectious etiologies, such as sarcoidosis. Common anterior mediastinal lesions include thymomas, teratomas (also called *teratoid* lesions), lymphomas, and thyroid lesions (2).

1. **Thymoma**. This is the most common neoplasm of the mediastinum, and it is often discovered incidentally. Besides thymomas, other tumors of the thymus include thymic carcinomas, thymic lymphomas, thymic cysts, and thymolipomas. Approximately 25% of all mediastinal masses are thymomas and around half of the anterior mediastinal masses are thymomas. Thymomas generally present in adult life, equally in men and women; they are rare in children. Most thymomas (about 80%) are benign lesions.

2. **Teratoma**. Frequently, anterior mediastinal masses are teratomas (also referred to as *teratoid lesions*). Teratomas are germ cell tumors that usually arise in young adults from abnormally derived embryonic layers. They are often asymptomatic but, if large, they may have a mass effect with compression of adjacent structures. Histologically, most teratomas contain ectodermal components (e.g., sebum, hair, teeth). Computed tomography (CT) scan shows the cystic component as well as regions of calcification. The treatment of teratoma is surgical excision, and the prognosis is excellent.

3. **Lymphomas.** These constitute approximately 10–20% of all anterior mediastinal masses. In children, lymphomas account for approximately 25% of mediastinal masses. In adolescents, acute lymphoblastic lymphoma may present as an anterior mediastinal mass, often with thymic involvement. In adults, most mediastinal lymphomatous masses are seen in patients between 20 and 40 years of age. One of the most common lymphomatous lesions in relatively young adults, especially women, that very often presents in the anterior mediastinum is Hodgkin lymphoma.

4. **Thyroid Lesions.** Presenting as mediastinal masses, these are usually substernal goiters extending into the anterior mediastinum. A thyroid mass here may be asymptomatic or, if large enough, may present with pain or dysphagia. Most patients are women, usually older than 40 years of age at presentation. Besides these, various other types of cystic neck masses may be present. These vary in their histology and embryogenesis. CT scan and radionucleotide studies are helpful in making a determination (3).

B. **Middle Mediastinum.** Approximately 20% of all mediastinal masses are located in the middle mediastinum. These include the heart, the great vessels to and from the heart; the bifurcation of the trachea into the bronchi; the pericardium; the phrenic nerve around the pericardium; portions of the vagus nerve; the esophagus; and the lymph nodes in this region, which include the paratracheal and the tracheobronchial lymph nodes. The lesions that may arise from the middle mediastinum include aortic aneurysms, dilation of the superior vena cava, dilation of the pulmonary artery, or dilation/enlargement of the azygos and the hemiazygos veins. Lymphomas, tumors of the heart, pericardial cysts, and metastatic lesions are other diagnostic considerations to be considered in this compartment.

C. **Posterior Mediastinum.** Approximately 20–25% of all mediastinal masses present in the posterior mediastinum whose contents include the esophagus, the descending portion of the thoracic aorta, the thoracic duct, portion of the vagus nerve, and lymph nodes. Neurogenic tumors predominate in the posterior mediastinum. These include neuroblastomas, ganglioneuromas, ganglioneuroblastomas, neurofibromas, schwannomas, and pheochromocytomas (4). Less frequently occurring lesions include paragangliomas, chemodectomas, and giant lymph node hyperplasia (Castleman disease). Benign mesenchymal lesions such as lipomas, fibromas, myxomas, and leiomyomas may also be seen. Malignant versions include liposarcomas, fibrosarcomas, and leiomyosarcomas.

D. **Mediastinal Widening.** Aortic dissection is an important cause of mediastinal widening. Other causes of mediastinal widening include aortic rupture, sternal fracture, pulmonary contusions, mediastinal masses, tumors of the lung, idiopathic mediastinal fibrosis, cardiac tamponade, and leaking aortic aneurysms. Also, lymphomas and metastatic lesions can lead to mediastinal widening. Sarcoidosis is an important autoimmune consideration. Infectious etiologies of hilar lymphadenopathy and/or mediastinal widening include mycobacterium tuberculosis, tularemia, pertussis, viral diseases (including human immunodeficiency virus [HIV] and Epstein-Barr virus), rickettsial infections, varicella pneumonia, fungal infections (including histoplasmosis, coccidioidomycosis), and tropical eosinophilia. Anthrax and plague are important infectious considerations in the age of bioterrorism. Other miscellaneous entities causing mediastinal widening include Goodpasture's syndrome, histiocytosis X, cystic fibrosis, and idiopathic pulmonary hemosiderosis. Finally, occupational lung diseases such as silicosis and berylliosis should also be considered.

III. **EVALUATION.** A carefully directed history and physical examination is essential before investigative studies are performed to determine the likely causes of a mediastinal mass.

A. **History.** A history of constitutional symptoms, including a documentation of fever, sweat, and weight loss, is important.

B. **Physical Examination.** Check vital signs at the time of examination. Check for skin lesions and evaluate for signs of skin pallor or conjunctival pallor. Examine the neck for thyromegaly, masses, or adenopathy. Auscultate the lungs for wheezes, rales, rhonchi, or pleural friction rubs. Listen for pericardial rubs. On abdominal examination, evaluate for liver or spleen enlargement. On genitourinary and pelvic examinations, evaluate for testicular and/or scrotal masses or ovarian masses. Significance should be attached to the presence of localized as well as generalized lymphadenopathy (due to metastatic disease, HIV or other viral infections, or when considering a diagnosis of lymphoma). One should recognize the significance of a "pathologic" lymph node (1 cm or larger, persisting for at least 4 weeks).

C. **Testing**

1. **Laboratory Tests.** Routine laboratory tests should include a complete blood count with differential, and an erythrocyte sedimentation rate, as well as specific tests to be performed, depending on the type of lesion suspected. These may include lactate dehydrogenase, α-fetoprotein, β fraction human growth hormone, serum calcium, parathormone, γ-globulins, serum antiacetylcholine receptor antibody, purified protein derivative skin test, and HIV antibody screening. Suspicious or pathologic peripheral lymph nodes should be biopsied.

2. **Diagnostic Imaging.** CT scan is a very useful and almost precise tool for localizing and characterizing mediastinal masses and can provide helpful clues as to their nature (5). CT scan is better than plain films at demonstrating calcification of lymph nodes that may follow tuberculosis and fungal infections (6). Magnetic resonance imaging (MRI) is less often used to evaluate mediastinal masses but may help in the evaluation of patients with superior vena caval obstruction, aortic aneurysms, and larger intrathoracic blood vessels as also neurogenic tumors. Chemical shift MRI may be used in the differentiation of varied thymic lesions (7). Transthoracic ultrasound is useful in evaluating the thymus in adults and children and can help distinguish cystic from solid mediastinal masses; it can also aid in distinguishing cardiac from paracardiac masses. Barium swallow and endoscopic ultrasound studies are useful adjuncts for evaluating masses within the middle mediastinum as well as for evaluating esophageal masses and lymph nodes adjacent to the esophagus (6).

3. **Biopsy.** Suspicious or pathologic peripheral lymph nodes should be biopsied.

IV. DIAGNOSIS

A. Widening of the mediastinum can be due to numerous conditions. When evaluating a suspicious lesion, look for clues that help differentiate a mediastinal origin from a lung, pleural, or chest wall origin. Masses with irregular, nodular, or spiculated borders tend to arise in the lung, whereas broad-based masses with smooth edges are more likely to arise in the mediastinum or mediastinal pleura.

B. To make a definitive diagnosis, a biopsy of the mediastinal mass may be necessary. Histologic diagnosis guides more specific laboratory and imaging studies. A tissue diagnosis is also important for disease staging and to inform treatment options for the specific condition.

REFERENCES

1. Davis RD Jr, Oldham HN Jr, Sabiston DC Jr. Primary cysts and neoplasms of mediastinum; recent change in clinical presentation, methods of diagnosis, management and results. *Ann Thorac Surg* 1987;44(3):229–237.
2. Suto Y, Araya S, Sakuma K, et al. Myasthenia gravis with thymic hyperplasia and pure red cell aplasia. *J Neurol Sci* 2004;224(1–2):93–95.
3. Lev S, Lev MH. Imaging of cystic lesions. Department of Radiology, Nassau County Medical Center, East Meadow, New York, USA. *Radiol Clin North Am* 2000;38(5):1013–1027.
4. Topcu S, Alper A, Gulhan E, et al. Neurogenic tumors of the mediastinum: a report of 60 cases. *Can Respir J* 2000;7(3):261–265.
5. Hoerbelt R, Keunecke L. The value of a noninvasive diagnostic approach to mediastinal masses. *Ann Thorac Surg* 2003;75(4):1086–1090.
6. Armstrong P, Padley S. *Grainger & Allison's diagnostic radiology: a textbook of medical imaging,* 5th ed. New York, NY: Churchill Livingstone, 2008.
7. Inaoka T, Takahashi K, Mineta M, Yamada T, Shuke N, Okizaki A, Nagasawa K, Sugimori H, Aburano T. Thymic hyperplasia and thymus gland tumors: differentiation with chemical shift MR imaging. *Radiology* 2007;243(3):869.

18.4 Osteopenia
Iriana Hammel

I. BACKGROUND. Osteopenia is the precursor of osteoporosis, a disease characterized by decreased bone mass and microarchitectural deterioration of bone tissue, leading to enhanced bone fragility and a consequent increase in fracture incidence (1).

Throughout life, older bone is periodically resorbed by osteoclasts at discrete sites and replaced with new bone made by osteoblasts. This process is known as remodeling. Remodeling is orchestrated and targeted to a particular site that is in need for repair by osteocytes (2, 3). An oversupply of osteoclasts relative to the need for remodeling and an undersupply of osteoblasts relative to the need for cavity repair are the main pathophysiologic changes in osteoporosis (2, 4, 5). Other factors contributing to decreased bone strength are small bone size, unfavorable macroarchitecture (such as increased length of the femoral neck), disrupted microarchitecture, compromised quality of the material, and decreased viability of osteocytes (2).

Osteoporosis increases the risk of bone fracture with subsequent diminished quality of life, decreased functional independence, and increased morbidity and mortality. Pain and kyphosis, height loss, and other changes in body habitus resulting from vertebral compression fractures diminish the quality of life in women and men (6).

Early identification and treatment of such patients reduces the individual and societal cost (1).

II. PATHOPHYSIOLOGY

A. Etiology. The imbalance of osteoclastic and osteoblastic activity can be caused by several age- and disease-related conditions, often classified as primary and secondary osteoporosis.

1. **Primary Osteoporosis.** Primary osteoporosis, the most common form of the disease, occurs in patients in whom a secondary cause of osteoporosis cannot be identified, including juvenile and idiopathic osteoporosis (7). Idiopathic osteoporosis can be further subdivided into postmenopausal (type I) and age-associated (type II) osteoporosis, as follows:

   a. Juvenile osteoporosis, a rare form of the disease, usually occurs in children or young adults of both sexes. These patients have normal gonadal function. The age of onset usually is 8–14 years. The hallmark characteristic of juvenile osteoporosis is sudden onset of bone pain and/or a fracture following trauma (7).

   b. Type I osteoporosis (postmenopausal osteoporosis) occurs in women aged 50–65 years and is characterized by a phase of accelerated bone loss. Occurring primarily from trabecular bone, fractures of the distal forearm and vertebral bodies are common (7).

   c. Type II osteoporosis (age-associated or senile) occurs in women and men older than 70 years and represents bone loss associated with aging. Fractures occur in cortical and trabecular bone. In addition to wrist and vertebral fractures, hip fractures are often seen in patients with type II osteoporosis (7).

2. **Secondary Osteoporosis.** Secondary osteoporosis occurs when an underlying disease, deficiency, or drug causes osteoporosis. Up to one-third of postmenopausal women, as well as many men and premenopausal women, have a coexisting cause of bone loss (8, 9). Conditions that may lead to osteoporosis include the following:

   a. Genetic (congenital): cystic fibrosis, Ehlers-Danlos syndrome, glycogen storage disease, Gaucher disease, hemochromatosis, homocystinuria, hypophosphatasia, idiopathic hypercalciuria, Marfan syndrome, Menkes steely hair syndrome, osteogenesis imperfecta, porphyria, Riley-Day syndrome, hypogonadal states (see below) (7).

   b. Hypogonadal states: androgen insensitivity, anorexia nervosa/bulimia nervosa, female athlete triad, hyperprolactinemia, panhypopituitarism, premature menopause, Turner syndrome, Klinefelter syndrome.

    c. Endocrine disorders: acromegaly, adrenal insufficiency, Cushing syndrome, estrogen deficiency, diabetes mellitus, hyperparathyroidism, hyperthyroidism, hypogonadism, pregnancy, prolactinoma (7, 10, 11).

    d. Deficiency states: calcium, magnesium, vitamin D and protein deficiencies (11, 12), Celiac disease, malabsorption, malnutrition, primary biliary cirrhosis, status postbariatric surgery, status postgastrectomy, or prolonged parenteral nutrition (7).

    e. Inflammatory diseases: inflammatory bowel disease, ankylosing spondylitis, rheumatoid arthritis, systemic lupus erythematosus (7).

    f. Hematologic and neoplastic disorders: hemochromatosis, hemophilia, leukemia, lymphoma, multiple myeloma, sickle cell anemia, systemic mastocytosis, thalassemia, metastatic disease (7).

    Medications known to cause or accelerate bone loss include anticonvulsants, antipsychotics, antiretrovirals, aromatase inhibitors, chemotherapeutic/transplant drugs, furosemide, corticotropin and glucocorticoids, such as prednisone (≥5 mg/d for ≥3 months), heparin (long term), hormonal/endocrine therapies (gonadotropin-releasing hormone agonists, luteinizing hormone-releasing hormone analogs), depot medroxyprogesterone, excessive thyroid supplementation, lithium, methotrexate, selective serotonin reuptake inhibitors (7, 10).

    Miscellaneous causes of osteoporosis include alcoholism, amyloidosis, chronic metabolic acidosis, congestive heart failure, depression, emphysema, chronic or end-stage renal disease, chronic liver disease, HIV/AIDS, idiopathic calciuria, idiopathic scoliosis, immobility, multiple sclerosis, ochronosis, organ transplantation, pregnancy/lactation, sarcoidosis, weightlessness (7).

B. Epidemiology. According to the National Osteoporosis Foundation, 10 million Americans have osteoporosis. Another 34 million have osteopenia, which leaves them at increased risk for osteoporosis (13). Each year in the United States, 1.5 million osteoporotic fractures occur. Of these, 700,000 occur in the spine, 300,000 occur in the hip, and 200,000 occur in the wrist. The remainder of fractures occur at other sites in the body. The cost associated with treatment of these fractures is also very high (estimated at $19 billion in 2012 and at $25 billion in 2025) (13). Risk factors for osteopenia and osteoporosis include age, Caucasian and Asian race, female gender, low calcium or vitamin D intake, high caffeine or salt intake, alcohol, smoking, falls, thin/frail body habitus, sedentary lifestyle, estrogen deficiency in women, and testosterone deficiency in men.

III. EVALUATION

A. History. A history of amenorrhea, pregnancy, lactation, oral contraceptive use, as well as a detailed menstrual history should be elicited from all female patients. A history of previous and chronic illnesses, falls, fractures, eating disorders, weight reduction surgery, calcium and vitamin D intake, alcohol, tobacco and caffeine use, sedentary lifestyle, family history of osteoporosis and certain prescription medications, such as steroids, anticonvulsants, proton pump inhibitors, antidepressants, and chemotherapeutic agents should be elicited from all patients. Male patients should be questioned about symptoms suggestive of testosterone deficiency. A history of decrease in height should be elicited from all patients, since it may be indicative of occult vertebral compression fractures.

B. Physical Examination. Patients should be evaluated for abnormal spinal curvature (kyphosis in particular), asymmetry of the paravertebral musculature, and skeletal bone deformities.

    Gait, posture, and balance evaluation should be performed, as should palpation over the vertebral processes, since tenderness may suggest vertebral fracture. All patients should be examined for signs of eating disorders and malnutrition, and male patients should be evaluated for signs of testosterone deficiency.

C. Diagnostic Testing

    1. Laboratory Testing. The following laboratory studies are used to establish baseline conditions or to exclude secondary causes of osteoporosis: complete blood count, electrolytes, calcium, phosphate, creatinine, liver function tests, thyroid-stimulating hormone level, and 25-hydroxy vitamin D level (7).

Other laboratory studies used to evaluate for secondary causes include 24-hour urine calcium (to assess for hypercalciuria), intact parathyroid hormone level, thyrotropin level, testosterone level, gonadotropin levels, erythrocyte sedimentation rate, C-reactive protein, urine cortisol, dexamethasone suppression tests, serum protein electrophoresis, urine protein electrophoresis, antigliadin and antiendomysial antibodies for Celiac disease, serum tryptase for mastocytosis, and bone marrow biopsy if a hematologic disorder is suspected (7).

2. **Imaging Tests.** Imaging options include plain radiography, densitometry, single-photon absorptiometry, dual-photon absorptiometry, dual-energy X-ray absorptiometry (DEXA), quantitative computed tomography (QCT) scanning, magnetic resonance imaging (MRI), bone scanning, and single-photon emission CT (SPECT) scanning (7).

Of all these imaging options, DEXA is currently the standard criterion for the evaluation of bone mineral density (BMD) (14, 15).

a. DEXA (Dual-Energy X-Ray Absorptiometry)

BMD has been shown to be the best indicator of fracture risk. The U. S. Preventive Services Task Force recommends measuring BMD in the following patients (16):

   i. Women aged 65 years and older without previous known fractures or secondary causes of osteoporosis (16).

   ii. Women younger than 65 years whose 10-year fracture risk[1] is equal to or greater than that of a 65-year-old white woman without additional risk factors (16).

b. Plain radiography may be indicated if a fracture is already suspected or if patients have lost more than 1.5 inches of height. It is not as accurate as BMD testing and it does not reveal osteoporotic changes until they affect the cortical bone. It is therefore considered an insensitive tool for diagnosing osteoporosis (7).

c. QCT scanning is more expensive, has relatively poor reproducibility, and requires a higher radiation dose than DEXA scanning. It is not an ideal technique when repeated measurements are needed to detect small changes in BMD. Consequently, QCT scanning is seldom used now (7).

d. SPECT is a bone imaging technique that offers better image contrast and more accurate lesion localization than planar bone scanning. SPECT scanning is helpful when accurate localization of skeletal lesions within large and/or anatomically complex bony structures is required (7).

e. Quantitative ultrasonography of the calcaneus is a low-cost portable screening tool. It has the advantage of not involving radiation, but it is not as accurate as other imaging methods (7).

f. MRI may be the imaging method of choice in the detection of acute fractures. It can be used to discriminate between acute and chronic fractures of the vertebrae and occult stress fractures of the proximal femur (7).

g. Bone scanning is a nonspecific modality, but it is very sensitive for detecting bony abnormalities, such as compression fractures (7).

3. **Biochemical Markers of Bone Turnover.** Biochemical markers of bone turnover reflect bone formation or bone resorption (7).

Serum markers of bone formation (osteoblast products) are currently available, such as bone-specific alkaline phosphatase or osteocalcin. Serum markers of bone resorption are also available, such as cross-linked C-telopeptide of type I collagen or tartrate-resistant acid phosphatase (7).

Urinary markers of bone resorption (osteoclast products) include hydroxyproline, free and total pyridinolines, N-telopeptide of collagen cross-links, and C-telopeptide of collagen cross-links (7).

---

[1] In 2008, a World Health Organization (WHO) task force introduced a Fracture Risk Assessment Tool, which estimates the 10-year probability of hip fracture or major osteoporotic fractures combined (hip, spine, shoulder, or wrist) for an untreated woman or man using easily obtainable clinical risk factors for fracture, with or without information on BMD (17).

The use of these biochemical markers is controversial due to concerns about intra-assay and inter-assay variability. Further studies are needed to determine the clinical utility of these markers in osteoporosis evaluation and management (7).

IV. DIAGNOSIS. Assessment of microarchitecture requires bone biopsy, which is not routinely used in clinical practice. Therefore, BMD assessment is the gold standard to diagnose osteoporosis (19).

The WHO has established the following definition and diagnostic criteria for osteopenia and osteoporosis, based on BMD measurements in white women:

A. Osteopenia—BMD between 1 and 2.5 SD below the mean for young adult women (T-score between −1 and −2.5)

B. Osteoporosis—BMD 2.5 SD or more below the normal mean for young adult females (T-score at or below −2.5)

The diagnostic finding of low BMD is nonspecific and can have a multitude of etiologies (see Section II Pathophysiology). An important fact to consider is that the clinical diagnosis of osteoporosis may be made in the presence of a fragility fracture, without BMD measurement (18).

REFERENCES

1. Duque G, Troen BR. Chapter 117. Osteoporosis. In: Halter JB, Ouslander JG, Tinetti ME, Studenski S, High KP, Asthana S, eds. *Hazzard's geriatric medicine and gerontology,* 6th ed. New York, NY: McGraw-Hill; 2009.

2. Manolagas SC. Pathogenesis of osteoporosis, Up-to-Date, August, 2012, Topic # 2044 version 8.0, http://www.uptodate.com/contents/pathogenesis-of-osteoporosis?source=search_result&search=pathogenesis+of+osteoporosis&selectedTitle=1%7E150

3. Xiong J, Onal M, Jilka RL, et al. Matrix-embedded cells control osteoclast formation. *Nat Med* 2011;17:1235–1241.

4. Manolagas SC. Birth and death of bone cells: basic regulatory mechanisms and implications for the pathogenesis and treatment of osteoporosis. *Endocr Rev* 2000;21:115.

5. Manolagas SC, Kousteni S, Jilka RL. Sex steroids and bone. *Recent Prog Horm Res* 2002;57:385.

6. Lindsay R, Cosman F. Chapter 354. Osteoporosis. In: Longo DL, Fauci AS, Kasper DL, Hauser SL, Jameson JL, Loscalzo J, eds. *Harrison's principles of internal medicine,* 18th ed. New York, NY: McGraw-Hill, 2012.

7. Dana Jacobs-Kosmin, MD, Sucharitha Shanmugam, MD; Chief Editor: Herbert S Diamond, MD. Osteoporosis (Medscape).

8. [Guideline] American Association of Clinical Endocrinologists medical guidelines for clinical practice for the prevention and treatment of postmenopausal osteoporosis: 2001 edition, with selected updates for 2003. *Endocr Pract* Nov-Dec 2003;9(6):544–564. [Medline].

9. Kelman A, Lane NE. The management of secondary osteoporosis. *Best Pract Res Clin Rheumatol* Dec 2005;19(6):1021–1037. [Medline].

10. Greenspan SL, Korytkowski M, Resnick NM. Chapter 23. Geriatric endocrinology. In: Gardner DG, Shoback D, eds. *Greenspan's basic & clinical endocrinology,* 9th ed. New York, NY: McGraw-Hill, 2011.

11. Mann GB, Kang YC, Brand C, Ebeling PR, Miller JA. Secondary causes of low bone mass in patients with breast cancer: a need for greater vigilance. *J Clin Oncol* Aug 1 2009;27(22):3605–3610. [Medline].

12. Holick MF. Vitamin D deficiency. *N Engl J Med* Jul 19 2007;357(3):266–281. [Medline].

13. National Osteoporosis Foundation. *Clinician's guide to prevention and treatment of osteoporosis.* Available at http://www.nof.org/professionals/clinical-guidelines. Accessed January, 2011.

14. Gosfield E 3rd, Bonner FJ Jr. Evaluating bone mineral density in osteoporosis. *Am J Phys Med Rehabil* May-Jun 2000;79(3):283–291. [Medline].

15. Curtis JR, Carbone L, Cheng H, Hayes B, Laster A, Matthews R, et al. Longitudinal trends in use of bone mass measurement among older Americans, 1999-2005. *J Bone Miner Res.* Jul 2008;23(7):1061–1067. [Medline]. [Full Text].

16. U.S. Preventive Services Task Force. Screening for Osteoporosis: U.S. Preventive Services Task Force Recommendation Statement. *Ann Intern Med* Jan 17 2011;[Medline].

17. Michael K. Screening for osteoporosis, Up-to-Date, August, 2012

18. Rosen H, Drezner C. Diagnosis and evaluation of osteoporosis in postmenopausal women, Up-to-Date, August, 2012.

19. Resnick D, Kransdorf M. Osteoporosis. In: Bone and Joint Imaging. 3rd ed. 2005:551.

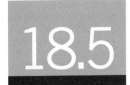

Solitary Pulmonary Nodule

Scott Ippolito

I. **BACKGROUND.** A solitary pulmonary nodule (also referred to as a coin lesion) is a common clinical problem (1). In lung cancer screening studies that enrolled individuals believed to be at high risk for neoplasms of the lung, the prevalence of solitary pulmonary nodules varied from 8% to 51% (2). It is usually detected incidentally on a chest X-ray or computed tomographic (CT) scan (3). A solitary pulmonary nodule is considered to be an isolated radiographic opacity that is spherical and well circumscribed. It measures less than 3 cm in diameter, is surrounded by aerated lung, and has no associated atelectasis, hilar enlargement, or pleural effusions. The size at which a nodule becomes a mass is arbitrary, although 3 cm is typically used. The major question that follows detection of a solitary pulmonary nodule is whether the lesion may be malignant. Toward that end, the physician needs to determine which of the following three approaches to use: observation with serial radiologic monitoring, biopsy, or immediate excision. The ideal approach would result in definitive resection of all malignant nodules, while avoiding resection of benign nodules that do not require therapy.

II. **PATHOPHYSIOLOGY.** Pulmonary nodules may be of either benign or malignant etiology. All types of lung cancer may present initially as a solitary nodule, including primary lung cancer, carcinoid tumors, and metastases. Benign causes include infections (i.e., granuloma, bacterial infection, abscess), benign neoplasms (i.e., hamartoma, hemangioma), congenital causes (i.e., bronchogenic cyst), and other causes (i.e., amyloid, sarcoidosis, rheumatoid arthritis, rib fracture) (4, 5).

III. **EVALUATION**

A. **History.** History is not definitive but can assist in moving the odds toward benign or malignant. The probability of a solitary pulmonary nodule being malignant rises with increasing patient *age*. Being younger than 40 years carries a less than 3% chance of malignancy, whereas being older than 60 years carries a greater than 50% chance of malignancy. Other *risk factors* for lung cancer include a history of smoking, asbestos exposure, family history, and previously diagnosed malignancy. *Radiographic features* can also be used to help predict whether a nodule is malignant. A lesion larger than 2 cm carries 50% likelihood that it is malignant (6). Review of prior imaging studies can reveal important information regarding growth. Lesions that are malignant tend to have a volume doubling time between 20 and 400 days, where volume doubling of a nodule corresponds to an approximately 30% increase in its diameter (3). Benign lesions either have a very rapid growth rate, with a doubling time of less than 20 days seen in infectious conditions, or extremely long doubling times. A nodule that has been present and unchanged for 2 years is almost certain to be benign.

B. **Physical Examination.** The presence of fever suggests a possible infectious etiology. Extrapulmonary manifestations of certain diseases, such as tuberculosis, sarcoidosis, or rheumatoid arthritis, may give some additional clues to the diagnosis. However, the contribution of physical diagnosis is limited.

C. **Testing.** If the nodule is detected on plain X-ray, then subsequent additional studies can include CT scan, fiber-optic bronchoscopy, percutaneous needle aspiration or biopsy, positron emission tomography (PET), and thoracoscopy (also called video-assisted thoracic surgery [VATS]) or thoracotomy for excision. Magnetic resonance imaging is not indicated in the evaluation of a solitary pulmonary nodule (5).

1. A *CT scan* can be useful in that a small nodule not seen on plain X-ray may be detected by it. The presence of multiple nodules favors a benign cause, except with the history of prior neoplasm, in which case metastatic disease is more likely. A stippled or eccentric

pattern of calcification within the nodule favors malignancy, whereas other characteristic patterns may favor a benign etiology (5). Malignant lesions tend to have more irregular and spiculated borders, whereas benign lesions often have relatively smooth and discrete borders. Nodules that have a ground glass appearance on CT are frequently malignant, with studies of such nodules indicating that approximately 20–60% are malignant (5). Benign lesions tend to have higher Hounsfeld units on CT scan, a measure of density, although there is no distinct cutoff point between benign and malignant lesions.

2. *Fiber-optic bronchoscopy* is a useful procedure for the diagnostic evaluation of large, central nodules and masses; however, it is much less useful for small solitary pulmonary nodules and for peripheral masses. The yield for diagnosing peripheral lesions smaller than 2 cm by brushing or transbronchial biopsy is 33%, whereas the yield for peripheral lesions greater than 2 cm is 62%. Fluoroscopy or endobronchial ultrasound, where available, can be used to optimize localization of the lesion and increase the yield to greater than 70%.

3. *Percutaneous needle aspiration* (also called fine needle aspiration) can be performed through the chest wall using either fluoroscopy or CT scanning to guide the placement of the needle within the lesion. Material for cytology is obtained, but there is no biopsy of a core of tissue. It has a diagnostic yield of 60% for peripheral nodules smaller than 2 cm and 64% for peripheral nodules smaller than 3 cm. It is more helpful for confirming malignancy rather than establishing a specific benign diagnosis and can be complicated by pneumothorax (7).

4. *Percutaneous needle biopsy* can be performed to obtain a core of tissue by using a cutting needle, thereby improving the diagnostic yield of benign nodules. An increasing number of centers are performing this procedure, but complications include hemorrhage and pneumothorax, which occur in 1% and 15% of biopsies, respectively (8).

5. *PET*, with flurodeoxyglucosse (FDG) used as a biological marker, can help distinguish malignant and benign lesions because cancers are metabolically active and take up FDG avidly. False-positive results can be seen in metabolically active nodules such as infectious granulomas and inflammatory conditions (9). False-negative results can occur because of the limited resolution of PET, which can form an image only down to approximately 8 mm, thereby possibly not detecting malignancies smaller than about 1 cm. In addition, some tumors, such as carcinoid and bronchoalveolar carcinoma, have very low metabolic rates and can be missed (10). An added benefit of PET is the acquisition of staging data if the nodule is malignant.

6. *VATS* can be performed as a method of surgical excision if the lesion is located close enough to the pleural surface. Alternatively, thoracotomy, which has greater morbidity, can be performed. The advantage of VATS and thoracotomy is that the procedures are both diagnostic and therapeutic. However, they are more invasive with inherent complications of hemorrhage and pneumothorax.

IV. DIAGNOSIS. The initial diagnosis of solitary pulmonary nodule is usually made through plain X-ray or CT. The differential diagnosis includes primary or metastatic lung malignancy. Further evaluation and monitoring depends on the clinical setting. Wherever possible, obtain old imaging studies for comparison. A nodule that has clearly grown on serial imaging tests should be excised (5). A nodule unchanged over a period of 2 years is almost certain to be benign. There is significant variation regarding what is considered optimal initial management; however, there is general consensus that management should be individualized. One approach uses the designation of low, intermediate, or high probability of malignancy based upon the clinician's overall impression, after consideration of all clinical and radiographic features.

A. A nodule that has a low probability of being malignant can be followed with serial CT scans. (CT scans are preferable to chest X-rays because growth is more readily detectable. Specifically, 3 to 5 mm of growth is necessary for detection on a chest X-ray, compared with only 0.5 mm on a high-resolution CT [3]).

B. A nodule that is smaller than 1 cm and has an intermediate probability of being malignant can be followed by serial CT scans.

C. A nodule that is 1 cm or larger and has an intermediate probability of being malignant should be evaluated by PET. Nodules that are negative on PET can be followed with serial CT scans, while nodules that are positive should be excised.

D. A nodule that has a high probability of being malignant should be excised.

The following guidelines, proposed by the Fleischner Society, advocate different frequencies for serial CT scans based upon the size of the nodule and the patient's risk for lung cancer (6). Patients are considered low risk if they have no history or minimal history of smoking and other risk factors; otherwise, they are considered high risk.

1. For nodules less than 4 mm, serial CT scans are not required if the patient is of low risk. Patients who are of high risk should have a CT performed at 12 months, with no further follow-up if the nodule is unchanged.

2. For nodules of 4–6 mm, a CT should be performed at 12 months if the patient is of low risk, with no further follow-up if the nodule is unchanged. Patients who are of high risk should have a CT performed at 6–12 months and at 18–24 months if the nodule is unchanged.

3. For nodules 6–8 mm, a CT should be performed at 6–12 months and at 18–24 months if the nodule is unchanged and the patient is of low risk. Patients who are of high risk should have a CT at 3–6, 9–12, and 24 months if the nodule remains unchanged.

4. For nodules greater than 8 mm, a CT should be performed at 3, 6, 9, and 24 months if the nodule remains unchanged, regardless of whether the patient is of low or high risk.

Consultation with a pulmonologist is warranted to decide whether and how the nodule should be sampled if the clinical features and radiologic features do not provide sufficient evidence that a lesion is either benign or malignant. Sampling of the nodule can be performed through the airway (bronchoscopy) or through the chest wall (percutaneous needle aspiration or biopsy).

REFERENCES

1. Libby DM, Smith JP, Altori NK, et al. Managing the small pulmonary nodule discovered by CT. *Chest* 2004;125:1522.

2. Wahidi NM, Govert JA, Goudar RK, et al. Evidence for the treatment of patients with pulmonary nodules: when is it lung cancer? *ACCP evidence-based clinical practice guidelines*, 2nd ed. *Chest* 2007;132:94S.

3. Ost D, Fein AM, Feinsilver SH. Clinical practice. The solitary pulmonary nodule. *N Engl J Med* 2003;348:2535

4. Winer-Muram HT. The solitary pulmonary nodule. *Radiology* 2006 Apr;239(1):34–49.

5. Gould MK, Fletcher J, Iannattoni MD, et al. American College of Chest Physicians. Evaluation of patients with pulmonary nodules: when is it lung cancer? ACCP evidence based clinical practice guidelines, 2nd ed. *Chest* 2007;132:108S–130S.

6. MacMahon H, Austin JH, Gordon G, et al. Guidelines for management of small pulmonary nodules detected on CT scans: a statement from the Fleischner Society. *Radiology* 2005;237:395.

7. Ost D, Fein A. Evaluation and management of the solitary pulmonary nodule. *AM J Respir Crit Care Med* 2000:162:782.

8. Wiener RS, Schwartz LM, Woloshin S, Welch HG. Population-based risk for complications after transthoracic needle lung biopsy of a pulmonary nodule; an analysis of discharge records. *Ann Intern Med* 2011;155:137.

9. Vansteenkiste JF, Stroobants SS. PET scanning in lung cancer: current recommendation and innovation. *J Thorac Oncol* 2006;1:71.

10. Gould MK,, Maclean CC, Kushner WG, et al. Accuracy of positron emission tomography in the diagnosis of pulmonary nodules and mass lesions: a meta-analysis. *JAMA* 2001;21:914–924.

Index

Note: Page numbers followed by *f* indicate figures; those followed by *t* indicate tables.